To my sons Clément and Amaury.
May I never disappoint you.

To my parents. Life did not allow them
to see this book published.

To Pang-Mei for supporting and inspiring me.

"… non c'è altra poesia che
l'azione reale."– Pier Paolo Pasolini

Arthur Atchabahian, MD

To my new baby daughter, Hema Leela.

To my wife Supurna whose unwavering
love and confidence in me continue to be
my source of strength through the tough times.

Ruchir Gupta, MD

The Anesthesia Guide

NOTICE

Medicine is an ever-changing science. As new research and clinical experience broaden our knowledge, changes in treatment and drug therapy are required. The authors and the publisher of this work have checked with sources believed to be reliable in their efforts to provide information that is complete and generally in accord with the standards accepted at the time of publication. However, in view of the possibility of human error or changes in medical sciences, neither the authors nor the publisher nor any other party who has been involved in the preparation or publication of this work warrants that the information contained herein is in every respect accurate or complete, and they disclaim all responsibility for any errors or omissions or for the results obtained from use of the information contained in this work. Readers are encouraged to confirm the information contained herein with other sources. For example and in particular, readers are advised to check the product information sheet included in the package of each drug they plan to administer to be certain that the information contained in this work is accurate and that changes have not been made in the recommended dose or in the contraindications for administration. This recommendation is of particular importance in connection with new or infrequently used drugs.

The Anesthesia Guide

EDITORS

Arthur Atchabahian, MD
Associate Professor of Clinical Anesthesiology
Department of Anesthesiology
New York University School of Medicine
New York, New York

Ruchir Gupta, MD
Assistant Professor of Anesthesiology
Department of Anesthesiology
North Shore–Long Island Jewish/
Hofstra Medical School
Syosset, New York

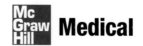

New York Chicago San Francisco Lisbon London Madrid
Mexico City Milan New Delhi San Juan Seoul Singapore Sydney Toronto

The Anesthesia Guide

1 2 3 4 5 6 7 8 9 0   CTP/CTP   18 17 16 15 14 13 12

ISBN 978-0-07-176049-2
MHID 0-07-176049-0

This book was set in Minion Pro by Thomson Digital.
The editors were Brian Belval and Robert Pancotti.
The production supervisor was Jeffrey Herzich.
The illustration manager was Armen Ovsepyan.
Project management was provided by Kunal Mehrotra, Thomson Digital.
The text designer was Alan Barnett.
China Translation & Printing Services, Ltd. was printer and binder.

Library of Congress Cataloging-in-Publication Data

Atchabahian, Arthur.
   The anesthesia guide / Arthur Atchabahian, Ruchir Gupta.
       p. ; cm.
   Includes bibliographical references and index.
   ISBN-13: 978-0-07-176049-2 (pbk.)
   ISBN-10: 0-07-176049-0 (pbk.)
   1. Anesthesia—Handbooks, manuals, etc. I. Gupta, Ruchir. II. Title.
   [DNLM: 1. Anesthesia—methods—Handbooks. WO 39]
   RD82.2.A83 2013
   617.9′6—dc23
                                                                        2012017520

CONTENTS

PART III. Monitoring

PART IV. General Anesthesia

PART V. Specific Procedures

PART VI. Cardiovascular and Thoracic

PART IX. Acute Pain (Postoperative)

PART X. Pediatrics

PART XII. Critical Care

PART XIII. Rapid Reference

CONTRIBUTORS

Yakub Abrakhimov, MD
Resident
Department of Anesthesiology
New York University School of
    Medicine
New York, New York

Frantzces Alabre, FNP-C, DNP
Pain Management-C
Pain Management Nurse Practitioner
New York University Hospital for
    Joint Diseases
New York, New York

Brooke Albright, MD
Captain, US Air Force
Assistant Professor of Anesthesiology
Department of Anesthesia and
    Pain Management
Landstuhl Regional Medical Center
Landstuhl, Germany

Nasrin N. Aldawoodi, MD
Critical Care Fellow
Department of Anesthesiology
Duke University Medical Center
Durham, North Carolina

Jennifer Alt, MD
Resident
Department of Anesthesiology
New York University
    School of Medicine
New York, New York

Zirka H. Anastasian, MD
Assistant Professor of Anesthesiology
Department of Anesthesiology
Columbia University
    College of Physicians and Surgeons
New York, New York

Megan Graybill Anders, MD
Assistant Professor of Anesthesiology
    and Critical Care Medicine
Department of Anesthesiology
University of Maryland School of
    Medicine
Baltimore, Maryland

Michael Anderson, MD
Assistant Professor of Anesthesiology
Department of Anesthesiology
Mount Sinai School of Medicine
New York, New York

Michael H. Andreae, MD
Assistant Professor of Anesthesiology
Department of Anesthesiology
Montefiore Medical Center
Albert Einstein College of Medicine
Bronx, New York

Harendra Arora, MD
Associate Professor
Department of Anesthesiology
Program Director, Anesthesiology
    Residency
Section Head, Vascular and
    Transplant Anesthesia
University of North Carolina at
    Chapel Hill
Chapel Hill, North Carolina

Erica A. Ash, MD
Resident
Department of Anesthesiology
New York University
    School of Medicine
New York, New York

Arthur Atchabahian, MD
Associate Professor of Clinical
    Anesthesiology
Department of Anesthesiology
New York University School of
    Medicine
New York, New York

Candra Rowell Bass, MD
Clinical Instructor
Department of Anesthesiology
University of North Carolina-Chapel Hill
Chapel Hill, North Carolina

**Adel Bassily-Marcus, MD,
FCCP, FCCM**
Assistant Professor
Department of Surgery
Mount Sinai School of Medicine
New York, New York

Marc Beaussier, MD, PhD
Professor and Chair
Department of Anesthesiology and
    Intensive Care
St-Antoine Hospital
Assistance Publique—Hôpitaux de Paris
University Pierre et Marie Curie
Paris, France

Lucie Beylacq, MD
Staff Anesthesiologist
Department of Anesthesiology and
    Intensive Care
François Xavier Michelet Center and
    Pellegrin University Hospital
Bordeaux, France

Ann E. Bingham, MD
Assistant Professor
Department of Anesthesiology and
    Perioperative Medicine
Oregon Health and Science University
Portland, Oregon

Jan Boublik, MD, PhD
Assistant Professor
Department of Anesthesiology
New York University
    School of Medicine
New York, New York

Caroline Buhay, MD
Instructor
Department of Anesthesiology
Weill-Cornell Medical College
New York, New York

Eric Cesareo, MD
Head of the Anesthesiology
    Department
Hopital Marc Jacquet
Melun, France

**Jean Charchaflieh, MD,
DrPH, FCCM, FCCP**
Associate Professor
Department of Anesthesiology
Yale University School of Medicine
New Haven, Connecticut

Wanda A. Chin, MD
Assistant Clinical Professor of
    Anesthesiology
Department of Anesthesiology,
    Pediatric Anesthesia Division
New York University
    School of Medicine
New York, New York

Manuel Corripio, MD
Chief Resident
Department of Anesthesiology
New York University
    School of Medicine
New York, New York

Ananda C. Dharshan, MBBS
Assistant Professor
Department of Oncology
Roswell Park Cancer Institute
Buffalo, New York

Lisa Doan, MD
Assistant Professor
Department of Anesthesiology
New York University School of Medicine
New York, New York

Adrienne Turner Duffield, MD
Resident Physician
Department of Anesthesiology
University of North Carolina
    at Chapel Hill
Chapel Hill, North Carolina

Ryan Dunst, MD
Resident
Department of Anesthesiology
Mount Sinai School of Medicine
New York, New York

Brian J. Egan, MD, MPH
Assistant Professor of Anesthesiology
Department of Anesthesiology
Columbia University
    College of Physicians and Surgeons
New York, New York

Elisabeth Falzone, MD
Staff Anesthesiologist
Department of Anesthesiology and
    Intensive Care Medicine
Percy Teaching Military Hospital
Clamart, France

Meghann M. Fitzgerald, MD
Instructor
Department of Anesthesiology
Weill Cornell Medical College
New York, New York

Oriane Gardy, MD
Fellow
Department of Emergency Medicine
Saint Antoine Hospital
Paris, France

John G. Gaudet, MD
Neuroanesthesiology Clinical Fellow
Department of Anesthesiology
Columbia University College of
    Physicians and Surgeons
New York, New York

Christopher Gharibo, MD
Associate Professor of Anesthesiology
    and Orthopedics
Medical Director of Pain Medicine
New York University
    School of Medicine
New York, New York

Ronaldo Collo Go, MD
Critical Care Fellow
Department of Critical Care
Mount Sinai Hospital
New York, New York

Nicolai Goettel, MD, DESA
Fellow
Department of Anesthesia
University of Toronto, University
    Health Network, Toronto Western
    Hospital
Toronto, Ontario, Canada

Amit Goswami, MD
Pain Management Specialist
Epic Pain Management
Wayne, New Jersey

Sumeet Goswami, MD, MPH
Assistant Professor of Anesthesiology
Department of Anesthesiology
Columbia University College of
    Physicians and Surgeons
New York, New York

Ruchir Gupta, MD
Assistant Professor of Anesthesiology
Department of Anesthesiology
North Shore–Long Island Jewish/
    Hofstra Medical School
Syosset, New York

Anjali Fedson Hack, MD, PhD
Assistant Professor
Department of Anesthesiology
Montefiore Medical Center
Albert Einstein School of Medicine
New York, New York

Brad Hamik, MD
Attending Physician
Department of Anesthesiology
Anesthesia Associates of Morristown
Morristown Memorial Medical Center
Morristown, New Jersey

M. Lee Haselkorn, MD
Fellow, Adult Cardiothoracic
    Anesthesiology
Department of Anesthesiology
Columbia University College of
    Physicians and Surgeons
New York, New York

Alan W. Ho, MD
Fellow
Department of Anesthesiology
Columbia University
    College of Physicians and Surgeons
New York, New York

Clément Hoffmann, MD
Staff Anesthesiologist
Department of Anesthesiology and
    Intensive Care Medicine
Percy Teaching Military Hospital
Clamart, France

Philipp J. Houck, MD
Assistant Professor of Clinical
    Anesthesiology
Department of Anesthesiology
Columbia University
    College of Physicians and Surgeons
New York, New York

Ghislaine M. Isidore, MD
Assistant Professor (Clinical) of
    Anesthesiology
Department of Anesthesiology
New York University
    School of Medicine
New York University Hospital for
    Joint Diseases
New York, New York

Elena Reitman Ivashkov, MD
Assistant Professor of Clinical
    Anesthesiology
Department of Anesthesiology
Columbia University College of
    Physicians and Surgeons
New York, New York

Zafar A. Jamkhana, MD, MPH
Assistant Professor of Internal Medicine
Division of Pulmonary, Critical Care,
    and Sleep Medicine
St Louis University
St. Louis, Missouri

Denis Jochum, MD
Anesthesiologist
Department of Anesthesiology
Albert Schweitzer Hospital
Colmar, France

Albert Ju, MD
Attending Anesthesiologist
New Jersey Anesthesia Associates
Florham Park, New Jersey

Bessie Kachulis, MD
Assistant Professor of Anesthesiology
Division of Cardiothoracic
  Anesthesiology
Department of Anesthesiology
Columbia University College of
  Physicians and Surgeons
New York, New York

Sumit Kapoor, MD
Fellow, Critical Care Medicine
Department of Surgery
Mount Sinai Hospital
New York, New York

Robert N. Keddis, MD
Cardiothoracic Anesthesia Fellow
Department of Anesthesia
New York University School of
  Medicine
New York, New York

Samir Kendale, MD
Resident
Department of Anesthesiology
New York University School of
  Medicine
New York, New York

M. Fahad Khan, MD, MHS
Assistant Professor
Center for the Study & Treatment
  of Pain
Department of Anesthesiology
New York University School of
  Medicine
New York, New York

Roopa Kohli-Seth, MD
Associate Professor of Surgery
Mount Sinai Medical Center
New York, New York

F. Wickham Kraemer III, MD
Section Chief, Acute and Chronic
  Pain Management
Department of Anesthesiology and
  Critical Care
Children's Hospital of Philadelphia
Perelman School of Medicine,
  University of Pennsylvania
Philadelphia, Pennsylvania

Priya A. Kumar, MD
Associate Professor
Department of Anesthesiology
University of North Carolina
Chapel Hill, North Carolina

Yan Lai, MD, MPH
Assistant Professor
Department of Anesthesiology
Mount Sinai School of Medicine
New York, New York

Jason Lau, MD
Resident
Department of Anesthesiology
New York University School of
  Medicine
New York, New York

Alexandra P. Leader, MD
Resident
Department of Pediatrics
Mount Sinai School of Medicine
New York, New York

Edward C. Lin, MD
Clinical Assistant Professor
Department of Anesthesiology
New York University School of
  Medicine
New York, New York

Sanford M. Littwin, MD
Division of Cardiothoracic and
  Pediatric Anesthesia
Director CA 1 Education
Department of Anesthesiology
St. Luke's-Roosevelt Hospital Center
Assistant Professor of Clinical
  Anesthesiology
Columbia University College of
  Physicians and Surgeons
New York, New York

Sansan S. Lo, MD
Assistant Professor of Clinical
    Anesthesiology
Division of Cardiothoracic Anesthesia
Department of Anesthesiology
Columbia University College of
    Physicians and Surgeons
New York, New York

Clara Alexandra Ferreira de Faria Oliveira Lobo, MD
Staff Anesthesiologist Anesthesiology
    and Pain Therapy Department
Centro Hospitalar de Trás-os-Montes e
    Alto Douro, Vila Real
Vila Real, Portugal

Christopher Lysakowski, MD
Consultant
Division of Anesthesiology
University Hospitals of Geneva
Geneva, Switzerland

Seth Manoach, MD, CHCQM
Assistant Chief Medical Officer for
    Inpatient Clinical Services
Attending Physician: Medical/Surgical
    ICU, Neurocritical Care,
    Emergency Medicine
State University of New York,
    Downstate Medical Center
Brooklyn, New York

Sonali Mantoo, MD
Intensivist
Critical Care Medicine
St. Vincent's Medical Center
Bridgeport, Connecticut

Donald M. Mathews, MD
Associate Professor of Anesthesiology
University of Vermont College of
    Medicine
Anesthesiologist, Fletcher Allen
    Health Care
Burlington, Vermont

Claude McFarlane, MD, MA
Associate Professor
Department of Anesthesiology
University of North Carolina Hospitals
Chapel Hill, North Carolina

Nirav Mistry, MD
Intensivist
Department of Medicine
JFK Medical Center
Edison, New Jersey

Satyanarayana Reddy Mukkera, MD, MPH
Critical Care Intensivist
Critical Care Medicine
Springfield Clinic
Springfield, Illinois

Teresa A. Mulaikal, MD
Cardiothoracic and Critical Care
    Anesthesia Fellow
Department of Anesthesiology
Columbia University College of
    Physicians and Surgeons
New York, New York

Neelima Myneni, MD
Fellow, Regional Anesthesia
Department of Anesthesiology
Hospital for Special Surgery
New York, New York

Harsha Nalabolu, MD
Instructor
Department of Anesthesiology
New York University School of
    Medicine
New York, New York

Jennie Ngai, MD
Assistant Professor
Director, Adult Cardiothoracic
    Anesthesiology Fellowship
Department of Anesthesiology
New York University School of
    Medicine
New York, New York

Ervant Nishanian, PhD, MD
Assistant Clinical Professor
Department of Anesthesiology
Columbia University College of
    Physicians and Surgeons
New York, New York

Tanuj P. Palvia, MD
Resident
Department of Anesthesiology
New York University School of
    Medicine
New York, New York

Leila Mei Pang, MD
Ngai-Jubilee Professor of Clinical
    Anesthesiology
Columbia University College of
    Physicians and Surgeons
New York, New York

Rita Parikh, MD
Staff Anesthesiologist
Department of Anesthesiology
Somnia, Inc.
New Rochelle, New York

Constantin Parizianu, MD
Pulmonary/Critical Care Attending
  Physician
Department of Critical Care
Good Samaritan Hospital
West Islip, New York

Krunal Patel, MD
Attending Physician
Nephrology Department
Mount Sinai Elmhurst
Mount Sinai Medical Center
New York, New York

Amit Poonia, MD
Fellow in Pain Management
Department of Anesthesiology
New York University School of
  Medicine
New York, New York

Sauman Rafii, MD
Resident
Department of Anesthesiology
New York University School of
  Medicine
New York, New York

Chaturani Ranasinghe, MD
Assistant Professor
Department of Anesthesiology/Division
  of Pain Management
University of Miami Miller School
  of Medicine
Miami, Florida

Imre Rédai, MD, FRCA
Assistant Professor of Anesthesiology
Department of Anesthesiology
New York University School of
  Medicine
New York, New York

J. David Roccaforte, MD
Assistant Professor
Bellevue Hospital Surgical ICU
Department of Anesthesiology
New York University School of
  Medicine
New York, New York

Amit H. Sachdev, MD
Resident
Department of Internal Medicine
University of Southern California
Los Angeles, California

Molly Sachdev, MD, MPH
Assistant Professor of Clinical Medicine
Division of Cardiology
Ohio State University Wexner
  Medical Center
Columbus, Ohio

Adam Sachs, MD
Resident
Department of Anesthesiology
New York University School of
  Medicine
New York, New York

Kriti Sankholkar, MD
Anesthesiologist
Department of Anesthesiology
Phelps Memorial Hospital
Sleepy Hollow, New York

David Sapir, MD
Attending Physician
Centre Hospitalien Sud Francilien
Corbeil Essonnes, Essonne, France

Nicholas B. Scott, FRCS(Ed), FRCA
Head of Clinical Anaesthesia
Hamad Medical Corporation
Doha, Qatar

Nitin K. Sekhri, MD
Pain Medicine Fellow
Department of Anesthesiology
Columbia University College of
  Physicians and Surgeons
New York, New York

Shahzad Shaefi, MD
Instructor in Anaesthesia
Department of Anesthesia, Critical
  Care, and Pain Medicine
Beth Israel Deaconess Medical Center
Boston, Massachusetts

Arif M. Shaik, MD
Neurointensivist
Neuro-Critical Care/Intensive
  Care Unit
St. Joseph Hospital
St. Paul, Minnesota
Aurora Bay Care Medical Center
Green Bay, Wisconsin

Naum Shaparin, MD
Director of Pain Service, Assistant
 Professor of Anesthesiology,
 Assistant Professor of Family and
 Social Medicine
Department of Anesthesiology
Montefiore Medical Center–Albert
 Einstein College of Medicine
Bronx, New York

Awais Sheikh, MD
Intensivist
Critical Care Medicine
SSM St. Clare Health Center
Fenton, Missouri

Kathleen A. Smith, MD
Assistant Professor
Department of Anesthesiology
University of North Carolina
Chapel Hill, North Carolina

Sarah C. Smith, MD
Assistant Professor
Department of Anesthesiology
Columbia University College of
 Physicians and Surgeons
New York, New York

Jamaal T. Snell, MD
Instructor
Department of Anesthesiology
New York University School of
 Medicine
New York, New York

Jamey J. Snell, MD
Chief Resident
Department of Anesthesiology
New York University School of
 Medicine
New York, New York

Jessica Spellman, MD
Assistant Professor
Department of Anesthesiology
Columbia University College of
 Physicians and Surgeons
New York, New York

Karim Tazarourte, MD
Head of the Emergency Department
Hôpital Marc Jacquet
Melun, France

Elrond Yi Lang Teo, MBBS
Fellow
Cardiothoracic Anesthesiology and
 Critical Care Medicine
Columbia University College of
 Physicians and Surgeons
New York, New York

Janine L. Thekkekandam, MD
Staff Anesthesiologist
Commonwealth Anesthesia Associates
Richmond, Virginia

Mark S. Tinklepaugh, MD
Instructor
Department of Anesthesiology
State University of New York Upstate
 Medical University, Clinical Campus
 at Binghamton
Our Lady of Lourdes Hospital
Binghamton, New York

Toni Torrillo, MD
Assistant Professor
Department of Anesthesiology
Mount Sinai School of Medicine
New York, New York

Jean-Pierre Tourtier, MD
Professor and Chair
Emergency Medical Service
Fire Brigade of Paris
Paris, France

Tony P. Tsai, MD
Attending Anesthesiologist
Department of Anesthesiology
Beth Israel Medical Center, Petrie
 Division
New York, New York

Aditya Uppalapati, MD
Assistant Professor
Pulmonary Critical Care and
 Sleep Medicine
St. Louis University
St. Louis, Missouri

Vickie Verea, MD
Chief Resident
Department of Anesthesiology
New York University School of
 Medicine
New York, New York

Lisa E. Vianna, DO
Attending Physician
Division of Cardiothoracic and
  Thoracic Surgery
North Shore Long Island Jewish Health
  System
New Hyde Park, New York

Yann Villiger, MD, PhD
Associate Professor
Department of Anesthesiology
Geneva University Hospital
Geneva, Switzerland

Lucia Daiana Voiculescu, MD
Assistant Professor
Department of Anesthesiology
New York University School of
  Medicine
New York, New York

Gebhard Wagener, MD
Associate Professor of Clinical
  Anesthesiology
Department of Anesthesiology
Columbia University College of
  Physicians and Surgeons
New York, New York

Mark Weller, MD
Assistant Professor
Department of Anesthesiology
Columbia University College of
  Physicians and Surgeons
New York, New York

Eric P. Wilkens, MD, MPH
Assistant Professor
Department of Anesthesiology
Albert Einstein College of Medicine
Montefiore Medical Center
New York, New York

Jennifer Wu, MD, MBA
Assistant Professor
Department of Anesthesiology
The University of Texas Medical School
Houston, Texas

Victor Zach, MD
Director of Stroke and
  Neurocritical Care
Neurology and Neurosurgery
John C. Lincoln Health Network
Phoenix, Arizona

FOREWORD

The spectrum of knowledge in the field of anesthesiology has expanded substantially in the last decade. A plethora of information is published on a monthly basis in seminal anesthesiology journals, which increases the need to synthesize the maze of information and to present it in a lucid, straightforward manner for a practicing anesthesiologist. A quick glance at the contents and organization of *The Anesthesia Guide* affirms its raison d'etre. *The Anesthesia Guide* does not seek to "dethrone" the mammoth textbooks or the densely packed review books and manuals. Instead, it synthesizes information for a busy clinician in an innovative format that will help guide everyday clinical decision-making. As a bonus, it offers numerous tips, techniques, and tricks of the trade that are not featured in most anesthesiology books that I have examined.

For *The Anesthesia Guide*, the editors have selected a highly practical combination of illustrations, clinical images, diagrams, and decision-making flowcharts in a uniquely didactic, simplified, and clinically relevant format. Clearly, weighty decisions had to be made regarding the selection of the material to be included in a relatively small volume that attempts to span the vast landscape of the clinical practice of anesthesiology. Having had a chance to preview several of the chapters, I can verify that the editors have chosen the most "bang-for-the buck" practical information. They have created a superbly attractive, all-encompassing, and invaluable "how to" compendium that is uniquely well suited for trainees and practicing anesthesiologists alike, who need a quick refresher on specific case management. The material is organized in more than 220 short chapters that cover preoperative evaluation, considerations of coexisting diseases, monitoring, management of specific and challenging anesthesia subspecialty cases, and concise and practical descriptions of common anesthesia procedures. It is particularly worthwhile to note the useful section on regional anesthesia, contributed by internationally renowned instructors in the field, one of whom is Dr. Atchabahian himself.

I warmly welcome and endorse *The Anesthesia Guide* as a daringly practical, no-nonsense manual of applied anesthesiology. The editors deserve praise for taking a bold step in departing from the classical textbook approach of amassing information, as well as avoiding the cramming that is so often present in manuals. Instead, they have opted to present material that truly matters in clinical practice. Consequently, I am convinced that *The Anesthesia Guide* will find its place in operating rooms, on anesthesia machines, in perioperative areas, in the pockets of residents and practicing clinicians, and on the office desks of many practitioners of anesthesiology worldwide.

Admir Hadzic, MD
Professor of Clinical Anesthesiology
College of Physicians and Surgeons, Columbia University
Senior Anesthesiologist, St. Luke's and Roosevelt Hospitals
New York, New York

PREFACE

Anesthesiology is a science. Anesthesia, at its best, is a craft, comparable with making violins or restoring antique cars. This dichotomy is actually true of all medical and surgical specialties. Research is indispensable; in a few decades, anesthesia will probably look nothing like our current specialty. However, as practitioners and educators, our main interest is to understand how to emulate our best colleagues *in the current state of science*, those whose patients emerge comfortable, and at least as healthy as before, from the most complex surgeries, and to transmit that knowledge while keeping in mind that anesthesiologists are physicians; they are not technicians who apply "one-size-fits-all" recipes.

When faced with a specific patient or case, extracting from most textbooks the information that will be useful in the operating room can be difficult and time-consuming. *The Anesthesia Guide* is an attempt to focus on a practical rather than theoretical approach. This book is not intended as a comprehensive textbook. We endeavored to keep the book small enough that it can be carried into the operating room. We used pictures, diagrams, tables, algorithms, and bulleted points rather than lengthy blocks of text. The book will allow a trainee to be fully prepared for a case and will "remind" an experienced clinician how a specific case should be handled. Thus, we made every attempt to include drug dosages, infusion rates, needed monitoring, possible complications, and troubleshooting of common intraoperative problems. Choices had to be made, and not everyone will agree with our selections, but we feel that deciding is preferable to providing a multitude of possible approaches and leaving the reader puzzled as to which one to choose.

We also strongly believe that anesthesiology encompasses all of perioperative medicine, and as a result the Acute Postoperative Pain and Critical Care parts of the book are heftier than in most American anesthesia textbooks.

Reader feedback will help to improve this book in subsequent editions. Please send us your thoughts and criticisms to theanesthesiaguide@gmail.com. We are looking forward to hearing from you.

ACKNOWLEDGMENTS

Brian Belval, without whose help and patience this project would never have been completed.

To all the contributors, who spent hours toiling and revising chapters with no reward except for the satisfaction of helping their fellow anesthesiologists.

Thanks to the models for the regional anesthesia pictures: Katie Riffey, Elizabeth Rennie, and Joseph Palmeri, MD.

PART I

PREOPERATIVE

CHAPTER 1
Preoperative Evaluation

Sansan S. Lo, MD

PURPOSE

- Establish relationship
- Familiarize self with patient, their medical problems and need for further evaluation, and the planned surgical procedure
- Assess anesthetic risk and develop perioperative plan (preoperative medications, intraoperative management, postoperative care)
- Discuss pertinent anesthetic risks, answer questions, and obtain informed consent
- Document the above

Should be done as early as possible before the day of surgery for high-risk patients.

Institutional differences in requirements and role of preoperative anesthesia evaluation clinics.

HISTORY

- Past medical history:
  - Disease processes, symptoms, treatment, severity
  - Degree of optimization
  - Need for further consultation/testing
  - ASA classification correlates well with outcomes

ASA Physical Status Classification System	
I	Normal, healthy patient
II	Mild systemic disease without functional limitations
III	Systemic disease with functional limitations
IV	Severe systemic disease that is constant threat to life
V	Moribund patient who will not survive without surgery
VI	Brain-dead patient for organ retrieval
E	All emergency procedures

- Past surgical history
- Past anesthetic history: general, MAC, spinal, epidural, peripheral nerve blocks
- Past history of anesthetic complications: allergic reactions, severe postoperative nausea and vomiting, delayed awakening, prolonged paralysis, neuropathy, intraoperative awareness, hoarseness, difficult intubation, postdural puncture headache

- Family history of anesthetic complications: malignant hyperthermia, prolonged paralysis
- Current medications:
  - Updated list and what patient took/to take day of surgery
  - Implications regarding intraoperative hemodynamics, drug interactions, tolerance to anesthetic drugs, bleeding tendencies, electrolyte abnormalities
  - See below for role of beta-blockers
  - Herbs or supplements, while not considered medications, can have significant side effects or drug interactions and the patient must be asked about their use (see chapter 10)
- Allergies:
  - Allergy versus adverse effects
  - Medications, latex (associated risk factors: see chapter 35), adhesives, egg, soy

SPECIFIC CONSIDERATIONS BY SYSTEMS

- Neuro:
  - Seizures, strokes and residual symptoms, TIA, other neurological disease
  - Paresthesias, preexisting neuropathies
  - Cervical spine disease
- Pulmonary:
  - Asthma (obtain peak flow), emphysema, dyspnea/orthopnea
  - Exercise tolerance and whether due to pulmonary etiology
  - Aggressive preoperative interventions may benefit patients with COPD: bronchodilators, physical therapy, incentive spirometers, smoking cessation, corticosteroids
  - Regional versus general anesthesia in patients at high risk for pulmonary complications
- OSA:
  - See chapter 13 for STOP-BANG score if patient suspect for OSA but not diagnosed
  - Presence and severity
  - Use of CPAP/BIPAP and settings
- Cardiovascular:
  - Angina, CAD, past MI, CHF, valvular disease, arrhythmias
  - Pacemaker/AICD
  - Exercise tolerance and whether functional capacity limited by cardiac causes.
  - Percutaneous coronary intervention (PCI), stents: see chapter 22
  - Revised Cardiac Risk Index and risk factors associated with perioperative cardiac events (high-risk surgery, ischemic heart disease, congestive heart failure, cerebrovascular disease, diabetes mellitus requiring insulin, preoperative serum creatinine >2.0 mg/dL) predict moderate (7%) to high (11%) risk of major cardiac complications for patients with two to three variables
  - ACC/AHA Task Force 2007 guidelines on perioperative cardiovascular evaluation and care for noncardiac surgery: see chapter 7
  - Beta-blockers per 2009 ACCF/AHA focused update on perioperative beta-blockade:
    - Continue chronic beta-blocker therapy
    - Initiation recommended in patients undergoing vascular surgery with high cardiac risk (CAD, ischemia on preoperative testing)
    - Initiation reasonable in patients undergoing vascular surgery if more than one clinical risk factor (as defined above)
    - Initiation reasonable in patients undergoing intermediate-risk surgery if CAD or more than one clinical risk factor
    - Always titrate to heart rate and blood pressure
  - Acute effects of beta-blockade decrease myocardial oxygen demand; possible anti-inflammatory benefit with plaque stabilization observed after prolonged use. Should be started days to weeks prior to elective surgery

- Hepatic:
  ‣ Hepatitis, coagulation abnormalities
- Renal:
  ‣ Renal insufficiency/failure
  ‣ Dependence on dialysis and last session
- Endocrine/metabolic:
  ‣ Obesity, diabetes, thyroid, adrenal
- Hematology:
  ‣ Hereditary coagulopathies/anemias, anticoagulant therapy, history DVT/PE
  ‣ Elicit h/o bleeding following minor trauma, tooth brushing, dental extraction or surgery
- GERD/risk of aspiration:
  ‣ Triggers, severity, optimization of GERD
  ‣ Hiatal hernia
  ‣ Delayed gastric emptying, obesity, long-standing DM; see chapter 50
- Recent URI:
  ‣ No guidelines on how long to wait. Consider age of patient, urgency of surgery, URI versus LRI, symptoms (cough/sputum, fevers, wheezing), comorbidities (asthma, COPD)
- EtOH/tobacco/other substances:
  ‣ Smoking/EtOH history
  ‣ Acute/chronic use of other substances
- Pregnancy:
  ‣ Possibility of, number of weeks, intraoperative implications
  ‣ Each institution has a policy regarding systematic testing or not of women of childbearing age

PHYSICAL EXAM

- Airway exam: Mallampati score, thyromental distance, jaw mobility, neck range of motion. Also consider prominent teeth, small chin, large neck, absence of teeth, beard, and obesity as other possible indicators of difficult mask ventilation or intubation
- Other considerations: dentures, removable bridges, loose/chipped teeth; hearing aids; contact lenses; potential OSA risk
- Height and weight
- Baseline VS including O_2 saturation. FSBG for diabetics. Abnormal values necessitate clinical correlation. May indicate need for further optimization
- Baseline physical exam including mental status and assessment for undetected murmurs, auscultation lung sounds

PREOPERATIVE TESTING

- Should not be routinely performed
- Pursue if clinically indicated for individual patient/procedure and if findings will affect perioperative care/plan/outcome
- Age-based criteria controversial; may be institution specific
- Tests:
  ‣ CBC:
    ▪ Consider in extremes of age, bleeding, hematologic disorders, liver disease, and surgery with possible blood loss
  ‣ Chemistry/liver function tests:
    ▪ Consider in endocrine/renal/liver disorders, perioperative therapies, use of certain medications
  ‣ Coagulation profile:
    ▪ Consider in bleeding/renal/liver disorders and surgery type

- Pregnancy tests:
  - History and exam may be insufficient
  - Maintain low threshold as positive results have significant anesthetic implications
- EKG:
  - Per ACC/AHA 2007 guidelines:
    - Recommended in patients with at least one clinical risk factor, high-risk surgery. Recommended in patients with known CAD, peripheral arterial disease, or cerebrovascular disease, intermediate-risk surgery
    - Reasonable in patients with no clinical risk factors, high-risk surgery. Reasonable in patients with at least one clinical risk factor, intermediate-risk surgery
    - Not indicated in asymptomatic patients, low-risk procedures regardless of age
  - Although routine EKG may have limited utility, might be useful baseline; MIs may be silent, may modify ASA classification
- TEE, stress tests:
  - Consider cardiovascular risk factors and type of surgery per ACC/AHA 2007 guidelines
- CXR:
  - No indications but consider if history of smoking, COPD, URI, cardiac disease
- PFTs/ABGs:
  - Rarely indicated
  - Consider for lung resection or to discern cause of reported decreased functional capacity
- Insufficient evidence to specify timing of tests. Per ASA Task Force on Preanesthesia Evaluation, tests within 6 months generally acceptable if no significant changes unless recent values needed for specific anesthetic techniques

REFERENCES

For references, please visit **www.TheAnesthesiaGuide.com**.

CHAPTER 2
Predicting Difficult Mask Ventilation and Intubation

Adam Sachs, MD

PREDICTING DIFFICULT AND IMPOSSIBLE MASK VENTILATION

- Overall incidence of difficult mask ventilation (DMV) is 1.4% with impossible mask ventilation (IMV) 0.15%
- Obesity, snoring, and lack of teeth can probably be overcome with simple airway maneuvers, which is why they are not risk factors for IMV:
  - Lack of teeth actually makes DL and intubation easier
- Neck circumference (> 50 or 60 cm at the level of the cricoid cartilage) is the most predictive factor of IMV
- Patients with three or more risk factors have a much higher likelihood of being IMV (odds ratio 8.9)
- Most patients (75%) who are IMV will be easy to intubate

Risk Factors Associated with Difficult versus Impossible Mask Ventilation	
Difficult mask ventilation	Impossible mask ventilation
Neck circumference	Neck circumference
Male sex	Male sex
Sleep apnea	Sleep apnea
Mallampati class 3 or 4	Mallampati class 3 or 4
Beard	Beard
BMI >26	
Snoring	
Lack of teeth	

PREDICTING DIFFICULT INTUBATION

- Overall incidence of difficult intubation (DI) is 5.2% (obstetric: 3.1%, obese: 15.8%) with failed tracheal intubation 0.15%
- A combination of tests tends to be a better predictor of DI than individual tests

Reliability of Different Characteristics Associated with Difficult Intubation				
Characteristics associated with difficult intubation	Definition	Sensitivity (%)	Specificity (%)	Positive predictive value or positive likelihood (PL)
Interincisor gap	<4 cm	30	97	28
Range of neck extension	Head extension ≤80°	10	93	18
Retrognathia	>90°	7	99	20
Thyromental distance	<6.5 cm	48	79	9.4 (<4 cm)
Mentohyoid distance	<4.5 cm	16	91	6
Sternomental distance	<12.5 cm	44	87	11
Neck circumference	>43 cm	92	84	37
Mallampati classification	Grade 3 or 4 view	49	86	3 (PL)
BMI	>30	83	50	14
Indirect laryngoscopy	Grade 3 or 4 view	69	98	31
Upper lip bite test	Class 3 (lower incisors cannot bite upper lip)	8	97	8

Tests Predicting Difficult Intubation		
Combinations of tests	Sensitivity (%)	Specificity (%)
Wilson risk score	46	89
Arné multivariate risk index	93	93
Simplified predictive intubation difficulty score	65	76

Arné Multivariate Simplified Score	
Risk factor	Points
Previous difficult intubation	
• No	0
• Yes	10
Pathologies associated with difficult intubation (facial malformation, acromegaly, cervical spondylosis, occipitoatlantoaxial disease, airway tumors, DM with "stiff joint syndrome")	
• No	0
• Yes	5
Clinical symptoms or airway pathology (dyspnea due to airway compression, dysphonia, dysphagia, sleep apnea syndrome)	
• No	0
• Yes	3
Interincisor gap (IG) and mandible luxation (ML)	
• IG ≥5 cm or ML >0	0
• 3.5 cm < IG < 5 cm and ML = 0	3
• IG <3.5 cm and ML <0	13
Thyromental distance	
• ≥6.5 cm	0
• <6.5 cm	4
Maximum range of head and neck movement	
• 100°	0
• 90 ± 10°	2
• <80	5
Mallampati	
• Class 1	0
• Class 2	2
• Class 3	6
• Class 4	8
Total possible	48

A score >11 predicts difficult intubation with a 93% sensitivity and a 93% specificity.

REFERENCES

For references, please visit **www.TheAnesthesiaGuide.com**.

CHAPTER 3
Preoperative Fasting Guidelines

Edward C. Lin, MD

Preoperative Fasting Guidelines	
Minimum fasting time	Material ingested
2 h	Clear liquids (e.g., water, fruit juice without pulp, soda, tea without milk, black coffee)
4 h	Breast milk
6 h	Infant formula Nonhuman milk Light meal (e.g., tea and toast)
>6 h	Intake of fried/fatty foods may delay gastric emptying. The individual practitioner should consider this and make a determination of the appropriate fasting period

- In addition to the above guidelines, practitioners must also take into consideration factors that may prolong gastric emptying (e.g., emergent procedure, pregnancy, diabetes, hiatal hernia, GERD, ileus, bowel obstruction, obesity [controversial])
- There is no evidence that smoking one cigarette prior to surgery increases the risk of aspiration
- It is generally accepted that trauma or acute illness slows gastric emptying. These patients are considered "full stomach" even if >8 hours have elapsed since the last meal

REFERENCE

For references, please visit **www.TheAnesthesiaGuide.com**.

CHAPTER 4
Pulmonary Function Tests

Ruchir Gupta, MD

FIGURE 4-1. Normal spirogram

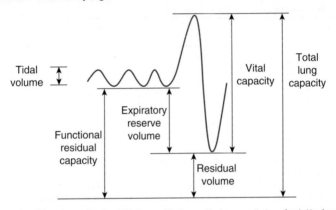

FIGURE 4-2. Normal lung volumes

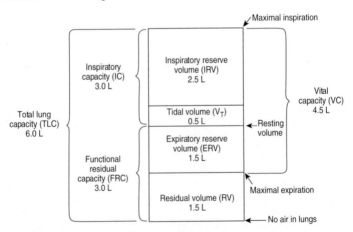

Pulmonary Function Tests in Disease States		
Respiratory variable	Obstructive (i.e., asthma, COPD)	Restrictive (i.e., pulmonary fibrosis, pneumonia)
Vital capacity	N or ↓	↓
Total lung capacity	↑	↓
FEV$_1$/FVC ratio	↓	N or ↓
Mid-maximal expiratory flow	↓	N
Maximum breathing capacity	↓	N
DLCO	Asthma: N or ↓ COPD: ↓↓	↓↓↓

N, normal; ↓, decreased; ↑, increased.

FIGURE 4-3. Components of the flow–volume loop

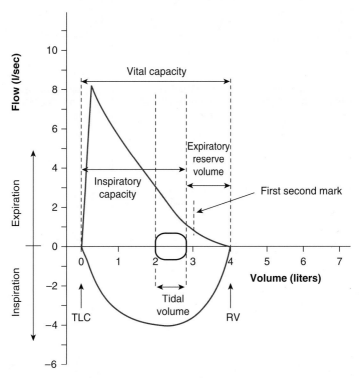

By convention, expiration is up and inspiration is down.

FIGURE 4-4. Alterations of flow–volume loop in disease states

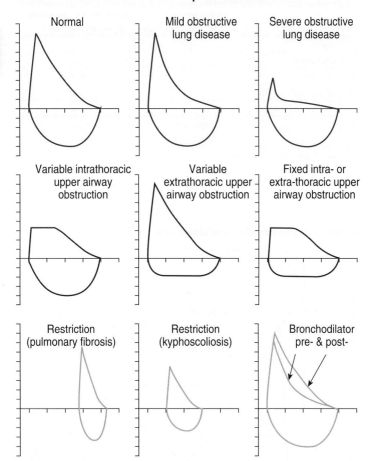

Normal

Mild obstructive lung disease

Severe obstructive lung disease

Variable intrathoracic upper airway obstruction

Variable extrathoracic upper airway obstruction

Fixed intra- or extra-thoracic upper airway obstruction

Restriction (pulmonary fibrosis)

Restriction (kyphoscoliosis)

Bronchodilator pre- & post-

FIGURE 4-5. Preoperative testing algorithm to predict surgical outcome for pneumonectomy

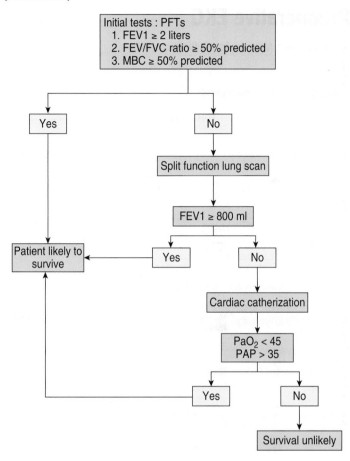

CHAPTER 5
Preoperative EKG

Bessie Kachulis, MD and Ann E. Bingham, MD

FIGURE 5-1. EKG waves and segments

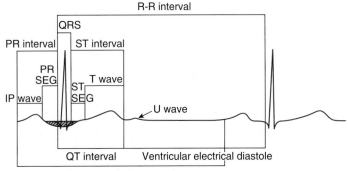

Reproduced from Fuster V, Walsh RA, Harrington RA. *Hurst's The Heart*. 13th ed. Figure 15-1.
Available at: www.accessmedicine.com. Copyright © The McGraw-Hill Companies, Inc. All rights
reserved.

Waves, Intervals, and Common Pathologies	
Time and voltage scale	When the ECG machine rate is 25 mm/s, each small box represents 0.04 s horizontally and 0.1 mV vertically
P wave	Represents: atrial depolarization Duration: 80–120 ms Amplitude: 2.5 mV in leads II and III Morphology (see Figure 5-2): • Biphasic in the right precordial leads (V_1 and V_2) • Upright in the lateral leads (I, aV_L, V_5, V_6), reflects right to left spread of the activation front Axis: 0–90° Pathology: atrial enlargement–P wave height greater than 2.5 mV

PR (or PQ) interval	Represents: impulse propagation from the atria throughout the AV node, bundle of His, bundle branches, and Purkinje fibers until the ventricular myocardium begins depolarization
	PR duration: 120–200 ms
	Pathology:
	    Long PR interval–slow AV nodal conduction (see section "First-Degree Heart Block")
	    Short PR with a delta wave–Wolff–Parkinson–White syndrome or preexcitation
	Note:
	    PR interval: beginning of P to the beginning of the QRS
	    PR segment: end of P to the beginning of the QRS

(continued)

Waves, Intervals, and Common Pathologies (*continued*)	

Q wave	Represents the negative deflection of the QRS before the R wave present in one or more inferior leads in more than 50% of normal adults, but is present in leads I and aV_L in less than 50% of normal adults
	Duration: less than 30 ms in limb leads, less than 50 ms in lead III, less than 30–40 ms in leads I, aV_L, V_5, and V_6
	Amplitude:
	    Less than 0.4 mV in all limb leads except the amplitude may be up to 0.5 mV in lead III
	    Depth of the Q wave should be less than 25% of the R wave height except in lead III

QRS	Represents: ventricular activation
	Duration: 70–110 ms (measured in the lead with the widest QRS complex)
	Amplitude: increases through V_5 (commonly referred to as "R wave progression"); see LVH
	Morphology: usually upwardly deflected in leads I and II, may be negative in aV_L, usually downwardly deflected in aV_R and V_1; chest leads V_2–V_3 are transition leads and are usually isoelectric in appearance, variable in lead III
	Axis: −30 to +90:
	    More negative than −30°: left-axis deviation
	    Greater than 90°: right-axis deviation
	Pathology: wide QRS—increased duration of ventricular depolarization: bundle branch block, LVH, ventricle depolarized by an ectopic focus

QT interval	Represents: duration of ventricular systole
	Duration: less than 460 ms for men and less than 470 ms for women; decreases with increasing heart rate, necessitating use of the QT corrected for heart rate, QTc
	    Bazett formula for the QTc: $QTc = QT/\sqrt{RR}$, where RR = R–R interval in seconds (=60/HR)
	    Upper limit of QTc $= \kappa \sqrt{RR}$, where $\kappa = 0.397$ for men and 0.415 for women
	Pathology:
	    Short QTc syndrome: less than 340 ms
	    QTc prolongation: medications, myocardial ischemia, infarction, cardiac surgery, hypokalemia, hypocalcemia, hypothermia, hypothyroidism, congenital long QT, severe bradycardia, and AV block

T wave	Represents: ventricular repolarization Duration: variable Amplitude: less than 0.6 mV in limb leads and at least 0.05 mV in leads I and II Morphology: normally asymmetric; the slope of initial portion is more gradual than that of the terminal portion, may be diphasic (a positive to negative deflection is more likely to be normal) Axis: leftward, inferiorly, and anteriorly; upright in leads I, II, V_5, and V_6 and inverted in aV_R Common normal variant: persistent juvenile pattern of T wave inversion in two or more of the right precordial leads (V_1–V_2) in a normal adult, resembling the pattern occurring in normal children and adolescents Pathology: T wave inversion may be a sign of ischemia. Perioperative T wave changes such as flattening, or even inversion, are common and are more likely to be due to changes in sympathetic tone, electrolytes, than ischemia

(*continued*)

Waves, Intervals, and Common Pathologies (*continued*)	
U wave	Diastolic deflection of unclear origin Duration: 90–110 ms Amplitude: less than 0.21 mV or 5–25% the height of the T wave Morphology: usually monophasic, positive or negative. Usually positive in all leads except aVR Axis: directed similarly to the T wave. The U wave can be confused with the second peak of a notched T wave Pathology: hypokalemia, bradyarrhythmias, hypothermia, LVH, drugs that can cause a prominent U wave

ST segment (see Figure 5-3)	Represents: depolarized ventricle
	Pathology:
	   ST depression: subendocardial injury or reciprocal depression in contralateral leads, but fails to localize the coronary lesion
	   ST elevation: transmural injury. The commonly accepted criterion for ischemia is a 0.1 mV (1 mm) ST segment elevation lasting at least 40 ms measured 60–80 ms after the J point in contiguous leads
	   Less common causes of ST elevation (usually global instead of regional): include pulmonary embolism, postmitral valvuloplasty, pericarditis, hyperkalemia, after transthoracic cardioversion or ICD discharge
	   J point elevation:
	     Normal variant (early repolarization)
	     ST segment elevation at the junction of the QRS and ST segment
	     Usually it involves leads V_2–V_5
	     Concave ST segment elevation
	     Notching of the downstroke of the R wave
	     Tall peaked T waves without reciprocal ST depression

FIGURE 5-2. Causes of abnormal P wave morphology

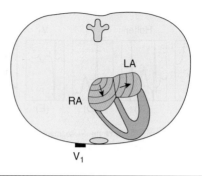

	Normal	Right	Left
II	RA LA	RA LA	RA LA
V₁	RA LA	RA LA	RA LA

Right atrial (RA) overload may cause tall, peaked P waves in the limb or precordial leads. Left atrial (LA) abnormality may cause broad, often notched P waves in the limb leads and a biphasic P wave in lead V₁ with a prominent negative component representing delayed depolarization of the LA. Reproduced with permission from Park MK, Guntheroth WG. *How to Read Pediatric ECGs.* 4th ed. St. Louis: Mosby, 2006. © Elsevier.

FIGURE 5-3. Normal variants of ST segment and T wave in the absence of heart disease

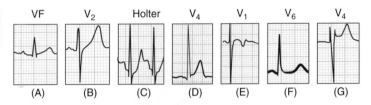

| VF | V₂ | Holter | V₄ | V₁ | V₆ | V₄ |
| (A) | (B) | (C) | (D) | (E) | (F) | (G) |

Different morphologies of normal variants of the ST segment and T wave in the absence of heart disease. (A and B) Normal variants. (C) Sympathetic overdrive: ECG of a 22-year-old male obtained with continuous Holter monitoring during a parachute jump. (D) Early repolarization. (E) Normal repolarization of a 3-year-old child. (F) ECG of a 75-year-old man without heart disease but with rectified ST/T. (G) ECG of a 20-year-old man with pectus excavatus. Normal variant of ST elevation (saddle morphology). Reproduced from Fuster V, Walsh RA, Harrington RA. *Hurst's The Heart.* 13th ed. Figure 15-17. Available at: www.accessmedicine.com. Copyright © The McGraw-Hill Companies, Inc. All rights reserved.

FIGURE 5-4. Acute pericarditis

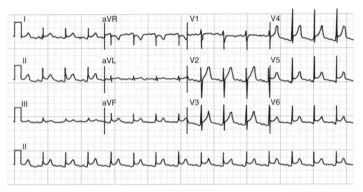

Diffuse ST elevations in I, II, III, aV$_F$, V$_3$–V$_6$, without T wave inversions. Also note concomitant PR-segment elevation in aVR and PR depression in the inferolateral leads. Reproduced from Longo DL, Fauci AS, Kasper DL, Hauser SL, Jameson JL, Loscalzo J. *Harrison's Principles of Internal Medicine.* 18th ed. Figure e28-13. Available at: www.accessmedicine.com. Copyright © The McGraw-Hill Companies, Inc. All rights reserved.

EKG AND MYOCARDIAL ISCHEMIA (FIGURE 5-5)

The leads that show changes can help localize the coronary lesion (keeping in mind the variability of coronary perfusion, especially in patients with CAD who may have extensive collateralization, and in post-CABG patients).

FIGURE 5-5. Myocardial infarction types with correlating infarction area

	Name	Type	ECG pattern	Infarction area (CE-CMR)	Most probable place of occlusion
Anteroseptal zone	Septal	A1	Q in V_1–V_2 SE: 100% SP: 97%	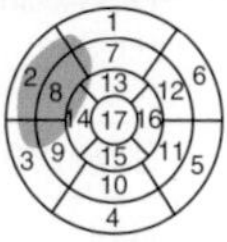	LAD S1 D1 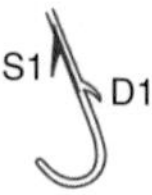
	Apical anterior	A2	Q in V_1–V_2 to V_3–V_6 SE: 85% SP: 98%	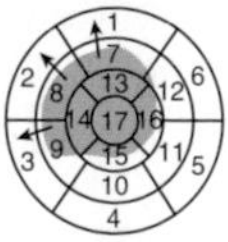	LAD S1 D1 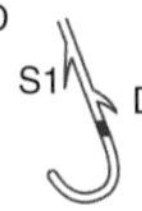
	Extensive anterior	A3	Q in V_1–V_2 to V_4–V_6, I and aVL SE: 83% SP: 100%	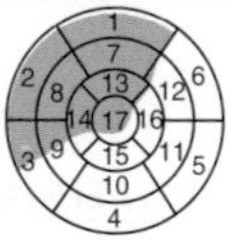	LAD S1 D1 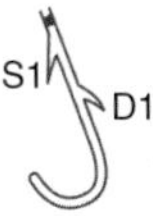
	Mid-anterior	A4	Q (qs or qr) in aVL (I) and sometimes in V_2–V_3 SE: 67% SP: 100%	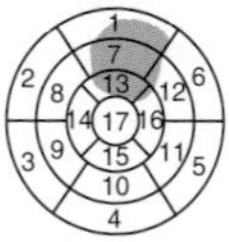	LAD S1 D1 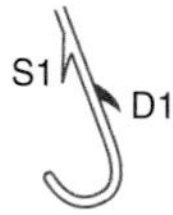
Inferolateral zone	Lateral	B1	RS in V_1–V_2 and/or Q wave in leads I, aVL, V_6 and/or diminished R wave in V_6 SE: 67% SP: 99%	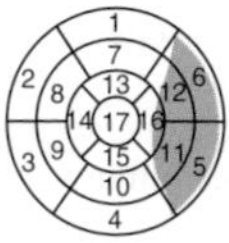	LCX 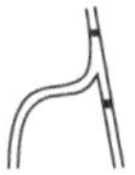
	Inferior	B2	Q in II, III, aVF SE: 88% SP: 97%	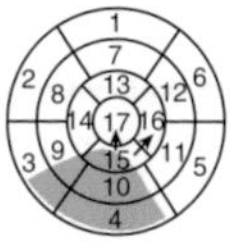	RCA LCX 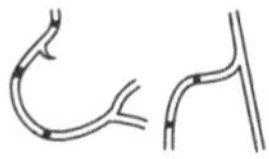
	Infero-lateral	B3	Q in II, III, Vf (B2) and Q in I, VL, V_5–V_6 and/or RS in V_1 (B1) SE: 73% SP: 98%	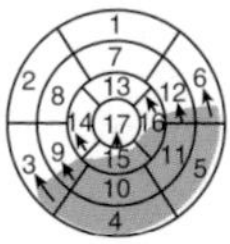	RCA LCX 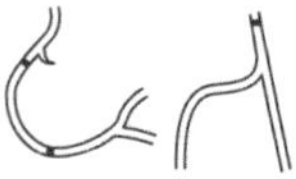

Correlations between the different myocardial infarction (MI) types with the infarction area assessed by contrast-enhanced cardiovascular magnetic resonance (CE-CMR), ECG pattern, name given to the infarction, and the most probable place of coronary artery occlusion. Because of frequent reperfusion treatment, usually the coronary angiography performed in the subacute phase does not correspond to the real location of the occlusion that produced the MI. The gray zones seen in the bull's eye view correspond to infarction areas, and the arrows correspond to their possible extension. D1, first diagonal; LAD, left anterior descending; LCX, left circumflex artery; RCA, right coronary artery; S1, first septal. Reproduced from Fuster V, Walsh RA, Harrington RA. *Hurst's The Heart*. 13th ed. Figure 15-66. Available at: www.accessmedicine.com. Copyright © The McGraw-Hill Companies, Inc. All rights reserved.

TABLE 5-1	Leads with ST Segment Elevations and Their Corresponding Coronary Arteries and Myocardium	
Lead(s)	Coronary artery/arteries	Corresponding myocardium
I, aV$_L$, and V$_1$–V$_4$	LAD (V$_2$ and V$_3$ most sensitive)	Medial half of LV wall, apex, anterior two thirds of intraventricular septum
aV$_L$	Diagonal branches	Anterolateral portion of LV
V$_3$R, V$_4$R, V$_5$R, III, and aV$_F$	RCA	RV
II, III, aV$_F$	RCA or circumflex (III and aV$_F$ most sensitive for RCA)	Inferior wall
V$_7$–V$_9$ (reciprocal ST depression in leads V$_2$ or V$_3$)	Left circumflex	Anterior and posterior aspect of lateral wall of LV
V$_5$ or V$_6$	Left circumflex	Anterior and posterior aspect of lateral wall of LV

STAGES OF ISCHEMIA AND ST ELEVATION MI (FIGURES 5-6 AND 5-7)

- Transient tall and peaked (hyperacute) T waves
- ST segment upwardly convex elevation (although it is also possible to have a non-ST elevation MI)
- Within days pathologic Q waves, and possibly decrease in amplitude of R waves, occur along with resolution of ST elevation
- A phase of pseudonormalization of the ECG appearance may occur after several days
- Usually the ST eventually returns to baseline with symmetric T wave inversion and a prolonged QT interval
- Q waves with ST elevation persisting 4 weeks or longer after MI correlate strongly with mechanical dysfunction or ventricular aneurysm

FIGURE 5-6. Acute anterior wall myocardial infarction

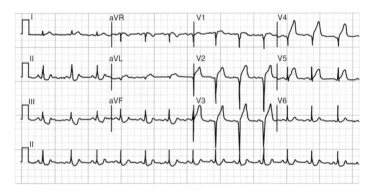

ST elevations and Q waves in V$_1$–V$_4$ and aV$_L$ and reciprocal inferior ST depressions. Reproduced from Longo DL, Fauci AS, Kasper DL, Hauser SL, Jameson JL, Loscalzo J. *Harrison's Principles of Internal Medicine*. 18th ed. Figure e28-6. Available at: www.accessmedicine.com. Copyright © The McGraw-Hill Companies, Inc. All rights reserved.

FIGURE 5-7. Extensive prior MI involving inferior, posterior, and lateral walls

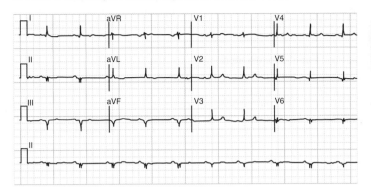

Q waves in leads II, III, aV$_F$, tall R waves in V$_1$, V$_2$, and Q waves in V$_5$, V$_6$. T wave abnormalities in leads I and aV$_L$, V$_5$, and V$_6$. Reproduced from Longo DL, Fauci AS, Kasper DL, Hauser SL, Jameson JL, Loscalzo J. *Harrison's Principles of Internal Medicine*. 18th ed. Figure e28-9. Available at: www.accessmedicine.com. Copyright © The McGraw-Hill Companies, Inc. All rights reserved.

ASSESSMENT OF LEFT VENTRICULAR HYPERTROPHY (FIGURE 5-8)

ECG changes seen with LVH include:
- Increased voltage of QRS complex (see voltage criteria, below); tall R waves in left sided-leads I, aV$_L$, V$_5$, and V$_6$ and deep S waves in right-sided leads V$_1$ and V$_2$
- ST segment abnormalities such as T wave inversion and depressed J point with downsloping ST depression
- QRS duration >110 milliseconds, reflecting longer time of activation for thickened ventricle

Voltage criteria for determining the presence of LVH:
- Sokolow–Lyon criteria: S in V$_1$ + (R in V$_5$ or R in V$_6$) >3.5 mV or R in aV$_L$ >1.1 mV
- Cornell criteria: R in aV$_L$ + S in V$_3$ = 2.8 mV in males and 2.0 mV in females

FIGURE 5-8. Left ventricular hypertrophy

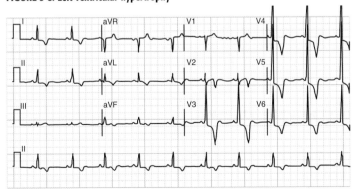

LVH with deep T wave inversions in limb leads and precordial leads. Striking T wave inversions in mid-precordial leads suggest *apical HCM* (Yamaguchi syndrome). HCM: hypertrophic cardiomyopathy. Reproduced from Longo DL, Fauci AS, Kasper DL, Hauser SL, Jameson JL, Loscalzo J. *Harrison's Principles of Internal Medicine*. 18th ed. Figure e28-19. Available at: www.accessmedicine.com. Copyright © The McGraw-Hill Companies, Inc. All rights reserved.

CONDUCTION ABNORMALITIES

The best leads for rhythm evaluation are II, III, and aV_F (the P wave morphology is most visible in these leads). With difficult diagnoses consider the use of esophageal leads for increased sensitivity.

A. Right bundle branch block

Delayed activation of the right ventricle (Figure 5-9).

Diagnostic criteria for RBBB:
- QRS duration >120 milliseconds
- rsr', rsR', rSR' in lead V_1 or V_2 and occasional wide and notched R waves
- S wave longer than 40 milliseconds or longer than the duration of the R wave in leads V_6 and I
- Normal R peak time in leads V_5 and V_6 but ≥50 milliseconds in lead V_1

FIGURE 5-9. Right bundle branch block

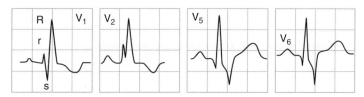

Reproduced from Patel A. *EKGs and Cardiac Studies: Essential Evidence-Based Data for Common Clinical Encounters*. Figure 7-1.

B. Left bundle branch block

Delayed activation of the left ventricle (Figure 5-10).

Diagnostic criteria of LBBB:
- QRS duration >120 milliseconds
- Monophasic R (no q) in I, V_5, V_6
- QS or rS in V_1 and notched (M shaped) R in I, V_5, V_6
- ST and T wave opposite to QRS, ST elevation and positive T in V_1 and V_2, ST depression and inverted T in I, V_5, V_6

FIGURE 5-10. Left bundle branch block

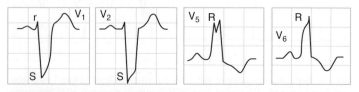

Reproduced from Patel A. *EKGs and Cardiac Studies: Essential Evidence-Based Data for Common Clinical Encounters*. Figure 7-3.

FIGURE 5-11. Acute MI in the presence of a right bundle branch block

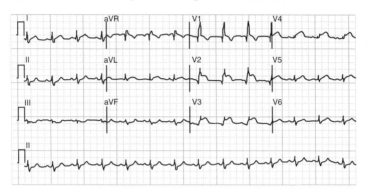

Acute anteroseptal MI (Q waves and ST elevations in V_1–V_4) with *RBBB* (note terminal R waves in V_1). Reproduced from Longo DL, Fauci AS, Kasper DL, Hauser SL, Jameson JL, Loscalzo J. *Harrison's Principles of Internal Medicine*. 18th ed. Figure e28-8. Available at: www.accessmedicine.com. Copyright © The McGraw-Hill Companies, Inc. All rights reserved.

RBBB does not interfere with the diagnosis of myocardial infarct (Figure 5-11).

LBBB obscures the ECG features, and increases the mortality, of an acute MI (Figure 5-12A and B).

Features of new AMI with preexisting LBBB include:
• More pronounced ST segment elevation
• ST segment deviations opposite to those of an uncomplicated LBBB
• Q waves in leads I or aV_L, V_5 or V_6, III and aV_F
• Notching of the S wave in leads V_3–V_5

The Sgarbossa criteria for new MI in the presence of LBBB:
• ST elevation ≥1 mm in leads with a positive QRS (5 points)
• ST depression ≥1 mm in V_1–V_3 (3 points)
• ST elevation ≥5 mm in leads with a negative QRS (2 points)

These criteria are specific (90% if score ≥ 3), but not sensitive, and are used for ruling in MI for thrombolytic therapy.

FIGURE 5-12. Acute MI in the presence of a left bundle branch block

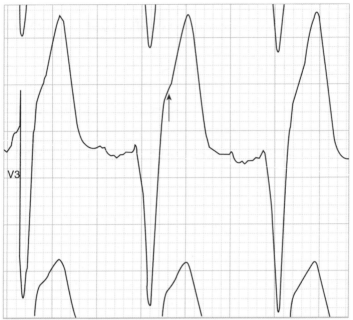

A

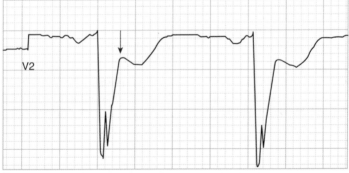

B

(A) The ST elevation is greater than 5 mm discordant from the primary QRS deflection (arrow). Reproduced from Knoop KJ, Stack LB, Storrow AB, Thurman RJ. *The Atlas of Emergency Medicine*. 3rd ed. Figure 23-6C. Available at: www.accessmedicine.com. Copyright © The McGraw-Hill Companies, Inc. All rights reserved. (B) The ST depression is greater than 1 mm concordant to the primary QRS deflection (arrow). Reproduced from Knoop KJ, Stack LB, Storrow AB, Thurman RJ. *The Atlas of Emergency Medicine*. 3rd ed. Figure 23-6B. Available at: www.accessmedicine.com. Copyright © The McGraw-Hill Companies, Inc. All rights reserved.

ATRIOVENTRICULAR CONDUCTION BLOCKS

A. First-degree heart block

PR interval greater than 200 milliseconds (Figure 5-13).

Etiology: beta-adrenergic blockers, calcium channel blockers, amiodarone, digitalis, quinidine, general anesthesia with inhalational agents, athletes, myocarditis.

FIGURE 5-13. First-degree heart block

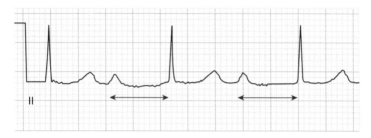

The PR interval is fixed (double arrows) and is longer than 0.2 seconds, or five small blocks. Reproduced from Knoop KJ, Stack LB, Storrow AB, Thurman RJ. *The Atlas of Emergency Medicine.* 3rd ed. Figure 23-14B. Available at: www.accessmedicine.com. Copyright © The McGraw-Hill Companies, Inc. All rights reserved.

B. Second-degree heart block

Some P waves are conducted through the ventricle and others are not.

Second-degree heart block type I, Mobitz type I (Wenckebach) (Figure 5-14):
- The PR interval progressively lengthens until there is nonconduction of a P wave
- It is relatively benign unless associated with hypotension or bradycardia
- Typically occurs in young healthy patients with high vagal tone

Second-degree heart block type II, Mobitz type II (Figure 5-15):
- P waves are occasionally not followed by a QRS complex, but the PR interval of conducted beats is constant and normal
- The QRS is wide in 80% of cases
- Commonly progresses to complete heart block and may indicate serious underlying heart disease

FIGURE 5-14. Second-degree AV block Mobitz type I (Wenckebach)

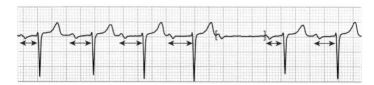

The PR interval gradually increases (double arrows) until a P wave is not followed by a QRS and a beat is "dropped" (brackets). The process then recurs. P waves occur at regular intervals, although they may be hidden by T waves. Reproduced from Knoop KJ, Stack LB, Storrow AB, Thurman RJ. *The Atlas of Emergency Medicine.* 3rd ed. Figure 23-15B. Available at: www.accessmedicine.com. Copyright © The McGraw-Hill Companies, Inc. All rights reserved.

FIGURE 5-15. Second-degree AV block Mobitz type II

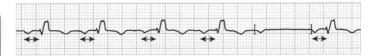

The PR interval is constant (double arrows) until the dropped beat (brackets). Reproduced from Knoop KJ, Stack LB, Storrow AB, Thurman RJ. *The Atlas of Emergency Medicine*. 3rd ed. Figure 23-16B. Available at: www.accessmedicine.com. Copyright © The McGraw-Hill Companies, Inc. All rights reserved.

C. Third-degree (complete) heart block

In *third-degree (complete) heart block* (Figure 5-16), the P wave and QRS complexes have separate and independent rates. The QRS morphology is usually wide. Its sudden appearance during anesthesia may cause profound hypotension and circulatory collapse and is an indication for immediate pacing.

FIGURE 5-16. Third-degree heart block

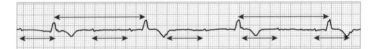

The P–P interval is uniform (lower double arrows) and the R–R interval is uniform (upper double arrows), but the P waves and QRS complexes are disassociated. Reproduced from Knoop KJ, Stack LB, Storrow AB, Thurman RJ. *The Atlas of Emergency Medicine*. 3rd ed. Figure 23-17B. Available at: www.accessmedicine.com. Copyright © The McGraw-Hill Companies, Inc. All rights reserved.

INDICATIONS FOR TEMPORARY PACING

Symptomatic bradycardia, new bundle branch block with transient complete heart block, complete heart block, Mobitz type II with anterior myocardial infarction, new bifascicular block, bilateral bundle branch block and first-degree atrioventricular block, postdefibrillation bradycardia, perioperative pharmacologic treatment causing hemodynamically significant bradycardia.

A. Antitachycardia/overdrive pacing

May prevent or terminate a tachyarrhythmia and is used for bradycardia-dependent VT, torsades de pointes, long QT syndrome, and treatment of recurrent SVT or VT.

B. Prophylactic temporary pacing

Pulmonary artery catheter placement in patients with left bundle branch block, new atrioventricular block or bundle branch block in acute endocarditis, cardioversion in the setting of sick sinus syndrome, AF prophylaxis after cardiac surgery, and after heart transplantation.

FIGURE 5-17. Dual-chamber pacemaker

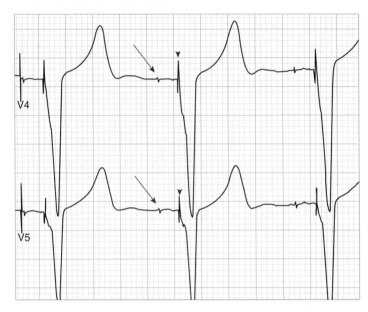

Tiny pacer spikes (arrows) precede the P waves, and somewhat larger pacer spikes precede the QRS complexes (arrowheads). The QRS complexes are wide, with discordant T waves. Reproduced from Knoop KJ, Stack LB, Storrow AB, Thurman RJ. *The Atlas of Emergency Medicine*. 3rd ed. Figure 23-26B. Available at: www.accessmedicine.com. Copyright © The McGraw-Hill Companies, Inc. All rights reserved.

EKG CHANGES WITH ELECTROLYTE ABNORMALITIES

(See chapter 36 on electrolyte abnormalities for EKG tracings.)

- Hyperkalemia:
  - ‣ Narrowing and peaking of T waves
  - ‣ Shortening of the QT interval
  - ‣ Widening of the QRS complex
  - ‣ Low P wave amplitude
  - ‣ Possible AV nodal block
  - ‣ With severe hyperkalemia, a sine-wave pattern of ventricular flutter occurs, followed by asystole
- Hypokalemia:
  - ‣ ST depression
  - ‣ Flattened T waves
  - ‣ Prominent U waves
  - ‣ Long QT interval predisposing to torsades de pointes
- Hypercalcemia:
  - ‣ Decreased QT interval. If serum calcium exceeds 15 mg/dL, T wave changes may occur
- Hypocalcemia:
  - ‣ Prolonged QT interval
- Hypermagnesemia:
  - ‣ Complete heart block and cardiac arrest (Mg^{2+} >15 mEq/L)
- Hypomagnesemia:
  - ‣ Long QT and torsades de pointes (Figure 5-18)

FIGURE 5-18. EKG in torsades de pointes

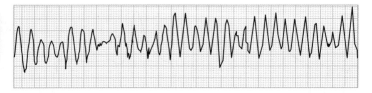

Very rapid wide complex tachycardia with sine-wave appearance and fluctuations in the amplitude of the QRS complexes consistent with torsades de pointes. Reproduced from Knoop KJ, Stack LB, Storrow AB, Thurman RJ. *The Atlas of Emergency Medicine*. 3rd ed. Figure 23-34B. Available at: www.accessmedicine.com. Copyright © The McGraw-Hill Companies, Inc. All rights reserved.

REFERENCES

For references, please visit **www.TheAnesthesiaGuide.com**.

CHAPTER 6
Preoperative Echocardiography

Sanford M. Littwin, MD

INDICATIONS

- Determine the overall health and "fitness" of the patient:
  ‣ If cardiomyopathy, assess function
  ‣ If valvular disease, assess status
- Ascertain if medical optimization has been achieved
- Stratify the patient's risk, and decide on needed interventions/invasive monitors that can ensure optimal outcome for the patient

ASSESSMENT OF PATIENTS WITH EITHER

- Transthoracic echo (TTE): gold standard for preoperative evaluation
- Transesophageal echo (TEE): if TTE suboptimal (e.g., body habitus, emphysema)

MODES

- Two-dimensional echo visualization of anatomic structures
- Color flow Doppler: visualization of blood flow and direction of flow; useful to assess, for example, regurgitant flow from valve (mnemonic BART: blue, away from probe; red, toward)
- Spectral Doppler (continuous/pulse wave) for determination of flow velocities
- Contrast imaging to determine presence of anatomic defects (e.g., PFO)

FIGURE 6-1. Views obtained by transthoracic echocardiography

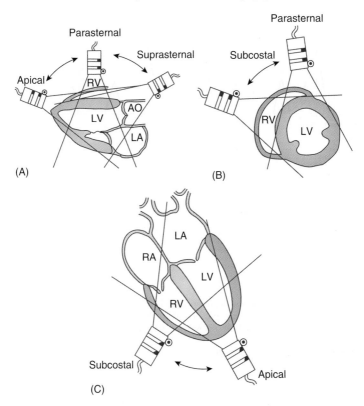

(A)

(B)

(C)

Visualization of the heart's basic tomographic imaging planes by various transducer positions. The long-axis plane (A) can be imaged in the parasternal, suprasternal, and apical positions; the short-axis plane (B) in the parasternal and subcostal positions; and the four-chamber plane (C) in the apical and subcostal positions. Reproduced from Fuster V, Walsh RA, Harrington RA. *Hurst's The Heart.* 13th ed. Figure 18-13. Available at: www.accessmedicine.com. Copyright © The McGraw-Hill Companies, Inc. All rights reserved.

ECHO PREOPERATIVELY CAN IDENTIFY

- Global LV function, cardiac performance
- Regional wall motion abnormalities (RWMA), areas that are likely underperfused or at risk for reversible ischemia
- Valvular dysfunction, type, and severity
- Related pathologies, PFO, masses, pericardial effusion
- Cardiopulmonary pressure calculations, chamber size, and valve areas

REPORT INTERPRETATION

- EF (normal around 65%)
- Diastolic function:
  - ▸ Flow velocities measured across the mitral valve during diastole. Three patterns of diastolic dysfunction are generally recognized based on isovolumetric relaxation time, the ratio of peak early diastolic flow (E) to peak atrial systolic flow (A), and the deceleration time (DT) of E (DT_E) (Figure 6-2)

FIGURE 6-2. Velocity patterns of diastolic dysfunction

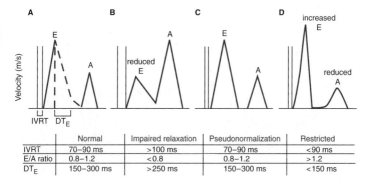

	Normal	Impaired relaxation	Pseudonormalization	Restricted
IVRT	70–90 ms	>100 ms	70–90 ms	<90 ms
E/A ratio	0.8–1.2	<0.8	0.8–1.2	>1.2
DT_E	150–300 ms	>250 ms	150–300 ms	<150 ms

Doppler echocardiography of diastolic flow across the mitral valve. (A–D) Increasing severity of diastolic dysfunction. E, early diastolic flow; A, peak atrial systolic flow; IVRT, isovolumic relaxation time; DT_E, deceleration time of E. Reproduced from Morgan GE, Mikhail MS, Murray MJ. *Clinical Anesthesiology*. 4th ed. Figure 19-11. Available at: www.accessmedicine.com. Copyright © The McGraw-Hill Companies, Inc. All rights reserved.

- Valve pathology: mild, moderate, severe (see chapter 88 on valvular disease):
  - MR: decreased forward flow out of aortic valve in systole, with concomitant regurgitant flow into LA during systole, LA enlargement, pulmonary HTN, falsely elevated EF
  - MS: decreased forward flow into LV, smaller LV volume, greater percent of LV volume ejection during systole
  - AR: regurgitant filling of LV during diastole, increased LV volume (volume overloaded heart)
  - AS: increased impedance to flow out of LV, concentric LV hypertrophy, possible decrease in LVEF
- Chamber size:
  - Enlargement indicative of either volume overload or pressure overload on heart
- Flow abnormalities and calculation of pressure gradients:
  - PA systolic pressure can be estimated if the patient has at least mild TR by measuring the peak velocity (v) of the regurgitant flow, which is a function of the pressure gradient between RV and RA. A certain RA value (~CVP) is assumed, typically 5–8 mm Hg unless there is a clinical reason to think it is higher. Modified Bernoulli (continuity) equation: $PASP = 4v^2 + RA$ pressure
- RWMA—visual examination of heart, performed in midesophageal four-chamber, midesophageal two-chamber, midesophageal long axis, and transgastric short axis:
  - Qualitatively graded as (Figure 6-3):
    - 1: normal (>30% thickening)
    - 2: mild hypokinesis (thickening between 10% and 30%)
    - 3: severe hypokinesis (<10% thickening)
    - 4: akinesis (no visible thickening)
    - 5: dyskinesis (paradoxical motion)
- Stress echo determination of reversible ischemic areas of heart as cardiac work is performed:
  - Simulated stresses on heart as would be seen during operation
  - Can compare visualized RWMA with EKG changes indicative of ischemia

FIGURE 6-3. Grading of wall motion abnormality on a short-axis view

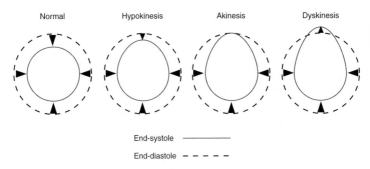

| Normal | Hypokinesis | Akinesis | Dyskinesis |

End-systole ——————

End-diastole — — — — —

CHAPTER 7
Cardiac Risk Stratification for Noncardiac Surgery, Lee's Score, NYHA Classification

Sumeet Goswami, MD, MPH and Amit Goswami, MD

RISK STRATIFICATION

TABLE 7-1 Lee's Revised Cardiac Risk Index
High-risk type of surgery
History of ischemic heart disease
History of congestive heart failure
History of cerebrovascular disease
Preoperative treatment with insulin
Preoperative serum creatinine >2 mg/dL

Rates of major cardiac complications in the validation cohort with 0, 1, 2, or ≥3 of these factors were 0.4%, 0.9%, 7%, and 11%, respectively.

Based on the American College of Cardiology/American Heart Association guidelines on perioperative evaluation for noncardiac surgery, cardiac risk factors can be segregated into two categories: *active cardiac conditions* (formerly known as major risk factors) and *clinical risk factors* (formerly known as intermediate risk factors) (Tables 7-2 and 7-3). Noncardiac surgical procedures are also stratified based on cardiac risk (Table 7-4).

TABLE 7-2	Active Cardiac Conditions
Conditions	Examples
Unstable coronary syndrome	Unstable or severe angina
	Recent myocardial infarction (within 30 days)
Decompensated heart failure	NYHA functional class IV; worsening or new-onset heart failure
Significant arrhythmias	High-grade atrioventricular block (Mobitz type II or third degree)
	Symptomatic ventricular arrythmias
	Supraventricular arrhythmias with uncontrolled ventricular rate (HR greater than 100 bpm at rest)
	Symptomatic bradycardia
Severe valvular disease	Severe aortic stenosis (mean gradient >40 mm Hg, valve area <1 cm^2 or symptomatic)
	Symptomatic mitral stenosis

TABLE 7-3	Clinical Risk Factors
History of ischemic heart disease	
History of compensated heart failure	
History of cerebrovascular disease	
Diabetes mellitus	
Renal insufficiency	

TABLE 7-4	Cardiac Risk Stratification for Noncardiac Surgical Procedures
Risk stratification	Procedure examples
Vascular (reported cardiac risk often more than 5%)	Aortic and other major vascular surgery
	Peripheral vascular surgery
Intermediate (cardiac risk generally 1–5%)	Intraperitoneal and intrathoracic surgery
	Carotid endarterectomy
	Head and neck surgery
	Orthopedic surgery
	Prostate surgery
Low (cardiac risk generally less than 1%)	Endoscopic procedures
	Superficial procedures
	Cataract surgery
	Breast surgery
	Ambulatory surgery

STEPWISE APPROACH TO PERIOPERATIVE CARDIAC ASSESSMENT

The stepwise approach to perioperative cardiac assessment is based on the presence of cardiac risk factors, risk stratification of the surgical procedure, and patient's functional capacity (Figure 7-1). Diagnostic evaluation and treatment is indicated for patients with active cardiac conditions (Table 7-2) such as unstable angina or decompensated heart failure. Additional diagnostic testing such as a stress test should also be considered in patients undergoing vascular procedures (Table 7-4) who suffer from three or more clinical risk factors (Table 7-3) and have poor functional capacity.

PATIENTS WHO BENEFIT FROM PREOPERATIVE CORONARY REVASCULARIZATION

Coronary revascularization (either CABG or PCI) is indicated (class I, benefit >>> risk; level of evidence A) in the following groups of patients undergoing noncardiac surgery:
- Stable angina with significant left main disease
- Stable angina with three-vessel disease
- Stable angina with two-vessel disease:
  ‣ With significant proximal LAD stenosis
  ‣ Either LVEF <50% or demonstrable ischemia on noninvasive testing
- High-risk unstable angina or non-ST elevation MI
- Acute ST elevation MI

TABLE 7-5	NYHA Classification: Stages of Heart Failure
Class	Patient symptoms
Class I (mild)	No limitation of physical activity. Ordinary physical activity does not cause undue fatigue, palpitation, or dyspnea
Class II (mild)	Slight limitation of physical activity. Comfortable at rest, but ordinary physical activity results in fatigue, palpitation, or dyspnea
Class III (moderate)	Marked limitation of physical activity. Comfortable at rest, but less than ordinary activity causes fatigue, palpitation, or dyspnea
Class IV (severe)	Unable to carry out any physical activity without discomfort. Symptoms of cardiac insufficiency at rest. If any physical activity is undertaken, discomfort is increased

FIGURE 7-1. Stepwise approach to perioperative cardiac assessment

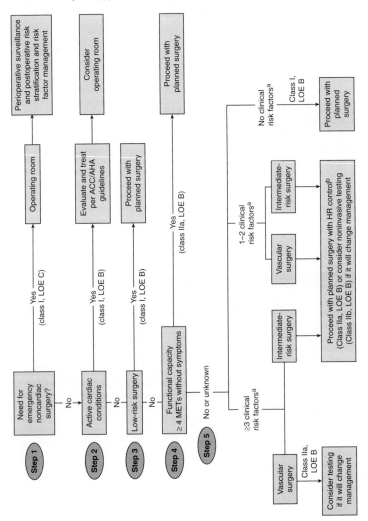

(A) See Table 7-3. (B) consider perioperative beta-blockade. Reprinted with permission from Fleisher LA , Beckman JA, Brown KA, et al. 2009 ACCF/AHA Focused Update on Perioperative Beta Blockade Incorporated Into the ACC/AHA 2007 Guidelines on Perioperative Cardiovascular Evaluation and Care for Noncardiac Surgery. *Circulation*. 2009;120:e169-e276. © 2009 American Heart Association, Inc.

REFERENCES

For references, please visit **www.TheAnesthesiaGuide.com**.

CHAPTER 8
Infective Endocarditis Prophylaxis

Edward C. Lin, MD

In 2007, the AHA published revised guidelines for the prevention of infective endocarditis.

TABLE 8-1	Conditions where it is Reasonable to Give Antibiotics to Prevent Infective Endocarditis (IE)

- Prosthetic cardiac valve or prosthetic material used for cardiac valve repair
- History of IE
- Unrepaired cyanotic CHD (including palliative shunts and conduits)
- For the first 6 months after completely repairing a congenital heart defect with prosthetic material or device
- Repaired CHD with residual defects at the site or adjacent to the site of a prosthetic patch or prosthetic device
- Valvulopathy after cardiac transplantation

TABLE 8-2	Procedures for which it is Reasonable to Give Antibiotics to Patients with the Conditions Given in Table 8-1	
Location	**Caveats**	
Dental	• Give only for procedures involving manipulation of the gingival tissue or the periapical region of teeth or perforation of the oral mucosa	
Respiratory tract	• For procedures involving incision or biopsy of mucosa • If procedure is to treat infection, use antibiotic that covers *Streptococcus* viridans, or, if infection known/suspected to be secondary to *S. aureus*, give antibiotic that covers *S. aureus* (use vancomycin if MRSA)	
Infected skin/skin structure/MSK	• Ensure that the antibiotic given will cover staphylococci and beta-hemolytic *Streptococcus*	

GI or GU tract procedures	• Antibiotics not recommended if only given to prevent infective endocarditis
	• Coverage for enterococci reasonable if:
	   (1) Patient has an established GI or GU infection
	   (2) Patient on antibiotics to prevent sepsis/wound infection from a GI or GU procedure
	   (3) Cystoscopy or urinary tract manipulation in a patient with an existing urinary tract enterococcal infection or colonization
	   (4) Urinary tract procedure is not elective	

TABLE 8-3	Antibiotic Regimen for Dental Procedures		
	Antibiotic	Adult dose	Pediatric dose (mg/kg)
Oral	Amoxicillin	2 g	50
Oral + allergic to PCN	Cephalexin	2 g	50
	Clindamycin	600 mg	20
	Azithromycin/ clarithromycin	500 mg	15
Intravenous/ intramuscular	Ampicillin	2 g	50
	Cefazolin/ceftriaxone	1 g	50
Intravenous/ intramuscular + allergic to PCN	Cefazolin/ceftriaxone	1 g	50
	Clindamycin	600 mg	20

REFERENCE

For references, please visit **www.TheAnesthesiaGuide.com**.

PART II

COEXISTING DISEASE

CHAPTER 9
Management of Chronic Medications in the Perioperative Period
Yakub Abrakhimov, MD

Of note, this chapter does not include the perioperative management of anticoagulants, antiplatelets, glucocorticoids, and anticonvulsants, which are treated in separate chapters.

GENERAL PRINCIPLES

- Understand pathophysiology of patient's various comorbidities and deduce if discontinuation of a particular drug would lead to disease progression
- Consider the possibility of withdrawal with an abrupt cessation of a particular drug
- Consider possible drug–drug interactions perioperatively
- Understand anticipated type of surgery, anesthesia, as well as the postoperative course

PERIOPERATIVE MANAGEMENT OF CARDIOVASCULAR AGENTS

See Table 9-1.

TABLE 9-1 Perioperative Management of Cardiovascular Agents

Medication	Two days prior to surgery	One day prior to surgery	Morning of surgery	Perioperative considerations
Beta-blockers	Yes *(do not stop)*	Yes *(do not stop)*	Yes *(do not stop)*	• Abrupt cessation may lead to hypertension, tachycardia, and myocardial ischemia • If needed (and enough time), adjust dose for HR 60–70 without hypotension • Shown to decrease perioperative risk of myocardial ischemia in patients with cardiac disease. *Perioperative initiation not recommended* (because of possible increased risk of CVA and mortality) • Can bridge patient to IV forms
Calcium channel blockers	Yes	Yes	Yes	• Stop if patient hypotensive • Abrupt cessation will not result in withdrawal effects • Can bridge patient to IV forms
Angiotensin-converting enzyme inhibitors/ angiotensin II receptor blockers (ACEI/ARB)	Yes	Yes	Yes, if used to treat hypertension No, if used for other indications	• Continuation may lead to hypotension perioperatively • Abrupt cessation may lead to rebound postoperative hypertension • Intraoperative use of IV angiotensin to treat refractory hypotension has been reported • No clear evidence of adverse effects of continuation; it might be less confusing for patients to take all HTN medications; however, this is controversial
Alpha-blockers	Yes	Yes	Yes	• Known to cause orthostatic hypotension and dizziness
Clonidine	Yes	Yes	Yes	• Abrupt cessation may lead to severe rebound hypertension • If patient is anticipated to restart PO clonidine within 12 h of preoperative dose, then clonidine should be continued up to and including day of surgery • If patient will be unable to restart PO dose within 12 h of preoperative dose, then he or she should be bridged to patch form of clonidine 3 days prior to surgery • PO dose should be tapered while patch form is initiated

Diuretics	Yes	Yes	No	Continuation may lead to hypovolemia and electrolyte disturbances
Statins	Yes	Yes	Yes	• In combination with perioperative risk of muscle injury, may contribute to development of myopathy • Perioperative use as cardioprotective agent still under investigation • Administer postoperatively by NGT if unable to swallow
Non-statin cholesterol lowering agents	Yes	No	No	• Cholestyramine/colestipol binds bile acids in GI tract and hinders absorption of various medications • Niacin/folic acid may lead to myopathy and rhabdomyolysis
Nitrates	Yes	Yes	Yes	• Transdermal forms may have decreased efficacy if skin perfusion is compromised
Digoxin	Yes	Yes	Yes	• Perioperative physiologic changes such as change in pH, hypoxia, electrolyte disturbances and use of other drugs may lead to digoxin toxicity • Extended half-life of 36–48 h (assuming normal renal function); thus, patient can miss dose with minimal loss in pharmacologic effect • Preoperative and Postoperative levels may be measured and IV form may be administered
Class I antiarrhythmics for A-Fib (quinidine, procainamide, disopyramide)	Yes	No	No	
Amiodarone, sotalol	Yes	Yes	Yes	

TABLE 9-2 Perioperative Management of Pulmonary, Gastrointestinal, and Immunosuppressive Medications

Medication	Two days prior to surgery	One day prior to surgery	Morning of surgery	Perioperative considerations
Beta-agonists/anticholinergics	Yes (do not stop)	Yes (do not stop)	Yes (do not stop)	• None
Theophylline	Yes	Yes	No	• Narrow therapeutic range • Interactions with other drugs • May obtain serum level of drug preoperatively and adjust dose accordingly
H2 blockers	Yes	Yes	Yes	• Can bridge patient to IV forms
Proton pump inhibitors	Yes	Yes	Yes	• Can bridge patient to IV forms
Cyclosporine Tacrolimus	Yes	Yes	Yes No cyclosporine if GA	• Monitor plasma levels and renal function
Methotrexate	Yes	Yes	Yes	• Hematologic and renal toxicity
Cyclophosphamide, azathioprine, mycophenolate mofetil	Yes	Yes	Yes	
Anti-TNF antibodies	No	No	No	• Hold × 7 days (increases infection risk) • Continue if colon surgery in Crohn's or ulcerative colitis patient

Oral contraceptives	Yes (do not stop) for surgery with low risk of venous thromboembolism (VTE) No for surgery with high risk of VTE	Yes (do not stop) for surgery with low risk of VTE No for surgery with high risk of VTE	Yes (do not stop) for surgery with low risk of VTE No for surgery with high risk of VTE	• Continuation may increase risk of perioperative VTE • Risk of VTE is increased with orthopedic surgery and surgery with extended postoperative period of immobility • Estrogens have to be discontinued for 3–4 weeks for coagulation profile to return to baseline (which may lead to unwanted pregnancies) • For surgery with high risk of VTE, discontinue at least 4 weeks prior to date of surgery
Postmenopausal hormone replacement	As above	As above	As above	• As above
Selective estrogen receptor modulators (SERMs)	As above	As above	As above	• When SERMs are used for breast cancer therapy, patient's oncologist should be consulted to evaluate for risks and benefits of continuing therapy in perioperative period
Levothyroxine	Yes	Yes	Yes	• Levothyroxine half-life is 6–7 days; thus, dose may be missed perioperatively without significant untoward events
Antithyroid medications	Yes	Yes	Yes	• Monitor for thyroid storm that may present as fever, tachycardia, and mental status changes • Consider administering through gastric tube if prolonged NPO status is anticipated
Metformin	No	No	No	• Continuation may lead to lactic acidosis if renal function is compromised or IV contrast is to be utilized during time of surgery • Discontinue 48 h prior to surgery

TABLE 9-3	Perioperative Management of Medications Involving the Endocrine System			
Medication	Two days prior to surgery	One day prior to surgery	Morning of surgery	Perioperative considerations
Sulfonylureas	Yes	Yes	Yes	• Continuation of sulfonylureas may lead to hypoglycemia • Hold sulfonylureas during fasting period
Thiazolidinediones	No	No	No	• Continuation of thiazolidinediones may lead to fluid retention • Hold thiazolidinediones a few days prior to surgery
GLP-1 agonists	Yes	Yes	No	• Continuation may delay gastric motility and contribute to a prolonged course of time prior to return of bowel function after major surgery
DPP-4 inhibitors	Yes	Yes	Yes	• Mostly used to control postprandial glucose levels, thus may not be indicated if patient is NPO
Insulin	Yes	Yes	Yes	• Hyperglycemia is associated with poor wound healing • Intermediate-acting insulin should be reduced to one half to two thirds of evening and morning doses • Full dose of glargine may be given • Consider initiating insulin infusion for major surgeries for tighter glucose control

For more details on medications to treat diabetes mellitus, see chapter 25.

TABLE 9-4   Perioperative Management of Psychotropic and Neurological Medications

Medication	Two days prior to surgery	One day prior to surgery	Morning of surgery	Perioperative considerations
Selective serotonin reuptake inhibitors (SSRIs)	Yes (do not stop)	Yes (do not stop)	Yes (do not stop)	• Risk of perioperative HTN • Use of SSRIs may lead to reduction of serotonin in platelets, which may increase risk of bleeding • Discontinue 3 weeks prior to high-risk surgeries such as procedures that involve the CNS
Tricyclic antidepressants	Yes	Yes	Yes	• Continuation may promote arrhythmias and augment response to sympathomimetics
MAO inhibitors	No	No	No	• Concomitant use with indirect sympathomimetics (ephedrine) may lead to a potentiated response secondary to massive release of stored catecholamines • Concomitant use with meperidine or dextromorphan may lead to serotonin syndrome • Typically used for major depression unresponsive to other treatments; discuss interruption with psychiatrist; if needed, continue throughout the perioperative period and avoid drugs that can interact
Antipsychotics	Yes	Yes	Yes	• Known to prolong QT interval, which may promote arrhythmias • Neuroleptic malignant syndrome may mimic signs/symptoms of malignant hyperthermia
Lithium	Yes	Yes	Yes	• Continuation may lead to prolongation of paralytic agents • Toxic levels may lead to arrhythmias and mental status changes • If continued perioperatively, serum levels and electrolytes should be closely monitored
Benzodiazepines	Yes	Yes	Yes	• Abrupt cessation may lead to agitation, seizures, and elevated blood pressure • Patient will have high tolerance to benzodiazepines, and possibly to other agents acting on the GABA receptor (e.g. propofol)
Parkinson disease medications	Yes	Yes	Yes	• See chapter 29 on Parkinson disease
Cholinesterase inhibitors (MG)	Yes	Yes	Yes	• Possible prolongation of NMB following SCh
Cannabis, cocaine	No	No	No	• No demonstrated medical concern with cannabis use and anesthesia (but common advice is to avoid use prior to surgery) • No cocaine × 7 days required preoperatively

REFERENCES

For references, please visit **www.TheAnesthesiaGuide.com**.

CHAPTER 10
Herbal Medicines and Supplements

Sansan S. Lo, MD

- Preoperative assessment of potential herbal medicine use is important for preoperative instruction and understanding of perioperative risks and complications
- Dietary supplements and alternative medicines are exempt from FDA regulation:
  ‣ Increasing usage, but are significantly underreported and often not addressed
  ‣ Significant biological effects including:
    ▪ Direct effects
    ▪ Drug interactions: pharmacodynamic and pharmacokinetic
  ‣ Ease of access without prescriptions
  ‣ Variable manufacturing quality control standards (potency, contaminants)
  ‣ Limited clinical studies
- Of note, this chapter does not include nonherbal supplements such as vitamins, minerals, amino acids, or hormones
- Many herbal medications have cardiovascular, coagulation, and sedative effects that may be associated with perioperative complications including MI, strokes, bleeding, and transplant rejection

TABLE 10-1	Herbal Medicines, Effects, and Anesthetic Implications	
Name of herb/ supplements	Common uses and pharmacologic effects	Perioperative concerns
Dong quai	"Health-promoting" and estrogen effects	• May increase INR, PT, aPTT • May be associated with photosensitivity
Echinacea	URIs, arthritis, open wounds	• Immunostimulatory effects with short-term use, thus contraindicated in autoimmune disease and immunosuppressive regimens • Immunosuppression with long-term use with implications on wound healing, opportunistic infections • Inhibitor of cytochrome P450 3A4 (see below) • Possible hepatotoxicity • Possible allergic reactions
Ephedra	Weight loss, energy increase/stimulant, respiratory tract conditions	• Dose-dependent sympathomimetic effects with increased BP, HR, vasoconstriction with many reported cases of cardiac and CNS complications including death • Increased risk of ventricular arrhythmias with concomitant use of agents that sensitize myocardium such as halothane

(continued)

TABLE 10-1	Herbal Medicines, Effects, and Anesthetic Implications (*continued*)	
Name of herb/ supplements	Common uses and pharmacologic effects	Perioperative concerns
		• Long-term use depletes endogenous catecholamines; associated with tachyphylaxis with potential perioperative hemodynamic instability (use direct-acting sympathomimetic agents intraoperatively) • Concomitant use with MAOIs can result in life-threatening hyperpyrexia, hypertension, coma • Should discontinue at least 24 h prior to surgery
Feverfew	Primarily migraine treatment. Also headaches, arthritis	• Inhibits platelet activity
Garlic	Antimicrobial, immunostimulatory, decreases blood pressure, lowers cholesterol	• Decreases blood pressure • Likely irreversible inhibition of platelets and may potentiate other platelet inhibitors • Discontinue at least 7 days prior to surgery
Gingko	Cognitive disorders, peripheral vascular disease, age-related macular degeneration, vertigo, tinnitus, erectile dysfunction, altitude sickness	• Inhibits platelet-activating factor • Discontinue at least 36 h prior to surgery
Ginseng	Protects against stress, restores homeostasis, lowers blood glucose	• Hypoglycemia • Platelet inhibition, possibly irreversible • Interference with efficacy of warfarin-induced anticoagulation • Discontinue at least 7 days prior to surgery
Kava	Anxiolytic, sedative	• May potentiate sedation • Potential for abuse, addiction, tolerance, and withdrawal unknown • Possible association with hepatic dysfunction • Discontinue at least 24 h prior to surgery
Saw palmetto	BPH	• Anti-inflammatory effects that may cause platelet dysfunction
St. John's wort	Mild anxiety and depression, wounds and burns	• Unknown mechanism; inhibits serotonin, norepinephrine, dopamine reuptake • Potential MAOI and SSR inhibitor. Discontinue in patients taking these medications • Induces photosensitivity. Avoid photosensitive drugs and laser treatments • Induces cytochrome P450 3A4 (decreasing activity of warfarin, cyclosporin, oral contraceptive, digitalis, midazolam, lidocaine, calcium channel blockers) • Affects digoxin pharmacokinetics (decreases levels) • Discontinue at least 5 days prior to surgery
Valerian	Insomnia treatment	• Produces sedation and hypnosis (GABA) • Potentiates sedation • Abrupt discontinuation may lead to benzodiazepine-like withdrawal symptoms • May increase anesthetic requirements with long-term use

Resources:
- National Center for Complementary and Alternative Medicine, National Institutes of Health (http://nccam.nih.gov)
- HerbMed (http://www.herbmed.org)

REFERENCES

For references, please visit **www.TheAnesthesiaGuide.com**.

CHAPTER 11
Patient on Corticosteroids

Clément Hoffmann, MD and Jean-Pierre Tourtier, MD

PHYSIOPATHOLOGY

- Corticosurrenal production under control of the hypothalamic–pituitary axis of:
  - Glucocorticosteroids (cortisol [=hydrocortisone] and corticosterone)
  - Mineralocorticosteroids (aldosterone)
- Basal corticosteroid production in an adult patient = 5–10 mg/m^2 per day of cortisol (equivalent to 5–7 mg prednisone or 20–30 mg hydrocortisone for an average adult)
- If extrinsic steroid therapy administered, negative feedback to the hypothalamic–pituitary axis and inhibition of the corticoadrenal production
- In case of stress (such as surgery, disease, physical exertion, pregnancy), the normal protective surge in systemic cortisol will be inhibited, thus putting the patient at risk of acute adrenal insufficiency
- Normal daily secretion of cortisol in the perioperative period (about 72 hours):
  - Minor surgery: 25 mg
  - Moderate surgery: 50–75 mg
  - Major surgery: 100–150 mg
- Stress-dose steroid replacement should be commensurate to the need; if excessive, risk of infectious complications, delayed wound healing, and disturbed metabolic regulation (hyperglycemia)

PREOPERATIVE

Corticosteroids as chronic therapy = major reason for adrenal insufficiency.

Even possible for short therapy (5 days) or low dose (5 mg per day of prednisone).

TABLE 11-1	Corticosteroid Equivalent Doses		
	Glucocorticosteroids		
	Equivalence to 20 mg hydrocortisone	Half-life (min)	Duration of action (h)
Hydrocortisone *Cortef®, Solu-Cortef®*	20	100	8
Prednisone *Generic only*	5	200	24
Prednisolone *Predacort®*	5	120–300	24
Methylprednisolone *Medrol®, Solu-Medrol®*	4	120–180	36

Note that dexamethasone should not be used to replace intrinsic steroid production, as it has no mineralocorticoid effect.

PERIOPERATIVE MANAGEMENT OF PATIENT ON CHRONIC STEROID THERAPY

A. Minor surgical stress (e.g., hand surgery, hernia)

Take the usual steroid therapy on the morning of surgery.

Possibly, on induction: 25 mg hydrocortisone IV or 5 mg methylprednisolone IV.

B. Moderate surgical stress (e.g., hysterectomy, cholecystectomy)

- *Elective surgery*: usual corticotherapy on the morning of surgery, 25 mg hydrocortisone IV q8 hours for 48 hours at the most
- *Emergency surgery*: on induction, 25–50 mg hydrocortisone IV, and then 25–50 mg hydrocortisone IV q8 hours

After surgery, usual therapy or equivalence with hydrocortisone IV q8 hours if unable to take po.

C. Major surgical stress (e.g., major trauma, prolonged surgery, or surgery where there is delayed oral intake, such as esophagectomy, cardiac surgery)

- *Elective surgery*: usual steroid therapy on the morning of surgery, 50 mg hydrocortisone IV on induction, and then 50 mg hydrocortisone IV q8 hours until patient able to resume usual therapy
- *Emergency surgery*: 100 mg hydrocortisone IV on induction, and then 50 mg hydrocortisone IV q8 hours until patient able to resume usual therapy

PERIOPERATIVE MANAGEMENT OF THE PATIENT WITH CHRONIC ADRENAL INSUFFICIENCY

Usual treatment: hydrocortisone and fludrocortisone (glucocorticosteroids and mineralocorticosteroids).
- *The day before*: usual therapy
- *The morning of surgery*:
  ‣ Premedication with 9-α-fludrocortisone 50 μg po
  ‣ During surgery: hydrocortisone 50 mg IV, and then 10–20 mg/h
- *After surgery if NPO*:
  ‣ Hydrocortisone 50 mg IV q8 hours

- *After surgery if can take po meds*:
  - ▸ Hydrocortisone 50 mg on POD1, then 40 mg on POD2, and then 30 mg q day for 2–3 days
  - ▸ 9-α-Fludrocortisone 50 µg po q day
- *Surveillance and precautions*:
  - ▸ Every day: blood and urine electrolytes, BP:
    - • Overdose: hypertension, low natriuresis, weight gain, edema
    - • Underdose signs: hypotension, hyponatremia, hyperkalemia, weight loss

SEPSIS

Sepsis = relative adrenal insufficiency. See chapter 212.

For patients with hypotension poorly responsive to fluid resuscitation and vasopressor therapy, administer hydrocortisone 200–300 mg per day for 7 days in three or four divided doses, or continuous infusion.

It is no longer recommended to use an ACTH stimulation test to identify nonresponders.

REFERENCES

For references, please visit **www.TheAnesthesiaGuide.com**.

CHAPTER 12
Anticoagulation, Antiplatelet Medications

Tony P. Tsai, MD

NB: For anticoagulation and neuraxial anesthesia, please see the chapter 119 on safety in regional anesthesia.

PERIOPERATIVE MANAGEMENT OF PATIENTS ON VITAMIN K ANTAGONISTS (VKA)

Pharmacology:
- VKAs block the carboxylation of factors II, VII, IX, and X as well as proteins C and S (coagulation inhibitors)
- Equilibrium is reached only after about 5 days as factors have different half-lives
- Initial hypercoagulable state as protein C has the shortest half-life

TABLE 12-1 Indications and Therapeutic Targets of VKAs	
Indications for target INR of 2.5; range 2–3	Indications for target INR of 3; range 2.5–3.5
• Atrial fibrillation (AF) • Rheumatic mitral valve disease and AF or a history of previous systemic embolism • St. Jude Medical aortic bileaflet valve • Bioprosthetic valves: VKA for first 3 months after aortic or mitral valve insertion • AF and a recent CVA or TIA	• Tilting disk valves and bileaflet mechanical valves in the mitral position • Caged ball or caged disk valves; give VKA in combination with aspirin, 75–100 mg/day

The following procedures do not warrant VKA discontinuation if INR 2–3:
- Cataract surgery without retrobulbar block
- EGD without biopsy, colonoscopy without biopsy/polypectomy, ERCP without sphincterotomy
- Minor dental procedures
- Joint and soft tissue injections and arthrocentesis

For AF, assess thromboembolic risk based on the CHADS2 score (0–6 points).

TABLE 12-2	CHADS2 Score for Assessment of Thromboembolic Risk
CHF	1 point
HTN	1 point
Age >75 years	1 point
DM	1 point
History of stroke	2 points

- 0 points: no indication for chronic anticoagulation; discontinue warfarin 5 days before surgery; do not resume unless other indication
- 1–2 points: discontinue warfarin 5 days before surgery; resume 5 days after surgery
- 3 points or more: discontinue warfarin 5 days before surgery; LMWH, or IV UFH relay

For valve replacements:
- Discontinue warfarin at least 5 days before elective procedure, or longer if INR >3.0
- Assess INR 1–2 days before surgery; if INR >1.5, consider 1–2 mg of oral vitamin K
- Reversal for urgent surgery: consider 2.5–5 mg of oral or intravenous vitamin K
- Immediate reversal for emergent surgery: consider fresh frozen plasma, *prothrombin complex concentrate, or recombinant factor VIIa*

Patients at high risk for thromboembolism:
- For patients who have a mechanical valve, high risk includes those who have mitral valve prostheses, older aortic valve prostheses, or had a CVA or TIA in the past 6 months
- For patients who have atrial fibrillation, high risk includes a CHADS2 score of 5–6, a CVA or TIA within the past 3 months, or rheumatic valvular heart disease
- For patients who had a venous thromboembolism (VTE), high risk includes a VTE within the past 3 months, severe thrombophilia
- Bridge with therapeutic subcutaneous low-molecular-weight heparin (LMWH), which is preferred (Lovenox 1 mg/kg every 12 hours or dalteparin 100 IU/kg every 12 hours), or intravenous unfractionated heparin (UFH) (especially if acute arterial/VTE within 1 month)
- Last dose of preoperative LMWH administered 24 hours before surgery; administer half of daily dose

No bridging necessary for patients at low risk for thromboembolism:
- For patients who have a mechanical valve, low risk includes patients with bileaflet aortic valve prostheses without atrial fibrillation and those who do not have other risk factors for CVA
- For patients who have atrial fibrillation, low risk includes CHADS2 score of 0–2
- For patients who had a VTE, low risk includes patients who had a single VTE more than 1 year before surgery and no other risk factors

NB: Despite discontinuation or reversal, bleeding risk probably increased, especially in thoracic surgery

TABLE 12-3	Management of a Bleeding Patient on VKA
Patient's status	What to do
5 > INR > 3, no significant bleeding	Decrease dose or omit dose, monitor INR frequently, and resume VKA at lower dose when INR is therapeutic; if only minimally above therapeutic range, no dose reduction may be required
9 > INR > 5, no significant bleeding	Omit one to two doses; monitor INR frequently; resume VKA at an adjusted dose when INR is therapeutic. For increased risk of bleeding, can omit dose and give 1–2.5 mg vitamin K po. If rapid correction of INR is needed, give 5 mg vitamin K po 24 h before surgery and add 1–2 mg vitamin K po if necessary
INR >9, no significant bleeding	Hold VKA, give 2.5–5 mg vitamin K po, wait 24–48 h, and add 1–2 mg vitamin K po if necessary. Resume VKA at an adjusted dose when INR is therapeutic
Any INR elevation, serious bleeding	Hold VKA and give 10 mg vitamin K IV (slow infusion); supplement with FFP, prothrombin complex concentrate, or recombinant factor VIIa. IV vitamin K can be repeated q 12 h
Life-threatening bleeding	Hold VKA and give FFP, prothrombin complex concentrate, or recombinant factor VIIa. Supplement with 10 mg vitamin K IV (slow infusion). IV vitamin K can be repeated q 12 h

PERIOPERATIVE MANAGEMENT OF PATIENTS RECEIVING UNFRACTIONATED HEPARIN OR LOW-MOLECULAR-WEIGHT HEPARIN

Pharmacology:
- Heparin binds to antithrombin (AT), which inactivates thrombin (factor IIa), factor Xa, and factor IXa
- LMWH also binds to AT but has less anti–factor IIa activity than UFH
- UFH activity is routinely monitored by aPTT, but this test is not very accurate
- LMWH can be monitored with the plasma anti-Xa level, which should be measured 4 hours after subcutaneous administration of a weight-adjusted dose of LMWH; this should only be done in patients with severe renal failure, in those who are pregnant, or in those who are at the extremes of body weight (should not be routine)
- UFH is rapidly reversed by protamine; 1 mg of protamine reverses 100 U of IV UFH. However, subcutaneous UFH may require a prolonged infusion of protamine

Indications and therapeutic targets:
- For UFH the target aPTT should be 1.5–2 times the baseline level
- For LMWH, subcutaneous dosing can be either once or twice daily (Lovenox 1 mg/kg every 12 hours or 1.5 mg/kg every day or dalteparin 100 IU/kg every 12 hours or 200 IU/kg every day)
- LMWH or UFH should be given for patients with DVT with or without PE, for AF <48 hours and no contraindications to anticoagulation, for prevention of DVT, for unstable angina and non-Q-wave myocardial infarction, and for treatment of acute ST-segment elevation myocardial infarction

TABLE 12-4	Stopping and Resuming UFH and LMWH	
UFH	**LMWH**
• Stop 4 h before planned surgery (approximately five elimination half-lives) • Resume 12–24 h after procedure if there is adequate hemostasis • For major surgery or a high bleeding risk surgery/procedure, use a low dose if possible and wait 48–72 h after surgery if there is adequate hemostasis	• For SQ, last dose should be 24 h before surgery (approximately five elimination half-lives) and should be half the total daily dose • Resume 24 h after procedure if there is adequate hemostasis • For major surgery or a high bleeding risk surgery/procedure, use a low dose if possible and wait 48–72 h after surgery if there is adequate hemostasis

PERIOPERATIVE MANAGEMENT OF PATIENTS ON ANTIPLATELET THERAPY

Patients with coronary stents:
  Elective surgery postponed if aspirin and thienopyridine (e.g., clopidogrel) therapy must be discontinued for the surgery:
  • Bare metal stents: 4–6 weeks
  • Drug-eluting stents: 12 months
  If surgery cannot be postponed, continue aspirin throughout perioperative period (see chapter 22 on patient with a coronary stent).

Patients at high risk for cardiac events (does not include coronary stents):
  Continue aspirin throughout perioperative period.
  Discontinue clopidogrel at least 5 days (preferably 10 days) before surgery.
  Resume clopidogrel 24 hours postoperatively.

Patients at low risk of cardiac events:
  Discontinue antiplatelet therapy 7–10 days before surgery.
  Resume antiplatelet therapy 24 hours postoperatively.

TABLE 12-5	Other Medications Affecting Blood Clotting	
Drug/half-life	**Mechanism of action**	**Side effects**
ASA 3.5–3.5 h	Low doses (60–325 mg/day): inhibits platelet COX Larger doses (1.5–2 g/day): also inhibits prostacyclin production and results in paradoxical thrombogenic effect	GI: nausea, vomiting, diarrhea, gastrointestinal bleeding and/or ulceration, dyspepsia, and heartburn Ear: tinnitus, vertigo, and hearing loss Hematologic: leukopenia, thrombocytopenia, purpura, and anemia Dermatologic and hypersensitivity: urticaria, angioedema, pruritus, skin eruptions, asthma, and anaphylaxis Miscellaneous: mental confusion, drowsiness, sweating, and thirst
Acetaminophen 1–2.5 h	Selective inhibition of COX-3 in the brain and spinal cord	GI: abdominal pain, nausea, and vomiting Hematologic: anemia, hemolysis, hemolytic anemia, hypoprothrombinemia, leucopenia, methemoglobinemia, neutropenia, pancytopenia, and thrombocytopenia Hepatic: elevated hepatic enzymes and hepatic necrosis Renal: renal papillary necrosis and renal tubular necrosis

(continued)

TABLE 12-5	Other Medications Affecting Blood Clotting (*continued*)	
Drug/half-life	Mechanism of action	Side effects
Fondaparinux 17–21 h, 77% eliminated unchanged through urine after 3 days	Binds to antithrombin to selectively inhibit factor Xa, but does not affect thrombin	Hematologic: major bleeding, anemia, purpura, thrombocytopenia, postoperative hemorrhage, and hematoma Hepatic: elevated AST and ALT GI: nausea, vomiting, constipation, diarrhea, abdominal pain, and dyspepsia Nervous system: headache, insomnia, dizziness, and confusion Dermatologic: rash, pruritus, and bullous eruption Cardiovascular: hypotension, hypertension, and edema GU: UTI and urinary retention Metabolic: hypokalemia
Clopidogrel (thienopyridine) 6 h, duration of action approximately 5 days	Inhibits platelet activation and aggregation through irreversible binding of platelet ADP receptors	Hematologic: major bleeding and thrombotic thrombocytopenic purpura GI: nausea, vomiting, constipation, diarrhea, and abdominal pain Nervous system: insomnia, dizziness, and confusion Cardiovascular: hypotension and edema
Abciximab (glycoprotein IIb/IIIa receptor binder) 10–30 min, platelet function recovers over 48 h	Interferes with platelet–fibrinogen and platelet–vWF binding and blocks final common pathway to platelet aggregation	Hematologic: major bleeding, thrombocytopenia, and anemia GI: nausea, vomiting, dyspepsia, diarrhea, and abdominal pain Nervous system: headache, dizziness, and anxiety Cardiovascular: chest pain, hypotension, bradycardia, tachycardia, and edema

HERBAL MEDICATIONS (SEE ALSO CHAPTER 10)

TABLE 12-6	Herbal Medications with Effects on Coagulation
Garlic	Platelet aggregation inhibitor, normal hemostasis 7 days after D/C
Ginkgo biloba	Platelet-activating factor inhibitor, normal hemostasis 36 h after D/C
Ginseng	Platelet aggregation inhibitor, normal hemostasis 24 h after D/C
St. John's wort	Induction of P450 drug metabolism, normal hemostasis 5 days after D/C

When used alone, garlic, *G. biloba*, ginseng, and St. John's wort are no contraindication for neuraxial anesthesia; however, when used with other medications affecting clotting, they may increase the risk of bleeding. Use clinical judgment.

REFERENCES

For references, please visit **www.TheAnesthesiaGuide.com**.

CHAPTER 13
Obstructive Sleep Apnea

Edward C. Lin, MD

PHYSIOLOGY

- Syndrome characterized by sleep-induced relaxation of pharyngeal muscle tone leading to upper airway obstruction
- Risk factors include obesity, tonsillar hypertrophy, craniofacial abnormalities (e.g., micrognathia), ingestion of alcohol/sedatives, male gender, and middle age
- Signs and symptoms: snoring, observed apnea during sleep, daytime somnolence, difficulty concentrating, morning headache
- Associated findings may include episodic hypoxemia, hypercarbia, polycythemia, hypertension, pulmonary hypertension, RV failure
- "Gold standard" test is polysomnography
- Severity may be measured by the apnea/hypopnea index (AHI), the number of apneic or hypopneic events per hour:
  - ▸ Mild—5–20
  - ▸ Moderate—21–40
  - ▸ Severe—>40
- Treatment is essentially medical (nasal CPAP) and reduces the incidence and severity of CV complications. Surgical treatment (UPPP, turbinectomy, septoplasty, etc.) is only an adjuvant

PREOPERATIVE

- Focused history and physical examination to evaluate patient's likelihood of having OSA
- Consider use of STOP-BANG questionnaire, a validated scoring system to assess risk of obstructive sleep apnea

TABLE 13-1   STOP-BANG Questionnaire
1. Do you **snore** loudly (louder than talking or loud enough to be heard through closed doors)?
2. Do you often feel **tired**, fatigued, or sleepy during daytime?
3. Has anyone **observed** you stop breathing during your sleep?
4. Do you have or are you being treated for high blood **pressure**?
5. **BMI** more than 35?
6. **Age** over 50 years old?
7. **Neck** >40 cm?
8. Male **gender**?

Three or more "yes" answers indicate a high risk for sleep apnea.

- If likelihood of sleep apnea is high:
  - ▸ Decide to either manage patient based on clinical criteria alone or have patient obtain additional workup or treatment (typically takes several weeks)
  - ▸ Decide whether procedure should be performed on an outpatient or an inpatient basis
  - ▸ Assess for difficult airway and obtain specialized airway equipment if deemed necessary
  - ▸ Use preoperative sedation cautiously if at all
  - ▸ Consider gabapentin premedication (900 mg po preoperatively) followed by 300 mg every 6 hours for at least 24 hours to reduce analgesic requirements

INTRAOPERATIVE

- If possible, completely avoid benzodiazepines
- Preoxygenate thoroughly as these patients are more prone to desaturation
- Have video laryngoscope (i.e., GlideScope, McGrath laryngoscope, etc.) and/or fiber-optic available to aid in intubation because majority of OSA patients are obese with difficult airways
- Avoid nitrous oxide if patient has history of pulmonary hypertension
- If general anesthesia, extubate fully awake and with full muscle strength
- Consider the use of regional or local techniques when appropriate
- Consider limiting opioids and instead relying on local/regional analgesia (field block, epidural catheter)
- If moderate sedation is used, continuously monitor adequacy of ventilation
- Dexmedetomidine might be a better option for sedation (MAC) than propofol
- Consider use of CPAP during sedation

POSTOPERATIVE

- Consider use of nonopioid postoperative analgesia (e.g., regional techniques, NSAIDs)
- Especially avoid continuous infusion of opioids
- Continue CPAP if feasible
- Consider discharge of patient from PACU into a monitored setting (step-down)
- Avoid discharge of patient from PACU to home/unmonitored setting until patient is no longer at risk of postoperative respiratory depression

REFERENCE

For references, please visit **www.TheAnesthesiaGuide.com**.

CHAPTER 14
Obesity

Edward C. Lin, MD

BASICS

A. Classification

TABLE 14-1	Obesity Categories Based on the Body Mass Index (BMI)
BMI	Category
<18.5	Underweight
18.5–24.9	Normal
25–30	Overweight
>30	Obese
>40	Morbidly obese
>55	Superobese

$$BMI = \frac{weight\ (kg)}{[height\ (m)]^2}$$

BMI may overestimate the severity of obesity in muscular individuals.
Ideal body weight (IBW): many formulas; easiest is to use weight for BMI of 23:
IBW (kg) = 23 × [height (m)]²

B. Physiologic effects

TABLE 14-2	Physiologic Effects of Obesity
Organ system	Associated physiologic effects
Respiratory	Restrictive lung disease (decreased FRC, ERV, TLC) Normal to decreased lung compliance, with significantly decreased chest wall compliance due to adipose tissue deposition Increased oxygen consumption and minute ventilation Increased work of breathing OSA Obesity hypoventilation syndrome V/Q mismatch CO_2 values are either low or normal unless have Pickwickian syndrome (defined as morbid obesity, hypersomnolence, hypoxemia, hypercapnia, pulmonary hypertension, polycythemia)
Cardiovascular	Hypertension Increased cardiac output secondary to increased ECF and hypervolemia Pulmonary hypertension, RV failure Ischemic heart disease LVH, heart failure

(continued)

TABLE 14-2	Physiologic Effects of Obesity (*continued*)
Organ system	Associated physiologic effects
Gastrointestinal	Fatty infiltration of the liver Hiatal hernia GERD Larger gastric volume Decreased gastric emptying (controversial) Increased defluorination of volatile anesthetics Cholelithiasis
Endocrine	DM, dyslipidemias
Vascular	DVT
Other	Osteoarthritis Increased risk of cancer, especially GI

PREOPERATIVE

- Focused history and physical examination to detect and to assess the severity of any obesity-related comorbidities:
  - ▸ Exercise tolerance, CAD, HTN, NIDDM, cardiomyopathy
  - ▸ Presence of snoring at night (may suggest undiagnosed hypoventilation syndrome); formal diagnosis of OSA not needed: in doubt, treat as such
  - ▸ Assess for difficult airway and prepare specialized airway equipment as necessary (i.e., awake fiber-optic):
    - ▪ Assess for difficult mask ventilation (morbid obesity with redundant tissue, OSA, beard, edentulous)
    - ▪ Special focus on:
      - ◆ Mallampati class
      - ◆ TM distance
      - ◆ Neck range of motion
      - ◆ Size of tongue
      - ◆ Redundancy of soft tissue in and around airway
      - ◆ Neck circumference at the level of thyroid cartilage >60 cm^2
- Elicit history of past diet medication use (fenfluramine with risk of valve thickening and pulmonary hypertension, amphetamines)
- Chem 7, CBC (polycythemia), EKG, and CXR (cardiomyopathy); consider TTE (although often poor quality)
- Ensure medical equipment appropriately sized (e.g., blood pressure cuff)
- OR table certified for patient's weight (if needed, use special table, or two tables)
- Ensure personnel available for positioning
- Consider aspiration prophylaxis
- Discuss increased anesthetic risk with patient

INTRAOPERATIVE

A. Induction

- Vascular access:
  - ▸ Potentially very difficult; consider use of ultrasound
- Preoxygenation:
  - ▸ Decreased FRC leads to rapid desaturation during even brief periods of apnea
- Mask ventilation:
  - ▸ May be difficult/impossible
  - ▸ Use two-person mask, oral airway, head strap
  - ▸ Use head of bed elevation, CPAP

- Intubation:
  ‣ Position in head-elevated laryngoscopy position (HELP) using pillows/towels: align tragus with sternum (Figure 14-1)
  ‣ Large chest may necessitate use of short-handle laryngoscope
  ‣ Advanced airway techniques/rescue devices (e.g., video laryngoscopy, LMA) should be readily available
  ‣ If difficult airway anticipated, consider awake airway management or RSI
  ‣ Avoid "burning bridges"

FIGURE 14-1. Head-elevated laryngoscopy position (HELP) for intubation of obese patients

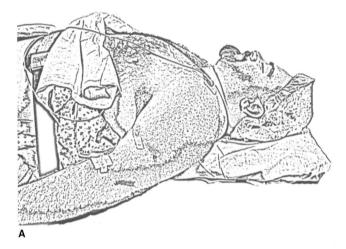

A

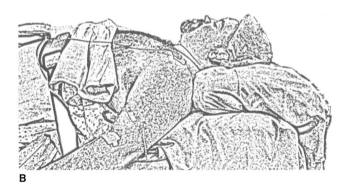

B

(A) Patient lying flat. (B) The patient's head and shoulders are propped up with pillows and towels to align the tragus with the sternum, aligning airway axes. (Drawing by Arthur Atchabahian, MD.)

B. Monitoring

- Invasive monitoring as dictated by medical comorbidities
- NIBP may be difficult to impossible; use arterial catheter for such patients
- Consider the use of anesthesia depth monitoring

C. Ventilation

- Use Vt around 8–10 mL/kg of IBW; adjust based on $PetCO_2$ and ABG
- Avoid high airway pressures if possible (PIP >35–40); consider use of pressure control ventilation
- Recruitment maneuvers as needed (sustained PIP of 40 cm H_2O for 30–60 seconds)
- Reverse Trendelenburg position may improve ventilatory parameters

D. Drugs/maintenance

- Initial dosing of medications is based on IBW (except for succinylcholine and cisatracurium); subsequent dosing is titrated to effect
- Increased uptake of volatile anesthetics
- Increased fat storage of medications may lead to accumulation with multiple doses
- Antibiotics: if BMI >35, use double beta-lactam doses, 900 mg clindamycin, 5 mg/kg gentamycin (maximum 500 mg)
- Careful positioning and padding of pressure points
- If using regional anesthesia, dosage of medication for neuraxial anesthesia is *decreased* (usually 20–25%)
- Consider limiting opioids intraoperatively and postoperatively and relying on regional anesthesia (epidural catheter) for pain control if possible

E. Extubation

- Extubate *fully awake* and at full strength
- Consider head-up position during extubation

POSTOPERATIVE

- Supplemental oxygen and monitored setting (SDU, ICU) until patient no longer at risk of respiratory compromise. Maximal reduction in blood oxygenation in obese patients occurs approximately 2–3 days postoperatively. It takes 7–10 days before reductions in FRC, VC, and FEV1 normalize
- Risk of unrecognized abdominal compartment syndrome with renal failure. Monitor closely
- Dose postoperative opioids according to IBW; morphine IV PCA
- Consider use of regional anesthesia for postoperative pain control to limit post-operative opioid use
- Labs: glucose, CK to r/o rhabdomyolysis if long surgery
- Insulin therapy if hyperglycemia
- Increased risk of wound infection
- Initiate thromboprophylaxis as soon as feasible

REFERENCES

For references, please visit **www.TheAnesthesiaGuide.com**.

CHAPTER 15
Conduction Abnormalities

Amit H. Sachdev, MD and Molly Sachdev, MD, MPH

NB: See chapter 5 on preoperative EKG for sample EKG strips.

PHYSIOPATHOLOGY

- Conduction blocks can occur at any point along the pathway (Figure 15-1)
- The lower the level of block along the electrical system, the worse the prognosis
- That is, block in the His–Purkinje system carries a much higher risk of sudden cardiac death, as compared with block at the level of the AV node

For most patients the level of block can be determined using the surface EKG findings (see preoperative EKG chapter 5 for examples of EKG tracings).

FIGURE 15-1. Pathway of electrical impulses in the heart

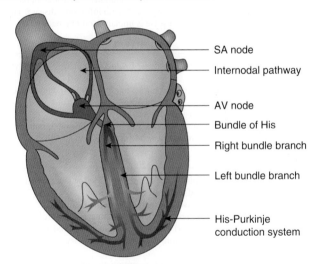

SA node

Internodal pathway

AV node

Bundle of His

Right bundle branch

Left bundle branch

His-Purkinje
conduction system

In the normal heart, electrical impulses originate in the SA node, travel through the AV node, and then to the His–Purkinje system as depicted in the figure. Reproduced from Fuster V, Walsh RA, Harrington RA. *Hurst's The Heart*. 13th ed. Figure 43-1. Available at: www.accessmedicine.com. Copyright © The McGraw-Hill Companies, Inc. All rights reserved.

TABLE 15-1	Determining Level of Block Based on Surface EKG	
Location of disease	Name of disorder	EKG findings
1. SA nodal disease	Sinus pause	No P waves
2. AV nodal disease	First-degree AV block	Prolonged PR interval
	Second-degree, type I (Wenckebach)	PR interval gets longer until a nonconducted P wave is seen
	Third-degree (complete) w/narrow escape rhythm	P's and QRS's are dissociated. However, QRS complex is narrow
3. Infranodal disease	Second-degree, type II	PR interval constant with intermittent nonconducted P waves
	Third-degree (complete) w/wide escape rhythm	P's and QRS's are dissociated. However, QRS complex is wide

- The conduction system is autonomically innervated until the level of the His-Purkinje system. Increased vagal or parasympathetic tone will lead to slowing of sinus rhythm and of the conduction through the SA node and AV node, while sympathomimetics or vagolytics will improve or hasten sinus node and AV nodal conduction
- However, if the block is infranodal, then drugs that target the autonomic nervous system will not allow for better conduction. They may lead to an increased supranodal heart rate but will not improve the infranodal rate. The degree of block may worsen if sympathomimetics are given to patients with infranodal disease. The only therapy for patients with infranodal disease is implantation of a pacemaker

PREOPERATIVE

- Obtain thorough history and baseline EKG. Ensure that plasma electrolytes are normal
- If symptomatic (unexplained syncope, fatigue, lightheadedness), consider evaluation by an electrophysiologist
- Longer recordings should be considered
- Patients with evidence of infranodal disease will likely need implantation of either a temporary or permanent pacemaker prior to surgery

ANESTHESIA

- Routine precautions with special attention to succinylcholine. Succinylcholine can trigger bradycardia, specifically if a second dose is given:
  ▸ Likely due to stimulation of muscarinic receptors in the sinus node
  ▸ May be prevented by vagolytic premedication (atropine, glycopyrrolate)
- IV opioid analgesics such as fentanyl are also known to cause bradycardia
- Significant hypoxemia, hypoventilation, vagal reflexes, and laryngospasm can lead to bradycardia
- When a patient develops a significant symptomatic intraoperative bradycardia, atropine 0.5 mg IV can be given; if ineffective, consider dopamine drip at 2–10 μg/kg/min or epinephrine drip at 2–10 μg/kg/min
- Transcutaneous pacing can be tried and if necessary emergent transvenous pacing

POSTOPERATIVE

- Consider electrophysiologist consultation for patients who developed significant bradycardias

PEARLS AND TIPS

- Patients with block in the His–Purkinje system usually do not respond to medications and will likely need pacemaker placement
- Electrolyte abnormalities (hyperkalemia) can lead to significant rhythm disturbances and should be evaluated if de novo conduction system abnormalities arise

CHAPTER 16
Tachyarrythmias

Amit H. Sachdev, MD and Molly Sachdev, MD, MPH

PHYSIOPATHOLOGY

- Tachycardias are classically divided into narrow QRS and wide QRS complex
- Narrow complex tachycardias (QRS <120 milliseconds) usually originate above the ventricle and are referred to as "supraventricular tachycardia" (SVT)

A. SVT

- SVT differential includes sinus tachycardia, atrial tachycardia, multifocal atrial tachycardia, junctional tachycardia, atrial fibrillation, atrial flutter, AV nodal reentrant tachycardia (AVNRT), orthodromic reentrant tachycardia (ORT), or paroxysmal junctional reciprocating tachycardia (PJRT)
- AVNRT (Figure 16-1) is a reentrant rhythm that utilizes dual AV nodal physiology or conduction via a slow and a fast pathway in the AV node. Typical AVNRT travels down the slow pathway node and up the fast pathway. Atypical AVNRT travels down the fast pathway and up the slow pathway
- ORT is a reentrant arrhythmia that utilizes an accessory pathway for retrograde conduction
- PJRT is also a reentrant arrhythmia that utilizes a slowly conducting retrograde pathway
- Identification and characterization of atrial activity (P waves) is central to the diagnosis of SVT (Figure 16-2):
  - If there are no P waves but rather a fibrillatory baseline, then the rhythm is atrial fibrillation. A sawtooth baseline implies atrial flutter
  - If the P waves are regular and fast, then the "RP interval" or the relationship of the P wave to the preceding R wave is critical to the diagnosis
  - If the diagnosis is not clear based on surface EKG characteristics alone, an EP study needs to be done

TABLE 16-1 EKG Appearance of Different Types of Tachycardias	
Narrow complex tachycardia	EKG appearance
Sinus tachycardia	Sinus P waves at rate >100 bpm
Atrial flutter	Classic sawtooth pattern on EKG
Atrial fibrillation	No clear P waves with irregularly irregular rhythm
AV nodal reentrant tachycardia (AVNRT)	Narrow complex tachycardia with no obvious P waves (short RP)
Orthodromic reciprocating tachycardia (ORT)	Narrow complex tachycardia. P waves often not visible. But if visible, then (mid RP)
Atrial tachycardia	Narrow complex tachycardia (long RP)
Paroxysmal junctional reciprocating tachycardia (PJRT)	Narrow complex tachycardia (long RP)

FIGURE 16-1. EKG of typical AVNRT, the most common type of SVT

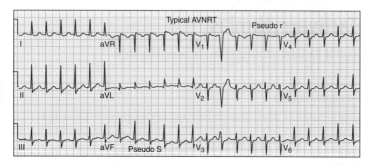

FIGURE 16-2. Algorithm for determining the etiology of narrow complex tachycardia (QRS <120 milliseconds)

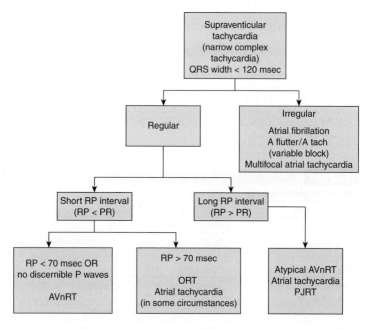

B. Wide complex tachycardias

- Wide QRS because electrical impulses either originate or travel outside the normal conduction system
- Differential for wide complex arrhythmias includes ventricular tachycardia, SVT with aberrancy, or conduction via an accessory pathway (antidromic reciprocating tachycardia)
  ‣ SVT with aberrancy implies a rhythm that originates above the ventricle but is conducted aberrantly through the ventricle; usually this is secondary to bundle branch block
  ‣ Antidromic reciprocating tachycardia is a reentrant tachycardia that utilizes an accessory pathway for conduction
- Torsades de Pointes is a specific type of WCT in which patients have an underlying long QT interval and develop polymorphic ventricular tachycardia
- Often, it is difficult to differentiate VT from SVT based on surface EKG alone. In unclear cases, it is best to assume VT. The Brugada criteria can be used to differentiate SVT from VT. However, they are neither very sensitive nor specific:
  ‣ Atrioventricular dissociation
  ‣ Absence of RS complex in all precordial leads
  ‣ R to S interval >100 milliseconds in at least one precordial lead
  ‣ Fusion beats
  ‣ Extreme left-axis deviation
  ‣ Different QRS morphology during tachycardia compared with baseline in patient with preexisting bundle branch block
  ‣ QRS appearance different from a typical bundle branch block appearance

PREOPERATIVE

- Obtain thorough history
- If patient has a history of frequent palpitations or documented SVT, consider referral to an electrophysiologist for EP study and ablation prior to presentation to OR
- AVNRT, ORT, ART, atrial flutter have a very high cure rate and low complication rate with ablation

ANESTHESIA

A. Inhalation agents

- Desflurane can lead to a moderate increase in heart rate at higher doses. This effect can be attenuated by concurrent use of fentanyl or esmolol
- Sevoflurane leads to little change in heart rate
- Neither desflurane nor sevoflurane sensitizes the heart to the arrythmogenic effects of epinephrine (contrary to halothane) and therefore can be administered concurrently

B. SVT therapy (Figure 16-3)

Vagal maneuvers and carotid sinus massage may be effective in terminating regular, narrow complex SVT and should be tried first if possible. Adenosine 6 mg, followed by another 6 mg, and then 12 mg pushed via a central line can be given if these measures fail. Cardioversion should be also considered if necessary (see Figure 16-3).

FIGURE 16-3. Algorithm for treating SVT

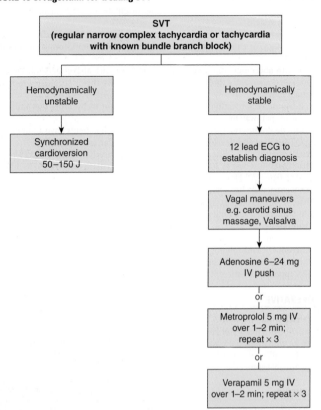

C. Atrial fibrillation and flutter (Figure 16-4)

- The first decision that needs to be made is that of rate control or rhythm control. If the arrhythmia is present for <48 hours, either approach can be used
- If the patient has been in atrial fibrillation or flutter for >48 hours, caution should be used in considering electrical or pharmacologic cardioversion, unless the patient has been on therapeutic anticoagulation for at least 3 weeks, or TEE is negative for thrombi. It should only be considered in emergent cases where rate control is not an option
- In patients for whom a rate control strategy is employed, nodal blockers such as diltiazem, verapamil, or metoprolol can be given. To maintain control, a diltiazem or esmolol drip can be initiated. In hemodynamically unstable cases, synchronized cardioversion should be considered
- In patients for whom a rhythm control strategy is opted, cardioversion is favored. However, multiple antiarrhythmic drugs are also known to acutely convert AF and are listed below

- Propafenone or flecainide should only be used for acute cardioversion in patients without known structural heart disease
- If ibutilide is given, the QT interval should be closely monitored for at least 4 hours, or until QTc is back to baseline
- In patients with structural heart disease, amiodarone can be used for both rate control and possible rhythm control. An effective dose is 150 mg IV bolus over 10 minutes, followed by 1 mg/min × 6 hours, and then 0.5 mg/min × 18 hours
- If antiarrythmic drugs are to be used chronically, expert opinion is advised given high potential for proarrythmia and other side effects

FIGURE 16-4. Acute therapy of recent-onset atrial fibrillation or flutter

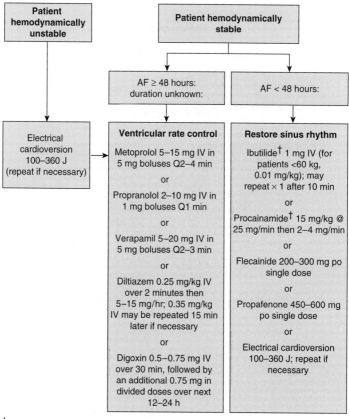

† Procainamide or ibutilide is the drug of choice for Wolff-Parkinson-White syndrome.

D. Wide complex tachycardia

- Patients with wide complex tachycardias should not be given nodal blockers or adenosine (potential to exacerbate hypotension and lead to hemodynamic compromise)
- Hemodynamically unstable VT should be cardioverted
- In patients who develop VT intraoperatively, electrolytes should be checked and consideration given to evaluate and avoid ischemic insult
- Therapy is different for monomorphic VT (Figure 16-5) and polymorphic VT (Figure 16-6)

FIGURE 16-5. Treatment of monomorphic VT

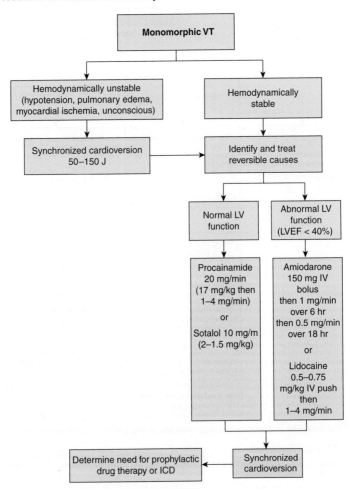

FIGURE 16-6. Treatment of polymorphic VT

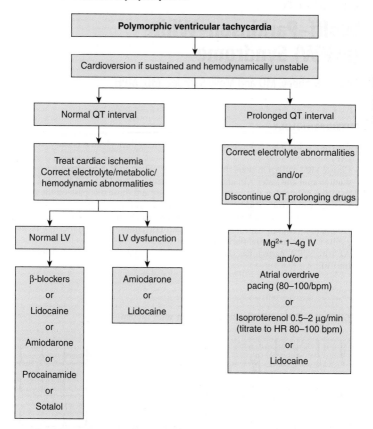

Reproduced from Hall JB, Schmidt GA, Wood LDH. *Principles of Critical Care*. 3rd ed. Figure 24-4.
Available at: www.accessmedicine.com. Copyright © The McGraw-Hill Companies, Inc. All rights
reserved.

POSTOPERATIVE

- Patients who develop intraoperative SVT or VT may be candidates for ablation or
  further therapies postoperatively. Consider expert consultation

PEARLS AND TIPS

- Cardiovert all tachyarrhythmias if patient is hemodynamically unstable
- Avoid nodal blockers or adenosine in patients with wide complex tachycardias

CHAPTER 17
Wolff–Parkinson–White (WPW) Syndrome

Amit H. Sachdev, MD and Molly Sachdev, MD, MPH

PHYSIOPATHOLOGY

- Aberrant connection from the atria to the ventricles through an accessory pathway (AP)
- Classic EKG pattern in sinus rhythm (Figure 17-1): short P–R interval (due to conduction over the faster AP) and a slurred upstroke of the QRS—"delta wave" (due to fusion of impulses that pass through AV node and those that pass via the AP)
- Patients with Wolff–Parkinson–White (WPW) syndrome can present in sinus rhythm or with reentrant narrow complex tachycardias (orthodromic reciprocating tachycardia [ORT]), wide complex tachycardias (antidromic reciprocating tachycardia [ART]), and atrial fibrillation (AF)
- AF with WPW pattern has classic EKG pattern (Figure 17-2) and can degenerate into VF

FIGURE 17-1. Classic WPW pattern on EKG in sinus rhythm

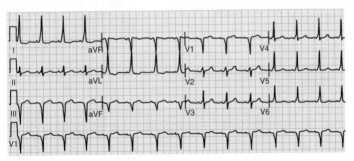

Slurring of the upstroke of the QRS. Reproduced from Knoop KJ, Stack LB, Storrow AB, Thurman RJ. *The Atlas of Emergency Medicine*. 3rd ed. Figure 23-42A. Available at: www.accessmedicine. com. Copyright © The McGraw-Hill Companies, Inc. All rights reserved.

FIGURE 17-2. Atrial fibrillation in a patient with WPW

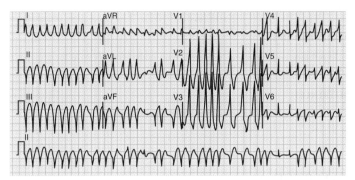

Note wide, bizarre, and irregular QRS complexes. Reproduced from Longo DL, Fauci AS, Kasper DL, Hauser SL, Jameson JL, Loscalzo J. *Harrison's Principles of Internal Medicine*. 18th ed. Figure E30-21. Available at: www.accessmedicine.com. Copyright © The McGraw-Hill Companies, Inc. All rights reserved.

PREOPERATIVE

- Perform EKG: WPW is diagnosed by history and EKG findings
- Consider referral to electrophysiologist for possible preoperative ablation

ANESTHESIA

- Management of paroxysmal tachycardia associated with WPW is similar to that of other SVTs. Treatment is required when there is clinical poor tolerance
- Be cautious when administering anesthetics that cause an increase in sympathetic tone or the production of extrasystoles that may precipitate tachycardia:
  ▸ Desflurane is sympathomimetic and can increase AV nodal conduction time, which may result in greater conduction via the AP and tachycardias
  ▸ Atropine, glycopyrrolate, ketamine can resulting in PSVT or AF and should be avoided
  ▸ Neostigmine slows AV nodal conduction and facilitates AP conduction. Therefore, it should be avoided
- Patients who develop an atrial arrhythmia intraoperatively (AF or atrial flutter) and have underlying WPW should *not* be given nodal blockers (including adenosine, calcium channel blockers, beta-blockers, or digoxin) or carotid sinus massage. Nodal blockers slow AV nodal conduction and allow for greater conduction through the faster conducting AP. This promotes degeneration of AF to VF:
  ▸ Cardioversion and/or sodium channel blockers (i.e., procainamide) are first-line therapy for patients with AF and WPW. Sodium channel blockers block the AP
  ▸ However, patients who develop a *narrow* complex arrhythmia such as ORT can be given nodal blockers to slow the rate

TABLE 17-1	Drugs to be Avoided in WPW
• Desflurane	
• Atropine	
• Glycopyrrolate	
• Ketamine	
• Neostigmine	
• Nodal blockers (e.g., diltiazem, verapamil, metoprolol, adenosine, digoxin)	

POSTOPERATIVE

- Catheter ablation may be considered postoperatively

PEARLS AND TIPS

- Do not give nodal blockers to patients with underlying WPW in the presence of an atrial arrhythmia

REFERENCES

For references, please visit **www.TheAnesthesiaGuide.com**.

CHAPTER 18
Pacemakers

Sanford M. Littwin, MD

- In the United States >500,000 pacemakers are implanted each year, with more than 6 million patients today having a pulse generator device
- Almost 100% of pacemakers are placed for a specific disease process rather than prophylactically
- Most patients have concomitant diseases: HTN, CAD, DM, pulmonary disease

INDICATIONS FOR PACEMAKER

- Symptomatic SA node dysfunction:
  ‣ Bradycardia, pauses
- Symptomatic AV node dysfunction:
  ‣ Third-degree (complete) heart block
  ‣ Second-degree heart block:
    ▪ With symptomatic bradycardia
    ▪ After AV node resection or following valve surgery
    ▪ Secondary to muscular disease
- Post-MI heart block (≥Mobitz II)
- Sick sinus syndrome
- Long QT syndrome
- Biventricular pacing for resynchronization in CHF

POSSIBLE CAUSES OF PACER MALFUNCTION

- *All implanted devises (pacemakers) are contraindicated in MRI suite*
- Possible other causes of interference:
  ‣ Electrocautery (Bovie)
  ‣ RF ablation
  ‣ Lithotripsy
  ‣ Electrolyte/acid–base abnormalities
  ‣ Medications:
    ▪ Succinylcholine (fasciculations can inhibit PM; not an absolute contraindication)
    ▪ Cardiac medications modifying detection or stimulation thresholds (e.g., sotalol, verapamil)
  ‣ Rare: orthopedic saw, telemetric devices, mechanical ventilators

PREOPERATIVE

- Determine type of pacemaker:
  - ‣ Manufacturer's identification card or ID bracelet
- Obtain EKG, and if needed CXR
- Determine if patient is pacer dependent:
  - ‣ Patient history
  - ‣ Postablative procedures
  - ‣ Rhythm strip with no spontaneous ventricular activity
- Determine when PM last interrogated and battery life
- Have available:
  - ‣ External defibrillator/transcutaneous pacer, transvenous pacer
  - ‣ Magnet
  - ‣ Isoprenaline and/or dopamine
- Make preparations to have pacemaker company representative available (or other qualified personnel):
  - ‣ Interrogation of device in holding area (or in OR if necessary to change device settings only after patient is anesthetized):
    - ▪ Turn PM to asynchronous mode (DOO or VOO)
    - ▪ Turn off any other option (rate-adaptive, antitachycardia, etc.)
  - ‣ If not possible (or if PM inappropriately inhibited by cautery), place magnet over device (must be kept in place for length of procedure); magnets will typically change pacing into asynchronous mode at a preprogrammed rate
- Minimize electromagnetic interference(s):
  - ‣ Place grounding pad away from pacer, and in such a position that the current from the cautery to the pad will not flow through the pacemaker or the heart
  - ‣ Use bipolar cautery if possible
  - ‣ If monopolar needed, advise surgeon to use short (<1 second) bursts
- Avoid dysrhythmia-triggering situations:
  - ‣ Electrolyte imbalance
  - ‣ Ischemia
  - ‣ Hypovolemia

INTRAOPERATIVE

- Intraoperative monitoring:
  - ‣ Special attention to EKG (capable of detecting pacer-generated spikes)
- Applicable alternatives to intrinsic (pacer): external pacer pads, defibrillator, and transvenous pacer
- Avoid inserting PAC if PM in place <4 weeks (risk of dislodgement)
- If PM malfunction:
  - ‣ Stop any electrical device in use (especially cautery)
  - ‣ Evaluate clinical impact
  - ‣ If poorly tolerated bradycardia:
    - ▪ Apply magnet
    - ▪ If ineffective, start isoprenaline/dopamine infusion; use transcutaneous and/or transvenous pacer
  - ‣ If cardiac arrest, initiate CPR; use transcutaneous and/or transvenous pacer
  - ‣ If tachycardia and DDD pacer, apply magnet; otherwise, treat as appropriate (see chapter 16 on tachyarrhythmias)

POSTOPERATIVE

- Reevaluation (by qualified personnel) of pacer
- Restore preoperative settings
- Removal of magnet:
  - ‣ Pacer should return to normally functioning mode
  - ‣ Interrogation of device by qualified personnel and/or admittance for observation until proper function can be determined

TABLE 18-1	Generic Pacemaker Code (NGB) for All Companies Manufacturing Pulse Generators			
Position I (pacing chamber(s))	Position II (sensing chamber(s))	Position III (response(s) to sensing)	Position IV (programmability)	Position V (multisite pacing)
0: none	0: none	0: none	0: none	0: none
A: atrium	A: atrium	I: inhibited	R: rate modulation	A: atrium
V: ventricle	V: ventricle	T: triggered	P: programmable	V: ventricle
D: dual	D: dual	D: dual	C: communicating	D: dual

REFERENCES

For references, please visit **www.TheAnesthesiaGuide.com**.

CHAPTER 19
Implantable Cardiac Defibrillators (ICDs)

Sanford M. Littwin, MD

More than 75% implantable cardiac defibrillators (ICDs) are placed as a prophylactic measure for risk of sudden cardiac death (SCD) from specific disease states (e.g., HCM).

Many patients who receive a pacemaker for specific causes (see chapter 18) will have dual-function devices, also capable of defibrillation.

All implanted devices, ICD as well as pacemakers, are contraindicated in the MRI suite.

INDICATIONS FOR ICD

- Prior cardiac arrest
- NYHA class II or III nonischemic dilated CM, EF <30%
- Prior MI (>40 days), EF <30%
- Structural heart disease or inherited arrhythmia syndromes (long QT, Brugada):
  - Genetic disorder that is characterized by right bundle branch block, ST segment elevation in V1 to V3, and sudden death in patients with a structurally normal heart. EKG pattern with J point elevation
- Syncope of unknown origin

CHARACTERISTICS

- Larger than pacemakers; therefore, often implanted under pectoralis muscle under GA (VF induction for testing)
- Functions:
  - *Overdrive pacing* if *monomorphic VT*
  - *Cardioversion or defibrillation* if *polymorphic VT or VF*
  - *Pacing function* if *pause* (especially after cardioversion or defibrillation)
- Four-letter code

TABLE 19-1	Code for ICD Devices		
Defibrillation	Antitachycardia	Tachycardia detection	Pacemaker
O: none	O: none	E: EKG	O: none
A: atrial	A: atrial	H: hemodynamic	A: atrial
V: ventricular	V: ventricular		V: ventricular
D: dual	D: dual		D: dual

ICD MALFUNCTION

- Rarely absence of response to VT/VF
- Most often inappropriate electric shock
- Causes:
  ‣ Electrocautery (Bovie) essentially
  ‣ RF ablation
  ‣ Lithotripsy
  ‣ ECT
  ‣ Electrolyte/acid–base abnormalities
  ‣ Medications:
    ▪ Succinylcholine (fasciculations can inhibit PM or trigger ICD; not an absolute contraindication)
  ‣ Other (rare): orthopedic saw, telemetric devices, mechanical ventilators, nerve stimulator (anesthesia or SSEP/MEP)

PREOPERATIVE

- Determine type of ICD functions through manufacturer's identification card and/ or ID bracelet
- Determine battery function and when the device was last interrogated
- Turn ICD functions off:
  ‣ Interrogation and disabling of device by company representative or qualified personnel
  ‣ If not possible, magnet application to be kept on for duration of procedure (usually done in OR):
    ▪ ICDs manufactured by CPI are deactivated after 30 seconds of magnet application (beeping sound) but magnet reapplication can reactivate device; therefore, do not use magnet (except in emergency) if type/brand of device not known
    ▪ Reevaluation of device postmagnet therapy

INTRAOPERATIVE

- Need to monitor HR by another device than EKG: pulse oximeter and/or A-line
- Deactivate device (if not done preoperatively in holding area):
  ‣ Defibrillator function
  ‣ Antitachycardia function
- Place external defibrillator pads connected to defibrillator:
  ‣ Anterior/posterior position, not apex/right upper thorax
  ‣ Not overlying implanted device
- Place cautery return pad as far from ICD as possible:
  ‣ Advise surgeon to use short <1 second bursts of electrocautery
  ‣ Use bipolar cautery if possible, regardless of device deactivation, to minimize risk of device damage from EMI
- Avoid/correct any cause of dysrhythmia: electrolyte imbalance, ischemia, hypovolemia
- If malfunction:
  ‣ Turn off all electrical devices
  ‣ If VT/VF without ICD response, use external defibrillator

▸ If inappropriate shocks, evaluate clinical tolerance:
  ▪ If poorly tolerated, apply magnet
  ▪ Otherwise, have company representative or qualified personnel come into OR to interrogate/deactivate device

POSTOPERATIVE

- Reactivate AICD function by qualified personnel
- Remove magnet if used to deactivate device:
  ▸ Interrogate function to ensure proper function
- If unable to interrogate device, admit to telemetry or similar-type unit until proper function confirmed

REFERENCES

For references, please visit **www.TheAnesthesiaGuide.com**.

CHAPTER 20
Hypertrophic Cardiomyopathy (HCM)

Sanford M. Littwin, MD

Also called Idiopathic Hypertrophic Subaortic Stenosis (IHSS).

BASICS

A. Etiology
- Autosomic dominant with variable genetic penetrance
- Highest incidence in 13–22 years old
- Males = females
- Highest incidence of sudden cardiac death (SCD) in all patients
- Features (Figure 20-1):
  ▸ Hypertrophy of left ventricle involving intraventricular septum
  ▸ Enlargement of one or both papillary muscles
  ▸ Septal bulging into the LVOT:
    ▪ Partial or complete LVOT outflow obstruction
  ▸ Paradoxical motion of anterior leaflet of mitral valve (systolic anterior motion [SAM]):
    ▪ Worsens LVOT obstruction
    ▪ Causes MR in 30%
  ▸ Exceptional RV involvement
- Diagnosis of exclusion based on echo findings

FIGURE 20-1. Comparison of normal heart and heart with HCM

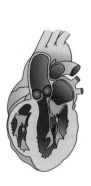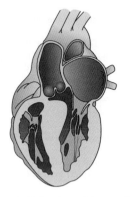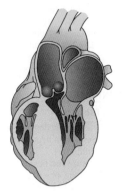

Normal heart (on left) compared with two types of hypertrophic cardiomyopathy (center and right). Note bulging of the septum into the LVOT. Reproduced from Fuster V, Walsh RA, Harrington RA. *Hurst's The Heart*. Figure 33-11. Copyright © The McGraw-Hill Companies, Inc. All rights reserved.

B. Diagnosis

- Most common symptoms are dyspnea, angina, dizziness, and syncope:
  - ‣ May be late signs or nonapparent in older patients
- Abnormal S4 heart sounds, systolic flow murmur
- Misplaced apical impulse
- Nonspecific EKG changes (atrial enlargement, LVH, inferolateral Q waves, PVCs)
- Echo findings:
  - ‣ Pressure gradient through the LVOT:
    - ▪ This varies widely between patients
  - ‣ SAM of mitral valve:
    - ▪ Dynamic outflow obstruction
    - ▪ Due to following conditions:
      - ♦ Anterior position of the mitral valve in the LV
      - ♦ Altered LV geometry due to septal bulge (hypertrophy)
      - ♦ Chordal slack
      - ♦ Venturi forces in the outflow tract (drop in pressure because of narrowed channel attracts anterior leaflet of mitral valve)
    - ▪ Described as closure of LVOT during systole
  - ‣ Mitral regurgitation

C. Treatment

- Medical:
  - ‣ Focused on HR control and negative inotropy:
    - ▪ Beta-blockers
    - ▪ Calcium channel blockers
  - ‣ Often works for nonsymptomatic patients
  - ‣ ICD implantation for avoidance of sudden cardiac death (SCD)
- Surgical:
  - ‣ Surgical myomectomy
  - ‣ Ablative procedures:
    - ▪ Decrease in mass of the ventricular hypertrophy
    - ▪ May be combined with corrective procedures to change aberrant anatomical problems with mitral valve

PREOPERATIVE

- Rule out associated myopathy
- Know the patients' functional status and the disease progression (i.e., symptoms they have had ongoing)
- ICD often present to prevent SCD (see chapter 19 on ICD) must be deactivated prior to surgery (interrogation by company representative, or magnet if not possible)
- Premedicate as appropriate to avoid anxiety-related tachycardia

INTRAOPERATIVE

A. Monitors

- Arterial line, depending on:
  - ‣ Severity of hypertrophic cardiomyopathy (HCM) (i.e., symptomatic vs. incidental finding)
  - ‣ Nature and invasiveness of surgical procedure
- TEE (and practitioner able to interpret) available to diagnose cause of hemodynamic deterioration

B. Hemodynamic principles

- Avoid factors that worsen obstruction:
  - ‣ Tachycardia (sympathetic stimulation, vagolysis)
  - ‣ Positive inotropes
  - ‣ Peripheral vasodilators
  - ‣ Hypovolemia
- Have immediately available:
  - ‣ Esmolol, diltiazem
  - ‣ Phenylephrine

C. Induction

- Balanced technique:
  - ‣ Avoid induction agents that decrease afterload (e.g., propofol) or increase HR (e.g., ketamine):
    - ▪ Etomidate and/or midazolam + fentanyl
  - ‣ NMB: avoid pancuronium (tachycardia) and succinylcholine
- Avoid intubating under light anesthesia
- Have esmolol and phenylephrine available to maintain HR and SVR
- Avoid neuraxial blockade because of vasodilation
- Peripheral nerve blocks: avoid epi in local anesthetic solution

D. Maintenance

- Volatile agents:
  - ‣ Use caution with desflurane (possible tachycardia)
- Treat arrhythmia aggressively (beta-blocker, calcium channel blocker)
- SAM and LVOT obstruction can lead to hypotension and arrhythmias. Treatment is centered on:
  - ‣ Decreasing HR and contractility: esmolol
  - ‣ Maintaining afterload: phenylephrine
  - ‣ Increasing LV volume: IV fluids

E. Emergence
- Tight HR control
- Avoid sympathetic stimulations:
  ‣ Smooth emergence
  ‣ Well-controlled pain

POSTOPERATIVE

- Adequate pain control essential

PEARLS

Hemodynamics:
- Keep preload and afterload high
- Avoid tachycardia
- Avoid inotropes

ICD often present to prevent SCD (see chapter 19 on ICDs); must be deactivated prior to surgery.

REFERENCES

For references, please visit **www.TheAnesthesiaGuide.com**.

CHAPTER 21
Angioedema

Kathleen A. Smith, MD and Adrienne Turner Duffield, MD

- Localized swelling of subcutaneous and submucosal tissues secondary to increased permeability of postcapillary venules:
  ‣ Asymmetric, nonpitting swelling of face, tongue, extremities, bowel wall
  ‣ Laryngeal edema has high mortality (25–40%)
- Females > males

CLASSIFICATION/PATHOPHYSIOLOGY OF ANGIOEDEMA

See table on following page.

Classification/Pathophysiology of Angioedema

Classification			Pathophysiology	Common triggers	Time course
Hereditary angioedema (HAE)	Type I (85%)		• C1 esterase inhibitor (C1-INH) deficiency • AD inheritance • C1-INH regulates complement, fibrinolytic, and coagulation pathways • Unregulated activity → release of vasoactive mediators	• Inflammation • Infection • Minor trauma (dental procedure, intubation, local trauma from snoring)	• Usually presents in childhood • Onset in hours • Lasts 2–4 days
	Type II (15%)		C1-INH present, but dysfunctional		
	Type III		• Coagulation factor XII mutation • Estrogen dependent • Elevated kinin		
Nonhereditary	Allergic		IgE mediated	Type I hypersensitivity reaction → mast cell degranulation	Requires prior sensitization NSAIDs, ASA, antibiotics, narcotics, oral contraceptives, latex, food	Onset in minutes → 1 h
	Idiopathic		• Unknown • Most common			Recurrent
	Acquired		• C1-INH consumption from antibody or excessive complement activation	Associated with malignancy (B-cell lymphoma, monoclonal gammopathy)		
	ACE inhibitor induced		• Elevated bradykinin • 0.1–2.2%	• Produces ↑ bradykinin, vasodilation		• Weeks to years after starting drug • Often misdiagnosed

PREOPERATIVE (PROPHYLAXIS)

- Thorough history:
  - Allergies
  - History of angioedema and known triggers
  - Current symptoms (stridor, dysphagia, dysphonia, dyspnea, abdominal pain, vomiting, diarrhea)?

TABLE 21-1	Suggested Prophylaxis Based on Type of Angioedema
Type	Prophylaxis
HAE	1. Attenuated androgens (danazol 10 mg/kg/day, maximum 600 mg/day), 4 days before and after surgery: • ↑ liver production C1-INH 2. Antifibrinolytics (ε-aminocaproic acid 1 g TID, tranexamic acid 50–75 mg/kg/day): • If unable to take androgens 3. C1-INH concentrate (500–1,000 U), given 1 h before surgery, second dose available 4. FFP (1–4 U) immediately before surgery 5. Ideally, C1-INH levels ≥50% of normal
Allergic	Avoid allergen, no medication proven helpful for prevention
Idiopathic	Daily antihistamine, glucocorticoids are second line given long-term side effects

INTRAOPERATIVE (TREATMENT)

- *Regardless of etiology, have a low threshold for SECURING AIRWAY; remember ABCs*

TABLE 21-2	Treatment of Angioedema Based on Type
Type	Treatment
All	• Secure airway, surgical airway if necessary • Treat associated hypotension (fluids, vasopressors) and bronchospasm (beta-agonists, epinephrine)
HAE	• Plasma-derived C1-INH (may require repeat dose) • FFP (second line) • *Not* responsive to epinephrine, antihistamines, or steroids
Allergic	• Antihistamines (H1 + H2) • Glucocorticoids • Epinephrine (laryngeal edema)
Acquired	• C1-INH concentrate, FFP • Treat underlying malignancy
Idiopathic	• Glucocorticoids
ACE inhibitor induced	• Discontinue ACE inhibitor • FFP, C1-INH • Steroids, antihistamines, epinephrine have limited effectiveness

- Avoid endotracheal intubation/LMA if possible in HAE
- Choice of induction agent unchanged
- Consider monitoring cuff pressures of intubated patients to identify rapid airway swelling

POSTOPERATIVE

- Ensure adequate cuff leak prior to extubation. *Do not* extubate if concerned
- Consider Cook exchange catheter when extubating
- Monitor in ICU setting
- If cause unknown, RAST skin testing or IgE-specific antibody testing may be indicated

PEARLS

FIGURE 21-1. Algorithm for treatment of laryngeal edema in patients with angioedema

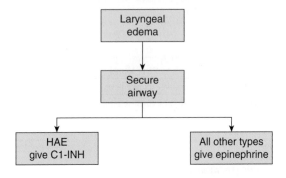

REFERENCES

For references, please visit **www.TheAnesthesiaGuide.com**.

CHAPTER 22
Patient with a Stent (or Following PCI)

Ghislaine M. Isidore, MD

- Stents implanted in >80% of percutaneous coronary intervention (PCI) following balloon angioplasty to decrease acute and long-term restenosis
- However, until reendothelialization, the risk of thrombosis is increased, and the patient must be maintained on dual antiplatelet therapy (typically ASA + clopidogrel [Plavix®])

TABLE 22-1	Duration of Antiplatelet Therapy Following PCI or Stent Implantation	
Procedure	Duration of dual antiplatelet therapy	Then, continue ASA
PCI without stent	2–4 weeks	Indefinitely
Bare metal stents (BMS)	30–45 days	Indefinitely
Drug-eluting stents (DES)	12 months	Indefinitely

The issue is the balance between:
- **Bleeding risk** of proposed surgery (to be assessed by surgeon and anesthesiologist) under antiplatelet therapy:
  ‣ *Low risk* (minor ophthalmologic, endoscopic, superficial procedures, dermatologic)
  ‣ *Intermediate risk* (orthopedic, urologic, uncomplicated abdominal, thoracic, or head and neck surgeries)
  ‣ *High risk* (aortic, vascular, anticipated prolonged surgical procedures associated with large fluid shifts or blood loss, emergency procedure)
  ‣ Also consider the site of surgery: intracranial and some ophthalmologic procedures where even minor bleeding is intolerable
- Likelihood and importance of **possible stent thrombosis** (assess in conjunction with a cardiologist, ideally the one who implanted the stent). Higher risk if:
  ‣ Noncardiac surgery <6 weeks for BMS and <1 year for DES
  ‣ Types of lesions:
    ▪ Ostial lesions
    ▪ Bifurcation lesions
    ▪ Small (<3 mm) stent diameter
    ▪ Multiple or long (>18 mm) lesions, overlapping stents
  ‣ DM
  ‣ Renal insufficiency
  ‣ Advanced age
  ‣ Low EF
  ‣ Prior brachytherapy (intracoronary irradiation to prevent reocclusion)
  ‣ Indication for stenting was acute MI or acute coronary syndrome

In most cases, the risk of thrombosis if antiplatelet therapy is interrupted is higher than the added risk of bleeding (even if transfusion is needed).

PERIOPERATIVE MANAGEMENT

- Discuss whether surgery can be safely performed in a hospital where a cath lab is not immediately available (if that is the case)
- If *emergent surgery*: proceed under antiplatelet therapy; manage bleeding as needed
- If *semi-urgent surgery*:
  ‣ Implant BMS
  ‣ Complete dual antiplatelet therapy as indicated (30–45 days)
  ‣ Then proceed to surgery on ASA
- If *elective surgery*:
  ‣ Patient with *DES*:
    ▪ Usual case: defer procedure until completion of appropriate course of dual antiplatelet therapy (12 months), and then perform procedure on ASA:
      ♦ If ASA is not recommended for that type of surgery (e.g., spinal fusion), discontinue ASA preoperatively and restart as soon as possible
    ▪ If patient is still taking clopidogrel after 12 months (because deemed high thrombosis risk by cardiologist):
      ♦ Discontinue clopidogrel and have surgery on ASA, if possible; restart clopidogrel as soon as possible

▸ Patient with *BMS*:
  ▪ Delay procedure for 30–45 days (until completion of dual antiplatelet therapy), and then perform procedure on ASA if possible
  ▪ If ASA not recommended, d/c ASA preoperatively and resume postoperatively as soon as possible

TABLE 22-2	Management Recommendation Depending on Risk of Surgical Bleeding and Risk of Stent Thrombosis		
Risk of stent thrombosis	Risk of surgical bleeding		
	High	Moderate	Low
High	• Stop all OAAs • Consider short-acting IV antiplatelet agents while off OAAs* • Proceed with surgery • Restart OAAs as soon as possible after surgery	• Continue at least one OAA if possible • Consider short-acting IV antiplatelet agents while off OAAs* • Proceed with surgery • Restart OAAs as soon as possible after surgery	• Continue all OAAs • Proceed with surgery
Moderate	• Stop all OAAs • Proceed with surgery • Restart OAAs as soon as possible after surgery	• Continue at least one OAA if possible • Proceed with surgery • Restart OAAs as soon as possible after surgery	• Continue all OAAs • Proceed with surgery
Low	• Stop all OAAs • Proceed with surgery • Restart OAAs as soon as possible after surgery	• Stop all OAAs • Proceed with surgery • Restart OAAs as soon as possible after surgery	• Continue at least one OAA if possible • Proceed with surgery • Restart OAAs as soon as possible after surgery

*Short-acting IV antiplatelet agent, for example, tirofiban (Aggrastat®); controversial; discuss indication and dosage with cardiologist.

CENTRAL NEURAXIAL ANESTHESIA FOR PATIENTS WITH STENTS

• CNB attenuates the postoperative hypercoagulable state
• Unclear how much this reduces the risk of stent thrombosis
• CNB contraindicated with antiplatelet drugs other than ASA, but potential for stent thrombosis with discontinuation of antiplatelet drugs
• ASA alone does not appear to increase the risk of neuraxial hematoma

STENT THROMBOSIS

• Presents as an STEMI or a sudden malignant arrhythmia
• Immediate transfer to cath lab for reperfusion to avoid a transmural MI

REFERENCES

For references, please visit **www.TheAnesthesiaGuide.com**.

CHAPTER 23
Preoperative Coagulation Assessment

Gebhard Wagener, MD and Ruchir Gupta, MD

PHYSIOPATHOLOGY

FIGURE 23-1. Classic model of coagulation

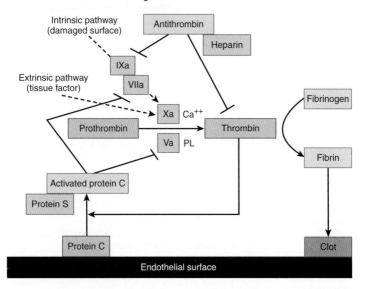

Classic coagulation cascade. Reproduced from Tintinalli JE, Stapczynski JS, Ma OJ, Cline DM, Cydulka RK, Mckler GD. *Tintinalli's Emergency Medicine: A Comprehensive Study Guide*. 7th ed. Figure 229-1. Available at: www.accessmedicine.com. Copyright © The McGraw-Hill Companies, Inc. All rights reserved.

- *Initiation*:
  ‣ Endothelial injury
  ‣ Subendothelial tissue factor (TF) exposed
  ‣ TF + circulating plasma FVII builds TF–FVII complex
  ‣ TF–FVII complex activates F-X, F-IX and a small amount of thrombin forms
- *Amplification*:
  ‣ Thrombin activates platelets via glycoprotein IIb/II a receptors
  ‣ F-Va binds to platelets
  ‣ More F-VIIa is released
- *Propagation*:
  ‣ Positive feedback:
    • F-Va leads to more release of F-IXa:
      ◆ F-IXa leads to formation of thrombin activatable fibrinolysis inhibitor (TAFI) that prevents fibrin breakdown

- F-IXa–F-VIII complex activates more F-X:
  - Thrombin burst
  - Fibrin production
  - Fibrin polymerization
- *Clot formation*

Assessment of Coagulation and Coagulation Tests	
Platelet count	• Automated counting cannot detect the presence of small or extremely large platelets • Manual smear can exclude the presence of pseudothrombocytopenia due to in vitro platelet agglutination
Bleeding time	• Evaluate platelet–vascular endothelium interaction • Prolonged bleeding time may occur in thrombocytopenia (<50,000), qualitative platelet abnormalities (e.g., uremia), von Willebrand disease (vWD), and severe fibrinogen deficiency • Does not predict surgical bleeding and is of limited usefulness in clinical bleeding
Prothrombin time (PT)	• Measures the efficiency of the fibrin production through the extrinsic pathway and the final common pathway: • Tissue factor, factor VII (extrinsic pathway), and factors X, V, prothrombin (factor II), and fibrinogen • Factors VII, X, and prothrombin are dependent on vitamin K and affected by coumadin; therefore, PT is used to monitor anticoagulation with coumadin
International normalized ratio (INR)	• Compensates for differences in PT reagents: • INR = patient PT/control PT
Activated partial thromboplastin time (aPTT)	• Measures the intrinsic (factors XII, XI, IX, VIII) and common pathway (factors II, V, X, and fibrinogen) • Used to monitor heparin effect and to evaluate deficiencies of all coagulation factors except factors VII and XIII
Thrombin time (TT)	• Measures the time it takes for a clot to form in the plasma of a blood sample to which an excess of thrombin has been added • If a patient is receiving heparin, a substance derived from snake venom called reptilase (not inhibited by heparin) is used instead of thrombin • Normal TT: 10–15 s or within 5 s of the control. Normal reptilase time: between 15 and 20 s • TT can be prolonged by heparin, fibrin degradation products, factor XIII deficiency, and fibrinogen deficiency/abnormality
Activated clotting time (ACT)	• An activating agent such as Celite or kaolin is added to a blood sample and the time to clot formation is measured • Used to confirm and monitor heparin effect as a point-of-care test during cardiac or vascular surgery

Thromboelastography	• Thromboelastography measures clinical clot formation and lysis not specific to coagulation pathways
	• TEG reflects clinically significant hemostasis and can guide transfusion and factor therapy
	• Coagulation is activated by adding calcium to a sample of citrated blood in a rotating cup. A rod is inserted into the cup and the deflection of the rod over time is measured
	• Parameters:
	  ▸ *R* value (~clotting time [CT]): the time for the first signs of a clot to appear
	  ▸ *k* value: time period from end of *R* until amplitude = 20 mm

(*continued*)

Assessment of Coagulation and Coagulation Tests (*continued*)

Thromboelastography	▸ α angle (~fibrin cross-linking): angle between the middle of the TEG tracing and the tangent of graph ▸ Maximum amplitude (MA) of the graph (~final strength of the clot) • Use of TEG is able to predict surgical hemorrhage, guide transfusion therapy in trauma, and reduce transfusion requirements, for example, during cardiac surgery
Rotational thromboelastometry (ROTEM)	• Similar to TEG but an oscillating rod is inserted in a cup of blood (the cup is not rotating). The machine is more resilient to shocks and vibrations • Parameters: ▸ CT: time from beginning to 2 mm amplitude–affected by fibrin formation, clotting factors, or anticoagulants ▸ Clot formation time (CFT): time from 2 to 20 mm amplitude–speed of clot formation affected by platelet function and fibrinogen ▸ Maximum clot firmness (MCF): MA (in mm)–clot firmness and quality: affected by platelets, fibrinogen, factor XIII, and fibrinolysis ▸ Maximum lysis (ML): amplitude at 30 min as percent of MCF–affected by fibrinolysis

Bleeding Disorders and Coagulation Tests

Condition	Prothrombin time (PT)	Partial thromboplastin time (PTT)	Bleeding time	Platelet count	Thrombin time (TT)
Vitamin K deficiency/warfarin	⇑	⇑	⇒	⇒	⇒
Disseminated intravascular coagulation	⇑	⇑	⇑	⇓	⇑
von Willebrand disease	⇒	⇑	⇑	⇒	⇒
Hemophilia	⇒	⇑	⇒	⇒	⇒
Early liver failure	⇑	⇒	⇒	⇒	⇒
End-stage liver failure	⇑	⇑	⇑	⇓	⇑
Uremia	⇒	⇒	⇑	⇒	⇒
Congenital afibrinogenemia	⇑	⇑	⇑	⇒	⇑
Factor V deficiency	⇑	⇑	⇒	⇒	⇒
Factor X deficiency as seen in amyloid purpura	⇑	⇑	⇒	⇒	⇒
Glanzmann thrombasthenia	⇒	⇒	⇑	⇒	⇒
Bernard–Soulier syndrome	⇒	⇒	⇑	⇓	⇒

FIGURE 23-2. Prolonged PT

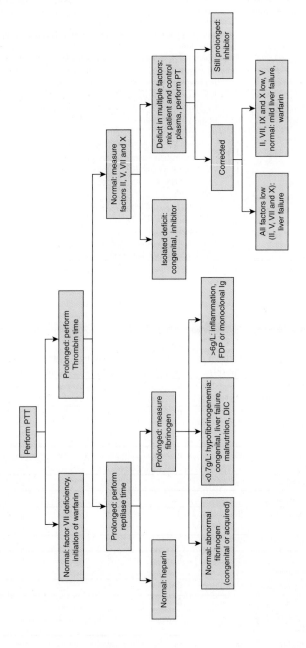

FIGURE 23-3. Prolonged PTT

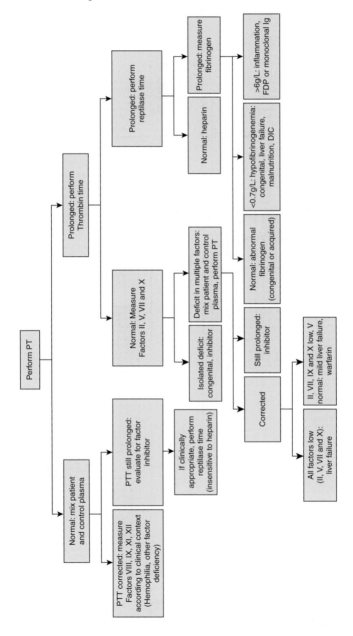

FIGURE 23-4. Prolonged bleeding time

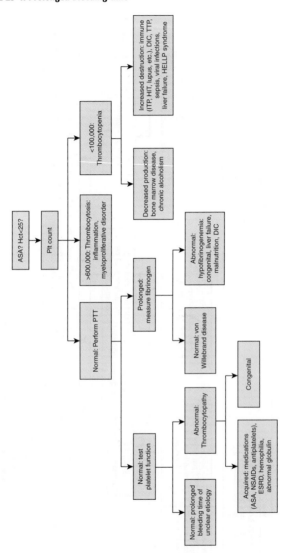

BLEEDING DIATHESIS

A. Inherited bleeding disorders
Hemophilias

See table on following page.

Disorder	Pathophysiology	Preoperative	Intraoperative	Postoperative	Treatment
Hemophilia A (X-linked)	Factor VIII deficiency • Severe: <1% • Moderate: 2–5% • Mild: >6%	Factor VIII level should be brought to ~100% for elective major surgery • Initial infusion of 50–60 U/kg in adult • Repeat infusion of 25–30 U/kg every 8–12 h	• Repeat infusion of 25–30 U/kg every 8–12 h	Continue therapy to maintain factor VII level >30% for up to 2 weeks to avoid postoperative bleeding. For bone or joint surgery, 4–6 weeks of replacement therapy needed	Factor VIII concentrate FFP or cryoprecipitate if FVIII unavailable Always evaluate for anti-FVIII antibodies (if refractory to FVIII, the only therapy may be activated FVII[1])
Hemophilia B (Christmas disease) (X-linked)	Factor IX deficiency • Severe: <1% • Moderate: 2–5% • Mild: >6%	Factor IX level should be brought to ~100% for elective major surgery • Initial infusion of 100 U/kg in adult • Repeat infusion of 50 U/kg every 12–24 h	• Repeat infusion of 50 U/kg every 12–24 h	Continue therapy to maintain factor IX level >30% for up to 2 weeks to avoid postoperative bleeding. For bone or joint surgery, 4–6 weeks of replacement therapy needed	Recombinant factor IX FFP or cryoprecipitate if FIX unavailable Always evaluate for anti-FIX antibodies (if refractory to FIX, the only therapy may be activated FVII[1])

[1]Activated factor VII in case of refractory hemophilia with anti-factor VIII or factor IX antibodies: 120–150 μg/kg 15 minutes prior to incision, and then 90–120 μg/kg q 2 hours. Discuss tapering with hematologist.

Types of von Willebrand Disease

Type	Pathophysiology	Bleeding time	vWF Ag	vWF:Rco	FVIIIc activity	Multimers	RIPA (time)	Treatment
1	Quantitative deficiency of vWF	↑	↓	Normal	Normal	Normal	↑	Desmopressin, vWF concentrate
2A	Abnormal platelet-dependent vWF function with no large multimers	↑↑	Normal	↓	Normal	None	↑↑	vWF concentrate (first choice) Desmopressin
2B	Heightened affinity of vWF for GP Ib-IX Thrombopenia	↑↑	Normal	↓	Normal	↓	↑↑	vWF concentrate
2M	Decreased affinity of vWF for GP Ib-IX Normal multimers	↑↑	Normal	↓	Normal	Normal	↑↑	vWF concentrate (first choice) Desmopressin
2N	Abnormal vWF binding to factor VIII	Normal	Normal	Normal	↓	Normal	Normal	vWF concentrate (first choice) Desmopressin
3	Severe–complete vWF deficiency and factor VIII deficiency	↑↑↑	None	None	<5%	None	↑↑↑	vWF concentrate (first choice) Desmopressin

vWF dose (surgical prophylaxis): 40–75 IU/kg IV, followed by repeat doses of 40–60 IU/kg in 8–12 h intervals.
DDAVP: 0.3 μg/kg IV in 50 mL saline slowly over 10–20 min.

Acquired Bleeding Disorders		
Disorder	Pathophysiology	Treatment as management
Vitamin K deficiency Warfarin overdose	• Vitamin K is essential to synthesize factors II, VII, IX, and X • Vitamin K deficiency can be due to malabsorption syndromes (intestinal diseases, primary biliary cirrhosis, primary sclerosing cholangitis) or coumadin (warfarin) therapy • Tests: increased prothrombin time (PT) and international normalized ratio (INR)	Approach to the coagulopathic patient on warfarin (also see chapter 12): • Need to resume/continue warfarin therapy ASAP (e.g., mechanical valve): avoid vitamin K; use FFP • INR therapeutic: • <5 (no bleeding): decrease/hold warfarin • INR 5–9 (no bleeding): hold warfarin; consider 1–2.5 mg vitamin K PO • INR >9 (no bleeding): hold warfarin and give 2.5–5 mg vitamin K PO • Significant bleeding or awaiting surgery: 10 mg vitamin K (slow IV); repeat once daily for three doses; give FFP if bleeding is serious
Liver failure	• Advanced liver disease and cirrhosis will cause decreases of circulating procoagulant factors • Portal hypertension will cause sequestration of platelets in the spleen • May also cause increased thrombosis and hypercoagulability due to deficiency of anticoagulant factors (i.e., proteins C and S) even if coagulation tests are increased	• Do not transfuse FFP for elevated INR unless clinical bleeding is evident (or needs surgery) • Consider vitamin K 10 mg (slow IV) daily for 3 days prior to surgery • If rapid normalization of INR needed for surgery/procedure, give FFP
Idiopathic thrombocytopenic purpura (ITP)	Increased platelet destruction due to an unknown cause	Elective surgery should be delayed in severe cases For emergency procedures, IVIg and platelet transfusion Routine monitoring, with special attention to bleeding on the surgical field, which may necessitate more platelet infusions

Anesthetic management:
- GA or IVRA; peripheral nerve blocks only if benefit >risk; central neuraxial blocks contraindicated
- Avoid A-line unless formally indicated
- Vein sparing. If CVL needed, use IJ (avoid femoral; subclavian contraindicated)
- Need for atraumatic intubation: risk of airway hematoma
- Avoid gastric tube, esophageal stethoscope, Foley unless necessary
- Avoid hemodilution
- No IM injection
- Avoid ASA. Discuss NSAIDs with hematologist

von Willebrand disease
- Evaluate for MVP (15%)

REFERENCES

For references, please visit **www.TheAnesthesiaGuide.com**.

CHAPTER 24
G6PD Deficiency

Ruchir Gupta, MD

BASICS

X-linked recessive deficiency in glucose-6-phosphate dehydrogenase enzyme leading to RBC hemolysis:
- Abnormally low levels of metabolic enzyme involved in pentose phosphate pathway
- Important in RBC metabolism
- Causes nonimmune hemolytic anemia (direct Coombs negative)
- Neonatal jaundice with kernicteris
- Hemolytic crisis in response to triggers
- More frequent in patients with African, southern European, Middle Eastern, southeast Asian, or central and southern Pacific Island descent

Information to Elicit in H & P in Patient with G6P Deficiency	
History	Physical exam
Previous crisis with treatment	Cyanosis
Medication for G6P deficiency	Jaundice
Recent history of fatigue	Dark urine
History of dark urine	
Complaint of lumbar/substernal pain	
Review medication history (especially recent initiation of any offending agent)	

PREOPERATIVE

- Thorough H & P
- Avoid triggers:
  ‣ Illness:
    ▪ Infection (hyperthermia)
    ▪ Stress
    ▪ Acidosis
    ▪ Hyperglycemia (thus DKA can trigger hemolysis)
  ‣ Foods: broad beans (also known as fava beans)
  ‣ Drugs:
    ▪ Antimalarial drugs: primaquine, pamaquine, chloroquine
    ▪ Sulfonamides: sulfanilamide, sulfamethoxazole mafenide, thiazolesulfone, dapsone
    ▪ Methylene blue, toluidine blue
    ▪ Drugs causing methemoglobinemia: benzocaine, lidocaine, articaine, prilocaine
    ▪ Certain analgesics: aspirin, phenazopyridine acetanilide
    ▪ Nalidixic acid, nitrofurantoin
    ▪ TNT
    ▪ Naphthalene (a chemical compound used for industrial strength removal of grease) should also be avoided by people with G6PD deficiency
- Administer benzodiazepine to prevent/treat anxiety

INTRAOPERATIVE

A. Monitors

Temperature probe:
- Avoid hyperthermia

At least two IVs in case transfusion necessary.

Foley: monitor urine closely for signs of hemolytic anemia (dark urine).

B. Induction

- Routine anesthetic care with no restrictions on GA versus MAC versus regional
- Avoid local anesthetics that can lead to methemoglobinemia (prilocaine, benzocaine, lidocaine [rare])

C. Maintenance

- Continue to avoid triggering agents
- Antibiotics, strict aseptic precautions to prevent infection
- Opioids or nerve block to provide adequate analgesia (as stress is a trigger)

POSTOPERATIVE

- Adequate analgesia
- Clinical signs (fatigue, cyanosis) will arise 24–72 hours after initiation of offending agent
- Labs:
  ‣ Peripheral blood smear: "schistocytes" and reticulocytes
  ‣ Denatured hemoglobin inclusions within RBCs = Heinz bodies
  ‣ LDH elevated
  ‣ Unconjugated bilirubin elevated
  ‣ Haptoglobin levels decreased
  ‣ Direct Coombs result should be negative (as hemolysis is not immune)
  ‣ Hemosiderin and urobilinogen in the urine indicate chronic intravascular hemolysis
- Patients being discharged home should be counseled to seek medical attention if signs and symptoms arise
- Treat acute hemolytic anemia by discontinuing the offending agent and maintaining adequate urine output with fluid replacement and diuretics
- Blood transfusions in more severe cases

PEARLS AND TIPS

Signs of hemolytic anemia from G6PD deficiency difficult to notice during GA: monitor for signs and symptoms closely postoperatively.

REFERENCES

For references, please visit **www.TheAnesthesiaGuide.com**.

CHAPTER 25
Diabetes Mellitus

Jennifer Wu, MD, MBA and Arthur Atchabahian, MD

Pathophysiology			
	Type 1	Type 2	Gestational
Incidence	0.4% of population in 2005	7% of population in 2005	4% of pregnant women
Onset	Typically before age 30	Increases with increasing age	
Risk factors	Genetics, environmental	Obesity, genetics	Obesity
Pathophysiology	Autoimmune destruction of beta cells, resulting in insulin deficiency	Insulin resistance, increased glucose production	Somatomammotropin causes insulin resistance
Complication	Diabetic ketoacidosis (DKA)	Hyperglycemic–hyperosmolar nonketotic coma	Congenital abnormalities, stillbirth
Outcome	• Ocular: cataracts, retinopathy, blindness • Vascular: coronary artery disease, peripheral vascular disease • Renal: leading cause of renal failure in the United States • Neurologic: peripheral neuropathy, autonomic neuropathy • GI: delayed gastric emptying • NB: HTN accelerates microangiopathy and macroangiopathy		• Most resolve postpartum • 30–60% chance of developing diabetes postpregnancy later in life

TREATMENT

See table on following page.

Treatment

	Insulin	Sulfonylurea	Metformin (a biguanide)	Acarbose (an intestinal alpha-glucosidase inhibitor)	Thiazolidinediones (troglitazone, rosiglitazone, and pioglitazone)	Meglitinides (repaglinide and nateglinide)
Mechanism of action	Anabolic hormone	Stimulates endogenous insulin secretion	• Inhibits gluconeogenesis • Increases glucose uptake in skeletal muscle	Decreases carbohydrate absorption	Activate peroxisome proliferator-activated receptors	Increase secretion of insulin
Hypoglycemia	Yes	Rare	No	No	No	Yes
Complications	Hypoglycemia, high dose may be atherogenic	Hypoglycemia	Risk of perioperative lactic acidosis; renal clearance	GI upset	Fluid retention	Weight gain
What to do preoperatively?	Administer half the dose of long-acting insulin; monitor blood glucose perioperatively; IV insulin has more reliable absorption than subcut	Hold while NPO to avoid hypoglycemia	Hold 1–2 days preoperatively to avoid lactic acidosis	Hold while NPO; no benefit while NPO	Consider holding 2 days preoperatively to avoid fluid retention	

Complications			
	Diabetic ketoacidosis (DKA) (see chapter 210 for more details)	Nonketotic hyperosmolar coma (NKHC) (see chapter 211 for more details)	Hypoglycemia
Precipitated by	• Poor patient compliance with insulin • Stress state, such as sepsis or myocardial infarction • Stress leads to an increase in counterregulatory hormones, which cause insulin resistance	• Patients with NIDDM do not suffer from DKA because circulating insulin levels are sufficient to prevent ketogenesis, but instead are at risk for NKHC • Precipitated by stress or drugs, including corticosteroids	Insulin and/or oral medications in the absence of glucose intake Counterregulatory hormones secreted in response to hypoglycemia include epinephrine, glucagon, growth hormone, and cortisol
Diagnosis	• Metabolic acidosis and hyperglycemia present in a patient with IDDM • Confirmation by urinalysis for ketones	Extreme hyperglycemia (>1,000 mg/dL) is sufficient for diagnosis Serum osmolality >320 mOsm/kg Urine ketones absent	
Signs and symptoms	• Nausea, vomiting, abdominal pain • Tachycardia and hypotension caused by dehydration • Somnolence	Elderly individual with type 2 DM Nausea/vomiting Muscle weakness and cramps Polyuria, and then oliguria Slight hyperthermia Confusion, lethargy, seizures, hemiparesis, and coma	Often occurs when blood glucose falls below 30–50 mg/dL Diaphoresis, tachycardia, altered mental status, seizures
Treatment	See chapter 210	See chapter 211	Oral 15 g carbohydrates (180 mL orange juice) Fluid resuscitation (1–2 L of NS over 1–2 h) 25 mL 50% glucose (each milliliter of 50% glucose will raise BS of 70-kg patient by ~2 mg/dL) 1 mg glucagon IV or IM— response in 15–30 min

PREOPERATIVE

• Airway evaluation:
  ‣ Stiff joint syndrome is a result of glycosylation of tissue; atlanto-occipital joint and TMJ stiffness may make laryngoscopy difficult; *prayer sign* to evaluate (inability to completely close gaps between opposed palms and fingers when pressing hands together as if to pray)

- Labs:
  - CBC, metabolic panel, urinalysis
  - Baseline finger-stick glucose
  - Glycosylated hemoglobin (HbA1c):
    - Goal <7.5%
    - An indication of the mean blood glucose concentration over 60 days
    - Higher levels are associated with the development of retinopathy, nephropathy, and neuropathy
- Cardiac evaluation:
  - HTN (risk of hemodynamic lability)
  - Ischemic heart disease is the most common cause of perioperative morbidity
  - Get EKG; consider further workup for CAD, as ischemia often silent
- Autonomic neuropathy, gastroparesis:
  - BP and HR orthostatic change:
    - Orthostatic change is a decrease in BP greater than 20/10 mm Hg
    - Symptom consistent with orthostatic changes is dizziness or loss of consciousness when standing
  - QT variability
- In patients with DKA, stabilize preoperatively if procedure not emergent
- Medications:
  - Continue oral hypoglycemic agents until the night before surgery
  - Metformin should be discontinued 2 days prior to surgery due to the risk of lactic acidosis
  - Small amounts of SQ regular insulin can be used to treat hyperglycemia. Regular insulin has peak effect in 2–4 hours
  - Insulin pump may be continued for short procedures. Insulin administration should be converted to IV insulin with perioperative blood glucose monitoring for long or complicated procedures

ANESTHESIA

- Consider giving nonparticulate antacid (Bicitra 30 mL) before induction if gastroparesis suspected
- Intraoperative hyperglycemia adversely affects wound healing and recovery from ischemic neurologic events; *maintain normoglycemia intraoperatively* (but avoid hypoglycemia); ideally insulin infusion on a dedicated line adjusted to FS
- Patients with autonomic neuropathy will not have the normal expected sympathetic response to hypoglycemia, are less able to maintain core body temperature, and may not have pain with acute myocardial infarction
- Sudden death syndrome can occur in patients with autonomic neuropathy; responds to epinephrine

POSTOPERATIVE

- Postoperative finger-stick glucose, SQ insulin coverage as needed (see below)
- If NPO, consider dextrose-containing IV fluids to prevent hypoglycemia

PROPOSED MANAGEMENT PROTOCOLS FOR HOSPITALIZED DIABETIC PATIENTS

A. Basal–bolus regimen (preferred):

- Discontinue oral antidiabetic drugs
- Start total daily insulin dose:
  - 0.4 U/kg per day if the admission blood glucose is 140–200 mg/dL
  - 0.5 U/kg per day if the admission blood glucose is between 201 and 400 mg/dL
  - Give one half of total daily dose as insulin glargine (long-acting) and one half as insulin glulisine (immediate-acting)
  - Give insulin glargine once daily at the same time of the day
  - Give insulin glulisine in three equally divided doses before each meal. Hold insulin glulisine if patient is not able to eat

- Supplemental insulin:
  - ▸ Measure blood glucose before each meal and at bedtime (or every 6 hours if NPO)
  - ▸ Give supplemental insulin glulisine following the "sliding scale" protocol for blood glucose >140 mg/dL
  - ▸ If a patient is able and expected to eat all or most of his or her meals, give supplemental glulisine insulin before each meal and at bedtime following the "usual" column
  - ▸ If a patient is not able to eat, give supplemental glulisine insulin every 6 hours (6–12–6–12), following the "insulin-sensitive" column
- Insulin adjustment:
  - ▸ If the fasting or mean blood glucose during the day is >140 mg/dL in the absence of hypoglycemia, increase insulin glargine dose by 20% every day
  - ▸ If patient develops hypoglycemia (<70 mg/dL), decrease glargine daily dose by 20%

B. Sliding scale regimen with regular insulin (simpler but poorer control):

- Discontinue oral antidiabetic drugs on admission
- If patient is able and expected to eat all or most of his or her meals, give regular insulin before each meal and at bedtime, following the "usual" column
- If patient is not able to eat, give regular insulin every 6 hours (6–12–6–12), following the "insulin-sensitive" column
- Insulin adjustment:
  - ▸ Measure blood glucose before each meal and at bedtime (or every 6 hours if NPO)
  - ▸ If fasting and premeal plasma glucose are persistently >140 mg/dL in the absence of hypoglycemia, increase insulin scale from the "insulin-sensitive" to the "usual" column or from the "usual" to the "insulin-resistant" column
  - ▸ If a patient develops hypoglycemia (blood glucose <70 mg/dL), decrease regular insulin from "insulin-resistant" to "usual" column or from the "usual" to "insulin-sensitive" column

Supplemental Insulin Scale			
Blood glucose (mg/dL)	Insulin sensitive	Usual	Insulin resistant
>141–180	2	4	6
181–220	4	6	8
221–260	6	8	10
261–300	8	10	12
301–350	10	12	14
351–400	12	14	16
>400	14	16	18

PEARLS AND TIPS

- Goals include avoiding hypoglycemia, extreme hyperglycemia, and electrolyte disturbances
- Overzealous glucose control can result in hypoglycemia

REFERENCES

For references, please visit **www.TheAnesthesiaGuide.com**.

CHAPTER 26
Liver Failure

Ruchir Gupta, MD

MAIN ETIOLOGIES

- ETOH
- Hepatitis B, C, and D
- Hemochromatosis, Wilson disease
- Autoimmune, inherited (biliary atresia, alpha-1 antitrypsin deficiency, etc.)

PREOPERATIVE

Assessment of Systemic Manifestations of Liver Disease	
System	Features
CV	Increased CO, increased TBW but relative hypovolemia, decreased SVR
Metabolic	Hypokalemia, hyponatremia, hypoalbuminemia, hypoglycemia Skeletal muscle wasting, poor skin turgor, loss of adipose tissue
Respiratory	Increased A-V shunts, decreased FRC, pleural effusions *Hepatopulmonary syndrome*—marked pulmonary HTN with prominence of A-V shunts. Orthodeoxia and platypnea (desaturation and dyspnea when upright)
GI	Ascites, portal HTN, esophageal varices, hypersplenism *Spontaneous bacterial peritonitis*—gram positive in asymptomatic patients but usually gram negative in symptomatic patients (*E. coli, Klebsiella*)
Renal	*Hepatorenal syndrome*—oliguric deterioration in renal function in patients with liver failure: • Cause unknown (may be caused by nephrotoxins not cleared by liver) • Resolves with liver transplantation • Intraoperative/postoperative dialysis may be necessary
Hematologic	Anemia, coagulopathy (decreased factors II, V, VII, X, increased PT), decreased platelets
Neurologic	Encephalopathy—etiology multifactorial: false neurotransmitters, inflammation Tx: lactulose (accelerates GI transit to reduce absorption of false neurotransmitters), neomycin (eliminates ammonia-producing bacteria), low-protein diet (lowers ammonia produced by protein breakdown) *West Haven criteria*: • Grade 1—trivial lack of awareness, euphoria or anxiety, shortened attention span, impaired performance of addition or subtraction • Grade 2—lethargy or apathy, minimal disorientation for time or place, subtle personality change, inappropriate behavior • Grade 3—somnolence to semistupor, but responsive to verbal stimuli; confusion; gross disorientation • Grade 4—coma (unresponsive to verbal or noxious stimuli) ▸ Transition from grade 1 to 2/3 may occur over a period of hours. Treatment should focus on relieving causes of increased ICP (head elevation, hyperventilation, osmotic diuretics)
Pharmacokinetic and pharmacodynamic	Increased Vd for most drugs Decreased protein binding with increased free drug fraction

- Assess overall severity of liver disease

Child–Pugh Classification of Severity of Liver Disease			
Variable	Absent (1 point)	Slight (2 points)	Moderate (3 points)
Ascites	None	Mild	Moderate
Bilirubin	<2	2–3	>3
Albumin	>3.5	2.8–3.5	<2.8
PT	<4	4–6	>6
Encephalopathy	None	Mild	Severe

Score	2-year survival (%)	Mortality risk of major abdominal surgery (excluding liver transplantation) (%)
5–6	85–100	10
7–9	60–80	30
10–15	35–45	50–70

- If elective surgery, optimize patient:
  - ▸ Reduce ascites
  - ▸ Correct electrolyte abnormalities (hypokalemia and hyponatremia)
  - ▸ Look for prerenal renal insufficiency (may need to have dialysis equipment intra-operatively/postoperatively if hepatorenal syndrome present)
  - ▸ Improve nutritional status:
    - ▪ If patient on TPN/feeds, continue intraoperatively and postoperatively
  - ▸ In patient with hemochromatosis or alcoholic dilated cardiomyopathy:
    - ▪ Assess cardiac function (TTE)
    - ▪ Possible conduction abnormalities
- Preoperative therapies:
  - ▸ Continue beta-blockers (if portal hypertension)
  - ▸ If premedication needed, prefer hydroxyzine to benzodiazepines; no premedication if encephalopathy

ANESTHESIA

GA preferred but regional can be considered in the absence of coagulation abnormalities. Superficial nerve blocks in "compressible" compartments (*not* infraclavicular, psoas compartment, or sciatic blocks) can be performed by an experienced practitioner even if coagulation abnormal.

A. Monitors

- A-line should be considered in major procedures (hemodynamic instability from low SVR)
- Large-bore IVs and/or CVL should be considered for rapid transfusion of blood products secondary to coagulation abnormalities
- Rapid transfusing device should be available on standby if rapid blood loss expected
- NGT relatively contraindicated, especially if esophageal varices are present

B. Induction
- Propofol or etomidate can be used but a vasoconstrictor (e.g., phenylephrine) should be on standby to avoid abrupt drops in BP
- Avoid benzodiazepines if possible

C. Intraoperative
- Antibiotherapy: avoid aminoglycosides
- Consider glucose-containing IV fluid; frequent monitoring of blood glucose and electrolytes
- Special care to prevent infection (immunosuppressed)
- Hepatitis precautions if applicable
- Prefer cisatracurium for NMB as elimination is organ-independent:
  ‣ Avoid histamine-releasing drugs (atracurium/mivacurium) to prevent further decreases in BP
- Minimize opioids as clearance decreased; remifentanil if minor procedure
- Monitor BIS/entropy and NMB to minimize drug doses and recovery time
- Maintain PT >40% and Fg >0.8 g/L with FFP and plts >50,000 (100,000 if craniotomy)
- Decreased sensitivity to vasoconstrictors. Use norepinephrine infusion if >50 mg ephedrine needed. Poor response to fluid administration b/o vasodilation

POSTOPERATIVE

- Special attention to electrolytes
- Consider delayed extubation if massive fluid shifts and transfusions have occurred
- Monitor coagulation to correct for any abnormality that can lead to postoperative bleeding
- Avoid acetaminophen (hepatotoxicity) and NSAIDs (renal toxicity)
- If severe liver failure, increase interval between morphine doses
- Consider DT prevention if alcoholic cirrhosis
- In the event of acute deterioration of hepatic function, urgent transplantation may be necessary (CI: severe CV disease, systemic infection, extrahepatic malignancy, severe psychiatric/neurologic disorders, absence of splanchnic venous inflow system)

PEARLS AND TIPS

- Hepatically cleared drugs may have prolonged effects due to impaired metabolism
- Drugs binding to albumin have higher free fraction (lower dose)
- Ascites decreases FRC and predisposes the patient to rapid desaturation

REFERENCES

For references, please visit **www.TheAnesthesiaGuide.com**.

CHAPTER 27
Chronic Renal Failure

Gebhard Wagener, MD

PHYSIOPATHOLOGY

Organ Systems Involved in Renal Failure	
Neuro	• Uremic encephalopathy • Depends on rate of rise of BUN, not absolute value • Peripheral and autonomic neuropathy
Cardiac	• Uremic pericarditis (rare) • Hypertension • Left ventricular hypertrophy and congestive heart failure (CHF)
Respiratory	• Volume overload and pulmonary edema
Gastrointestinal	• Delayed gastric emptying

Renal	• Acidosis:
	  ‣ Non-anion gap acidosis with renal bicarbonate loss and hyperchloremia
	  ‣ Anion gap acidosis due to hyperphosphatemia
	• Hyperkalemia:
	  ‣ Worsened by acute acidosis (pH $\Downarrow$ by 0.1 causes K^+ $\Uparrow$ by 0.5 mEq/L)

Hematology	• Normocytic, normochromic anemia
	• Uremic platelet dysfunction and coagulopathy:
	  ‣ Impaired von Willebrand factor (vWF) release from endothelium
	  $\Rightarrow$ impaired platelet activation
	  ‣ Can be treated with desmopressin (0.3 μg/kg) that releases
	  endogenous vWF

ID	• Immunosuppression due to myelodepression • Catheter-related infections • Peritonitis with peritoneal dialysis
Others	• Vascular access • Tunneled dialysis catheter • Double-lumen central venous catheters (Vas Cath) • Arteriovenous (AV) fistula and shunts

PREOPERATIVE EVALUATION

A. History

- How long has the patient been on dialysis?
- When was the last dialysis?
- How long was the last dialysis?
- Were there any problems during the last dialysis such as hypotension, impaired fluid removal, dizziness?
- Any recent fever, chills, or infections?
- In case of peritoneal dialysis: when was the abdomen filled or emptied the last time?

B. Physical exam
- Examine shunt site and auscultate the shunt
- Evaluate for signs of CHF and neuropathy
- Examine abdomen in case of peritoneal dialysis

C. Tests
- Complete blood count (anemia), serum chemistry (K^+, BUN, Mg^{2+}, phosphate), and coagulation profile
- ECG (cardiomyopathy, low voltage with uremic pericardial effusion)
- Chest x-ray (pulmonary edema and pleural effusions, catheter location, cardiomyopathy)

Schedule *dialysis 1 day prior to surgery*.

Schedule *RBC transfusion during hemodialysis if necessary*.

Continue peritoneal dialysis until surgery.

ANESTHESIA

A. Regional anesthesia
- Possible if no coagulopathy present
- Document preexisting neuropathy
- Sympathectomy may exacerbate autonomic dysfunction and hypotension

B. General anesthesia
- *Positioning*:
  - ‣ Careful positioning of arms with attention to fistula
- *Induction*:
  - ‣ Minimize sedative agents
  - ‣ Rapid sequence induction if delayed gastric emptying is suspected
  - ‣ Succinylcholine may be used if preoperative K^+ <5 mEq/L
  - ‣ Avoid rocuronium or vecuronium; preferred NMB is cisatracurium
- *Fluids*:
  - ‣ Minimize fluids for minor surgery
  - ‣ For major and intermediate surgery:
    - ▪ Replace fluid loss (blood loss and insensitive losses) with lactated Ringer (LR) or other balanced salt solutions, not normal saline (NS)
    - ▪ NS causes hyperchloremic acidosis that worsens hyperkalemia and may preclude extubation
- *Drugs*:
  - ‣ Normal metabolism (independent from renal function):
    - ▪ (Cis-) atracurium, succinylcholine, esmolol, remifentanil
  - ‣ Titrate all other drugs to effect:
    - ▪ Vecuronium, rocuronium, fentanyl, midazolam, hydromorphone
  - ‣ Avoid (or titrate carefully) drugs with renally eliminated metabolites:
    - ▪ Morphine, vecuronium, meperidine, midazolam
  - ‣ Sevoflurane is probably safe but avoid low fresh gas flow
- *Extubation*:
  - ‣ Check arterial blood gas prior to extubation for any longer cases
  - ‣ If there is significant metabolic (anion gap) acidosis: keep patient intubated and extubate after a treatment of HD:
    - ▪ Metabolic acidosis would cause hyperventilation to maintain a normal pH and lead to exhaustion and respiratory failure

POSTOPERATIVE

For minor (and some intermediate) surgery:
- Hemodialysis according to schedule
- No contraindication for discharge home on the day of surgery

For most intermediate and all major surgeries:
- Hemodialysis hours after surgery
- Observe closely for 24–48 hours
- Prevent fluid overload and pulmonary edema
- Monitor for hyperkalemia

PEARLS AND TIPS

Treatment of hyperkalemia (from fastest to slowest)

Calcium:
- No effect on K+ levels but antagonizes effects of hyperkalemia on myocardium
- Give through central venous access (extravasation can be catastrophic)
- One gram $CaCl_2$ IV over 2–5 minutes

Insulin–glucose:
- Drives K+ back into cell with ATPase pumps
- Boluses of 10 IU insulin combined with 25–50 g dextrose intravenous
- Check plasma potassium and glucose levels frequently and consider starting insulin infusion if hyperglycemia

Sodium bicarbonate:
- Osmotic volume load that may exacerbate pulmonary edema and CHF
- Give 50–100 mEq slowly over 15–20 minutes only in intubated and hyperventilated patients
- Produces CO_2 that diffuses intracellularly where it will be converted to carbonic acid and cause paradoxical intracellular acidosis
- Avoid if possible in patients with renal failure

Beta-2 agonists:
- Activate Na^+/K^+-ATPase and shift K+ into the cells (within 2 hours)
- Can cause substantial tachycardia
- Albuterol: 10–20 mg by nebulizer over 10 minutes
- Epinephrine infusion 0.05 µg/kg/min (response not predictable with advanced renal failure)

Hyperventilation:
- Hyperventilate to increase pH: decreasing H+ ion will force potassium intracellular
- Each increase of pH by 0.1 causes a decrease of K+ by 0.5 mEq

Kayexalate:
- Resin that exchanges sodium with potassium
- 0.5 g/kg as a rectal enema every 6 hours
- Not indicated for acute life-threatening hyperkalemia

Renal replacement therapy:
- Most effective removal of potassium
- Continuous renal replacement therapy may not be fast enough (lower blood and dialysate flows) but more feasible intraoperatively
- Intermittent hemodialysis can be safely done without hypotension if no fluid is removed and bicarbonate instead of acetate is used as a buffer

Avoid hyperkalemia associated with large-volume RBC transfusion:
- Prior to surgery, wash packed red blood cells using Cell Saver, which will remove extracellular potassium
- Refrigerate these washed cells near the operating room; transfuse if hyperkalemia is worsening but hemorrhage requires continued red blood cell transfusion

REFERENCES

For references, please visit **www.TheAnesthesiaGuide.com**.

CHAPTER 28
Acute Renal Injury

Elrond Teo, MBBS and Gebhard Wagener, MD

PHYSIOPATHOLOGY (FIGURES 28-1 TO 28-3)

FIGURE 28-1. Causes of acute kidney injury

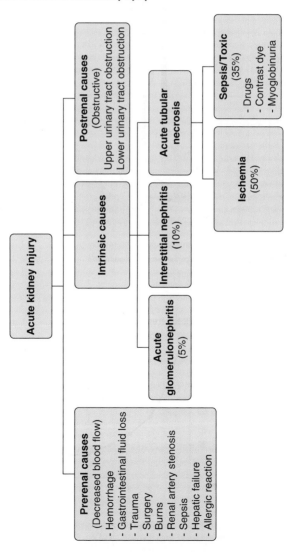

FIGURE 28-2. Renal anatomy and physiology

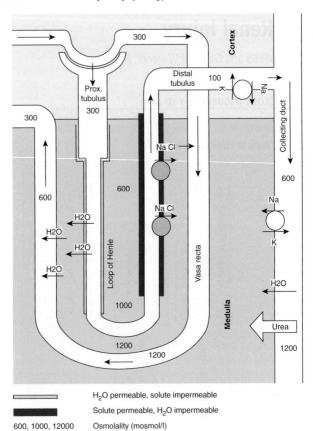

▭ (light bar)	H₂O permeable, solute impermeable
▬ (dark bar)	Solute permeable, H₂O impermeable
600, 1000, 12000	Osmolality (mosmol/l)

FIGURE 28-3. Relationship of GFR to serum creatinine

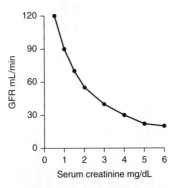

The relation between serum creatinine and glomerular filtration rate (GFR) is not linear. Small increases in serum creatinine can reflect large decreases in GFR.

PREOPERATIVE

A. Estimation of glomerular filtration rate

- Only valid in a stable situation, that is, not while in ARF
- If ARF, measure clearance; a 2-hour clearance is as good as a 24-hour measurement

Modification of Diet in Renal Disease Study (MDRD) Group formula:

Estimated creatinine clearance

$$= 186 \times \left[\frac{\text{creatinine}}{88.4}\right]^{-1.154} \times (\text{age})^{-0.203} \times \text{gender} \times \text{race}$$

Gender	Female (0.742)	Male (1)
Race	Black (1.21)	Non-black (1)

Cockroft–Gault formula:

Estimated creatinine clearance (mL/min)

$$= \frac{(140 - \text{age (years)}) \times \text{weight (kg)}}{0.814 \times \text{creatinine}} \times \text{gender}$$

Gender	Male (1)	Female (0.85)

Classification of Chronic Renal Disease		
Stage	Description	GFR (cm³/(min 1.73 m²))
1	Kidney damage with normal or increased GFR	>90
2	Kidney damage with mild decrease in GFR	60–89
3	Moderate decrease in GFR	30–59
4	Severe decrease in GFR	15–29
5	Kidney failure	<15 or dialysis

PRACTICAL MANAGEMENT OF THE PATIENT WITH ELEVATED SERUM CREATININE PRESENTING FOR SURGERY

A. Preoperative evaluation

- Estimate creatinine clearance:
  - Using either Cockroft–Gault or MDRD formula
- Acute or chronic?
  - Previous serum creatinine values
  - Sudden rise?
- Causes:
  - Low perfusion:
    - Cardiogenic shock
    - Sepsis and infection
    - Hypovolemia
  - Nephrotoxic insults:
    - Radiocontrast
    - Aminoglycosides
    - Calcineurin inhibitors (tacrolimus/FK-506 or cyclosporine)
  - Other causes
  - Urinary tract infections
  - Postrenal obstruction

B. Preoperative management

- Consider maintenance fluid while NPO
- Consider preventive strategies especially for radiographic procedures: no strategy has however been proven to be effective (see below):
  - ‣ Sodium bicarbonate
  - ‣ *N*-Acetylcysteine

C. Intraoperative management

- Consider invasive monitoring: urine output not necessarily reliable indicator of adequate perfusion:
  - ‣ Pulmonary artery catheter
  - ‣ Intraoperative transesophageal echocardiography
- Diligent fluid management:
  - ‣ Fluid deficit and maintenance and blood loss
  - ‣ Lactated Ringer will cause less acidosis (and hyperkalemia) than normal saline
- Avoid further insults:
  - ‣ Minimize amount of (low osmolar) radiocontrast
  - ‣ Avoid hypotension: maintain BP near baseline (not "normal") BP
- With marginal renal function/anticipated large blood loss and possibility for hyperkalemia:
  - ‣ Frequent monitoring of potassium and pH
  - ‣ Prepare insulin/glucose
  - ‣ Maintain adequate calcium levels
  - ‣ Consider intraoperative continuous venovenous hemodialysis (CVVHD)

ANESTHESIA

Causes of Renal Injury		
Preoperative	Intraoperative	Postoperative
Chronic renal insufficiency		
Concomitant liver disease		
Preoperative radiocontrast		
Preoperative nephrotoxic drugs		
Hypovolemia: NPO		
	Cardiopulmonary bypass	
	Aortic cross-clamp	
	Hypotension, hypovolemia	
	Vasopressors	
	Nephrotoxic drugs: aminoglycosides, NSAIDs	
		Nephrotoxic drugs Calcineurin inhibitors: Tacrolimus (FK-506) or cyclosporin

A. Postoperative

Diagnostic criteria for acute kidney injury (Figure 28-4).

An abrupt (within 48 hours) reduction in kidney function currently defined as an absolute increase in serum creatinine of more than or equal to 0.3 mg/dL ($\geq$26.4 μmol/L), a percentage increase in serum creatinine of more than or equal to 50% (1.5-fold from baseline), or a reduction in urine output (documented oliguria of less than 0.5 mL/kg/h for more than 6 hours).

FIGURE 28-4. Acute Kidney Injury Network (AKIN) criteria

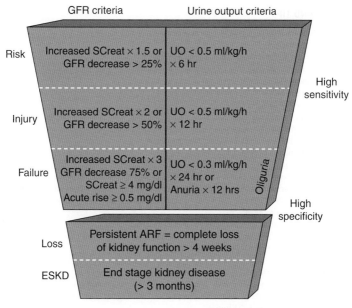

The Risk, Injury, Failure, Loss, and End-Stage Kidney Disease (RIFLE) criteria. The staging system proposed is a highly sensitive interim staging system and is based on recent data indicating that a small change in serum creatinine influences outcome. Only one criterion (creatinine or urine output) has to be fulfilled to qualify for a stage. Given wide variation in indications and timing of initiation of renal replacement therapy (RRT), individuals who receive RRT are considered to have met the criteria for stage 3 (Failure) irrespective of the stage they are in at the time of RRT. GFR, glomerular filtration rate; ARF, acute renal failure. Reproduced from Critical Care 2004, 8:R204. © 2004 Bellomo et al. This article is online at: http://ccforum.com/content/8/4/R204.

Urine Electrolytes and Low Urine Output		
	Acute tubular necrosis (ATN)	Prerenal azotemia
Urine osmolarity (mOsm/L)	250–300	>400
Urine/plasma osmolality ratio	1:1	>1.4:1
Urine/plasma creatinine ratio	<20:1	>50:1
Urine sodium (mEq/L)	>80	<20
Fractional excretion of sodium (FeNa) (%)	>3	<1

PEARLS AND TIPS

Strategies to prevent or ameliorate acute kidney injury:
- *Rule out postrenal causes*:
  ‣ Urinary catheter obstruction/misplacement:
    ▪ Bladder ultrasound
  ‣ Hydronephrosis caused by renal calculi or tumor:
    ▪ Renal ultrasound
- *Prevent further insults*:
  ‣ Maintain euvolemia
  ‣ Avoid nephrotoxic drugs
  ‣ Avoid unnecessary exams using radiocontrast
  ‣ Maintain blood pressure
- *Identify patients at risk*:
  ‣ Estimate preoperative GFR and flag patients with eGFR<60 mL/min
  ‣ Small changes of serum creatinine from normal may reflect large changes of GFR
- *Interventions: consider the following interventions; however, none, except hydration, has been proven to be effective*:
  ‣ Hydration, that is, 0.5 mL/kg/h for 24 hours prior to insult
  ‣ Loop diuretics/furosemide: 1–5 mg/h by intravenous infusion or a single intravenous bolus dose of 20–80 mg:
    ▪ No advantage on renal function but can cause toxicity. May convert oliguric into nonoliguric ARF with no proven effect on outcome
  ‣ Mannitol: likely not effective; 25 g IV over 60 minutes before insult
  ‣ Acetylcysteine: likely not effective; 100–150 mg/kg IV load followed by 10–20 mg/kg/h for 4–24 hours
  ‣ Sodium bicarbonate: likely effective to prevent radiocontrast injury: 154 mEq/L sodium bicarbonate in D5 water: 3 mL/kg/h for 1 hour prior to radiocontrast followed by 1 mL/kg/h during and 6 hours after the procedure
  ‣ Dopamine: not effective, plasma levels and heart rate response variable

REFERENCES

For references, please visit **www.TheAnesthesiaGuide.com**.

CHAPTER 29
Parkinson Disease

Mark S. Tinklepaugh, MD

BASICS

- Common neurodegenerative disease of the CNS characterized by loss of dopaminergic input in the basal ganglia
- *Cause*:
  ‣ Generally considered idiopathic with some evidence of genetic and environmental components
  ‣ Decreased incidence with exposure to cigarette smoking and increased with exposure to pesticides
- *Prevalence and incidence*:
  ‣ Affects 1 million people in the United States with approximately 50,000 new cases reported annually
  ‣ Average age of onset is 60
- *Main signs*:
  ‣ Resting tremor
  ‣ Rigidity
  ‣ Bradykinesia
  ‣ Festinating gait
  ‣ Postural instability
- *Other signs*:
  ‣ Autonomic dysfunction (orthostatic hypotension, GERD, sialorrhea, cramps)
  ‣ Pharyngolaryngeal involvement with aspiration (most common cause of death)
  ‣ Respiratory involvement (chest rigidity, mixed obstructive–restrictive syndrome, decreased response to hypoxemia)
  ‣ Dementia
  ‣ Depression
  ‣ Oculogyric crises
- *Treatment*:
  ‣ *Goal of treatment*: decrease cholinergic activity through anticholinergics or dopamine agonists
  ‣ *Levodopa*:
    ▪ Levodopa absorbed in proximal small bowel
    ▪ Converted to dopamine by DOPA decarboxylase
    ▪ Five to 10% levodopa crosses blood–brain barrier; remainder converted to dopamine peripherally
    ▪ Side effects are N/V, vasoconstriction, hypovolemia, hypotension, decreased myocardial NE stores
    ▪ Levodopa supplementation leads to decreased endogenous production of dopamine
    ▪ Peripheral decarboxylase inhibitor (carbidopa) in combination with levodopa (Sinemet®) decreases peripheral levodopa metabolism which decreases dopamine side effects
    ▪ Entacapone, a COMT inhibitor, used alone (Comtan®) or in combination with carbidopa and levodopa (Stalevo®) to decrease peripheral metabolism of levodopa
    ▪ Amantadine (Symadine®) releases DOPA in the striatum

- *Dopamine agonists*:
  - Bind to postsynaptic receptors in the brain
  - Preferred in younger patients since they delay motor complications
  - Side effects include somnolence, insomnia, nausea, hallucinations, and cardiac valvular fibrosis with pergolide (Permax®) and cabergoline (Dostinex®, Cabaser®)
  - Other dopamine agonists include bromocriptine (Parlodel®), pramipexole (Mirapex®), and ropinirole (Requip®)
  - Apomorphine (Apokyn®), another agonist, is the only injectable medication (SQ only, not IV)
- *MAO-B inhibitors*:
  - Increase peripheral bioavailability of levodopa. Selegiline (Eldepryl®, Emsam®, Zelapar®) and rasagiline (Azilect®) commonly used
- *Deep brain stimulation (DBS)*:
  - Used when drug therapy inadequate
  - Pacemaker implanted in brain to stimulate the subthalamic nucleus in the basal ganglia (see chapter 102, Awake craniotomy)

PREOPERATIVE

- Neuro evaluation preoperatively can be useful to establish baseline cognitive ability and to assist in perioperative management
- Parkinson disease medications and glycopyrrolate (Robinul®) (to decrease sialorrhea and vagal tone) should be administered preoperatively
- Levodopa half-life short (1–3 hours) and no IV form
- May consider levodopa via OGT for lengthy non-GI surgery
- Aspiration and laryngospasm are a significant concern secondary to GERD, sialorrhea, and dysfunction of upper airway musculature
- Phenothiazines, droperidol, and metoclopramide (Reglan®) are contraindicated as antidopaminergic effect exacerbates extrapyramidal symptoms

INTRAOPERATIVE

- Regional versus general:
  - Regional anesthesia may be preferred
  - Hypotension secondary to autonomic dysfunction and vasodilatory effect of dopamine agonists is a major concern
  - Regional allows decreased perioperative opioids in patients with increased likelihood (8-fold) of postoperative hallucinations and confusion
- General anesthesia:
  - Intubation may be difficult due to skeletal muscle rigidity
  - In patients receiving long-term levodopa therapy, induction may result in marked hypotension or HTN. Use direct-acting agent to treat hypotension (i.e., phenylephrine)
  - Increased airway resistance and increased chest wall rigidity may lead to clinically significant mixed obstructive/restrictive pattern
  - Induction: alfentanil and fentanyl associated with acute dystonic reactions. Sufentanil might be the safest opioid (limited evidence)
  - Propofol preferred for induction. Ketamine best avoided due to increased SNS response
  - Succinylcholine (although risk of hyperkalemia) and nondepolarizing muscle relaxants acceptable. Do not reverse NMB!
  - High-dose morphine can lead to akinesia
  - Combination of meperidine and selegiline has been associated with agitation, muscle rigidity, and hyperpyrexia
  - Avoid ephedrine in patients receiving MAO-I
  - Desflurane, sevoflurane, and isoflurane acceptable for maintenance. Monitor for excessive vasodilation. Possible dysrhythmias with association with levodopa

- ► DBS:
  - Typically off medications over 12 hours preoperatively
  - Either awake craniotomy (local for stereotaxic frame + MAC) or GA
  - Long procedure (up to 12 hours): very careful positioning

POSTOPERATIVE

- Parkinson medications should be resumed as soon as feasible. If stopped for >24 hours, resume at one third or one half of preoperative dose and increase
- Single or sequentially titrated SQ doses of apomorphine (Apokyn®) may assist in episodes of acute muscle rigidity or if unable to administer oral medications, even through gastric tube:
  - ► Doses range from 0.2 mL (10 mg/mL) SQ to maximum recommended dose of 0.6 mL (6 mg)
  - ► Contraindicated with HT5 antagonists such as ondansetron (Zofran®), dolasetron (Anzemet®), granisetron (Kytril®) secondary to profound hypotension and loss of consciousness
  - ► Caution urged with use of antihypertensives, vasodilators, and dopamine antagonists such as neuroleptics and metoclopramide (Reglan®)
- Patients may be more confused and disoriented up to 24 hours after surgery
- Airway obstruction, laryngospasm, and aspiration remain a concern
- Treat PONV with dexamethasone and HT5 inhibitors only
- Monitor renal function (levodopa inhibits the renin–angiotensin–aldosterone system)
- Do not give vitamin B_6 as it can interfere with levodopa metabolism

PEARLS AND TIPS

- Preoperative neurology evaluation may be helpful for perioperative care
- Preoperative meds should be given if feasible
- Regional may be preferred to GA to avoid airway and respiratory difficulties and to minimize potential postoperative confusion
- Hypotension is a concern with regional anesthesia secondary to autonomic dysfunction
- If GA selected, difficult airway, aspiration, and laryngospasm should be considered. Neurological consultation prudent if Apokyn® required postoperatively

REFERENCES

For references, please visit **www.TheAnesthesiaGuide.com**.

CHAPTER 30
Multiple Sclerosis

Arthur Atchabahian, MD

PHYSIOPATHOLOGY

- Autoimmune disease characterized by antibody-mediated demyelination in central nervous system, which leads to impaired nerve conduction. Peripheral nerves are not involved
- Combination of genetic and environmental factors
- 2F/1M
- Age of onset usually 20–40, but can be seen at any age
- Signs and symptoms related to site of CNS affected by demyelination
- Broad spectrum—relapses and remissions, or chronic and progressive
- Variety of triggers, such as stress and heat (fever)
- Many signs and symptoms are possible, but more commonly seen are visual symptoms from optic nerve involvement, skeletal muscle/spasms from spinal cord involvement, bowel/bladder dysfunction, lack of coordination, paresthesias, seizures, depression, autonomic disturbances in advanced disease. Lower extremities more frequently involved than upper extremities
- Diagnosis usually based on cerebrospinal fluid antibodies or magnetic resonance imaging
- MS patients can be treated with a wide variety of medications, some targeting the disease and some targeting specific symptoms:
  - ‣ Treatment with corticosteroids, interferons (Avonex, Betaseron, Rebif), glatiramer (Copaxone), azathioprine (Imuran), mitoxantrone (Novantrone; cardiotoxic), natalizumab (Tysabri), cyclophosphamide (Cytoxan), and methotrexate
  - ‣ Symptomatic treatment with baclofen (Lioresal), tizanidine (Zanaflex) for muscle spasms, cholinergic medications for urinary symptoms, or antidepressants for mood disturbances

PREOPERATIVE

- Thorough history with careful attention to history of relapses, remissions, triggers, typical complaints, and symptoms during exacerbations
- Complete list of medications should be reviewed prior to induction to delineate any potential interactions with anesthetic medications
- Elicit steroid use and potential for adrenal suppression
- Preoperative neurologic exam with focus on visual symptoms as well as skeletal muscle weakness should be performed to establish a baseline
- Elective surgery should not be performed during periods of relapse

ANESTHESIA

- Exacerbations during the perioperative period are possible due to surgical stress, regardless of anesthetic technique or medications
- Succinylcholine is best avoided due to possibility of increased potassium release
- Nondepolarizing NMB: both increased sensitivity and resistance have been described; judicious use with peripheral nerve stimulator is recommended
- Stress-dose steroids if indicated
- Increased temperature can precipitate symptoms, monitor body temperature; avoid hyperthermia
- Spinal anesthesia may increase risk of postoperative exacerbations, maybe because the demyelination makes the CNS more sensitive to LA neurotoxicity, but epidural and peripheral nerve block techniques appear safe

- No evidence that general anesthesia drugs, either injected or inhaled, exacerbate MS
- Autonomic dysfunction should be taken into consideration when monitoring hemodynamics and during fluid management

POSTOPERATIVE

- Reassess neurologic status
- Look for evidence of relapses, and assess for presence of any potential triggers that may be present in the postoperative environment
- Exercise vigilance with respect to postoperative temperature control
- Communication with surgeon, neurologist, and primary care physician is essential
- Baclofen withdrawal can occur, especially if long-standing therapy, with neuropsychiatric symptoms (hallucinations, anxiety, tremor), and possibly seizures, or even muscle rigidity and hyperthermia resembling neuroleptic malignant syndrome

PEARLS AND TIPS

- Perform both a thorough history of disease progression and neurologic exam prior to surgery
- Spinal anesthesia may increase risk of postoperative exacerbations, but no evidence that general anesthesia, epidural, or PNB exacerbates MS
- *Avoid hyperthermia*
- Platelet aggregation is increased in MH
- Increased risk of urinary retention
- Special considerations in parturients:
  - ‣ Risk of relapses decreases in third trimester, but increases postpartum
  - ‣ Judicious use of regional anesthesia for labor/cesarean section: discuss risks/benefits with patient

REFERENCE

For references, please visit **www.TheAnesthesiaGuide.com**.

CHAPTER 31
Myasthenia Gravis

Arthur Atchabahian, MD

OVERVIEW

- Autoimmune disease where antibodies are produced to the (postsynaptic) acetylcholine (ACh) receptor of neuromuscular junction (NMJ), possibly originating in thymus
- Ten percent of patients have congenital myasthenia with abnormal ACh receptors; cholinesterase inhibitors will be ineffective in these patients
- Results in functionally decreased (70–80%) number of postsynaptic receptors
- Incidence of about 1:10,000
- Before age of 40 years, 2F/1M, 40% thymus enlargement
- After age of 40 years, 1F/1M, 20% thymoma
- Most commonly affects ocular muscles, but can affect any skeletal muscle, including muscles of respiration
- Characterized by skeletal muscle weakness *that improves with rest*

Differences between Eaton–Lambert Syndrome and Myasthenia Gravis		
Syndrome	Myasthenia gravis	Eaton–Lambert syndrome
Association with cancer	Not associated with cancer	Usually small cell lung cancer (SCLC), but also non-SCLC, lymphosarcoma, malignant thymoma, or carcinoma of the breast, stomach, colon, prostate, bladder, kidney, or gallbladder Clinical manifestations often precede cancer diagnosis by 2–4 years
Pathophysiology	Autoimmune attack directed against the postsynaptic acetylcholine receptor, results in impaired ACh effect at the NMJ	Autoimmune attack directed against the voltage-gated calcium channels (VGCCs) on the presynaptic motor nerve terminal results in impaired ACh release Parasympathetic, sympathetic, and enteric neurons are all affected
Clinical diagnosis	Increasing weakness with repeated effort Improvement with rest	Increasing strength with repeated effort Reappearance of tendon reflexes after a period of muscle contraction by the patient
Epidemiology	Relatively common Bimodal distribution (see above)	Rare (~400 cases in the United States at any given time) Typically in >60 years old, but has been reported in children
Autonomic findings	None	Dysautonomia: dryness of the mouth, impotence, difficulty in starting the urinary stream, and constipation
Treatment (besides supportive)	See below	• Treatment of underlying neoplasm • Cholinesterase inhibitors • 3,4-Diaminopyridine • Immunosuppression with corticosteroids, IVIg, guanidine, aminopyridines, and azathioprine

- Clinical course often marked by periods of exacerbations and remissions
- Treatment:
  ‣ Cholinesterase inhibitors to increase amount of ACh at NMJ
  ‣ Corticosteroids
  ‣ Immunosuppression (mycophenolate mofetil, azathioprine, cyclosporine, tacrolimus, and occasionally cyclophosphamide)
  ‣ Plasmapheresis to remove antibodies, IVIg
  ‣ Thymectomy

Main Cholinesterase Inhibitors Used to Treat MG			
Medication	Onset/duration	Typical dosage	Side effects
Pyridostigmine (Mestinon)	PO: 15–30 min/3–4 h	PO: 60 mg qid	Muscarinic side effects (diarrhea, abdominal cramps, salivation, nausea), treated with atropine/ diphenoxylate or loperamide
Neostigmine (Prostigmin)	PO: 1 h/90 min IM: 30 min/1 h IV: immediate/20 min	PO: 15 mg IM: 1.5 mg IV: 0.5 mg	Same
Ambenonium (Mytelase)	PO: 20–30 min/3–8 h	PO: 5–25 mg qid	Same

Severity: Osserman–Genkins Classification	
Stage I	Ocular symptoms only (diplopia, ptosis)
Stage IIA	Mild generalized myasthenia with slow progression; no bulbar involvement
Stage IIB	Moderately severe generalized myasthenia: severe skeletal and bulbar involvement but no crises; drug response less than satisfactory
Stage III	Moderate generalized weakness
Stage IV	Late severe myasthenia; severe generalized weakness, respiratory dysfunction, or both

- Pregnancy:
  ‣ Worsening in first 4 months, at delivery, and postpartum (up to 3 weeks)
  ‣ Optimize therapy; immunosuppressants are contraindicated
  ‣ Epidural for delivery or c/s; avoid high level; consider ropivacaine (less motor block)
  ‣ Breastfeeding OK if well controlled
  ‣ Neonatal myasthenia (antibodies cross placenta) in 20–30%: weak cry, difficulty feeding, occasional respiratory distress; treat with cholinesterase inhibitors, plasmapheresis

PREOPERATIVE

- Possible associated autoimmune diseases (myocarditis, thyroiditis) should be ruled out
- Elective surgery should be deferred in periods of relapse and ideally performed in periods of remission—infection, surgery, pregnancy can all trigger exacerbations

- Laryngeal/pharyngeal involvement predisposes to inability to clear secretions and pulmonary aspiration
- Muscular groups affected, strength, and course of exacerbations/remissions should be assessed by thorough history and physical
- Many patients require postoperative ventilation, depending on:
  ‣ Preoperative vital capacity less than 15 mL/kg (PFTs may be necessary for risk stratification)
  ‣ Disease duration (greater than 6 years)
  ‣ Pyridostigmine dose greater than 750 mg per day
  ‣ Coexisting COPD
- Continuation of cholinesterase inhibitors during perioperative period is controversial, since these drugs can interfere with others used during the perioperative period (such as succinylcholine, nondepolarizing muscle relaxants, ester local anesthetics, or reversal agents); typically stop 6–12 hours before surgery if no respiratory involvement, but continue throughout if severe myasthenia. Coordinate with neurologist

INTRAOPERATIVE

- Use regional anesthesia if possible; avoid ester local anesthetics (prolonged half-life as metabolized by cholinesterase). Thymectomy under GA + high thoracic epidural has been described
- Sensitive to nondepolarizing muscle relaxants (use one tenth of the usual dose, NMB monitoring; *NB*: monitoring orbicularis oculi will overestimate NMB if ocular involvement)
- Resistant to depolarizing muscle relaxants, but may see longer duration of action of succinylcholine if patient taking cholinesterase inhibitors
- Decision to use paralytics, either depolarizing or nondepolarizing, should be made on a case-by-case basis
- Sometimes an induction agent combined with potent inhalation agent can facilitate endotracheal intubation; however, some patients may not be able to tolerate the hemodynamic effects of these agents
- Reduced doses of nondepolarizing muscle relaxants may be necessary to facilitate endotracheal intubation, or to optimize surgical conditions—in these cases peripheral nerve stimulation should be used

Medications to Avoid in Patients with MG	
Do not use	Use with caution
• Beta-blockers (even eye drops)	• Nondepolarizing NMB
• Chloroquine, quinine, quinidine, procainamide	• Benzodiazepines
• IV magnesium	• Phenothiazines, lithium, carbamazepine
• Phenytoin	• PO cycline antibiotics
• Dantrolene (except if MH)	• PO magnesium
• Antibiotics: aminoglycosides, quinolones, macrolides, colimycine, IV cycline antibiotics	• Local anesthetics in large amounts
• Botulinum toxin	• Penicillamine (unlikely to be used by anesthesiologist)

POSTOPERATIVE

- Extubation criteria: comparison of strength and respiratory parameters to preoperative values, such as PFTs and ABGs if available; VC >25 mL/kg, NIF >−30 cm H_2O; most stage III and IV patients will need postoperative ventilatory support; use low Vt (5 mL/kg), aggressive PT, or even fiber-optic bronchial toilet

- Other factors that can interfere with neuromuscular transmission, and therefore myasthenia gravis, include electrolyte levels, inhaled anesthetics, antibiotics, respiratory acidosis, local anesthetics
- Residual weakness may be related to residual neuromuscular block, or other factors
- There have been anecdotal reports of reversal of NMB in patients with MG using sugammadex (not available in the United States)
- Coordinate with neurologist for resumption of anticholinesterase treatment; steroids, plasmapheresis, and/or IV globulin can be necessary if unable to extubate
- When evaluating the postoperative myasthenia gravis patient suffering from weakness, cholinergic crisis, residual NMB, and myasthenic crisis need to be in the differential

Differentiating Cholinergic from Myasthenic Crisis		
Weakness in MG	Cholinergic crisis	Myasthenic crisis/residual NMB
Cause	Excess ACh at nicotinic and muscarinic receptors, usually from excess anticholinesterase administration	Lack of ACh receptors, or competitive antagonism of ACh
Clinical manifestations	Skeletal muscle weakness, miosis, increased secretions, bradycardia, airway constriction, vomiting/diarrhea (parasympathetic-mediated GI hyperreactivity)	Skeletal muscle weakness Ineffective cough, aspiration, dyspnea
Diagnosis/treatment	No improvement or even worsening with edrophonium 3–4 mg IV Hold cholinesterase inhibitors	Edrophonium improves symptoms

REFERENCES

For references, please visit **www.TheAnesthesiaGuide.com**.

CHAPTER 32
Preexisting Spinal Cord Injury

Candra Rowell Bass, MD and Priya A. Kumar, MD

BASICS

- Spinal cord injury (SCI) is common (~10,000–11,000 cases per year), occurring usually after trauma
- Degree of dysfunction is directly related to level of injury, especially severe if above T6
- Most common site of injury is lower cervical spine or upper lumbar region:
  ▸ Midthoracic injury less common due to rotational stabilization provided by the rib cage and intercostal muscles
- Pathophysiology:
  ▸ Upregulation of acetylcholine receptors from immobilization causes resistance to nondepolarizing neuromuscular blockers and increased potassium release with depolarizing neuromuscular blockers (e.g., succinylcholine)
  ▸ Sympathetic hyperreflexia:
    ▪ Nociceptive afferent circuits rebranch below the lesion and anastomose with sympathetic efferents, especially between T5 and L2
    ▪ Hyperreflexia mostly if lesion above T6, but possible even around T12
    ▪ Higher risk with:
      ◆ Urological surgery
      ◆ Complete cord section
      ◆ Chronic pain
      ◆ Maximal 1–6 months after injury, but can persist indefinitely
    ▪ Small stimuli can evoke exaggerated, unopposed sympathetic response:
      ◆ Extreme HTN with reflex bradycardia and other dysrhythmias
      ◆ Headache, anxiety
      ◆ Sweating
      ◆ Flushing or pallor
      ◆ Piloerection
    ▪ Complications:
      ◆ Myocardial ischemia
      ◆ Cardiac arrest
      ◆ Pulmonary edema
      ◆ Hemorrhagic CVA
  ▸ Reduced lower limb blood flow, but increased arterial and venous pooling leads to increased risk of thromboembolic disease
  ▸ Spasticity: similar mechanism as hyperreflexia
- Natural history of injury:
  ▸ Acute (<3 weeks from injury):
    ▪ Spinal shock: hypotension and bradycardia
    ▪ Loss of thoracic sympathetic outflow, with vasodilatation and pooling of blood
    ▪ Relative predominance of vagal stimulation to the heart
    ▪ Retention of urine/feces leading to diaphragm elevation, which may impair respiration
    ▪ Hyperesthesia above the lesion
    ▪ Reflexes and flaccid paralysis below the lesion
  ▸ Intermediate (3 days to 6 months):
    ▪ Hyperkalemic response to depolarizing NMB
  ▸ Chronic (after 6 months):
    ▪ Return of muscle tone
    ▪ Positive Babinski sign
    ▪ Hyperreflexia syndrome

PREOPERATIVE CONSIDERATIONS

System	Assessment	Test/intervention
Airway	• Cervical cord injury	• Early intubation with in-line stabilization
Pulmonary	• Respiratory muscle involvement • Diaphragm involved at C5 or above SCI • Atelectasis/pneumonia • Impaired handling of secretions	• Pulmonary function tests (FEV1/FVC) • ABG • Chest x-ray
Cardiac	• Myocardial conduction abnormalities • Hypotension (orthostatic) • Baseline BP may run lower than normal	• Electrocardiogram • Invasive BP monitoring
Renal	• Status of renal function • Urinary tract infections • Intravascular volume status • Bladder function	• BUN, Cr
Electrolytes/GI	• Electrolyte status • Bowel function • Full stomach from GI atony (mostly if cervical lesion)	• Na$^+$, K$^+$ • RSI
Neurological	• Mental status • Deficits (level of SCI) • Autonomic hyperreflexia	• Review imaging
Musculoskeletal	• Bone fractures • Decubitus ulcers	• Physical examination

NB:
- Creatinine does not correlate with renal function
- Intramuscular injections may have delayed absorption

INTRAOPERATIVE CONSIDERATIONS

- Gentle induction for GA (potential for severe hypotension) or neuraxial/regional anesthesia where indicated (less hemodynamic lability, but difficult to assess level; monitor carefully as diagnosis of high/total spinal might be delayed)
- Avoid succinylcholine from 24 hours after injury due to risk of hyperkalemia. Response typically seen if drug is given from 1 week to 6 months after the injury but may be seen before or after that period:
  ‣ If laryngospasm occurs, the benefits of giving a small dose of succinylcholine (20 mg) may outweigh the risk
- Careful padding of pressure points/decubitus ulcers
- Consider invasive BP monitoring because of potential for hemodynamic lability
- Watch for sympathetic excess or deficiency:
  ‣ Treat with vasoconstrictors (e.g., phenylephrine) or vasodilators (e.g., NTG, nitroprusside), beta-agonists (e.g., isoproterenol), or beta-blockers (e.g., esmolol; avoid long-acting beta-blockers because of risk of unopposed alpha constriction)
- Monitor temperature closely. Hypothermia may result from cutaneous vasodilation and inability to shiver. Hyperthermia may result from impaired sweating
- Ensure that the patient is receiving thromboembolic prophylaxis

POSTOPERATIVE CONSIDERATIONS

- Patients with high-level SCI may be difficult to extubate
- Aggressive pulmonary toilet to prevent atelectasis and pneumonia
- Monitor for AH in the PACU (e.g., stimulation from Foley placement)
- AH symptoms can result from distended bladder/bowel or surgical pain

REFERENCES

For references, please visit www.TheAnesthesiaGuide.com.

CHAPTER 33
Porphyria

Mark S. Tinklepaugh, MD

BASICS

- Pathophysiology:
  ‣ Autosomal dominant defect in heme synthesis; 90% of gene carriers are asymptomatic; 80% of symptomatic patients are women from puberty to menopause
  ‣ Heme is a porphyrin critical in the formation of hemoglobin and cytochrome P450 complex (drug metabolism)
  ‣ Aminolevulinic acid (ALA) synthase is the enzyme involved in the rate-limiting step of heme formation:

  $$\text{Glycine + succinyl CoA} \rightarrow \text{ALA}$$

  ‣ ALA synthase is induced by feedback inhibition when heme requirements increase
  ‣ Partial enzyme defect in heme pathway leads to buildup of ALA and other intermediaries leading to neurotoxicity, especially when need for heme (catabolism increased by menstrual hormones) or need for cytochrome P450 enzymes by inducing drugs
  ‣ Classified as:
    ▪ Erythropoietic porphyrias:
      ◆ Günther disease and protoporphyria
      ◆ Patients are children; no acute crises
    ▪ Hepatic porphyrias:
      ◆ Cutaneous porphyria
      ◆ Acute porphyrias with related symptomatology (most often problematic with anesthesia):
        ○ Acute intermittent porphyria (AIP), most common form
        ○ Variegate porphyria (VP), protoporphyrinogen oxidase deficiency
        ○ Hereditary coproporphyria (HC), coproporphyrinogen oxidase deficiency
        ○ Plumboporphyria (PP), ALA dehydrase deficiency
- Precipitating factors:
  ‣ *Clinical conditions*:
    ▪ Dehydration, fasting, infection, emotional stress, hormonal changes (menstruation/pregnancy), alcohol
  ‣ *Enzyme-inducing drugs*:
    ▪ Barbiturates, etomidate (Amidate®), ethanol, hydantoin anticonvulsants, phenytoin (Dilantin®), hormonal steroids (progesterone, estrogen)

TABLE 33-1	Signs and Symptoms of Acute Porphyria	
Abdominal pain Constipation, all the way through pseudoobstruction		95%
Dark urine From reddish to black, within 10–30 min		70%
N/V, autonomic dysfunction (tachycardia, HTN)		55–80%
Peripheral neuropathy, hemiplegia, quadriplegia, respiratory paralysis Transfer to ICU		60%
CNS–cranial nerves, mental status changes		30–55%
Electrolyte abnormalities (hyponatremia, hypokalemia, hyperchloremia)		30–50%
Seizures		20%
Cutaneous signs (in HC and VP) Vesicles or bullae on face and hands (photosensitization) + hyperpigmentation/ hypopigmentation		

- Lab diagnosis:
  - ▸ Urgently: urinary porphyrin precursors (delta-ALA and porphobilinogen)
  - ▸ Porphyrins in urine and stool (uroporphyrin, coproporphyrin, protoporphyrin)
  - ▸ Specialized lab: enzyme activities, gene mutation
  - ▸ Chem 7: Hyponatremia due to SIADH, more common if neuro involvement
- Treatment of crisis:
  - ▸ Analgesia (morphine), anxiolysis (benzodiazepine, phenothiazine)
  - ▸ D10% at 125 mL/h
  - ▸ Heme arginate 3–4 mg/kg per day IVSS over 30–40 minutes × 4 days; very effective on digestive symptoms; will prevent neurological symptoms, but not effective if already present. Possible thrombophlebitis
  - ▸ Other symptomatic treatment as needed (e.g., beta-blockers for tachycardia)

PREOPERATIVE

- Identify patients by personal and familial history
- Consider neurological evaluation to assess CNS/PNS and mental status
- Premedicate to alleviate stress; midazolam acceptable
- Avoid enzyme-inducing drugs
- Treat preexisting infection and assess volume and electrolytes

INTRAOPERATIVE

- *Regional anesthesia* not contraindicated; must consider autonomic instability, hypovolemia, and theoretical risk of exacerbation of peripheral neuropathies
- Bupivacaine acceptable for both spinal and epidural anesthesia
- *General anesthesia*: use safe drugs (see Table 33-2)

TABLE 33-2	Pharmacologic Considerations in Patients with Porphyria	
Drug type	Safe drugs	Drugs to avoid
Induction agent	Propofol	Barbiturates Etomidate
Inhalation agent	Nitrous oxide Sevoflurane Desflurane Isoflurane	Enflurane
Analgesic	Fentanyl Morphine Sufentanil Acetaminophen	
Neuromuscular blocking agents	Succinylcholine Pancuronium Vecuronium, rocuronium Cisatracurium, atracurium	
Reversal agents	Atropine Glycopyrrolate Neostigmine	
Local anesthetics	Bupivacaine Lidocaine	
Sedatives and antiemetics	Droperidol Phenothiazines Midazolam Ondansetron	Diazepam Ketamine
Cardiovascular	Propranolol Atenolol Epinephrine Procainamide	Hydralazine Verapamil Nifedipine Diltiazem

POSTOPERATIVE

- Study family further to identify porphyria patients
- Card to be carried by patient
- Education: avoid triggering events (dehydration, diet, alcohol, tobacco, stress, fatigue, infection, drugs [barbiturates, acetaminophen, sulfa drugs, BCP])

PEARLS AND TIPS

- Acute porphyria attacks rare, but 10% fatal due to underlying infection or respiratory failure
- Use safe drugs and avoid triggering agents (see Table 33-2)
- Tachycardia worsens as crisis progresses
- Develop short list of safe medications acceptable for GA
- *Do not use* barbiturates to treat seizures
- Regional anesthesia: discuss risk of exacerbating neuropathy; avoid in acute crises
- *AIP*—most severe form with HTN, renal dysfunction; life threatening
- *Variegate porphyria* (VP)—photosensitive skin lesions and neurotoxicity prominent; pad skin lesions
- *HC*—symptoms similar to VP, less severe
- *PP*—rare, presents at young age, little known regarding anesthesia

REFERENCES

For references, please visit **www.TheAnesthesiaGuide.com**.

CHAPTER 34
Geriatric Physiology

Janine L. Thekkekandam, MD and Harendra Arora, MD

People over 65 years of age are 3.5 times more likely to have surgery. Aging results in a progressive decline in the functional reserve of all organs; the rate at which function diminishes is highly variable between individuals.

PATHOPHYSIOLOGY OF AGING BY SYSTEM

Cardiovascular
- Decreased arterial elasticity:
  - Increased afterload
  - Left ventricular hypertrophy
  - Increased systolic blood pressure, mean arterial pressure, and pulse pressure
- Autonomic imbalance:
  - Increased vagal tone
  - Decreased sensitivity of adrenergic receptors
  - Decreased baroreceptor reflex
- Fibrosis of the conducting system and loss of sinoatrial node cells
- Sclerosis/calcification of valves
- High incidence of diastolic dysfunction

Respiratory
- Decreased lung tissue elasticity (due to reorganization of collagen and elastin):
  - Early collapse of small airways and overdistension of alveoli (V/Q mismatch)
  - Increased residual volume (total lung capacity unchanged)
  - Increased closing capacity
  - Decreased arterial oxygen tension
  - Loss of alveolar surface area (increased anatomic and physiologic dead space)
- Increased V/Q mismatch
- Increased chest wall rigidity leading to increased work of breathing
- Blunted response to hypercapnia, hypoxia, and mechanical stress
- Decreased protective reflexes (coughing and swallowing) increasing the risk for aspiration
- Increased pulmonary vascular resistance and pulmonary arterial pressure
- Blunted hypoxic pulmonary vasoconstrictive response

Renal
- Decreased renal mass:
  - Mostly renal cortex secondary to decreased functioning glomeruli
  - Progressive decline in creatinine clearance
  - Increased risk of perioperative acute renal failure
- Decreased renal blood flow:
  - Decreases 10% every decade of aging
  - Serum creatinine unchanged due to loss of muscle mass
- Decreased tubular function:
  - Altered sodium balance, urine concentrating ability, and drug excretion
  - Increased risk for dehydration and electrolyte abnormalities
- Decreased renin–aldosterone system resulting in impaired potassium excretion

Neurologic
- Decreased brain mass, particularly the cerebral cortex (frontal lobes)
- Cerebral blood flow decreases 10–20%, although autoregulation stays intact

(continued)

- Decreased neurotransmitter synthesis: GABA, serotonin, dopamine, norepinephrine, and acetylcholine system
- Variable degrees of cognitive function decline, especially short-term memory
- Decreased general anesthesia (MAC) and local anesthetic requirements

Gastrointestinal
- Decreased liver function secondary to reduced liver mass and hepatic blood flow:
  ‣ Reduced biotransformation
  ‣ Decreased albumin production
  ‣ Decreased plasma cholinesterase
- Delayed gastric emptying
- Increased gastric pH

Musculoskeletal
- Reduced muscle mass; atrophic skin; frail veins
- Increased body fat; total body water decreases
- Arthritis can affect various joints that can complicate positioning
- Degenerative changes of the cervical spine; intubation potentially more difficult

Endocrine/metabolic
- Atrophy of endocrine glands leading to impaired hormone function:
  ‣ Insulin, thyroxine, growth hormone, testosterone
- Blunted neuroendocrine stress response
- Decreased heat production and alteration in hypothalamic temperature-regulating center increases risk of hypothermia

Age-related pharmacologic effects
- Increased body fat and decreased total body water:
  ‣ Higher plasma concentration of water-soluble drugs
  ‣ Lower plasma concentration of fat-soluble drugs
- Reduced clearance secondary to decreased hepatic and renal function
- Altered protein binding:
  ‣ Reduced albumin affects binding of acidic drugs (opioids, barbiturates, benzodiazepines)
  ‣ Increased α_1-acid glycoprotein affects binding of basic drugs (local anesthetics)
- Pharmacodynamic changes:
  ‣ Drug effects may be intensified due to decreased number of available receptors
  ‣ Reduced anesthetic requirement (or MAC)

PREOPERATIVE EVALUATION

- Perform a thorough history and physical examination and determine appropriate preoperative testing (based on clinical correlate)
- Assess optimization of preexisting conditions such as CAD, hypertension, or diabetes
- Determine if patient has a living will, power of attorney, or advanced directive
- Review medication history as polypharmacy is common among the elderly, increasing the risk of medication interaction

INTRAOPERATIVE

- Monitoring based on procedure type and underlying organ involvement
- Careful titration of anesthetic agents with cardiac- and respiratory-depressant effects
- Careful attention toward fluid management to avoid fluid overload; at the same time maintain adequate hydration/tissue perfusion
- Age-related respiratory effects as well as coexisting pulmonary disease may necessitate vigorous preoxygenation
- Avoid hypothermia

- Regional anesthesia is a reasonable choice:
  - Local anesthetic dose requirement is typically reduced; reduce local anesthetic dose for spinal anesthesia by 40%
  - Increased risk of hypotension from the sympathectomy

AGE-RELATED EFFECTS ON ANESTHETIC AGENTS

Anxiolytics
- Dose of benzodiazepine should be minimized

Intravenous induction agents
- Reduced dose requirement of IV induction agents (propofol, thiopental, etomidate, ketamine)
- Propofol induction dose for 80-year-old = 50% dose for 20-year-old

Inhalational anesthetics
- MAC ↓ by 0.6% every year above 40 years
- Recovery from inhaled anesthetics delayed due to increased volume of distribution (↑ fat content) and decreased pulmonary gas exchange

Opioids
- 50% reduction in dose requirement between ages 20 and 89 years
- Enhanced sensitivity to opioids mostly due to pharmacodynamic changes rather than changes in pharmacokinetics
- Decreased elimination of active metabolites (morphine-3- and morphine-6-glucuronide)
- For morphine, reduce dose by 50%; adjust interval based on need
- For remifentanil, decrease bolus by 50%, and use one-third infusion rate compared with young patient

Muscle relaxants
- Onset of action is delayed due to decreased muscle blood flow and cardiac output
- Dose requirement for most water-soluble nondepolarizing agents reduced since total body water is decreased
- Prolonged elimination half-life for agents (pancuronium, vecuronium, rocuronium) that are eliminated by hepatic or renal excretion
- Duration of action of cisatracurium is unaffected in elderly; onset delayed
- Despite altered pseudocholinesterase levels in the elderly, no clinically significant prolongation in the effects of succinylcholine

Time to peak effect after IV bolus

Neuromuscular blocker	Young adult	Elderly patient
Succinylcholine (1 mg/kg)	1.2 min	1.5 min
Cisatracurium (0.1 mg/kg)	3.0 min	4.1 min
Rocuronium (1 mg/kg)	1.0 min	1.35 min

NSAIDs
- Reduce dose by 25–50%; increase interval between doses
- Contraindicated if CrCl <50 mL/min

POSTOPERATIVE MANAGEMENT

- Optimal pain management to improve respiratory effort, prevent delirium, and promote early ambulation
- Higher incidence of perioperative complications in the elderly due to age-related physiologic changes as well as associated comorbidities:
  - Infection
  - Thromboembolism
  - Respiratory: most common morbidity for reasons mentioned above

- Cardiovascular: MI and cardiac arrest more common in elderly
- Stroke: risk factors are age, atrial fibrillation, and history of previous stroke
- Postoperative confusion, delirium, or cognitive dysfunction common in elderly

---

Postoperative Cognitive Dysfunction (POCD)
- Incidence: 5–15%
- Multifactorial; possibly from low levels of certain neurotransmitters (acetylcholine)
- Risk factors: lower education, previous stroke, alcohol use, drug effects, underlying dementia, inpatients, metabolic derangements, and hypothermia
- Similar incidence with general and regional anesthetic techniques

---

PEARLS AND TIPS

- Aging results in reduced organ function; comorbidities further worsen the reserve
- Expect reduced anesthetic requirement of local and general anesthetic drugs

REFERENCES

For references, please visit **www.TheAnesthesiaGuide.com**.

CHAPTER 35
Latex Allergy

Mark S. Tinklepaugh, MD

BASICS

Three types:
- *Contact dermatitis*:
  - Eighty percent of all reactions to wearing latex gloves
  - Seen as dry, cracked skin worsened by powder and soap
  - Nonimmunological response
  - Treat by avoiding irritants and application of topical steroids
- *Type IV delayed hypersensitivity*:
  - Eighty percent of all immunological responses to latex
  - T-cell-mediated immunological response to latex allergen, usually chemical additive of latex manufacturing
  - Usually presents 6–72 hours after exposure; mild itch to oozing blisters much like poison ivy; may respond to topical steroids
- *Type I immediate hypersensitivity*:
  - IgE-mediated reaction to proteins found in latex
  - May be *localized* with immediate urticaria (hives)
  - May be *generalized* with hives, bronchospasm, airway obstruction, anaphylaxis, cardiovascular collapse

At-risk groups:
- *Health care workers*:
  ‣ Twenty-four percent of anesthesiologists/nurse anesthetists have contact dermatitis
  ‣ Prevalence of latex sensitization in anesthesiologists/nurse anesthetists is up to 15%, and that in general population is up to 6%
  ‣ Health care workers who are patients themselves involved in up to 70% of latex-related adverse events
  ‣ Rubber industry workers, greenhouse workers, and hair stylists at increased risk
- *Patients with multiple surgeries*:
  ‣ Frequent exposure to latex products experienced by patients with congenital urological anomalies and spina bifida can have incidence as high as 60%
- *Food allergies*:
  ‣ *Tropical fruit* (avocado, kiwi, banana), *chestnuts*, *stone fruit* (peach, nectarine, apricot, almond, plum, cherry). *Buckwheat*, a grain substitute used in gluten-free diets of patients with celiac disease, is known to have cross-reactivity with latex
- *Allergy history*:
  ‣ Atopic, asthma, rhinitis, hay fever, or eczema

PREOPERATIVE

- Identify at-risk patients by history and testing. Well-coordinated perioperative team approach to patient care critical
- *Skin prick* testing specific and sensitive, but reserved for inconclusive laboratory testing because of potential severe reaction in sensitized patient
- Radioallergosorbent test (RAST), an in vitro test for latex-specific IgE antibodies, recommended, but can have up to 30% false negatives
- Elective cases should be first case of day if possible
- Signs identifying the patient as latex allergic or at risk should be posted throughout the operating and recovery suites
- Pretreatment with antihistamines and/or systemic steroids not shown to prevent anaphylaxis or attenuate severity of Type I response

INTRAOPERATIVE

- Anesthesia (and surgical) equipment latex-free:
  ‣ Gloves, nasal/oral airways, endotracheal tubes, blood pressure cuffs, masks, bags, circuits, ventilator bellows, tourniquets, intravenous catheters, Swan–Ganz catheters (balloon: special PACs without a balloon are available), suction catheters, temperature probes
  ‣ Rubber stoppers removed from multidose vials; medications stored in syringes should be reconstituted every 6 hours
  ‣ Prepare dilute epinephrine (10 µg/mL) immediately available. See chapter 201 for treatment of anaphylaxis

POSTOPERATIVE

- Cart containing non-latex items and signs identifying patient as latex sensitive should remain with patient throughout hospital course. Medic alert bracelet recommended

PEARLS AND TIPS

- Key is to identify allergic patient by history/testing; if in doubt, treat as such
- Avoid antigen exposure intraoperatively and perioperatively

- Contact dermatitis and Type IV delayed hypersensitivity usually responds to avoiding the offending irritant (powder, soap, glove type, chemical additive) and topical steroids
- Type I immediate hypersensitivity:
  ‣ Mild reactions respond to antihistamines and systemic steroids
  ‣ Severe reaction may be life-threatening and may require anaphylaxis protocol
- Severity guides treatment. Prompt administration of dilute epinephrine (0.1 µg/kg) IV is paramount

REFERENCES

For references, please visit **www.TheAnesthesiaGuide.com**.

CHAPTER 36
Electrolyte Abnormalities (Na, K, Ca, Mg, PO$_4$)

J. David Roccaforte, MD

NORMAL VALUES

	Conventional units	Conversion	SI units
Sodium (Na)	136–144 mEq/L	mEq/L × 1.0 = mmol/L	136–144 mmol/L
Potassium (K)	3.3–5.0 mEq/L	mEq/L × 1.0 = mmol/L	3.3–5.0 mmol/L
Calcium (Ca) serum	8.5–10.5 mg/dL 4.25–5.25 mEq/L	mg/dL × 0.25 = mmol/L mEq/L × 0.5 = mmol/L	2.1–2.6 mmol/L
Calcium (Ca$_i$) Ionized	4.5–5.3 mg/dL 2.25–2.8 mEq/L	mg/dL × 0.25 = mmol/L mEq/L × 0.5 = mmol/L	1.12–1.4 mmol/L
Magnesium (Mg)	1.8–3.0 mg/dL 1.5–2.4 mEq/L	mg/dL × 0.411 = mmol/L mEq/L × 0.5 = mmol/L	0.74–1.23 mmol/L
Phosphate (PO$_4$)	2.5–4.5 mg/dL	mg/dL × 0.323 = mmol/L	0.81–1.45 mmol/L

CONSIDERATIONS FOR DELAYING A CASE TO CORRECT ABNORMALITIES

Delay and treat	Proceed and treat	Proceed and monitor
Elective case	Emergent or urgent case	Any case type
Acute change	Acute change	Chronic abnormality
Symptomatic patient	Symptomatic patient	Asymptomatic patient
Abnormal ECG	Abnormal ECG	Normal ECG

A. Perioperative management

- **Hypernatremia:** Na ≥145 mEq/L
  - ▸ *Critical value*: Na ≥ 160 mEq/L
  - ▸ Common causes: Hyperaldosteronism (excess mineralocorticoid), Cushing syndrome (excess glucocorticoid), excessive hypertonic saline or sodium bicarbonate administration, gastrointestinal losses, renal excretion, osmotic diuresis, diabetes insipidus
  - ▸ *Signs and symptoms*: Intense thirst, confusion, irritability, hyperreflexia, lethargy, coma, twitching, seizures
  - ▸ *Notes*:
    - ▪ Hypernatremia is always associated with a primary gain in Na or excess loss of water. Diagnosing the etiology hinges on assessment of the patient's volume status (see Figure 36-1)
    - ▪ A rapid rate of rise in Na is associated with worse neurologic outcomes (central pontine myelinolysis):

FIGURE 36-1. Algorithm for determining etiology of hypernatremia

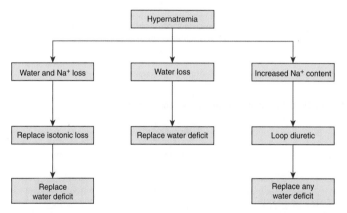

- ◆ Myelin sheath destruction in pons
- ◆ Always iatrogenic
- ◆ Very high mortality
- ◆ Earliest symptom is difficulty speaking and swallowing
- ◆ MRI is diagnostic; however, most cases are diagnosed at autopsy
- ▪ Gradual increases in Na, even to levels ≥160 mEq/L, are generally well tolerated
- ▸ *Treatment*: Calculate free water deficit (L) = {([measured Na] − 140)/140} × body weight (in kg) × 0.6 (men) or 0.5 (women)
  - ▪ If *Na is moderately elevated*:
    - ◆ Administer H_2O enterally provided the gut is functional; otherwise judiciously infuse isosmotic, hyponatremic IV solution (D5W) with close monitoring

- If treating *acute central diabetes insipidus (DI)*:
  - Begin vasopressin IV at 2 U/h and titrate to reduce urine output to ≤0.5 mL/kg/h
  - Administer 0.45% NaCl 1 mL IV for each 1 mL urine output
- *Caution*:
  - A decrease in serum sodium of >0.5 mEq/L/h can lead to cerebral edema. If the patient has elevated ICP, correct hyponatremia very slowly if at all
  - If the abnormality develops rapidly (over hours), the rate of correction can match the rate of acquisition even if it exceeds 0.5 mEq/L/h
- **Hyponatremia:** Na ≤135 mEq/L:
  - *Critical value:* Na ≤125 mEq/L
  - Common causes: Burns, sweating, vomiting, diarrhea, pancreatitis, diuretics, salt-wasting nephropathy, cerebral salt wasting, mineralocorticoid deficiency (Addison's disease), congestive cardiac failure, cirrhosis with ascites, nephrotic syndrome, chronic renal failure, syndrome of inappropriate antidiuretic hormone secretion (SIADH), hypothyroidism, hypopituitarism (glucocorticoid deficiency), primary polydipsia, iatrogenic (excessive administration of parenteral hypotonic fluids, post-transurethral prostatectomy)
  - *Signs and symptoms*: Nausea, headache, lethargy, hyporeflexia, confusion, seizures, coma
  - *Notes*:
    - Hyponatremia is always associated with a primary loss of Na or excess gain of water. Diagnosing the etiology hinges on assessment of the patient's volume status (see Figure 36-2)

FIGURE 36-2. Algorithm for determining etiology of hyponatremia

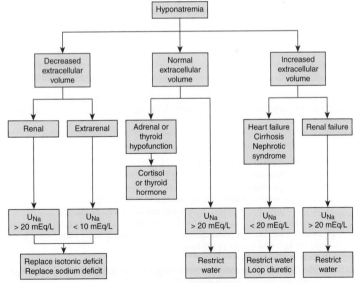

U_{Na} = Urinary sodium concentration

- A rapid drop in Na is associated with worse neurologic outcomes (cerebral edema)
- Gradual decreases in Na, even to levels ≤125 mEq/L, are generally well tolerated
▸ *Treatment*: Assess for hypovolemia and symptoms:
  - If *hypovolemic*:
    ♦ Correct hypovolemia with 0.9% NaCl IV and blood products as appropriate
  - If *symptomatic*:
    ♦ Restrict fluids; administer loop diuretic if Na <110; cautiously administer 3% NaCl IV (4–6 mL/kg) to raise serum Na 3–5 mEq/L or until symptoms improve. Hypertonic saline must be given cautiously because rapid infusion can lead to hypokalemia, pulmonary edema, and hyperchloremic metabolic acidosis
  - If *subarachnoid hemorrhage*:
    ♦ Avoid fluid restriction as it is associated with increased risk of cerebral infarction
  - In all *other* circumstances:
    ♦ Restrict IV and oral fluids
    ♦ Closely monitor intravascular volume status and rate of Na correction
▸ *Caution*:
  - Overly aggressive correction predisposes to central pontine myelinolysis (see above)
  - An increase in serum sodium of 0.5 mEq/L/h is considered safe in all circumstances
  - If the abnormality develops rapidly (over hours), the rate of correction can match the rate of acquisition even if it exceeds 0.5 mEq/L/h
- **Hyperkalemia:** K$^+$ ≥5.1 mEq/L:
  ▸ *Critical value*: K$^+$ ≥7.0 mEq/L
  ▸ Common causes: Renal failure, volume depletion, medications that block K$^+$ excretion (e.g., spironolactone, triamterene), hypoaldosteronism (due to adrenal disorders and hyporeninemic states [such as type IV RTA], NSAIDs, ACE inhibitors), long-standing use of heparin, digitalis toxicity, iatrogenic K$^+$ administration (see Figure 36-3)

FIGURE 36-3. Algorithm for determining etiology of hyperkalemia

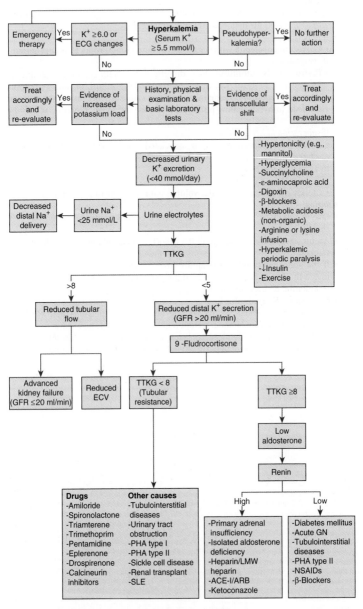

TTKG, transtubular potassium gradient; ECV, effective circulatory volume; PHA, pseudohypoaldosteronism. Reproduced with permission from Brenner BM, Rector FC III. *Brenner & Rector's The Kidney.* 8th ed. Philadelphia: Saunders; 2008:574. © Elsevier.

▸ *Signs and symptoms*: Cardiac arrhythmias, prolonged PR interval, peaked T waves and widened QRS complex on ECG, muscle weakness, hyperactive deep tendon reflexes, confusion (see Figure 36-4)

FIGURE 36-4. EKG changes in hyperkalemia

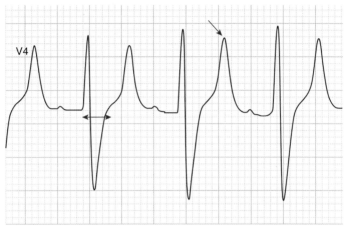

A

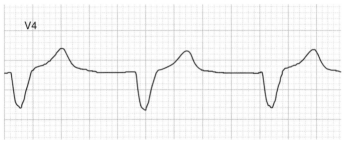

B

(A) Peaked T waves (arrow), widened QRS (double arrow), and subtle flattening of the P waves are seen in this patient with a serum K of 7.1. Reproduced from Knoop KJ, Stack LB, Storrow AB, Thurman RJ. *The Atlas of Emergency Medicine*. 3rd ed. Figure 24-45B. Available at: www. accessmedicine.com. Copyright © The McGraw-Hill Companies, Inc. All rights reserved. (B) Wide, blunted QRS with near sine wave appearance. No P waves visible. Serum K was 8.5 in this patient. Reproduced from Knoop KJ, Stack LB, Storrow AB, Thurman RJ. *The Atlas of Emergency Medicine*. 3rd ed. Figure 24-46B. Available at: www.accessmedicine.com. Copyright © The McGraw-Hill Companies, Inc. All rights reserved.

▸ *Notes*:
  ▪ Hyperkalemia causes cardiac abnormalities much more frequently than neurologic changes
  ▪ Gradual and chronic changes in K$^+$, even to levels ≥7 mEq/L, may be well tolerated
▸ *Treatment*: Assess for exogenous K$^+$, medications, and ECG abnormalities:
  ▪ If *ECG is abnormal* and patient is *unstable*:
    ◆ Monitor ECG and blood pressure continuously

- Administer calcium chloride (10%) 500–1,000 mg (5–10 mL) IV over 2–5 minutes; effect within 3 minutes; repeat if no effect after 5 minutes; duration of action: 30–60 minutes
- No effect on K^+ levels but antagonizes effects of hyperkalemia on myocardium
- Administer sodium bicarbonate 50 mEq IV over 5 minutes:
  ○ Osmotic volume load that may exacerbate pulmonary edema and CHF
  ○ Produces CO_2 that is converted in cells into carbonic acid, causing paradoxical intracellular acidosis
  ○ Avoid if possible in patients with renal failure
- Administer glucose 25 g (50 mL of D50) IV + 10 U regular insulin IV over 15–30 minutes (drives K^+ into cells; check K and glucose levels frequently; start insulin infusion if hyperglycemia)
- Administer nebulized albuterol: 10–20 mg over 15 minutes; effective in 60% of patients, unclear resistance mechanism (shifts K^+ into the cells [within 2 hours]; possible tachycardia)
- Give furosemide 40–80 mg IV
- Administer sodium polystyrene sulfonate (Kayexalate) 15–30 g in 50–100 mL of 20% sorbitol enterally or by retention enema (resin that exchanges Na for K)
- Provide emergent dialysis (CVVH may not be fast enough [lower blood and dialysate flows] but more feasible intraoperatively)

- If *ECG is abnormal* and patient is *stable*:
  - Monitor ECG continuously
  - Administer glucose 25 g (50 mL of D50) IV + 10 U regular insulin IV over 15–30 minutes
  - Administer sodium bicarbonate 50 mEq IV over 5 minutes
  - Administer nebulized albuterol: 10–20 mg over 15 minutes
  - Give furosemide 40–80 mg IV
  - Administer sodium polystyrene sulfonate (Kayexalate) 15–30 g in 50–100 mL of 20% sorbitol, enterally or by retention enema
  - Provide urgent dialysis, if CRF
- Discontinue exogenous K^+ administration (IV and enteral)
- If possible, discontinue medications associated with hyperkalemia (potassium-sparing diuretics, angiotensin-converting enzyme inhibitors, NSAIDs)
- If *ECG is normal*, consider:
  - ECG monitoring and observation
  - Sodium polystyrene sulfonate (Kayexalate) 15–30 g in 50–100 mL of 20% sorbitol enterally or by retention enema
  - Furosemide 40–80 mg IV
  - Regular dialysis as scheduled, if CRF

▸ *Caution*:
  - Avoid enteral Kayexalate in patients with gastroparesis, ileus, bowel obstruction, or risk of aspiration
  - Avoid hyperkalemia associated with large-volume RBC transfusion:
    - Prior to surgery, wash packed red blood cells using cell saver, which will remove extracellular potassium
    - Refrigerate these washed cells near the operating room; transfuse if hyperkalemia is worsening but hemorrhage requires continued red blood cell transfusion

- **Hypokalemia**: $K^+ \leq 3.2$ mEq/L:
  ▸ *Critical value*: $K^+ \leq 2.5$ mEq/L
  ▸ Common causes: Vomiting, diarrhea, ileostomy, villous adenoma, laxatives, thiazide and loop diuretics, Cushing syndrome, elevated aldosterone, renal tubular acidosis, hypomagnesemia, aminoglycosides, amphotericin B, prednisone (see Figure 36-5)

FIGURE 36-5. Algorithm for determining etiology of hypokalemia

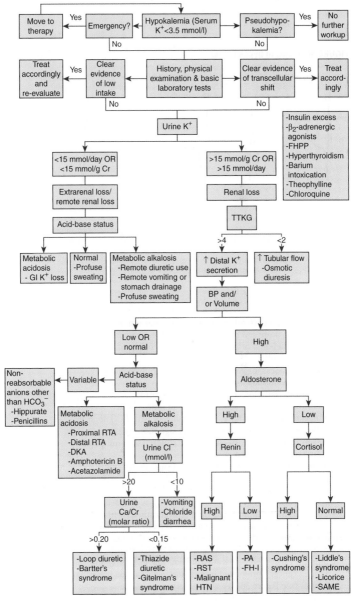

FHPP, familial hypokalemic periodic paralysis; TTKG, transtubular potassium gradient; RTA, renal tubular acidosis; RAS, renal artery stenosis; RST, renin-secreting tumor; PA, primary aldosteronism; FH-I, familial hyperaldosteronism type I; SAME, syndrome of apparent mineralocorticoid excess. Reproduced with permission from Brenner BM, Rector FC III. *Brenner & Rector's The Kidney.* 8th ed. Philadelphia: Saunders; 2008:565. © Elsevier.

▸ *Signs and symptoms*: Cardiac arrhythmias, U waves, T-wave flattening, muscle weakness, fatigue, constipation, leg cramps (see Figure 36-6)

FIGURE 36-6. EKG in hypokalemia

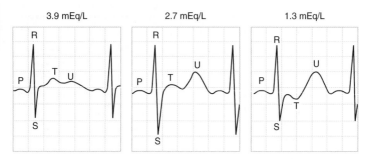

▸ *Notes*:
  ▪ Even mild hypokalemia may cause muscular symptoms. Cardiac abnormalities occur with more severe hypokalemia (unless patient is on digitalis therapy)
  ▪ Hypomagnesemia must be treated concurrently, or correction of hypokalemia will be difficult
▸ *Treatment*: Assess for symptoms and ECG abnormalities:
  ▪ If *hemodynamically unstable*:
    ◆ Provide continuous ECG and BP monitoring
    ◆ Administer KCl IV 10 mEq over 5 minutes (adults)
  ▪ If *hemodynamically stable, symptomatic*, or with *ECG abnormalities*:
    ◆ Provide continuous ECG and vital sign monitoring
    ◆ Administer KCl IV 10–20 mEq/h (children 0.25 mEq/kg/h)
  ▪ If *asymptomatic* with a *normal ECG*:
    ◆ Consider continuous ECG and vital sign monitoring
    ◆ Provide enteral supplementation: 1–2 mEq/kg per day divided in three doses
▸ *Caution*:
  ▪ Risk of cardiac arrhythmias is significantly augmented with digitalis therapy
  ▪ IV KCl is best administered via a central catheter with the tip outside the right heart. Peripheral venous KCl infusion is painful, and if infiltrated can be caustic
• **Hypercalcemia:** Serum Ca ≥10.6 mg/dL or Ca$_i$ ≥5.4 mg/dL:
  ▸ *Critical values*: serum Ca ≥13 mg/dL or Ca$_i$ ≥6.0 mg/dL
  ▸ Common causes: Hyperparathyroidism, malignancy (multiple myeloma, breast and lung cancer), prolonged immobility, renal failure, hyperthyroidism, thiazide diuretics (see Figure 36-7)

FIGURE 36-7. Algorithm for determining etiology of hypercalcemia

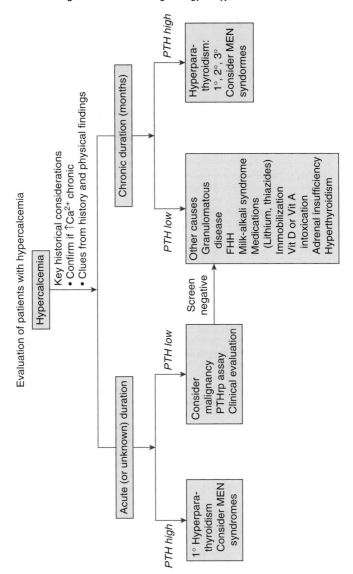

FHH, familial hypocalciuric hypercalcemia; MEN, multiple endocrine neoplasia; PTHrP, parathyroid hormone–related peptide. Reproduced from Longo DL, Fauci AS, Kasper DL, Hauser SL, Jameson JL, Loscalzo J. *Harrison's Principles of Internal Medicine*. 18th ed. Figure 353-6. Available at: www. accessmedicine.com. Copyright © The McGraw-Hill Companies, Inc. All rights reserved.

▸ *Signs and symptoms*: Muscle weakness, fatigue, disorientation, seizures, coma, cardiac arrhythmias, shortened QT interval, dysphagia, constipation. If major hypercalcemia, PR prolongation, AV block, T wave widening, VF (see Figure 36-8)

FIGURE 36-8. EKG changes in hypocalcemia and hypercalcemia

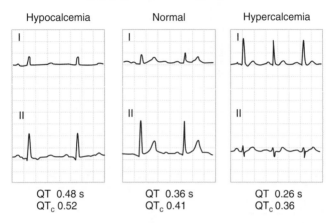

Hypocalcemia	Normal	Hypercalcemia
QT 0.48 s	QT 0.36 s	QT 0.26 s
QT_C 0.52	QT_C 0.41	QT_C 0.36

Prolongation of the Q-T interval (ST segment portion) is typical of hypocalcemia. Hypercalcemia may cause abbreviation of the ST segment and shortening of the QT interval. Reproduced from Longo DL, Fauci AS, Kasper DL, Hauser SL, Jameson JL, Loscalzo J. *Harrison's Principles of Internal Medicine*. 18th ed. Figure 228-17. Available at: www.accessmedicine.com. Copyright © The McGraw-Hill Companies, Inc. All rights reserved.

▸ *Notes*:
  ▪ Most hypercalcemia is associated with primary hyperparathyroidism and malignancy (>90%)
  ▪ Albumin-corrected serum calcium *inaccurately* predicts ionized calcium levels in 38% of critically ill patients. Follow measured ionized calcium levels whenever possible
▸ *Treatment*: Assess ECG and intravascular volume status:
  ▪ Discontinue Ca-containing IV (lactated Ringer's) and enteral solutions
  ▪ Discontinue medications that increase calcium (lithium, HCTZ, vitamins A and D)
  ▪ If *symptomatic*, with an *abnormal ECG* and *not hypervolemic*:
    ◆ Continuously monitor ECG until normalized
    ◆ Administer 0.9% NaCl IV, 300–500 mL/h until urine output increases to ≥200 mL/h, and then reduce NaCl infusion to 100–200 mL/h
    ◆ Consider chelation agents (PO_4 or EDTA) or bisphosphonates in extreme conditions
    ◆ Consider calcitonin IV or SC 2–8 IU/kg q6–12 hours
  ▪ If *hypervolemic*:
    ◆ Give furosemide IV 1 mg/kg
    ◆ Monitor oxygenation continuously
    ◆ Consider emergent hemodialysis
  ▪ If *asymptomatic* with a *normal ECG* and *euvolemic*:
    ◆ Administer 0.9% NaCl IV, 100–200 mL/h
    ◆ Consider calcitonin IV or SC 2–8 IU/kg q6–12 hours
▸ *Caution*: Monitor K and Mg concentrations closely and supplement as appropriate during treatment

- **Hypocalemia:** Serum Ca ≤8.4 mg/dL or Ca$_i^{2+}$ ≤4.4 mg/dL:
  ▸ *Critical values*: Serum Ca ≤7 mg/dL or Ca$_i^{2+}$ ≤3.6 mg/dL
  ▸ Common causes: Hypoparathyroidism, renal failure, vitamin D deficiency, prolonged magnesium-containing laxative use, tumor lysis syndrome, pancreatitis (see Figure 36-9)

FIGURE 36-9. Algorithm for determining etiology of hypocalcemia

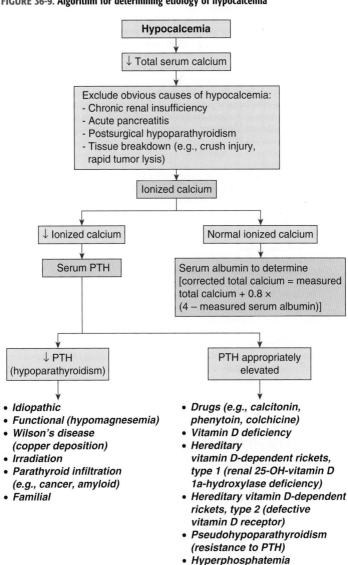

▸ *Signs and symptoms*: Anxiety, agitation, delirium, seizures, facial paresthesia, muscle cramps, hyperreflexia, tetany, stridor, prolonged QT, hypotension, heart failure (see Figure 36-8)

▸ *Notes*:
  ▪ Trousseau sign: A tourniquet inflated around the arm occludes arterial flow for 3 minutes. The hand and forearm are observed for spasm
  ▪ Chvostek sign: A tap to the facial nerve at the angle of the mandible elicits contraction of the ipsilateral facial muscles. Chvostek sign is considered less sensitive than the Trousseau sign
  ▪ Presentation of hypocalcemia can be indistinguishable from hypomagnesemia

▸ Treatment: Assess ECG for abnormalities and hemodynamics for stability:
  ▪ *IV calcium is contraindicated if digitalis treatment: risk of VF*
  ▪ If *hypotensive*:
    ◆ Continuously monitor ECG and blood pressure
    ◆ Push 1 g 10% calcium chloride (10 mL) IV over 3 minutes via central line, or in 50–100 mL D5W IV over 10 minutes via peripheral IV
    ◆ *Then* give 10% calcium gluconate (93 mg of elemental Ca/mL) or 10% calcium chloride (273 mg of elemental Ca/mL) IV, 1–2 mg elemental Ca/kg/h (in 500–1,000 mL D5W) for 6–12 hours or until ionized calcium normalizes, or symptoms abate
  ▪ If *symptomatic* and *normotensive*:
    ◆ Continuously monitor ECG
    ◆ Administer 100–200 mg of elemental Ca as 10% calcium gluconate (93 mg of elemental Ca/mL) *or* 10% calcium chloride (273 mg of elemental Ca/mL) in 50–100 mL D5W IV over 10 minutes
    ◆ *Then* give 10% calcium gluconate (93 mg of elemental Ca/mL) or 10% calcium chloride (273 mg of elemental Ca/mL) IV, 1–2 mg elemental Ca/kg/h (in 500–1,000 mL D5W) for 6–12 hours or until ionized calcium normalizes, or symptoms abate
  ▪ If *asymptomatic*:
    ◆ Consider enteral calcium supplementation,
    ◆ Administer 10% calcium gluconate or 10% calcium chloride 500–1,000 mg IV over 6 hours

▸ *Caution*:
  ▪ Avoid infusing Ca-containing solutions in the same line as a blood transfusion as the EDTA may chelate with the Ca and allow the blood to clot
  ▪ Untreated hypomagnesemia will make hypocalcemia refractory to therapy

• **Hypermagnesemia:** ≥3.1 mg/dL or ≥2.5 mEq/L:
  ▸ *Critical values*: ≥10 mg/dL or ≥8.2 mEq/L
  ▸ *Common causes*: Renal failure, hyperparathyroidism, iatrogenic magnesium administration (for preeclampsia, or as enemas)

Symptoms and Signs of Hypermagnesemia	
Magnesium level	Signs/symptoms
4–6 mEq/L (4.8–7.2 mg/dL)	Hyporeflexia–deep tendon reflexes disappear Nausea/vomiting/flushing
6–10 mEq/L (7.2–12 mg/dL)	Respiratory compromise/apnea Mental status changes/lethargy Hypotension EKG changes: prolonged PR, QRS, and QT intervals Hypocalcemia
>10 mEq/L (12 mg/dL)	Flaccid paralysis, complete heart block, coma, cardiac arrest/asystole

- *Signs and symptoms*: Decreased deep tendon reflexes, lethargy, confusion, muscle weakness, respiratory depression, vasodilation, hypotension, prolonged PR interval, widened QRS complex, bradycardia, arrhythmias, up to respiratory and cardiac arrest
- *Notes*:
  - Hypermagnesemia is most frequently associated with renal failure or Mg therapy for the treatment of preeclampsia
- *Treatment*: Assess ECG, symptoms, and respiratory status:
  - Discontinue exogenous sources of magnesium
  - If *severely symptomatic* with an *abnormal ECG* or *impaired renal function* or *hypervolemic*:
    - Consider securing the airway and providing respiratory support
    - Administer 500–1,000 mg 10% calcium chloride (5–10 mL) IV over 3–5 minutes via central line, or in 50–100 mL D5W IV over 10–20 minutes via peripheral IV
    - Give glucose 25 g (50 mL of D50) IV + 10 U regular insulin IV over 15–30 minutes
    - Consider furosemide IV 1 mg/kg
    - Consider emergent hemodialysis
  - If *mildly symptomatic* with a *normal ECG, normal renal function, not hypervolemic*:
    - Five hundred to 1,000 mL 0.9% NaCl IV over 30 minutes to 1 hour
    - Furosemide IV 1 mg/kg
  - If *asymptomatic* with a *normal ECG*:
    - Observe
- *Caution*: Dilution, diuresis, and dialysis may induce hypocalcemia, which will exacerbate the effect of hypomagnesemia
- **Hypomagnesemia:** ≤1.7 mg/dL or ≤1.4 mEq/L:
  - *Critical values*: ≤1.2 mg/dL or ≤1.0 mEq/L
  - *Common causes*: Diarrhea, pancreatitis, loop and thiazide diuretic use, hypercalcemia, renal failure, post-parathyroidectomy

Differentiation between Renal and Nonrenal Causes of Hypomagnesemia	
Test	Criteria for renal magnesium wasting
24-h urine collection for magnesium	>10–30 mg Mg/24 h
Fractional excretion of magnesium[1] (FeMg)	>2%
$$\frac{\text{Urine Mg} \times \text{plasma Mg}}{(0.7 \times \text{plasma Mg}) \times \text{urine Cr}} \times 100$$	

[1]Plasma magnesium concentration is multiplied by 0.7 since only 70% of the circulating magnesium is filtered because it is free (not bound to albumin).
Reproduced with permission from Lerma EV, Berns JS, Nissenson AR. *Current Diagnosis & Treatment: Nephrology & Hypertension.* New York: McGraw-Hill; 2009. Table 8-2. Copyright © The McGraw-Hill Companies, Inc. All rights reserved.

- *Signs and symptoms*:
  - Neuromuscular: muscle weakness and twitches, hyperreflexia, tetany, Chvostek and Trousseau signs (see "Hypocalcemia"), stridor, seizures, anxiety, depression, confusion, delirium, Wernicke encephalopathy
  - Cardiac: tachycardia, prolonged PR and QT intervals, torsades de pointes, HTN, coronary spasm
- *Note*: The presentation of hypomagnesemia can be indistinguishable from hypocalcemia

‣ *Treatment*: Assess for symptoms and ECG abnormalities:
  ▪ If *severely symptomatic or ECG is abnormal*:
    ◆ Continuously monitor ECG and BP
    ◆ Administer 10% magnesium sulfate IV, 2–4 g (20–40 mL) in 50–100 mL D5W over 5–10 minutes (can be repeated up to a total of 10 g $MgSO_4$)
  ▪ If *mildly symptomatic* with a *normal ECG*:
    ◆ Consider continuous ECG monitoring
    ◆ Administer 10% magnesium sulfate IV 1 g/h for 3–4 hours and reassess
  ▪ If *asymptomatic* with a *normal ECG*:
    ◆ Assess for ongoing GI or renal losses
    ◆ Supplement enterally if possible
    ◆ Anticipate diarrhea
‣ *Caution*:
  ▪ Hypokalemia in combination with hypomagnesemia significantly increases the risk of severe arrhythmias
  ▪ Magnesium potentiates nondepolarizing NMB and calcium channel blockers; monitor closely if renal failure or myasthenia gravis

- **Hyperphosphatemia:** ≥4.5 mg/dL:
  ‣ *Critical value*: None
  ‣ *Common causes*: Renal failure, tumor lysis syndrome, rhabdomyolysis, iatrogenic via phosphate-containing laxatives and enemas
  ‣ *Signs and symptoms*:
    ▪ Chronic: soft tissue calcifications, especially of blood vessels, causing ischemia
    ▪ Acute: hypocalcemia with tetany, massive soft tissue calcifications, neuropsychiatric symptoms
  ‣ *Notes*:
    ▪ Hyperphosphatemia is most often associated with renal failure, and is rarely an acute emergency
    ▪ Acute hyperphosphatemia is generally asymptomatic
    ▪ Hypocalcemia due to soft tissue precipitation is an associated finding when the $Ca \times PO_4$ product is chronically elevated (>55)
  ‣ *Treatment*: Assess for exogenous PO_4 intake:
    ▪ Discontinue phosphate supplementation
    ▪ Administer enteral phosphate-binding medications (calcium carbonate antacids, 500 mg po twice per day)
    ▪ Hemodialysis

- **Hypophosphatemia:** ≤2.4 mg/dL:
  ‣ *Critical value*: ≤1.0 mg/dL
  ‣ *Common causes*: Refeeding syndrome, post-parathyroidectomy, chronic diarrhea, hyperparathyroidism, Fanconi syndrome
  ‣ *Signs and symptoms*: Acutely asymptomatic
  ‣ *Notes*: Hypophosphatemia is associated with refeeding syndrome. Within days, severe hypophosphatemia can produce anorexia, muscle weakness, encephalopathy, seizures, coma, rhabdomyolysis, hemolysis, hypotension, coagulopathy, acute tubular necrosis, liver failure, severe arrhythmias, and CHF, all refractory to treatment
  ‣ *Treatment*: Assess renal function, serum potassium and calcium levels:
    ▪ Discontinue enteral and parenteral nutrition; restart nutrition at a lower rate once serum phosphate is normalized
    ▪ Discontinue phosphate-binding antacids and phosphate-wasting diuretics
    ▪ Correct hypomagnesemia
    ▪ If *severe* hypophosphatemia (≤2.16 mg/dL):
      ◆ Continuously monitor ECG and vital signs
      ◆ Administer K_3PO_4 or Na_3PO_4 solution IV, 15 mmol of PO_4 over 1 hour
      ◆ Monitor serum ionized calcium levels and treat hypocalcemia as appropriate
      ◆ Monitor serum phosphate levels closely and continue repletion until stabilized

- If *impaired renal function*:
  - ◆ Administer Na_3PO_4 solution IV, 0.16–0.25 mmol of PO_4/kg over 3–6 hours
- If *normal renal function*:
  - ◆ Administer K_3PO_4 solution IV, 0.16–0.25 mmol of PO_4/kg over 3–6 hours
- ▸ *Caution*: Because hypophosphatemia is relatively asymptomatic during the acute abnormality, it is tempting to defer treatment. Because phosphorus is a fundamental component of ATP, which is used in all vital cellular processes including RNA transcription and protein production, the catastrophic systemic manifestations of hypophosphatemia are delayed from the acute insult. For this reason, low serum phosphate levels should be treated with the same urgency and enthusiasm as one would treat equivalently low potassium levels

CHAPTER 37
HIV and Anesthesia

Harsha Nalabolu, MD

BASICS

- Normal CD4 count 500–1,200/mm^3
- Viral load low if <5,000/mL, high if >10,000

PREOPERATIVE

Assess organ systems; modify anesthetic plan as appropriate.

Assessment of Organ Systems	
CNS/PNS	• In early stages peripheral neuropathies are not uncommon, whereas in later stages central demyelinating neuropathies with dementia occur • Coexisting CNS infections can create mass effects increasing ICP
Pulmonary	• Opportunistic infections; most commonly pneumocystis carinii pneumonia (PCP) occurs when CD4 count is less than 200 • PCP can result in pneumatoceles that can rupture, leading to pneumothorax necessitating prolonged mechanical ventilation; CXR may be normal; however, CT chest scans reveal bilateral hazy infiltrates • Tuberculosis, nocardiosis, and lymphomas can also affect the lungs
Cardiac	• Patients with long-standing HIV infections develop myocarditis and up to 30% may develop dilated cardiomyopathy
Hematologic	• Some patients present with hypercoaguable state or idiopathic thrombotic thrombocytopenia • Antiretroviral agents such as AZT cause bone marrow suppression leading to coagulopathic state

A thorough medication review, and especially an understanding of each medication's side effects, is important.

Side Effects of HIV Medications	
Drug name (generic)	Common side effects
Nucleoside analog reverse transcriptase inhibitors (NRTIs)	
• Retrovir (zidovudine), AZT	Pancytopenia, neuropathy, myopathy
• Videx (didanosine), ddI	Peripheral neuropathy, pancreatitis, GI
• Zerit (stavudine), d4t	Peripheral neuropathy, pancreatitis
• Hivid (zalcitabine), ddC	Peripheral neuropathy, pancreatitis
• Epivir (lamivudine), 3Tc	Peripheral neuropathy, GI, rash
• Hepsera (adefovir)	Renal toxicity, increased LFTs, GI
• Ziagen (abacavir)	GI, rash, myalgia
Non-nucleoside reverse transcriptase inhibitors (NNRTIs)	
• Viramune (nevirapine)	GI, increased LFTs, rash, p450 induction
• Sustiva (efavirenz)	GI, increased LFTs, rash, teratogenicity
• Rescriptor (delavirdine)	GI, increased LFTs, rash
Protease inhibitors (PIs)	
• Invirase, Fortovase (saquinavir)	GI, hyperglycemia, inhibits p450 CYP$_3$A
• Crixivan (indinavir)	GI, hyperglycemia, inhibits p450 CYP$_3$A, renal
• Norvir (ritonavir)	failure, nephrolithiasis
• Viracept (nelfinavir)	GI, hyperglycemia, inhibits p450 CYP$_3$A,
• Agenerase (amprenavir)	increased LFTs
	GI, hyperglycemia, inhibits p450 CYP$_3$A
	Rash, inhibits p450 CYP$_3$A
Fusion inhibitor	
• Enfuvirtide	Bacterial pneumonia, injection site pain
Antipneumocystis antibiotic	
• Pentamidine	Arrhythmias, bronchospasm (aerosolized), electrolyte abnormalities

- CBC, electrolytes, renal function, LFTs, and coagulation profile
- CD4 count and viral load <3 months
- EKG as well as a TTE if long-standing disease or if symptoms suggest cardiac involvement
- CXR should be routinely performed, as well as a chest CT if CD4 count <200
- MRI of brain or spine if demyelinating neuropathy suspected
- Consider delaying an elective case if CD4 <200 due to an increased risk in postoperative infectious complications. If CD4 <50, increased 6-month mortality following surgery
- Do not stop HIV medications; discuss with ID specialist if patient unable to take PO postoperatively
- Transfusion relatively contraindicated: consider EPO if risk of high blood loss (see autologous transfusion chapter 66)

INTRAOPERATIVE

- Anesthetic technique based on patient's preoperative evaluation (systems affected)
- Regional anesthesia is preferred if possible due to lack of interactions between anesthetics and antiretroviral or antiopportunistic drugs or less potential immune system perturbation:
  - In HIV-infected parturients, less morbidity and mortality with neuraxial anesthesia
  - Besides usual contraindications to neuraxial block, some specific to the HIV population such as intracranial infections or spinal cord pathology need to be ruled out

- ‣ Epidural blood patches for PDPH are not contraindicated:
  - ▪ Epidural blood patch in patients with high viral load is not clearly contraindicated but advanced disease may be a contraindication due to risk of latent neurologic pathology
  - ▪ Epidural injection of a saline or dextran can be a reasonable alternative
  - ▪ Epidural injection of fibrin glue is another alternative; however, it has not been compared prospectively with standard epidural blood patch
- General anesthesia is considered to be safe but drug interactions and toxic effects of antiretroviral agents make administration of general anesthesia more challenging
- Anesthesia providers need to be cognizant of p450 inhibition or induction:
  - ‣ Protease inhibitors inhibit p450
  - ‣ Viramune (nevirapine) induces p450

Anesthetic Agents and p450 Interactions	
Examples of drugs metabolized by p450 (avoid)	Drugs not metabolized by p450 (prefer)
Midazolam	Propofol
Fentanyl	Etomidate
Ketamine	Cisatracurium
Quinidine	Desflurane
Amiodarone	Alfentanil, remifentanil

- Immunologic suppression from surgery, stress, anesthetic agents has been shown to be detrimental in terms of cancer recurrence but there are no data on HIV
- Allogeneic transfusions are immunomodulatory and blood transfusion in advanced HIV-infected patients may increase viral load through activation in small studies:
  - ‣ However, leukoreduced red blood cell transfusions showed no difference in levels of CMV, HIV, or cytokine activation
  - ‣ Autotransfusion is contraindicated
  - ‣ Use EPO preoperatively if risk of high blood loss

POSTOPERATIVE

- Resume treatment ASAP

PEARLS AND TRICKS

- Obtain CD4 and viral load within 3 months
- Do not stop HIV medications; know the side effects of the patient's medications
- Prefer anesthetic drugs not metabolized by p450: propofol, etomidate, alfentanil, remifentanil, desflurane
- Regional anesthesia preferred; however, rule out HIV-specific contraindication (intracranial infection, spinal cord pathology, etc.)
- Avoid transfusion (despite a lack of evidence that it is harmful). Use EPO preoperatively if risk of high blood loss

REFERENCES

For references, please visit **www.TheAnesthesiaGuide.com**.

CHAPTER 38
Coexisting Diseases with Anesthetic Implications

Kriti Sankholkar, MD

Disease	Disease characteristics	Anesthetic considerations
Achondroplasia	• Autosomal dominant • Most common cause of dwarfism • Odontoid hypoplasia, atlantoaxial instability, bulging discs, and severe cervical kyphosis • Central sleep apnea and OSA may be a feature • Pulmonary HTN • Cor pulmonale • Hydrocephalus	• Proportionately smaller airways • Potential airway difficulties, cervical spine instability, and the potential for spinal cord trauma with neck extension; obtain *cervical spine x-rays*. Consider FOB intubation • Consider PFTs • ETT size should be weight based • Relative contraindication to neuraxial blocks
Alport syndrome (hereditary nephritis)	• Ocular abnormalities and hearing loss • Disease culminates in systemic HTN and renal failure	• Intraglomerular pressure may be lowered by ACEI • Same anesthetic considerations as in renal failure and HTN
Ankylosing spondylitis	• Chronic, progressive, inflammatory disease spine articulations and adjacent soft tissues • Occurs more commonly in men • Spine exam reveals skeletal muscle spasm, loss of lordosis, and decreased mobility • Weight loss, fatigue, low-grade fever, conjunctivitis, and uveitis are systemic signs • Pulmonary involvement may reveal apical cavitary lesions with fibrosis and pleural thickening with ↓ pulmonary compliance and vital capacity secondary to arthritis; restrictive syndrome (30–45% of patients after 15 years) • Associated psoriasis • TMJ involvement with limitation of mouth opening • Cardiovascular: AI (up to 10% after 30 years), dysrhythmias, conduction abnormalities • Renal insufficiency: rare	• May need awake FOB intubation if cervical spine is involved (major kyphosis) • Restrictive lung disease may result in higher airway pressures • Spinal deformity and instability: careful positioning and padding • Neuraxial anesthesia is acceptable but may be difficult • Neurologic monitoring should be considered for corrective spine surgery

(*continued*)

Disease	Disease characteristics	Anesthetic considerations
Arthrogryposis	• One type, autosomal recessive, is a myopathy • Other type: polymalformative syndrome • Multiple extremity contractures due to periarticular fibrosis with muscular atrophy • Possible TMJ and spine involvement (cervical spine ⇒ intubation issues; thoracic spine ⇒ restrictive syndrome	• Plan for difficult intubation • Careful positioning • Sensitive to sedatives/anesthetics • Myopathy: avoid succinylcholine; monitor NMB • Possible MH • Monitor postoperatively for possible respiratory failure
Bartter syndrome	• Autosomal recessive renal disease • Hypokalemic, hypochloremic metabolic alkalosis • Normal blood pressure, no edema • Elevated plasma renin and aldosterone • Treatment aimed at prostaglandin synthetase inhibition with indomethacin	• Patients may be treated with indomethacin, β-blockers, and spironolactone • Monitoring of urine output (compensate for polyuria), arterial blood pressure, and CVP is indicated • Patients are resistant to effects of exogenous angiotensin and norepinephrine • Watch for hypokalemia and hypotonia
Bullous dermatitis (Lyell, Stevens–Johnson, pemphigus, bullous pemphigoid, etc.)	• Separation of epidermis • Skin and mucous membrane bullous lesions may lacerate • Most severe form is Stevens–Johnson syndrome • May be associated with viral infection, streptococci, cancer, autoimmunity, collagen vascular diseases or drug-induced • Tachycardia, high fever, and tachypnea may be features • Treatment may involve long-term corticosteroids • Associated diseases include porphyria, amyloidosis, multiple myeloma, DM, and hypercoagulable states • Malnutrition, anemia, electrolyte derangements, and hypoalbuminemia are common	• Upper airway and trachea may have lesions → airway management should be approached with caution • Regional anesthesia may be given if skin is intact • Pulmonary blebs may be present → ↑ risk of PTX • Avoid NO if blebs are suspected • Steroid supplementation may be necessary intraoperatively • Dehydration and hypokalemia may be present due to skin losses • Adequately protect skin at sites of taping, tourniquet, BP cuff, face mask • Suture in all lines
Dermatomyositis	• Inflammatory myopathy and skin changes • Proximal muscle weakness • Dysphagia, pulmonary aspiration, and pneumonia from pharyngeal and respiratory muscle weakness • Heart block, myocarditis, and left ventricular dysfunction may also be present	• Pulmonary aspiration is a risk • Normal response to both SCh and NDMRs has been shown

(continued)

Disease	Disease characteristics	Anesthetic considerations
Distal tubular acidosis	• Autosomal dominant • Inability to excrete H^+ (exchanged for K), with hyperchloremic hypokalemic acidosis • Renal Ca loss with secondary hyperparathyroidism • Hypercalcemia further increasing urinary Ca • Nephrocalcinosis, stones, rickets • Frequent infections	• Meticulous maintenance of electrolyte balance • Convert PO supplementation to IV form • Follow serum and urine electrolyte and compensate losses
Down syndrome (trisomy 21) Trisomy 13 (Patau syndrome) Trisomy 18 (Edwards syndrome)	• Variable clinical features including brachycephaly, a flat occiput, dysplastic ears, epicanthal folds, strabismus, enlarged tongue, midface hypoplasia, a high-arched palate, micrognathia, short, broad neck with occipitoatlantoaxial instability, hypermobile joints, and hypotonia • Patients have respiratory difficulties secondary to floppy soft palate, enlarged tonsils, laryngotracheal or subglottic stenosis, OSA, and recurrent pulmonary infections • Congenital cardiac defects include ASD, VSD, endocardial cushion defect, patent ductus arteriosus, or tetralogy of Fallot • Uncorrected cardiac defects may lead to pulmonary HTN • GERD, duodenal atresia, imperforate anus, and Hirschsprung disease occur with ↑ frequency	• May need IM ketamine preoperatively in an uncooperative patient • Preoperative neurologic evaluation should be thorough • Consider premedication with oral midazolam and guardian present for induction of anesthesia • May have difficult airway → use smaller ETT; consider awake FOB • Spinal cord compression is a concern secondary to occipitoatlantoaxial instability • Bradycardia during induction is more common • Strict asepsis is required since patients are immunocompromised • Endocarditis prophylaxis • OSA and stridor are not uncommon postoperatively
Ehlers–Danlos syndrome	• Autosomal dominant • Associated with skin fragility, easy bruisability, and osteoarthritis • Type IV (vascular)—mutations in the type III procollagen gene → ↑ risk of premature death • Type IV is most common clinical presentation with arterial dissection or intestinal rupture • Obstetric complications include premature labor and excessive bleeding • ↑ risk of spontaneous PTX, diaphragmatic hernia, aortic and/or mitral (MVP) regurgitation, cardiac conduction abnormalities • Possibly von Willebrand factor deficiency	• Evaluate hemostasis preoperatively; obtain echo • No IM injections • Avoid instrumentation of nose or esophagus • May have excessive hematoma during CVL or arterial line placement • IV extravasation may go unnoticed secondary to high skin laxity • Low airway pressure during CMV is recommended to avoid PTX • Regional anesthesia → ↑ risk of hematoma formation; evaluate risk/benefit ratio • Up to 25% maternal death (bleeding, uterine rupture, aorta or IVC rupture)

(*continued*)

Disease	Disease characteristics	Anesthetic considerations
Fanconi anemia	• Autosomal recessive • Pancytopenia progresses to acute leukemia	• May need transfusion prior to surgery • If immunocompromised, will need more specific antibiotic coverage
Guillain–Barré	• Sudden-onset skeletal muscle weakness starting in legs and spreading cephalad • Flaccid paralysis with diminished DTRs • Respiratory muscle weakness and impaired ventilation may occur • Autonomic nervous system dysfunction is a feature • Thromboembolism rate is increased	• May have exaggerated autonomic response → use invasive arterial monitoring • Do not use SCh → hyperkalemia may occur from denervation • NDMRs may be used (lower dose, monitoring) • Postoperative extubation may be delayed secondary to ventilatory depression and weakness
Hartnup disease (pellagra-like dermatosis)	• Autosomal recessive • Neutral aminoaciduria • Seizures, dermatitis, and mental retardation • Treated with high-protein diet, nicotinamide, and sunlight protection	• Maintain acid–base balance • Maintain adequate intravascular volume • Avoid seizure threshold lowering anesthetics
Hemochromatosis	• Autosomal recessive • Progressive iron deposition in body tissues • Incidence higher in men • May go on to develop DM and CHF • Hepatomegaly, portal HTN, and primary hepatocellular carcinoma may develop	• Preoperative evaluation of anemia, cirrhosis, electrolyte abnormalities, renal and cardiac dysfunction should be thorough • Coagulation studies should be obtained and preoperative vitamin K given if PT is prolonged • Thrombocytopenia may require platelet transfusion • Hypoglycemia should be treated preoperatively • Hypoalbuminemia → ↓ protein binding → ↓ drug dose • Cardiomyopathy may make patients more sensitive to depressant effects of volatile anesthetics and more sensitive to catecholamines

(continued)

Disease	Disease characteristics	Anesthetic considerations
Hemolytic anemia	• Includes sickle cell anemia, Hb C, β-thalassemia • Chronic progressive lung damage may occur • Splenomegaly, sometimes splenectomy needed to prolong RBC life span • Possible neurologic and muscle (myopathy) involvement • Low baseline O_2 saturation, elevated Cr, cardiac dysfunction, CNS defects, concurrent infection • Sickle cell disease, not trait, increases risk of perioperative complications. Avoid dehydartion, hypothermia, hypoxemia; do not use tourniquet	• Minor surgery: low risk; intra-abdominal, intracranial or intrathoracic surgery: high risk • Need to have preoperative Hct of 30% • Avoid succinylcholine if myopathy (or in doubt) • Avoid dehydration, acidosis, and hypothermia • Aggressive postoperative pain management required • Acute chest syndrome can develop 2–3 days postoperatively → treatment: oxygenation, analgesia, and blood transfusion • *Avoid oxidizing agents*
Hereditary jaundice (Rotor, Dubin–Johnson)	• Unconjugated hyperbilirubinemia (Gilbert syndrome and Crigler–Najjar syndrome) • Conjugated hyperbilirubinemia (Dubin–Johnson syndrome)	• Fasting should be minimized as this increases bilirubin accumulation • Morphine administration is not affected (metabolized by a different glucuronosyltransferase enzyme system)
Homocystinuria	• Autosomic dominant • Failure of transsulfuration of precursors of cystine • Dislocation of the lens, osteoporosis • Kyphoscoliosis, brittle light-colored hair, and malar flush • Seizures, mental retardation • Hypoglycemia • Increased risk of thromboembolism	• Minimize perioperative thromboembolism by administering pyridoxine, preoperative hydration, dextran infusion, anticoagulation, and early ambulation postoperatively • Monitor blood glucose • Risk of bone fracture
Horton's	• Panarteritis involving mostly middle-sized external carotid branches, possibly leading to blindness • Can occasionally involve aorta, coronary arteries	• Assess arterial involvement • Maintain high BP to avoid ischemia leading to tissue necrosis or blindness • Long-term steroid therapy
Hyperkalemic periodic paralysis	• Autosomal dominant • Intermittent acute attacks of skeletal muscle weakness or paralysis associated with hyperkalemia • Attacks usually last about an hour • Triggers: exercise, cold, shivering, NPO • GERD possible • Long-term treatment by procainamide	• Preoperative potassium depletion with diuretics • Give glucose infusion while NPO • Avoid potassium solutions, SCh, ketamine • Frequent electrolyte monitoring → treat hyperkalemia and EKG changes with calcium • Prevent hypothermia • Modified RSI with rocuronium

(continued)

Disease	Disease characteristics	Anesthetic considerations
Hypokalemic periodic paralysis	• Autosomal dominant • Intermittent acute attacks of skeletal muscle weakness or paralysis associated with hypokalemia • Attacks may last few hours to few days • Triggers: carbohydrates, sodium • Treatment: acetazolamide + potassium	• Avoid glucose and NS infusion, acidosis, hypothermia, β-agonists • NDMRs and SCh can be used safely (monitor) • Use mannitol for all infusion • Use potassium-sparing diuretic if diuresis is required intraoperatively • Frequent electrolyte monitoring → treat hypokalemia with potassium infusion up to 40 mEq/h
Kartagener syndrome	• Triad of chronic sinusitis, bronchiectasis, and situs inversus • Caused by impairment of cilia	• Treat any active pulmonary infection • EKG lead placement should be reversed • Left internal jugular should be considered for CVL cannulation • Double-lumen ETT positioning should be reversed according to anatomical changes • Nasal ETT should be avoided

Long QT syndrome (LQTS)	• Acquired versus congenital
	• Acquired:
	  ▸ Bradycardia
	  ▸ High-degree AV block
	  ▸ Hypokalemia, hypocalcemia, hypomagnesemia
	  ▸ Cirrhosis
	  ▸ Amiodarone, tricyclic antidepressants, phenothiazines, vasodilators
	• Congenital:
	  ▸ Isolated: autosomal dominant
	  ▸ Associated with deafness: autosomal recessive
	• Syncope associated with stress, emotion, exercise, or sympathetic stimulation
	• QTc exceeds 460–480 ms
	• Most common EKG finding during syncope is polymorphic ventricular tachycardia = torsades de pointes
	• Correction of electrolyte abnormalities (K or Mg) treats LQTS
	• Pacing with β-blocker therapy is also used
	• Incidence higher in women than in men
		• Preoperative EKG should be obtained in patients with family history of sudden death or unexplained syncope
		• Both Isoflurane and sevoflurane can prolong QTc–one is not better than the other
		• Droperidol and antiemetics should also be used with caution
		• Avoid sympathetic stimulation and hypokalemia (associated with hyperventilation)
		• Defibrillator should be readily available

(continued)

Disease	Disease characteristics	Anesthetic considerations
Lupus	• Multisystem chronic inflammatory disease • Typically affects young women • Stresses such as infection, pregnancy, or surgery worsen lupus • Symmetrical arthritis in the hands, wrists, elbows, knees, and ankles is common • Systemic manifestations appear in the central nervous system, heart, lungs, kidneys, liver, neuromuscular system, and skin	• Anesthetic management affected by organ system and extension of involvement • Patients may be on steroids → may need perioperative supplementation • Laryngeal involvement may occur in one third of patients → approach intubation with caution (cricoarytenoid dislocation)
Marfan syndrome	• Autosomal dominant connective tissue disorder • "Abe Lincoln" appearance • High-arched palate, pectus excavatum, kyphoscoliosis, and hyperextensibility of the joints • Early pulmonary emphysema, spontaneous PTX, lens dislocation may be features • Cardiac abnormalities → aortic dilation, dissection, or rupture, mitral valve prolapse • Cardiac conduction abnormalities	• Cardiac assessment should be thorough with echo • Avoid TMJ dislocation • Avoid sustained increase in systemic blood pressure → ↑ risk of aortic dissection • TEE should be considered • Maintain high suspicion for PTX
Menkes syndrome	• X-linked recessive • Abnormal copper absorption and metabolism • Neurologic: spasticity, seizures + bone involvement • Collagen disease (similar to Ehlers–Danlos) possible, with fragile tissues and valve involvement • Frequent upper airway infection	• Continue anticonvulsant treatment • Risk of regurgitation • Avoid succinylcholine (risk of hyperkalemia) • Infections can lead to upper airway stenosis; have small ETT available • Pharyngeal obstruction postoperatively (poor muscle tone): monitor like OSA
Mitochondrial myopathies	• Skeletal muscle energy metabolism dysfunction • Abnormal fatigability with sustained exercise, skeletal muscle pain, and progressive weakness • May affect brain, heart, liver, and kidneys	• Dilated cardiomyopathy and CHF • Susceptible to drug-induced myocardial depression, cardiac conduction defects, and hypoventilation • Preoperative respiratory function assessment, swallow evaluation for intact pharyngeal and laryngeal reflexes → impairment might lead to inability to clear secretions and aspiration

(*continued*)

Disease	Disease characteristics	Anesthetic considerations
Motor neuron disorders (ALS [Lou Gehrig's disease], progressive bulbar palsy, progressive muscular atrophy, primary lateral sclerosis, and progressive pseudobulbar palsy)	• ALS: upper and lower motor neuron deficits, progressive disease • Skeletal muscle atrophy, weakness, and fasciculations including the tongue, pharynx, larynx, and chest • Fasciculations of the tongue plus dysphagia lead to pulmonary aspiration • Autonomic nervous system dysfunction manifests as orthostatic hypotension and resting tachycardia • Ocular muscles are spared	• Exaggerated ventilatory depression with GA • Vulnerable to hyperkalemia following administration of SCh • Prolonged responses to NDMRs • Pharyngeal muscle weakness may lead to pulmonary aspiration; glycopyrrolate to reduce secretions • Epidural anesthesia has been used with success without neurologic impairment
Moyamoya disease	• Progressive stenosis of intracranial vessels with development of secondary capillary network for collateral flow • "Puff of smoke" finding on angiogram • Might be familial, but can develop following head trauma, or be associated with neurofibromatosis, tuberous sclerosis, and fibromuscular dysplasia • Higher incidence of aneurysms • Ischemia in children, hemorrhage in adults	• Treatment is directed at controlling ischemia • Extracranial–intracranial bypass is a surgical treatment • Preoperative neurologic deficits should be evaluated and noted • Place invasive blood pressure monitoring prior to induction • Avoid hypocapnia or vasoconstrictors (to avoid worsening ischemia) • Maintain hemodynamic stability • Avoid ketamine for induction and use SCh with caution in patients with neurologic deficits • Consider colloid or NS for maintenance IVF
Myopathies (Duchenne, Becker, Steinert, etc.)	• Duchenne: X-linked (males only), death before age of 20 years • Steinert: myotonia (impaired relaxation)—most common in adults • Hereditary pain degeneration and atrophy of skeletal muscle • Sensation and reflexes are intact • Cardiac muscle degeneration → cardiomyopathy and dysrhythmias • Respiratory muscle weakness → ↑ secretions, ↓ pulmonary reserve, more PNA • Worsened by pregnancy; uterine atony	• Preoperative: assess degree of weakness, triggers, obtain echo (Duchenne), Holter (Steinert), assess respiratory function (PFTs if needed) • SCh is contraindicated → ↑ risk of rhabdomyolysis, hyperkalemia, cardiac arrest • Gastric hypomotility → ↑ risk of aspiration • Response to NDMRs is normal; monitor, avoid neostigmine • Dantrolene should be readily available • Monitoring should be directed at detecting MH • Regional anesthesia preferred • Postoperative pulmonary dysfunction should be anticipated • Avoid myocardial depressants → use propofol and volatile anesthetics with caution

(continued)

Disease	Disease characteristics	Anesthetic considerations
Osteogenesis imperfecta (Lobstein disease)	• Autosomal dominant connective tissue disease affecting bones, sclera, and inner ear • "Brittle bone" disease • Affects females more than males • Blue sclera, impaired platelet function, and hyperthermia with hyperhidrosis may be features • Increased serum thyroxine is present in 50% of patients	• Desmopressin may help normalize platelet function • Neuraxial block OK if coagulation normal • BP cuff can cause humeral fracture • SCh-induced fasciculations can induce fractures • Usually have decreased cervical motion secondary to bone remodeling • DL should be approached with caution secondary to ↑ risk of fractures; protect teeth • Awake FOB should be considered if suspicion of difficult airway • Kyphoscoliosis and pectus excavatum may lead to ↓ vital capacity • Monitor temperature (risk of hyperthermia)
Paget disease (of bone)	• Might be familial, with more men affected • Abnormal osteoblastic and osteoclastic activity → weak and enlarged bones; increased blood flow to bone and overlying soft tissues; possible high cardiac output heart failure • ↑ alkaline phosphatase • Fractures, arthritis, nerve compression, paraplegia, hypercalcemia, and renal calculi may be present	• Surgical treatment involves joint replacement, osteotomies, or decompressive surgery • Evaluate cervical spine stability • Possible difficult neuraxial block
Phacomatoses (Bourneville, von Recklinghausen, von Hippel–Lindau, etc.)	• Autosomal dominant mutations • Benign tumors of different organ systems • Treatment and complications are determined by system involvement • Features include, for example, mental retardation, seizures, facial angiofibromas, cardiac rhabdomyoma, spinal cord or intracranial tumors, retinal angiomas, cancer, or endocrine abnormalities • Impaired renal function and cardiac arrhythmias may be present	• Evaluate upper airway, mediastinal, and spinal (especially cervical) abnormalities preoperatively • Have antiepileptic medications ready • Consider possibility of pheochromocytoma → tx with antihypertensives prior to surgery if known • Nervous system involvement may limit use of neuraxial anesthesia • Response to anesthetics is usually normal • Response to NDMRs and SCh may be exaggerated

(continued)

Disease	Disease characteristics	Anesthetic considerations
Pierre Robin syndrome	• Micrognathia with glossoptosis and cleft palate • Acute upper airway obstruction, difficulty feeding, failure to thrive, and cyanosis are features • Patients may develop chronic hypoxemia and pulmonary HTN from chronic airway obstruction • Occasionally associated with Stickler syndrome (progressive arthro-ophthalmopathy, neurosensory deafness)	• Evaluate upper airway carefully • Anticholinergics to ↓ airway secretions • Avoid opiates and sedatives prior to intubation • Emergency FOB, LMA, cricothyrotomy, tracheostomy supplies should be readily available at the bedside • Avoid use of muscle relaxants until airway is secured • Awake nasal or oral FOB intubation can be attempted after appropriate topicalization of the airway • Inhalation induction and FOB with jaw lift maneuver can be attempted after adequate depth of anesthesia is obtained • Extubation should only be undertaken when patient is fully awake and alert; risk of obstruction with hypoxemia and negative pressure pulmonary edema
Polyarteritis nodosa	• Vasculitis that most often occurs in women and in association with hepatitis B antigenemia and allergic reactions to drugs • Small- and medium-sized artery involvement resulting in HTN, glomerulitis, CAD and myocardial ischemia, peripheral neuropathy, and seizures • Asthma	• Coexisting renal disease, HTN, and cardiac disease should guide anesthetic management • Corticosteroid supplementation may be necessary • Titrate NMB carefully • Risk of pharyngolaryngeal edema
Polymalformative syndromes (Apert, Crouzon, Dandy Walker, etc.)	• Craniosynostosis, maxillary hypoplasia, relative mandibular prognathism • May have eye and ear, cardiac, spine defect • May have elevated ICP	• Careful airway evaluation • May have difficult mask fit, limited mouth opening, choanal atresia • Consider awake FOB intubation • Preoperative evaluation of concurrent abnormalities • Avoid muscle relaxants until airway is established • BP control is necessary to prevent uncontrolled intracranial hypertension

(continued)

Disease	Disease characteristics	Anesthetic considerations
Prader–Willi	• Chromosomal abnormality • Hypotonia at birth, associated with weak cough, swallowing difficulty, and airway obstruction; repeated aspiration leads to hypoxemia and pulmonary HTN • Hyperphagia, obesity, and DM develop as children get older • Pickwickian syndrome, mental retardation, micrognathia, a high-arched palate, strabismus, a straight ulnar border, congenital dislocation of the hip, dental caries, and seizures can all be present • Altered carbohydrate metabolism	• Intraoperative glucose monitoring and administration are necessary • Adjust anesthetic doses for ↓ skeletal muscle mass and ↑ fat content • SCh has been administered without adverse reaction in these patients • Increased incidence of perioperative aspiration; use RSI • Risk of hypothermia/hyperthermia; no association with MH
Pseudocholinesterase deficiency	• Plasma pseudocholinesterase deficiency will prolong the effect of succinylcholine, mivacurium, ester LAs, esmolol and ASA • Acquired deficit: liver failure, malnutrition, pregnancy • Genetic deficit: autosomal recessive	• Avoid succinylcholine; paralysis for several hours (homozygous), shorter if heterozygous. Often Phase 2 block • Mivacurium: also prolonged block • Supportive treatment; give cholinesterase if available, or FFP • Give card/letter; test family members
Psoriasis	• Very common (1–2% of population) • Accelerated epidermal growth resulting in inflammatory erythematous papules covered with loosely adherent scales • Skin lesions are remitting and relapsing • May be symmetrical or asymmetrical • High output cardiac failure may be present • Patients may be treated with coal tar shampoo, salicylic acid ointment, topical corticosteroids, topical retinoid or systemic therapy with methotrexate or cyclosporine or biologic therapy with monoclonal antibodies • Cirrhosis, renal failure, HTN, pneumonitis, and arthritis possible	• Anesthetic considerations should include treatment of side effects from psoriasis therapy • Skin trauma from IV may accelerate plaque development • Increased skin blood flow may alter thermoregulation • Do not insert lines or perform RA through lesions (frequent *Staphylococcus aureus*)

(continued)

Disease	Disease characteristics	Anesthetic considerations
RA, Still's disease (juvenile RA)	• Chronic inflammatory arthritis • Symmetrical polyarthropathy and significant systemic involvement • Atlantoaxial subluxation and cricoarytenoid arthritis are common • Systemically, vasculitis, pericarditis, myocarditis, coronary artery arteritis, accelerated coronary atherosclerosis, cardiac valve fibrosis, cardiac nodules, pericardial and/or pleural effusion may be present • Pericarditis, conduction abnormalities, valvular involvement with regurgitation • Restrictive syndrome, sometimes severe, more frequent in males; fibrosis; bronchiectasis; bronchiolitis; side effects (e.g., interstitial pneumonia from MTX, infection from immunosuppression, TB from anti-TNF) • Renal: amyloidosis or side effects of therapies • Anemia, hypersplenism • Peripheral nerve vasculitis, ocular involvement	• *Flexion–extension cervical x-rays*: >3 mm distance from anterior arch of the atlas to the odontoid process indicates atlantoaxial subluxation • Minimize head and neck movement during DL • Crycoarytenoid involvement causes airway narrowing: use small ETT • ↓ mouth opening → difficult DL; consider awake FOB intubation • Fragile skin, joint deformity: careful positioning and padding • If any doubt, get PFTs; the earliest abnormality is a decrease in DLCO • Get EKG and TTE • Neuropathies: evaluate clinically • Consider steroid supplementation • Platelet function may be affected secondary to NSAID or ASA use • Penicillamine can lead to prolonged NMB
Scleroderma	• Inflammation, vascular sclerosis, fibrosis of the skin and viscera • Pericarditis, dysrhythmias, conduction abnormalities • Pulmonary fibrosis, pleural effusion, pulmonary HTN • Glomerulonephritis • Raynaud • CREST syndrome (*c*alcinoses, *R*aynaud phenomenon, *e*sophageal hypomotility, *s*clerodactyly, *t*elangiectasia)	• Avoid SCh: risk of rhabdomyolysis • May need FOB intubation secondary to small mouth opening and taut skin • IV access may be difficult due to dermal thickening • May need invasive arterial monitoring → use caution secondary to ↑ risk of ischemia secondary to Raynaud • Avoid gastric tube (esophageal involvement) • Hypotension may occur secondary to intravascular volume depletion • ↑ risk of regurgitation secondary to LES hypotonia • Avoid hypoxia and acidosis → ↑ pulmonary vascular resistance • Patients may be particularly sensitive to opioids and need ventilator support postoperatively • Regional anesthesia may be difficult but would ↑ peripheral vasodilation

(continued)

Disease	Disease characteristics	Anesthetic considerations
Shy-Drager syndrome (multiple system atrophy)	• Multiple system atrophy: degeneration and dysfunction of various central nervous system structures (basal ganglia, vagus nucleus, brain stem, spinal cord tracts) • Autonomic nervous system dysfunction (CN IX and X) → orthostatic hypotension (BP drop >30 mm Hg without tachycardia), anhidrosis, urinary retention, bowel dysfunction, and sexual impotence • Upregulated expression of α-adrenergic receptors • Can be a feature of other diseases (advanced DM, syringomyelia, Parkinson)	• Preload with IV fluid, have pressors available (exaggerated response to ephedrine, phenylephrine preferred), as no adrenergic response to anesthesia or surgery; possible initial 50 µg phenylephrine, and then 5 µg/kg/min infusion to prevent hypotension • Can use neuraxial anesthesia but be vigilant about BP response • Exaggerated hypotension with volatile anesthetics • Treat bradycardia promptly with atropine or glycopyrrolate • Monitor temperature; risk of hyperthermia • Possible laryngospasm on extubation ⇒ reintubate with SCh; rarely need for tracheotomy
Sjögren's	• Chronic inflammatory disease • Keratoconjunctivitis sicca, xerostomia, and RA • Primarily affects women • May have parotid and submandibular gland enlargement	• Dry eyes and dry mouth: use artificial tears; rebreathing circuit to allow for added humidification • May have difficulty visualizing vocal cords secondary to gland enlargement • Avoid anticholinergic agents that further inhibit secretions
Spherocytosis	• Autosomal dominant • Defect in spectrin and ankyrin • Patients may be clinically silent • Symptoms include mild hemolytic anemia, splenomegaly, and easy fatigability • Hemolytic crisis can be precipitated by viral or bacterial infection • Aplastic crisis can be precipitated by parvovirus B19 infection	• Anesthetic consideration relates to degree of severity of anemia • Patients may complain of biliary colic secondary to pigment cholelithiasis
Spinal and cerebellar degenerative diseases (e.g., Friedreich's ataxia)	• Friedreich's ataxia: autosomal recessive • Cardiomyopathy and kyphoscoliosis are prominent • Ataxia, dysarthria, nystagmus, skeletal muscle weakness, spasticity, and diabetes mellitus may all be present • Usually fatal by adulthood secondary to cardiac failure	• If cardiomyopathy is present, avoid inotropy-reducing drugs • Response to muscle relaxants is normal • Kyphocoliosis may affect patient positioning and make epidural anesthesia more difficult; consider spinal anesthesia instead • Likelihood of respiratory failure is higher

(continued)

Disease	Disease characteristics	Anesthetic considerations
Storage disorders (glycogenoses, lipids, amino acids, mucopolysaccharides, etc.)	Glycogen storage diseases • Lack of enzymes leads to buildup of intermediate products • Hypoglycemia can be severe → need frequent feeding to maintain blood glucose • Chronic metabolic acidosis, osteoporosis, mental retardation, growth retardation, and seizures	• Arterial pH and glucose monitoring • Glucose administration intraoperatively if needed • Avoid LR → may worsen metabolic acidosis • Avoid hyperventilation to avoid respiratory alkalosis leading to skeletal muscle lactate release
	Impaired amino acid metabolism • Mental retardation, seizures, aminoaciduria, metabolic acidosis • Hyperammonemia, hepatic failure, and thromboembolism	• Maintain fluid balance and avoid acid–base imbalance • Avoid anesthetics that lower seizure threshold
	Lipids • Sphingolipidoses, gangliosidoses, leukodystrophies • Encephalopathy • Variable visceral involvement: kidney, liver, adrenal, blood vessels	• Assess visceral involvement
	Impaired purine metabolism • Lesch–Nyhan syndrome → increased uric acid production • Mental retardation, seizures, self-mutilation, renal failure	• Avoid renal toxic and renally cleared agents • Caution when using SCh • Caution when using catecholamines
	Mucopolysaccharosidases • Hurler, Hunter, San Filippo, pseudo-Hunter • Encephalopathy, ataxia, facial dysmorphia, liver, bones	• Assess visceral involvement
Systemic mastocytosis	• Mast cell proliferation in all organ systems except CNS • May have spontaneous degranulation with release of histamine, heparin, prostaglandins, and numerous enzymes • Pruritus, urticaria, flushing, severe hypotension, and tachycardia may result • Bronchospasm and bleeding are unusual	• Life-threatening anaphylactoid reactions with surgery are possible • Epinephrine should be readily available • Patients should undergo preoperative skin testing for anesthetic agents • Patients should be pretreated with an H_1 and an H_2 histamine receptor antagonist and glucocorticoid prior to dye contrast study

(continued)

Disease	Disease characteristics	Anesthetic considerations
Takayasu arteritis	• Idiopathic, chronic, progressive occlusive vasculitis affecting systemic and pulmonary arteries • Inflammatory changes in aorta and branches • Seen in young Asian women • Patients may exhibit HA, vertigo, visual disturbances, seizures, or a stroke with hemiparesis or hemiplegia • Loss of arm pulses and/or bruits • V/Q abnormalities, pulmonary HTN, myocardial ischemia, conduction system abnormalities, renal artery stenosis, ankylosing spondylitis, and rheumatoid arthritis may all be present • Treatment involves corticosteroids, antiplatelet/anticoagulant therapy, ACEI or calcium channel blockers, bypass surgery as needed	• Must consider patients' medications and systemic involvement of disease • Establish effect of head position on patients' symptoms prior to induction of anesthesia • Evaluate pulmonary and renal function • Neuraxial anesthesia may be difficult secondary to anticoagulant therapy, musculoskeletal changes and associated hypotension; advantageous b/o increased blood flow • Short-acting anesthetics during GA will allow prompt evaluation of neurologic status • Noninvasive BP monitoring may be difficult/impossible: radial and/or femoral A-line may be necessary • Maintain BP stable: risk of necrosis in the territory of involved arteries • PA catheter or TEE may be necessary for major surgery • Intraoperative EEG monitoring may be indicated for patients with severely compromised carotid artery flow
Weber–Christian disease	• Nodular nonsuppurative panniculitis, nodular fat necrosis • Chronic, febrile disease with painful nodules in fat of any area of the body • Constrictive pericarditis • Adrenal insufficiency	• Avoid trauma to subcutaneous fat • Lower temperature with acetaminophen, not ice • Anesthetic management is affected by involved organ systems (heart, adrenal)

(continued)

Disease	Disease characteristics	Anesthetic considerations
Wegener's granulomatosis	• Necrotizing granulomas in inflamed blood vessels in the central nervous system, airways, lungs, cardiovascular system, and kidneys • May have narrowed glottis or subglottic area secondary to granulation tissue • Vasculitis → pulmonary vascular occlusion, hemoptysis, pleural effusion • Progressive renal failure	• Patients on cyclophosphamide therapy may have ↓ plasma cholinesterase activity (avoid SCh, mivacurium) • No prolongation of paralysis after SCh has been observed • Avoid traumatic DL and use smaller ETT • If arteritis is present, invasive arterial monitoring might be needed • If cardiac involvement, use volatile anesthetics with caution secondary to myocardial depression • Renal disease may influence choice of anesthetic and muscle relaxant
Wilson disease	• Autosomal recessive • Total body copper deposition ⇒ cirrhosis, encephalopathy, cataracts, renal failure (tubulopathy), cardiomyopathy • Treatment may be with trientine or penicillamine • Side effects of penicillamine include nausea, vomiting, leukopenia, pseudocholinesterase deficiency, and myasthenia-like syndrome • Thrombocytopenia	• Preoperative evaluation of anemia, cirrhosis, electrolyte abnormalities, renal and cardiac dysfunction should be thorough • Coagulation studies should be obtained and preoperative vitamin K given if PT is prolonged • Thrombocytopenia may require platelet transfusion • Hypoglycemia should be treated preoperatively • Hypoalbuminemia → ↓ protein binding → need to ↓ drug dose • Cardiomyopathy may make patients more sensitive to depressant effects of volatile anesthetics and more sensitive to catecholamines • Penicillamine: avoid SCh and mivacurium; monitor NMB

REFERENCES

For references, please visit **www.TheAnesthesiaGuide.com**.

PART III

MONITORING

CHAPTER 39
Intraoperative EKG
Ann E. Bingham, MD and Bessie Kachulis, MD

INTRAOPERATIVE ISCHEMIA DETECTION

The most sensitive leads for ST segment monitoring are V_3, V_4, and V_5.

Sensitivity of Various Lead Combinations for Detecting Ischemia			
London et al.		Landesberg et al.	
$II + V_2 + V_3 + V_4 + V_5$	100%		
$V_4 + V_5$	90%	$V_3 + V_5$	97%
$II + V_5$	80%	$V_4 + V_5$	92%
$II + V_4 + V_5$	96%	$V_3 + V_4$	100%
Single leads V_5, V_4, and V_3	75%, 61%, and 24%, respectively	Single leads V_5, V_4, and V_3	75%, 83%, and 75%, respectively

- Cardiac events are the most common cause of death in the perioperative period
- Unstable angina, myocardial infarction, and heart failure are estimated to occur in 1–10% depending on the risk of the surgical procedure and the severity of patient's disease
- Overall, 4% of patients undergoing noncardiac surgery have significant cardiac events

INTRAOPERATIVE ARRHYTHMIAS

May occur in 84% of patients during surgery.

Etiology: ischemia, anesthetics, electrolyte abnormalities, endotracheal intubation, reflexes, vagal stimulation, central nervous stimulation, intracranial hemorrhage, autonomic nervous system dysfunction, central venous cannulation, surgical manipulation of cardiac structures, pericardial effusion, hypothermia, acute pericarditis, pulmonary embolus.

THREE-ELECTRODE SYSTEM

- Electrodes are placed on the right arm (RA), left arm (LA), and left leg (LL)
- For bipolar leads (I, II, and III), one pair is selected for monitoring and the other one is used as a ground (i.e., the electrodes are positive, negative, and ground)

- While the three-lead system is useful for arrhythmia detection, it is of limited utility when monitoring for myocardial ischemia

MODIFIED THREE-ELECTRODE SYSTEM (SEE FIGURE 39-1)

- The modified three-electrode system includes modified chest leads (MCL), CS_5, CM_5, CB_5, and CC_5
- P waves are maximized for atrial dysrhythmia monitoring and there is increased sensitivity for detecting anterior wall ischemia

FIGURE 39-1. Modified three-lead systems to detect ischemia

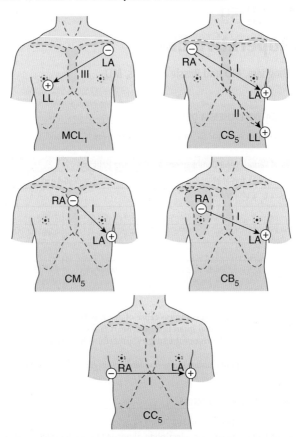

MCL_1: monitor lead III with LL electrode placed on right fifth intercostal space, on the medio-clavicular line; CS_5, monitor lead I with LA electrode placed on left fifth intercostal space on the anterior axillary line; monitor lead II with LL electrode in its normal position (for arrhythmia); CM_5, monitor lead I with RA electrode on sternal manubrium and LA electrode on left fifth intercostal space on the anterior axillary line; CB_5, monitor lead I with RA electrode over right scapula and LA electrode on left fifth intercostal space on the anterior axillary line; CC_5, monitor lead I with RA electrode on right fifth intercostal space on the anterior axillary line and LA electrode on left fifth intercostal space on the anterior axillary line. Reproduced with permission from Thys DM, Kaplan JA. *The ECG in Anesthesia and Critical Care*. New York: Churchill Livingstone, 1987. © Elsevier.

FIVE-ELECTRODE SYSTEM

- The five-electrode system allows the recording of the six limb leads (I, II, III, aVR, aVL, aVF) and a precordial unipolar lead, usually V_5
- Unlike the three-electrode systems, this allows monitoring several areas of the myocardium for ischemia, and distinguishing between atrial and ventricular arrhythmias

MONITOR SETUP

- Numerical values for the position of the ST may be displayed on screen. The measurement point is usually 60–80 milliseconds from J point but it can be adjusted
- Visual trend line may used to easily detect ST segment deviations
- On some monitors (Philips), ST segment and arrhythmia monitoring use a "fast learning algorithm" and 15 beats are required for rhythm recognition
- User selects primary and secondary ECG leads for single-lead or multilead arrhythmia analysis
- If the patient is paced, set the "Patient Paced" status to "Yes" so that pacer pulses are filtered out and not interpreted as QRS beats
- Filter selection limits artifacts (e.g., 60 Hz artifact from AC) but lowers the sensitivity

MONITOR LEARNING

According to Philips, the programmed algorithm "learns" the primary ECG lead when ECG monitoring is initiated, the relearn function is activated, a patient's paced status is changed, a "leads off" inoperative situation lasting longer than 60 seconds is corrected, or the ECG lead or lead label is changed. Do not set up learning when a ventricular rhythm is present. During the learning phase, the detection of asystole or ventricular fibrillation remains active.

ARTIFACTS

- Electrocautery
- Cardiopulmonary bypass
- SSEP/MEP monitoring

POSTOPERATIVE CONSIDERATIONS

- The majority of postoperative myocardial infarctions occur within 48 hours of surgery and the majority of those MIs are asymptomatic
- Changes in T wave or ST segment morphology are a common perioperative ECG finding in the general surgical population and are attributed to changes in catecholamines, ventilation, body temperature, electrolytes, or transient conduction abnormalities

REFERENCES

For references, please visit **www.TheAnesthesiaGuide.com**.

CHAPTER 40
Hemodynamic Monitoring

Seth Manoach, MD, CHCQM and
Jean Charchaflieh, MD, DrPH, FCCM, FCCP

INVASIVE MONITORING: PULMONARY ARTERY, CENTRAL VENOUS, AND RADIAL ARTERY CATHETERS

- Invasive hemodynamic monitoring relies on insertion of catheters into:
  - Systemic arteries: arterial catheter (*A-line*)
  - Central veins: central venous catheter (*CVC*)
  - The pulmonary artery: pulmonary artery catheter (*PAC*)
- These catheters allow clinicians to:
  - *Visualize waveforms* and measure pressures to perform continuous assessment of cardiac function
  - *Measure or derive cardiac output (CO)* and other key hemodynamic variables
  - *Sample and analyze oxygenation* of systemic arterial (SaO_2), central venous ($ScvO_2$), or mixed venous (pulmonary arterial) (SvO_2) blood from the catheters
  - Use this information to make diagnoses and guide treatment (Tables 40-1 and 40-2)

TABLE 40-1	Approximate Normal Ranges for Selected Hemodynamic Parameters in Adults
Parameter	Normal range
CVP	0–6 mm Hg
Right ventricular systolic pressure	20–30 mm Hg
Right ventricular diastolic pressure	0–6 mm Hg
PAOP	6–12 mm Hg
Systolic arterial pressure	100–130 mm Hg
Diastolic arterial pressure	60–90 mm Hg
MAP	75–100 mm Hg
CO	4–6 L/min
CI	2.2–4.2 L/min/m^2
SV	40–80 mL
SVR	800–1400 dyne s/cm^5
SVRI	1,500–2,400 dyne s/cm/m^2
PVR	100–150 dyne s/cm^5
PVRI	200–400 dyne s/cm^5/m^2
CaO_2	16–22 mL/dL
$C\overline{v}O_2$	~15 mL/dL
DO_2	400–660 mL/min/m^2
VO_2	115–165 mL/min/m^2

CaO_2, arterial oxygen content; $C\overline{v}O_2$, central venous oxygen pressure; CVP, mean central venous pressure; DO_2, systemic oxygen delivery; MAP, mean arterial pressure; PAOP, pulmonary artery occlusion (wedge) pressure; PVR, pulmonary vascular resistance; PVRI, pulmonary vascular resistance index; CO, cardiac output; CI, cardiac output indexed to body surface area (cardiac index); SV, stroke volume; SVR, systemic vascular resistance; SVRI, systemic vascular resistance index; VO_2, systemic oxygen utilization.

TABLE 40-2	Calculated Hemodynamic Parameters		
Variable	Formula	Normal	Units
Cardiac index	$\dfrac{\text{Cardiac output (L/min)}}{\text{Body surface area (m}^2)}$	2.2–4.2	L/min/m²
Total peripheral resistance	$\dfrac{(\text{MAP} - \text{CVP}) \times 80}{\text{Cardiac output (L/min)}}$	800–1400	dyne s/cm⁵
Pulmonary vascular resistance	$\dfrac{(\overline{\text{PA}} - \text{PAOP}) \times 80}{\text{Cardiac output (L/min)}}$	100–150	dyne s/cm⁵
Stroke volume	$\dfrac{\text{Cardiac output (L/min)} \times 1,000}{\text{Heart rate (beats/min)}}$	40–80	mL/beat
Stroke index (SI)	$\dfrac{\text{Stroke volume (mL/beat)}}{\text{Body surface area (m}^2)}$	20–65	mL/beat/m²
Right ventricular stroke work index	$0.0136 \, (\overline{\text{PA}} - \text{CVP}) \times \text{SI}$	30–65	g-m/beat/m²
Left ventricular stroke work index	$0.0136 \, (\text{MAP} - \text{PAOP}) \times \text{SI}$	46–60	g-m/beat/m²

$\overline{\text{PA}}$, mean pulmonary arterial pressure; g-m, gram meter; MAP, mean arterial pressure; CVP, central venous pressure; PA, mean pulmonary artery pressure; PAOP, pulmonary artery occlusion pressure.

- The *A-line* measures systemic systolic (*SBP*) and diastolic (*DBP*) blood pressure:
  ▸ Clinicians can use this to calculate perfusion pressures (cerebral, cardiac, and spinal cord)
  ▸ ABG, electrolytes, Hb, and *lactate* measurements from the *A-line* provide *downstream* or tissue bed perfusion indices and may help pinpoint "upstream" (e.g., cardiopulmonary or vascular) causes of ↓ oxygen delivery (DO_2)
  ▸ The *A-line* can also assess volume status and volume responsiveness:
    ▪ Patients must be sedated and/or pharmacologically paralyzed so they are synchronous with *mechanical positive pressure ventilation with Vt ≥8 mL/kg*. They must also be in sinus rhythm:
      ◆ Positive pressure ventilation causes ↓ right heart filling during inspiration, when intrathoracic pressures ↑, and ↑ filling during expiration
      ◆ Blood typically crosses the pulmonary vascular bed during half a respiratory cycle; thus, LV preload ↑ during inspiration, and vice versa. The timing can change depending on HR and RR
      ◆ This causes respiratory pulse pressure variation (*ΔPP*) in patients on the ascending part of the Starling curve
      ◆ Patients on the flat portion of the Starling curve (e.g., exacerbations of congestive heart failure, acute renal failure and volume overload, hypothermia) are preload insensitive and volume repleted or overloaded. *Stroke volume (SV) will not significantly change in these patients*
      ◆ *ΔPP >11–13% predicts relative hypovolemia and volume responsiveness*
      ◆ With severe intravascular volume depletion clinicians may observe gross ΔPP on the *A-line* tracing. Such patients may have significant ΔPP even when Vt <8 cm³/kg or during spontaneous respiration (Figure 40-1)
      ◆ *In spontaneous respiration, the respiratory RV–LV filling cycle and ΔPP is reversed, as inspiration causes a negative intrathoracic pressure and increases venous return and RV filling*

FIGURE 40-1. A-line tracing in hypovolemia

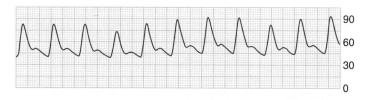

Radial artery tracing showing gross pulse pressure variation, indicating that the patient is very likely to be volume depleted/volume responsive. Reproduced from Longo DL, Fauci AS, Kasper DL, Hauser SL, Jameson JL, Loscalzo J. *Harrison's Principles of Internal Medicine.* 18th ed. Figure 267-4. Available at: www.Accessmedicine.com. Copyright © The McGraw-Hill Companies, Inc. All rights reserved.

- ‣ Some proprietary monitoring systems use ΔPP and complex age-adjusted analysis of *A-line* waveform to estimate CO
- ‣ New noninvasive systems use analogous respiratory cycle–based changes in the pulse oximetry waveform to predict volume responsiveness and estimate CO
- The *CVC*:
  - ‣ Measures *CVP*, which is ≈*RAP*:
    - ▪ Normal values for CVP are from 6 to 8, but rise with mechanical ventilation and PEEP
    - ▪ In patients with tricuspid regurgitation, primary right heart failure, or pulmonary hypertension this value may rise
    - ▪ In general, *low single-digit CVP values predict hypovolemia more accurately than elevated values predict volume overload*
  - ‣ *Can be used to measure ScvO$_2$* (central venous):
    - ▪ *ScvO$_2$* is typically ≈5% higher than $S\overline{v}O_2$ because it samples blood above the opening of the coronary sinus
    - ▪ Blood sampled from the SVC will be typically slightly more desaturated than blood from the IVC in an awake patient. The opposite is true when the patient is anesthetized
    - ▪ *ScvO$_2$* can be compared with SaO$_2$ to estimate oxygen extraction ratio (*O$_2$ER*) from the upper or lower VC territory:

$$O_2ER = \frac{VO_2}{DO_2} \times 100, \text{ usually } 20\text{–}30\%$$

- ▪ *O$_2$ER* usually rises if DO$_2$ (O$_2$ delivery) is insufficient to meet tissue demand, from a normal of 25% to 33%, to as low as to 67%. Beyond that, if DO$_2$ continues to fall, VO$_2$ falls and becomes delivery dependent
- ‣ Patients in sinus rhythm have a and v waves, with x and y descents in-between and a small c wave on the x descent (Figure 40-2)
- ‣ Mechanical events occur slightly later than electrical events, so the *a wave marking atrial contraction* follows the P wave and *occurs during the QRS* (Figure 40-2)
- ‣ *The v wave* shows an increase in atrial pressure as it fills during ventricular systole, when the tricuspid valve is closed. It *occurs during the T wave* (Figure 40-2)
- ‣ The x descent, between the a and v waves, marks falling pressure during atrial relaxation. The c wave may appear as the tricuspid valve closes during the x descent (Figure 40-2)

FIGURE 40-2. CVP tracing showing timing of a, c, and v waves, and x and y descents relative to EKG

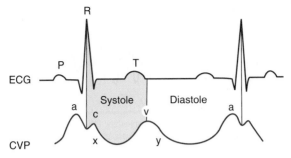

- ▸ During ventricular relaxation the tricuspid valve reopens, and the y descent marks the pressure drop as blood drains from the RA to the RV (Figure 40-2)
- ▸ Large a waves may occur with tricuspid stenosis or AV dissociation (cannon a waves), as the atrium contracts against a stenotic or closed TV, and large v waves may occur with tricuspid regurgitation
- The PAC:
  - ▸ Is most commonly inserted through the right internal jugular (RIJ) or left subclavian (LSC) veins
  - ▸ If the catheter is placed through the RIJ or LSC, SVC/RAP waves typically appear at 10–15 cm. The balloon is usually inflated at 20 cm mark with 1–1.5 mL of air
  - ▸ The balloon is *always inflated prior to advancing the catheter, and deflated before the catheter can be withdrawn*
  - ▸ As the catheter is advanced into the *RV* (20–30 cm), the *tracing becomes a single steep systolic wave that peaks on the T wave, descends steeply, and then slowly rises during diastolic RV filling* (Figure 40-3)
  - ▸ Because *RV passage can induce ventricular tachycardia*, the catheter is rapidly advanced into the PA (40–55 cm). The *PA systolic wave is also seen during the T wave, but pulmonic valve closure and arterial elasticity cause higher PA than RV diastolic pressures*

Distinguishing RV and PA

- During diastole, as blood flows into the LA, *PA pressure falls*, while *it rises in the RV during diastole* with RV filling (Figure 40-3).
- Higher diastolic pressure in the PA (*diastolic step-up*).
- Presence of *dicrotic notch* in the PA waveform.

- ▪ The catheter can be advanced in the PA until it wedges (Figure 40-3) in a *zone III* branch (Figure 40-4). The pulmonary artery occlusion pressure (PAOP), also known as the pulmonary wedge (pulmonary capillary wedge pressure [PCWP]), is measured when the intrathoracic pressure is closest to zero, that is, at end-expiration (bottom of the waveform if the patient is on PPV, top if breathing spontaneously)
- ▸ The proportion of the lungs that is zone III can be reduced by high airway pressures and PEEP, and especially by changes in patient position. A CXR showing the tip of the catheter located in spatial coordinates below the level of the left atrium on a lateral film if the patient is supine is usually sufficient

FIGURE 40-3. **Changes in PAC waveform as catheter is advanced**

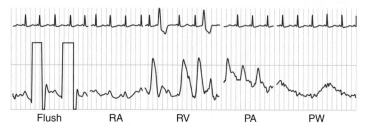

Flush   RA   RV   PA   PW

RA, right atrium; RV, right ventricle; PA, pulmonary artery; PW, pulmonary wedge (or PAOP).
Reproduced from Hall JB, Schmidt GA, Wood LDH. *Principles of Critical Care.* 3rd ed. Figure 13-4.
Available at: http://www.accessmedicine.com. Copyright © The McGraw-Hill Companies, Inc. All
rights reserved.

- The following characteristics suggest the tip is outside zone III:
  - "Smooth-looking" PAOP tracing with blunting of a and v waves
  - PADP <PAOP
  - Increase in PAOP >50% of change in alveolar pressure during PPV
  - Decrease in PAOP >50% of the reduction in PEEP
- The inflated balloon isolates the catheter tip from the right heart and LA pressure is transmitted by a continuous column of blood (Figure 40-4)
- The *PAOP waveform has the same features as the RAP tracing, but is phase shifted further right* because RAP is directly measured, while PAOP pressure waves pass from the LA, through pulmonary veins, alveolar capillaries, and distal PA branches
- As a result, the a wave falls after the QRS, and the v wave occurs after the T wave. When PA and PAOP pressures have similar appearances (e.g., in mitral regurgitation [MR]), *the phase shift allows the clinician to determine when the catheter is truly wedged*
- PAOP mean pressure is never ≥PA end-diastolic pressure (PAedp) and is typically ≈5 mm Hg lower than PAedp (Figures 40-3 and 40-5)
- *PAOP should be measured as the average height of the a wave during end-expiration, which is ≈LVedp when intrapleural pressure is closest to atmospheric pressure (Figure 40-5). The balloon should be left inflated for the shortest time possible and be reinflated only occasionally if there is a consistent relationship between PAOP and PAedp*
- In 1973, Swan and coworkers studied patients with myocardial infarction and identified 6–8 and 14–18 mm Hg for RAP and PAOP that corresponded to optimal ventricular preload. Despite assertions to the contrary, these values have proven to be remarkably consistent
- In MR, the v wave becomes prominent. When *LV myocardial ischemia leads to papillary muscle dysfunction and MR, pathognomonic new large v waves may appear on the PAOP tracing*
- The PAC has lumens that open into the right atrium and pulmonary arteries. By measuring O_2 saturation from sensors or from blood taken at the opening of each catheter lumen one can compare:
  - $ScvO_2$ to SvO_2:
    - If SvO_2 ≥5% higher than $ScvO_2$, intracardiac left-to-right shunt (e.g., a VSD or an ASD) should be ruled out with an echographic bubble study

FIGURE 40-4. Zones of the lung according to West

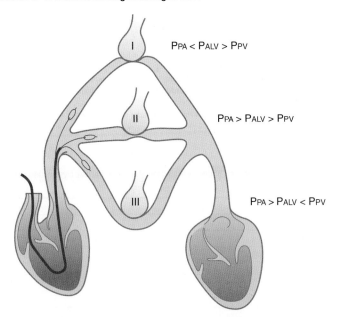

I $P_{PA} < P_{ALV} > P_{PV}$

II $P_{PA} > P_{ALV} > P_{PV}$

III $P_{PA} > P_{ALV} < P_{PV}$

P_{PA}, pulmonary artery pressure; P_{ALV}, alveolar pressure; P_{PV}, pulmonary vein pressure.
In zone I, there is (theoretically) no blood flow.
In zone II, blood flow happens only intermittently, when $P_{PA} > P_{ALV}$.
In zone III, blood flow is continuous.
Reproduced with permission from O'Quin R, Marini JJ. Pulmonary artery occlusion pressure: clinical physiology, measurement, and interpretation. *Am Rev Respir Dis.* 1983;128:319.

- SaO$_2$ from an *A-line* to SvO$_2$ from the PAC. This measures AVDO$_2$ or O$_2$ER. See chapter 220:
  - If $O_2ER \geq 1/3$ of SAO_2, DO_2 is likely to be inadequate. Typically, unless the patient is very hypoxemic or the CO is very low, the most efficient way to increase DO$_2$ is by transfusing RBCs. However, transfusion in itself might worsen outcomes
- To measure CO one injects room temperature saline into the RAP port of the PAC:
  - By measuring change in temperature over time at the distal port ($\int dT/dt$), one can calculate CO
  - *CO varies inversely with the area under the curve* described by $\int dT/dt$. This curve is usually displayed on the monitor when one performs *thermodilution*
  - Conceptually, with ↑ CO, the saline mixes with more warm blood, and moves more quickly past the distal port, so the change in temperature, $\int dT/dt$, falls as CO rises
  - Using cold saline decreases the signal noise, but is no longer used as it can trigger bradycardia
- One can theoretically plot LV filling pressures against corresponding SVs to derive a Frank–Starling curve
  - In practice, this translates into a key principle that is broadly applicable to other indices in hemodynamic monitoring: observation of an individual's optimal filling pressures and comparisons within a given individual over time are often much more important than tabulated normal values, that is, *trends in the same patient matter more than absolute values*

- With an *A-line*, PAC, and a single EKG tracing one can derive a comprehensive real-time hemodynamic profile. This includes CO; heart rate; oxygenation; and mean arterial, right atrial, pulmonary artery, and pulmonary artery occlusion (*PAOP* or *wedge*) pressures to calculate DO_2, VO_2, *SVR*, *PVR*, O_2ER, *SV*, and other indices (Tables 40-1 to 40-3):
  ▸ These data can be used to *determine whether a patient's DO_2 is adequate to meet end-organ demand* and if not:
    ▪ Diagnose problems with intravascular volume, valves, right or left ventricular performance, pulmonary or systemic vascular tone, or pulmonary function
    ▪ *Direct treatment accordingly*
  ▸ *Multiple studies have shown that many clinicians do not correctly interpret and act on hemodynamic data*

TABLE 40-3	Hemodynamic Changes in Common Shock and Cardiac Dysfunction States						
Disease state	RA	RV	PA	PCWP	CO	SVR	MAP
Cardiogenic shock	↑	↑	↑	↑	↓	↑	↓
Hypovolemic shock	↓	↓	↓	↓	↓	↑	↓
Cardiac tamponade	↑	↑	↑	↑	↓	↑	↓
Congestive heart failure (biventricular)	↑	↑	↑	↑	↓	↑	↓
Primary RV failure	↑	↑	↓	↓	↓	↑	↓
LV failure	↑	↑	↑	↑	↓	↑	↓
Septic shock	N or ↓	N or ↓	N or ↓	N or ↓	↑	↓	↓
ARDS	N or ↑	N or ↑	N or ↑	N or ↓	N, ↑, ↓	N, ↑, ↓	N, ↑, ↓
Acute pulmonary embolism	↑	↑	↑	↓	↓	↑	↓
Ventricular septal defect	↑	↑	↑	↑	↓	↑	↓
COPD	↑	↑	↑	N	↓	↑	↓
Constrictive pericarditis	↑	↑	↑	↑	↓	↑	↓
Restrictive pericarditis	↑	↑	↑	↑	↓	↑	↓
Primary pulmonary hypertension	↑	↑	↑	N	↓	N	↓

RA, right atrial pressure; RV, right ventricular pressure; PA, pulmonary artery pressure; PCWP, pulmonary capillary wedge pressure; CO, cardiac output; SVR, systemic vascular resistance; MAP, mean arterial pressure; ↑, increased; ↓, decreased; N, normal; ARDS, acute respiratory distress syndrome; COPD, chronic obstructive pulmonary disease.

Reproduced with permission from Hanley M, Welsh C. *Current Diagnosis & Treatment in Pulmonary Medicine.* New York: McGraw-Hill; 2003. Table 5-4. Copyright © The McGraw-Hill Companies, Inc. All rights reserved.

REFERENCES

For references, please visit **www.TheAnesthesiaGuide.com**.

CHAPTER 41
Noninvasive Cardiac Output Monitoring

Sarah C. Smith, MD

Comparison of Available Noninvasive Cardiac Output Monitors			
	Advantages	Limitations	Truly noninvasive?
CO_2 Fick principle, for example, NICO®	• Good agreement between NICO® and ultrasound transit time • Patient may be breathing spontaneously or on a ventilator	• Accuracy adversely affected by hyperventilation and V/Q mismatch (preexisting lung disease or postoperative atelectasis)	Yes; however, patient must be intubated
Esophageal Doppler, for example, CardioQ (single use), WAKIe TO (reusable)	• High validity for monitoring changes in cardiac output in critically ill patients • Using esophageal Doppler to optimize fluid management has been shown to improve outcomes	• Patient must be intubated and sedated • Small risk of injury to the esophagus • Limited agreement with thermodilution	No, requires placement of probe in the esophagus
Transpulmonary lithium dilution, for example, LiDCO	• High signal-to-noise ratio • Good agreement with thermodilution • Low risk of toxicity	• Not approved for patients <40 kg, pregnant women, or patients taking lithium • Accuracy reduced by aortic insufficiency, intra-aortic balloon pump, nondepolarizing NMB	No, requires an intra-arterial line
Arterial pulse contour analysis, for example, Vigileo®	• Good agreement with other methods of cardiac output determination • Continuous measurement of SV and CO • Also display SVV (SV variation) with a value >15% indicating fluid responsiveness • Easy to use	• Adversely affected by a poor arterial waveform (arrhythmia, intra-aortic balloon pump) • Older devices may not adequately compensate for changes in vascular tone • Newer devices have good agreement with thermodilution and esophageal Doppler	No, requires an intra-arterial line
Bioimpedance, for example, Cheetah NICOM®, BioZ Dx®	• Completely noninvasive • Impedance to high-frequency current between electrodes on chest; estimates thoracic blood volume	• Relative hemodynamic stability required • Accuracy reduced by arrhythmias, aortic insufficiency, intra-aortic balloon pump • Contraindicated in patients with pacemakers	Yes, adhesive surface electrodes only

CO₂ FICK PRINCIPLE

- The indirect Fick equation is defined as the following:

$$CO = \frac{\dot{V}_{CO_2}}{C_{vCO_2} - C_{aCO_2}}$$

where $\dot{V}_{CO_2}$ is the CO_2 produced, C_{vCO_2} is the central venous CO_2 content, and C_{aCO_2} is the arterial CO_2 content. $\dot{V}_{CO_2}$ is determined by the minute ventilation and instantaneous CO_2 content. C_{aCO_2} is estimated from the end-tidal CO_2.
- By combining measurements during rebreathing and during normal ventilation, C_{vCO_2} can be eliminated from the equation
- To improve accuracy, shunt fraction can be estimated from F_iO_2 and Pao_2 from blood gases

ESOPHAGEAL DOPPLER

- A Doppler transducer is inserted into the esophagus of an anesthetized intubated patient such that the characteristic waveform of blood flow in the *descending* aorta is displayed
- The area under the aortic velocity envelope is calculated as a velocity time integral (VTI) that is referred to as the stroke distance (SD)
- The monitor utilizes a computer algorithm to determine the stroke volume (SV) and CO by multiplying the SD by the cross-sectional area of the descending aorta (Figure 41-1)

FIGURE 41-1. Typical esophageal Doppler descending aortic waveform

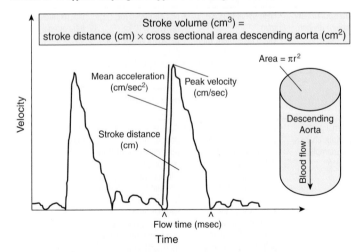

The area under the maximum aortic velocity envelope is calculated as a VTI (cm) and represents the SD. The monitor uses a proprietary algorithm to calculate the SV and CO based on the data labeled in the figure. The basic principle of this calculation is that assuming the cross-sectional area (CSA) of the aorta remains constant and that all blood cells are moving at maximum velocity during systole, stroke volume is the product of CSA and SD.

FIGURE 41-2. Spectral Doppler tracings of descending aorta blood flow

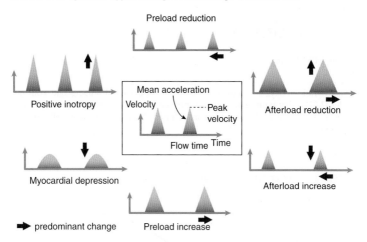

Changes in the velocity–time waveform shape result from alterations in contractility (mainly affect peak velocity and mean acceleration), preload (mainly affect systolic flow time corrected for heart rate [FTc]), and afterload (which affect FTc, mean acceleration, and peak flow velocity). Reproduced with permission from Singer M. Esophageal Doppler monitoring of aortic blood flow: beat-by-beat cardiac output monitoring. *Int Anesthesiol Clin*. 1993;31:99.

REFERENCES

For references, please visit **www.TheAnesthesiaGuide.com**.

CHAPTER 42
Pulse Oximeter

Ruchir Gupta, MD

Measures ratio of oxygenated to deoxygenated hemoglobin (Hb) using light-emitting diodes (LEDs) that emit light (red and infrared) of different wavelengths (660 and 940 nm). Oxygenated Hb absorbs more infrared light, whereas deoxy-Hb absorbs more red.

FIGURE 42-1. Oxygen Saturation Curve

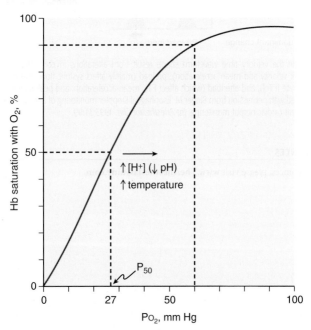

Oxyhemoglobin dissociation curve for whole blood.

An increase in temperature or a decrease in pH (as in working muscle) shifts this relationship to the right, reducing the hemoglobin saturation at the same Po_2 and thus aiding in the delivery of oxygen to the tissues.

P_{50} (Po_2 resulting in 50% saturation) = 27 mm Hg.

P_{90} = 60 mm Hg.

Reproduced from Brunton LL, Chabner BA, Knollmann BC. *Goodman & Gilman's The Pharmacological Basis of Therapeutics*. 12th ed. Figure 19-8. Available at: www.accessmedicine.com.

Causes of Erroneous Pulse Oximetry Readings	
Carboxy-Hb (HbCO)	Artificially higher reading than actual O₂ saturation
Met-Hb	Fixed at about 85%
IV methylene blue	Massive drop in measured saturation (artificial)
Poor perfusion (PVD, cold extremities)	Nonpulsatile waveform results in inaccurate measurement
Irregular rhythm (e.g., rapid atrial fibrillation)	Reading unreliable
Severe anemia (<5 g/dL)	Unreliable reading
Nail polish (black, blue, green)	Interferes with LED absorption by Hb causing lower reading or absence of reading
Onychomycosis	Interferes with LED absorption by Hb causing lower reading or absence of reading

MASIMO TOTAL HEMOGLOBIN (SPHB®)

- Proprietary system that uses "more than 7 wavelengths of light" to acquire data.
- Measures:
  - Total Hb (SpHb®)
  - Oxygen content (SpOC™)
  - Carboxyhemoglobin (SpCO®)
  - Methemoglobin (SpMet®)
  - Pleth Variability Index (PVI®)
  - Oxygen saturation (SpO₂), pulse rate (PR), perfusion index (PI)
- Estimates Hb concentration, and surrogates of tissue perfusion and cardiac output
- Time to loss of signal is longer and recovery time shorter with BP inflation if on same limb
- With good signal conditions, Masimo found to be more reliable than older oximeters
- In conditions of severe hypoxemia, Masimo found to be equivalent in accuracy to older oximeters

CO-OXIMETER

- Uses several different wavelengths to determine oxy-, carboxy-, and met-Hb percentages
- Can be used to accurately determine CO poisoning and methemoglobinemia
- "Fractional" saturation determined by:

$$\text{Fractional } S_{aO_2} = \frac{\text{oxyhemoglobin}}{\text{oxyhemoglobin} + \text{reduced Hb} + \text{HbCO} + \text{met-Hb}} \times 100$$

REFERENCES

For references, please visit **www.TheAnesthesiaGuide.com**.

CHAPTER 43
Capnography

Ruchir Gupta, MD

FIGURE 43-1. Normal capnogram

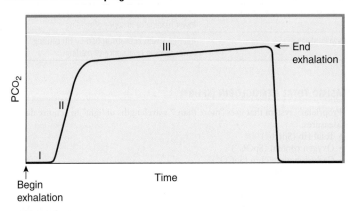

(I) Anatomic dead space.
(II) Transition from anatomic dead space to alveolar plateau.
(III) Alveolar plateau (typically slight upward slope).
Reproduced from Longnecker DE, Brown DL, Newman MF, Zapol WM. *Anesthesiology.* Figure 31-7.
Available at: http://www.accessanesthesiology.com. Copyright © The McGraw-Hill Companies, Inc.
All rights reserved.

GRADIENT BETWEEN EtCO₂ AND Paco₂

- Healthy lungs: 2–3 mm Hg awake, 5–8 mm Hg anesthetized
- COPD: up to 10 mm Hg awake, 15–20 mm Hg anesthetized
- Further increased by heat/moisture exchanger
- Further increased by V/Q mismatch: PE, hypovolemia, lateral position

Causes of Acute Changes in Capnogram	
Exponential decrease	Increased dead space (suspect PE or arrest)
Sudden drop to zero	Likely circuit disconnect
Gradual decrease but not to zero	Leakage or partial obstruction of airway
	Air embolism, PE
	Drop in CO: hypovolemia, IVC cross-clamping
	Decrease in metabolic rate: hypothermia, deep anesthesia
Gradual increase	Prolapse of expiratory valve or decreased minute ventilation
Sudden increase	Release of tourniquet, aortic unclamping, MH

FIGURE 43-2. **Changes in capnogram in different disease states**

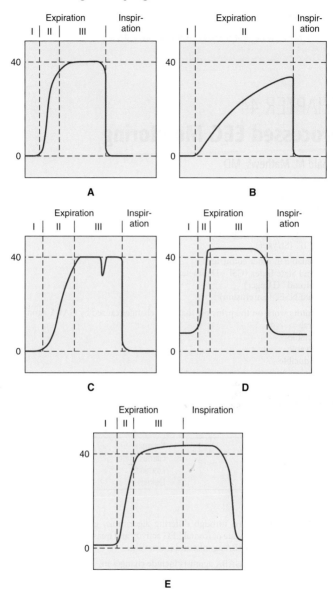

(A) A normal capnograph demonstrating the three phases of expiration: phase I—dead space; phase II—mixture of dead space and alveolar gas; phase III—alveolar gas plateau. (B) Capnograph of a patient with severe chronic obstructive pulmonary disease. No plateau is reached before the next inspiration. The gradient between end-tidal CO_2 and arterial CO_2 is increased. (C) Depression during phase III indicates spontaneous respiratory effort. (D) Failure of the inspired CO_2 to return to zero may represent an incompetent expiratory valve or exhausted CO_2 absorbent. (E) The persistence of exhaled gas during part of the inspiratory cycle signals the presence of an incompetent inspiratory valve. Reproduced from Morgan GE, Mikhail MS, Murray MJ. *Clinical Anesthesiology*. 4th ed. Figure 6-25. Available at: http://www.accessmedicine.com. Copyright © The McGraw-Hill Companies, Inc. All rights reserved.

REFERENCES

For references, please visit **www.TheAnesthesiaGuide.com**.

CHAPTER 44
Processed EEG Monitoring

Donald M. Mathews, MD

Currently available in the United States:
- Bispectral Index (BIS™, Covidien)
- SEDLine™ Patient State Index (PSI™, Masimo)
- M-Entropy™ (GE Healthcare)
- SNAP II™ (Stryker)

Also available in other countries:
- Cerebral State Index (CSI™, Danmeter)
- Narcotrend™ (Drager)
- NeuroSENSE™ (Carefusion)

All monitors work on the principle that EEG changes caused by GABA agonists are, in general:
- Predictable
- Observable
- Reproducible

Anesthetics and EEG	
Agents that correlate with processed EEG values	Agents that do not correlate with processed EEG values
Halogenated volatile gases	Ketamine
Propofol	Nitrous oxide
Benzodiazepines	Etomidate
Barbiturates	Opioids

Processed EEG monitors, through differing algorithms, generate an index value (0–100) that reflects the state of frontal EEG activity and quasi-linearizes the relationship between dose of GABA agonist and index value.

EEG changes seen with GABA agonists include changes in:
- Predominant frequencies
- Relative power distribution
- Phase relationship and randomness
- Pattern changes, such as burst suppression

EEG Waveform as a Function of Anesthetic Depth

Wave name	Associated frequencies (Hz)	Usual anesthetic state when prominent
γ (gamma) or β2	30–80	Conscious
β (beta)	12–30	Conscious or initial excitation with induction
ά (alpha)	8–12	Conscious with eyes closed and relaxed or general anesthesia (with spindles)
θ (theta)	4–8	General anesthesia
δ (delta)	0–4	Deep anesthesia

Pros and Cons of Using Processed EEG Monitors

Advantages	Disadvantages
• On average, less use of volatile agents or propofol • On average, faster emergence • On average, less time before eligible for PACU discharge • Potential to better identify unexpected outliers: those that require either more or less agent than average • Possible decrease in recall of unintended consciousness during surgery, particularly in the high-risk patient (but perhaps not better than utilizing end-tidal gas monitoring with alarms enabled) • Allow real-time display of one to four channels of raw frontal EEG	• Cost • Ideal use involves watching and interpreting raw EEG wave: most anesthesiologists do not have appropriate basic knowledge • No absolute value assures unconsciousness or consciousness • Values not real time: some processing time and smoothing functions cause a delay between change in state and change in index • In some patients, there appears to be a more quantal relationship between agent level and EEG than a linear one. In these patients with a "plateau," titrating agent levels down may result in a sudden state change with patient movement

Various EEG Monitors

Monitor	Recommended range for GA	Notes
BIS™	40–60	β ratio (related to activity in 30–47 Hz range) is component of upper range of index. Facial muscle EMG activity will increase this value and when EMG activity is present, BIS may be higher than expected. In this condition, BIS will decrease when NMB agents or antinociceptive medications given. Pediatric, bilateral sensor available
M-Entropy™	40–60	State entropy (SE, 0.5–32 Hz) range is 0–91; response entropy (RE, 0.5–47 Hz) range is 0–100. When RE is significantly higher than SE, facial EMG activity may be present and may represent opportunity to administer antinociceptive medications or NMBs. Unilateral sensor
SEDLine™ PSI™	25–50	Bilateral sensor. Four-channel EEG display. Monitor can display bilateral density spectral array (DSA)
SNAP II™	Not available	Index derived from 0 to 18 Hz and 80 to 420 Hz. Some comparative data in literature

Suggestions when using processed EEG monitors:

- Monitors are particularly helpful during propofol–TIVA anesthetics
- Display raw EEG whenever possible; learn usual EEG changes with drug administration, and during induction and emergence
- Learn to recognize sleep spindles (usually appropriate hypnotic state) and burst suppression (usually too deep hypnotic state)
- Use index value in the context of other information; do not make decisions based on this information alone
- If value seems incorrect, examine waveform to assure enough EEG power: often in the elderly patient these monitors have trouble due to inadequate EEG power
- Examine waveform for artifact, especially high-frequency artifacts: although artifact rejection is good, anything in OR environment that introduces signal and is not recognized as artifact can bias readings
- If agent is reduced significantly and the index value does not increase significantly, you may have patient in "plateau"
- Ketamine administration usually results in transient increase in index value, as do ephedrine and epinephrine
- Opioids and nitrous oxide do not grossly affect processed EEG per se; however, the chance of patient movement or somatic response at any particular processed EEG value decreases with increased use of these agents

PART IV

GENERAL ANESTHESIA

CHAPTER 45
Preoperative Anesthesia Checklist

Kriti Sankholkar, MD

BEFORE PATIENT ENTERS OPERATING ROOM

A. Machine checkout

The following monitors should be available for every anesthetic procedure:
- EKG leads (three- or five-lead)
- Pulse oximeter
- Noninvasive blood pressure monitor
- Temperature monitoring

Additional monitors depending on surgery type and patient history may include:
- Invasive arterial blood pressure monitoring
- Central venous pressure monitoring
- Pulmonary artery catheter monitoring
- Precordial Doppler
- EEG/BIS monitoring

The anesthesia machine should be checked every day and rechecked in between cases if different anesthesia equipment is used or if the anesthesia operator changes.

The following monitors should always be available:
- Oxygen analyzer
- Capnography
- Low- and high-pressure alarms
- Spirometer

Checkup procedure:
- Backup gas cylinders and Ambu-type bag valve mask device should be available in the room
- Turn on the machine master switch and all monitors
- A high-pressure system check should be performed with the oxygen cylinder supply and the central supply
- A value of 1,000 psi in an O_2 E cylinder indicates 340 L of O_2 (half-full) at atmospheric pressure, that is, it would last for 34 minutes at 10 L/min
- A low-pressure system leak test should be performed (tests for leaks from flow control valves to common gas outlet)
- Check flow meter function
- Calibrate the O_2 sensor
- Check leak test of breathing system
- Check manual ventilation and ventilator bellows
- Check integrity of unidirectional valves

- Check capnography function
- Check scavenging system and CO_2 absorber; change absorbent if necessary
- Ensure APL valve is in the open position and ventilator is set to "manual" prior to patient's arrival in OR

Additionally:
- Ensure that the MH box or cart is available and stocked
- Ensure defibrillator is in functioning condition and readily available
- If using local anesthetics, ensure lipid rescue is available and ready for use
- Ensure rapid transfuser is available and stocked for use if needed

B. Anesthesia setup

Can be remembered with the mnemonic **MSMAID**.

M—"machine"

- Perform machine check as indicated above

S—"suction"

- Ensure suction is available and attached to appropriate length of tubing to reach patient's head
- Attach Yankauer tip to end of tubing

M—"monitors"

- Ensure that monitors as indicated above are available, calibrated, and ready to be used
- All monitors should be of the appropriate size for the patient including blood pressure cuff size, arterial and central catheter sizes
- Ensure that disposable monitors are attached and ready to be used for the next patient such as EKG leads, pulse oximeter, and, in some cases, BP cuff
- A nerve stimulator should be readily available and functioning
- Fluid warmers and patient warming blankets and devices should also be readily available and functioning
- Have eye protection and lubricant ready

A—"airway"

- Check handle with light source and laryngoscope. Multiple functioning laryngoscope blade styles and sizes should be readily available in the OR
- Choose appropriate ETT size and style for procedure, with one size larger and one size smaller readily available
- Check ETT for cuff integrity. Stylet ETT or have stylets available
- Ensure appropriately sized oral and nasal airways and tongue depressors are available
- Have backup airway devices available such as GlideScope, fiber-optic bronchoscope, LMA
- Have stethoscope available
- Have devices or tape to secure ETT available
- Ensure vaporizers are adequately filled

I—"intravenous"

- Prepare IV line with appropriate choice of IV fluid and tubing setup
- Prepare IV start kit with gauze, alcohol swab, tourniquet, and appropriately sized catheters available
- Set up fluid warmer if necessary for the case
- Have rapid transfuser available if appropriate for procedure
- Have drug infusion pump ready if needed
- Have any IV medication drips ready if needed

D—"drugs"

At the minimum, emergency drugs and drugs needed for the case should be drawn up. These include:
- Sedative
- Induction agent
- Analgesic
- Neuromuscular blocker
- Antiarrhythmic (lidocaine)
- Vasopressor(s) (phenylephrine/ephedrine/epinephrine)
- Anticholinergic (atropine)
- Additional succinylcholine

Appropriate antibiotics should be available.

AFTER PATIENT ENTERS OR

- Confirm correct patient with at least two patient identifiers: name, date of birth, medical record number
- Confirm patient's procedure to be performed including side and site
- Confirm any allergies to medications or environment that patient may have
- When patient is lying on operating table, ensure appropriate patient positioning with regard to patient comfort
- Keep patient warm with blankets or warming device if possible
- Use sequential compression devices on lower extremities where indicated and place prior to induction of anesthesia
- After anesthesia induction, ensure that patient does not have undue pressure on any pressure points including head, eyes, ears, nose, elbows, knees, breasts, chest, abdomen, hips, or heels
- Ensure all bony prominences in contact with operating table are appropriately padded
- Do not hyperextend joints including arms at elbows and shoulder, knees, hips
- After intubation, ensure appropriate ventilator settings of tidal volume, peak inspiratory pressure, respiratory rate, F_iO_2, inhaled or intravenous anesthetic concentration, and flow meter rate
- Secure airway device with tape or holder
- Ensure eyes are adequately covered and protected
- Recheck patient's side and site of surgery and allergies prior to surgical incision

CHAPTER 46
Management of Total Intravenous Anesthesia (TIVA)

Donald M. Mathews, MD

- General anesthesia with intravenous agents requires administration of both hypnotic and antinociceptive medications

Agents Used for TIVA	
Hypnotic agents	Antinociceptive agents
Propofol	Opioids
Barbiturates	Ketamine
Benzodiazepines	Nitrous oxide
Etomidate	Alpha-2 agonists

- Total intravenous anesthesia (TIVA) usually accomplished with *propofol* and *opioid* agents, although other agents and combinations are possible

TIVA Using Propofol Compared with Balanced Anesthesia with Inhalational Agents	
	Comments
Advantages	
Less nausea	Multiple studies, true even with multimodal PONV prophylaxis
Better postoperative mood	Euphoria may be related to effect on internal cannabinoids
Less pain	Some suggestive data: low doses (0.1 MAC) of volatile agents are hyperalgesic (pain-worsening) in animal models
No malignant hyperthermia trigger	No need for dantrolene storage (assuming no succinylcholine usage)
No anesthesia machine	Highly portable anesthetic: just need monitors, delivery vehicles (pumps), and oxygen delivery equipment
Antioxidant properties	Free radical scavenging
No ambient gas in OR No greenhouse gases	Better for OR personnel, environment
Disadvantages	
More setup required	Must prepare agents
Possible propofol infusion syndrome	Rare: usually seen in prolonged ICU infusions in critically ill patients
Lipid overload	Only with prolonged infusion
No "ischemia-like" preconditioning	Volatile agents limit tissue damage from ischemia: whether this effect is more protective than propofol's antioxidant properties depends on experimental model

FIGURE 46-1. Schematic representation of synergistic relationship between propofol and opioids

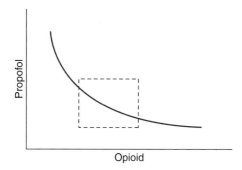

Dashed box represents "sweet spot" of interaction, combinations that allow adequate states of GA with relatively fast emergence.

PHARMACOKINETICS/DYNAMICS

- Propofol TIVA requires understanding of and attention to pharmacokinetic (Pk) and pharmacodynamic (Pd) principles
- Propofol infusions over time result in accumulation with increasing plasma levels: to maintain a stable level, rates must be decreased over time (see below)
- Context-sensitive half-time (time required for plasma level to fall 50%) of propofol is relatively predictable (approximately 20–40 minutes, depending on duration of infusion)
- Target-controlled infusion (TCI) pumps (not available in the United States) maintain stable predicted plasma or effect-site concentrations of propofol and opioids
- Propofol as a sole agent requires enormous doses to achieve state of general anesthesia
- Propofol infusion rates can be significantly decreased with the addition of moderate amounts of opioids because of a *synergistic* relationship

PROPOFOL DOSING STRATEGIES

Suggested Propofol Administration Schedules		
	"Low" schedule	"High" schedule
Bolus	2 mg/kg	2.5 mg/kg
First 15 min	100 µg/kg/min	150 µg/kg/min
15–45 min	80 µg/kg/min	125 µg/kg/min
After 45 min	70 µg/kg/min	100 µg/kg/min

- Propofol administration: with adequate opioid administration, most patients will have adequate propofol levels when infusions are delivered between the "low" and "high" dosing schedules (Figure 46-2)
- TCI targets of 2.5–4.0 µg/mL usually result in adequate dosing
- Processed EEG monitoring is useful in assisting with propofol titration: act as Pd monitor of adequacy of propofol level

FIGURE 46-2. Predicted plasma concentrations of propofol at "low" and "high" dosing schedules in the table

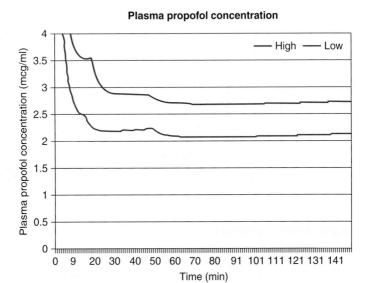

Note a need to decrease infusion rates to maintain stable levels. Also note some patients may require levels higher than these.

OPIOID DOSING STRATEGIES

- Usually accomplished with fentanyl congener (fentanyl, remifentanil, alfentanil, sufentanil) by bolus and infusion
- All but remifentanil require occasional decrement in infusion rate to prevent accumulation (decrease infusion rate by 10% every 45–60 minutes)
- Choose opioid based on desired speed of onset and offset characteristics (i.e., context-sensitive half-time). See Figure 58-1

Properties of Various Opioids			
Opioid	Onset time (min)	Context-sensitive half-time (min)	Comment about context-sensitive half-time with infusion greater than 2 h
Fentanyl	3.5–5	Variable	Quite prolonged. Disadvantage if levels are high; advantage if levels adequate for spontaneous respiration (prolonged postoperative analgesia)
Remifentanil	1–2	5	No change
Alfentanil	1–2	20–30	Slight increase
Sufentanil	5–6	20–40	Slight–moderate increase

- Remifentanil will require alternative opioids for postoperative pain
- Attempts should be made to deliver "just enough" for each patient to minimize the development of tolerance
- Ketamine 0.1–0.2 mg/kg may be effective in limiting development of tolerance

Suggested Doses of Various Opioids					
Opioid	Initial bolus (μg/kg)	Low infusion rate (μg/kg/min)	Average infusion rates (μg/kg/min)	High infusion rate (μg/kg min))	TCI target (ng/mL)
Fentanyl	2–3	0.015	0.02–0.033	0.04	1–2
Remifentanil	0.5–1	0.075	0.1–0.2	0.3	2–8
Alfentanil	20–50	0.4	0.5–1.0	1.5	50–150
Sufentanil	0.2–0.3	0.0025	0.0033–0.005	0.0067	0.2–0.3

"ONE-SYRINGE" TECHNIQUES

- Propofol and opioids can be combined in one syringe for infusion
- Physicochemical stability of these mixtures is not clear
- The combinations present in the following display table will place patients in the theoretical "sweet spot" of Figure 46-1. Note that some patients may require greater infusion rates
- Additional opioid for loading and episodic prn boluses required
- To begin case: propofol bolus 2 mg/kg (without added opioid) plus listed opioid loading dose, and then begin propofol–opioid mixture

Suggested Mixtures of Opioids with Propofol				
Opioid	Loading dose (μg/kg)	Add to 500 mg propofol	Propofol dosing (see above)	Notes (to prevent excessive accumulation of opioid)
Fentanyl	2	100 μg	Low–high	Syringe #3 and subsequent syringes should contain 75 μg
Alfentanil	20	2,500 μg	Low–high	Syringe #3 and subsequent syringes should contain 2,000 μg
Sufentanil	0.3	20 μg	Low–high	Syringe #3 and subsequent syringes should contain 15 μg
Remifentanil	0.5	500 μg	Low–high	No need to change based on length of infusion
Remifentanil	0.5	1000 μg	Low	No need to change based on length of infusion

REFERENCES

For references, please visit **www.TheAnesthesiaGuide.com**.

CHAPTER 47
Vasoactive Medications

Ruchir Gupta, MD

VASOPRESSORS AND INOTROPES

See table on following page.

Vasopressors and Inotropes

Drugs	Receptors activated	Hemodynamic effects	Dilution (in 250 mL)	Final concentration	IV infusion rate (µg/kg/min)	IV bolus (if applicable)	Special precautions/comments
Adrenergic agonists							
Epinephrine	α_1, α_2, β_1, β_2, β_3	HR ↑ MAP ↑ CO ↑ PVR ↑–	4 mg	16 µg/mL	0.02–0.3 (2–20 µg/min)	Variable, from 5 µg to 1 mg	
Norepinephrine (Levophed®)	α_1, α_2, β_1	HR ↓ MAP ↑↑ CO – PVR ↑↑	4 mg	16 µg/mL	0.05–0.5		
Phenylephrine (Neosynephrine®)	α_1, weak α_2, weak β_1	HR ↓ MAP ↑↑ CO ↓ PVR ↑↑	10 or 20 mg	40 or 80 µg/mL	0.15–0.75	40–80 µg	
Ephedrine	α_1 (indirectly), β_1, β_2	HR ↑ MAP ↑ CO ↑ PVR ±				5–10 mg	Repeated doses less effective (tachyphylaxis)

Dopamine	DA1, DA2	RBF ↑↑	200 mg	800 µg/mL	0.5–3 ("renal" dose)	
	β_1, β_2	HR ↑↑ MAP ↑ CO ↑↑ PVR –	400 mg	1.6 mg/mL	3–10 (β dose)	
	α_1, α_2, β_1, β_2	HR ↑↑ MAP ↑↑ CO ↑↑ PVR ↑↑	800 mg	3.2 mg/mL	10–20 ($\alpha + \beta$)	
Fenoldopam (Corlopam®)	DA1	HR == MAP ↓ CO ↑ PVR ↓↓	10 mg	40 µg/mL	0.1 Increase by 0.1 q15–20 min until target MAP reached	Renal vasodilator
Dobutamine (Dobutrex®)	β_1, weak β_2	HR ↑ MAP ↑ CO ↑↑ PVR ↓	250 mg	1 mg/mL	2–30	
Isoproterenol (Isuprel®)	β_1, β_2	HR ↑↑ MAP ↓ CO ↑↑ PVR ↓↓	2 mg	8 µg/mL	0.01–0.5	Photosensitive

(continued)

Vasopressors and Inotropes *(continued)*

Drugs	Receptors activated	Hemodynamic effects	Dilution (in 250 mL)	Final concentration	IV infusion rate (µg/kg/min)	IV bolus (if applicable)	Special precautions/ comments
Other							
Vasopressin (arginine vasopressin, Pitressin®)		HR 0 MAP ↑↑ CO ↓ PVR –	100 U in 100 mL	1 U/mL	0.1–0.4 U/min		
Milrinone (Primacor®)	Phosphodiesterase inhibitor	HR –↑ MAP 0 CO ↑↑ PVR ↓↓	50 mg	200 µg/mL	0.375–0.75	N/A	
Inamrinone (Inocor®)	Phosphodiesterase inhibitor	HR –↑ MAP 0 CO ↑↑ PVR ↓↓	100 mg	0.4 mg/mL	5–10	0.75 µg/kg (load)	
Levosimendan (Simdax®)	Weak PDE inhibitor, mainly calcium sensitizer	CO ↑↑ SV ↑↑↑ MAP ↓ PVR ↓	12.5 in 500 mL of D5	0.025 mg/mL	0.05–2 µg/kg/min		Photosensitive, but does not need to be kept from light during infusion

Medications Used to Lower the Blood Pressure					
Drugs	IV infusion (µg/kg/min)	Dilution (in 250 mL)	Final concentration	Bolus (if applicable)	Special precautions/comments
Vasodilators					
Nitroglycerin	0.1–7	50 mg	200 µg/mL	50–100 µg	
Nitroprusside (Nipride®)	0.1–10	50 mg	200 µg/mL		Photosensitive, protect from light during infusion. Can result in: • Thiocyanate toxicity (slurred speech, dizziness, stupor) • Cyanide toxicity (metabolic acidosis, tachyphylaxis, increased MVO$_2$)
Fenoldopam (Corlopam®)	0.1–0.2	10 mg	40 µg/mL		
Hydralazine (Apresoline®)				2.5–20 mg	Takes 15 min for full effect; do not administer more often than q15 min
Enalaprilat (Vasotec®)				0.625–1.25 mg	
Calcium channel blockers					
Diltiazem (Cardizem®)	1–3	100 mg	400 µg/mL		
Nicardipine (Cardene®)	1–4	25 mg	100 µg/mL		
Nifedipine (Procardia®)	1–3	50 mg	200 µg/mL		
Verapamil (Calan®)	1–5	50 mg	200 µg/mL		
Clevidipine (Cleviprex®)	1–2 mg/h	N/A (prepackaged lipid emulsion)	0.5 mg/mL		To avoid lipid overload, do not administer more than 1,000 mL/24 h or an average of 21 mg/h
β-Blockers					
Metoprolol (Toprol®)				2.5–5 mg	Selective (works on β$_1$ receptors)
Propranolol (Inderal®)				0.25–0.5 mg IV	Nonselective (works on β$_1$ and β$_2$ receptors)
Esmolol (Brevibloc®)	50–200	2,500 mg	10 mg/mL	0.5–1 mg/kg IV	Selective (works on β$_1$ receptors)
Labetalol (Trandate®)	2 mg/min (up to a total of 300 mg)	200 mg	2 mg/3 mL	5–20 mg (up to a total of 300 mg)	α- and β-blocker Ratio 1:3 PO and 1:7 IV

Adrenergic/Vasopressin Receptors and End-Organ Effects	
Receptor	End-organ effects
α_1	Constriction of blood vessels, increased myocardial contractility
α_2	Constriction of blood vessels, platelet aggregation, inhibition of lipolysis
α_3	Lipolysis, tachycardia, increased myocardial contractility
β_1	Stimulation of renin release in JGA, lipolysis, increased cardiac output, increased HR
β_2	Dilation of blood vessels, bronchial relaxation, stimulation of renin release, lipolysis
β_3	Lipolysis
D1	Dilation of vascular smooth muscle (renal, mesenteric, coronary), increased renin
D2	Inhibits release of NE, may constrict renal and mesenteric smooth muscle
V1	Vasoconstriction
V2	Causes water reabsorption in the collecting tubule

CHAPTER 48
Breathing Circuits

Jamaal T. Snell, MD

BASIC FUNCTIONS

- Oxygen delivery
- CO_2 removal
- Anesthetic agent administration

CIRCUIT CLASSIFICATIONS (OPEN VS. CLOSED OR REBREATHING VS. NON-REBREATHING)

See table on following page.

Circuit Classifications (Open vs. Closed or Rebreathing vs. Non-Rebreathing)		
Open	Insufflation • Blowing of oxygen or anesthetic gas over the patient's face via mask or head drape	No rebreathing
	Open drop • No longer used. Modern version is the drawover apparatus; useful when compressed gases are not available	
Semi-open	Mapleson breathing systems (A, B, C, D, E, F) • Portable, inexpensive but require high fresh gas flow (FGF) • Consist of a varied arrangement of FGF, breathing bag, reservoir tubing, expiratory/overflow valve • No unidirectional valves, so rebreathing *can* occur if FGFs are not appropriate • Mapleson A: most economic for spontaneous breathing • Mapleson D/Bain: most economic for controlled ventilation	
Semiclosed	Circle system • Most common arrangement used in modern anesthesia • Because air is rebreathed, CO_2 must be removed • Considered "semi-open" because there is only partial rebreathing since some gas is lost from the APL/scavenger system • Helps to maintain heat, humidity, decrease the required amount of FGF, decrease pollution of atmosphere	Rebreathing
Closed	Circle system • As above; however, there is total rebreathing of exhaled air (i.e., FGF is approximately equal to patient's basal O_2 requirement with anesthetics) • Makes quick changes in gas/anesthetics difficult	

MAPLESON SYSTEM CLASSIFICATION

See table on following page.

Mapleson System Classification

Mapleson class	Other names	Configuration[1]	Required fresh gas flows		Comments
			Spontaneous	Controlled	
A	Magill attachment		Equal to minute ventilation (≈80 mL/kg/min)	Very high and difficult to predict	Most efficient for spontaneous ventilation. Poor choice during controlled ventilation
B			2 × minute ventilation	2–2.5 × minute ventilation	**Not used in modern practice**
C	Water's to-and-fro		2 × minute ventilation	2–2.5 × minute ventilation	**Not used in modern practice**
D	Bain		2–3 × minute ventilation	1–2 × minute ventilation	Bain coaxial modification: fresh gas tube inside breathing tube (to warm fresh gas). Most efficient for controlled ventilation
E	Ayre's T-piece		2–3 × minute ventilation	3 × minute ventilation (I:E = 1:2)	Exhalation tubing should provide a larger volume than tidal volume to prevent rebreathing. Scavenging is difficult. Decreased resistance in circuit conducive to weaning
F	Jackson Rees		2–3 × minute ventilation	2 × minute ventilation	A Mapleson E with a breathing bag connected to the end of the breathing tube to allow controlled ventilation and scavenging. Commonly used for pediatric patients and transportation

[1]FGI, fresh gas inlet; APL, adjustable pressure limiting (valve).

Circle System: Essential Components		
	Characteristics	Potential hazard
Gas supply	• Carrier gases (O_2, N_2O, air) supplied to anesthesia machine via central supply of hospital or portable E cylinders	• Variable, high-pressure system from cylinders. Regulators decrease pressure to ~45 psi. Some machines employ a second regulator that further reduces the pressure to ~12–16 psi • Incorrect identification can be fatal • Color system for cylinders and hoses (i.e., O_2, green; N_2O, blue; air, yellow) • Central supply hoses outfitted with Diameter Index Safety System (DISS) • Cylinders outfitted with Pin Index Safety System (PISS) • Hypoxic mixtures prevented by fail-safe/oxygen supply safety devices that shuts off N_2O and other gases when the pressure of oxygen supply falls below a specific threshold • Potential for leaks
Valves	• Unidirectional valves: essential for circle system; prevent rebreathing CO_2 • APL • O_2 flush valve: delivers oxygen straight from the pipeline or cylinder regulator at ~45–50 psi. Flow rate between 35 and 75 L/min. For an O_2 flush flow rate of 60 L/min, 1 L of O_2 flows into the breathing circuit for every second that the O_2 flush button is held down	• Valve incompetency can be identified via abnormal capnograph waveforms (see chapter 39) • High pressure of O_2 flush (bypasses second high-pressure regulator)
Flow meters	• Downstream from pressure regulators • Needle valves regulate the flow of incoming fresh gas separately • Bobbins are read at the top/ball floats are read at the middle • Flow meter accuracy is affected by altitude. Especially with high flow rates, at elevated altitudes, the decreased density of the gas will cause the actual flow to be higher than what is indicated	• Inaccuracies due to cracks/leaks, static electricity, dirt, back pressure from ventilator • Hypoxic mixtures can result if several meters are in sequence and one forms a leak. Any flow meter placed before the leak will also lose gas; thus, O_2 is placed last in the sequence of flow meters • N_2O/O_2 proportional flow meters prevent the operator from selecting a combination of flows that can be hypoxic (typically set at 25–30% oxygen)

(continued)

Circle System: Essential Components (continued)

	Characteristics	Potential hazard

Vaporizers	• Different types: simple, low resistance, precision (found on most modern machines)
	• Calibrated based on each volatile gases' saturated vapor pressure (SVP)
	• SVP: halothane > isoflurane > enflurane > sevoflurane > methoxyflurane
	• The higher the SVP, the lower the chamber flow required (i.e., halothane has the lowest chamber flow)
	• Desflurane has a high SVP (close to atmospheric pressure) and a steep SVP versus temperature curve. This can cause unstable gas output; thus, the vaporizers are heated/pressurized to ~2 atm
	• Factors affecting output accuracy:
	  ▲ Altitude ▲ Gas flow rates
	  ▲ Time ▲ Temperature
		• Keyed fillers to prevent filling vaporizers with the wrong volatile. Filling a vaporizer calibrated for a gas with a *lower* SVP will result in much *higher* output than indicated on the chamber
		• Interlocks prevent the simultaneous administration of two volatile anesthetics
		• Leaks common because of constant refilling

Reservoir bag	• Reservoir of gas to provide extra gas above FGF during peak inspiratory flow and high tidal volumes • Accommodates increases in pressure in the breathing circuit (3 L bag can limit to ~40 cm H_2O even when fully inflated) • Provides ability to manually provide positive pressure and assist ventilation • Provides tactile feedback to user of patient's breathing pattern/lung compliance and visual confirmation of breathing	• Size of the bag must be appropriate for patient's size • Too small: bag will collapse, will not provide adequate gas above FGF when increased volume is required • Too large: can cause barotrauma with manual ventilation

CO$_2$ absorbing systems	• Essential for any circle system
	• CO$_2$ absorbents
	• *Soda lime* (most common)
	  ▸ 94% CaOH, 5% NaOH, and 1% KOH
	  ▸ Capable of absorbing up to 14–23 L of CO$_2$ per 100 g of absorbent
	• *Baralyme*
	  ▸ 20% barium hydroxide, 80% CaOH
	  ▸ Capable of absorbing up to 9–18 L of CO$_2$ per 100 g of absorbent
	• *Amsorb®* (newest absorbent)
	  ▸ Greater inertness than soda lime or barium hydroxide lime, thus less degradation of volatile anesthetics (i.e., sevoflurane into compound A or desflurane into carbon monoxide)
	  ▸ Capable of absorbing ~12 L of CO$_2$ per 100 g of absorbent
		• Improper function of valves with closed interface can expose the patient to negative pressure (from vacuum) or positive pressure/barotrauma and occupational exposure (e.g., from obstruction/occlusion of scavenging tubing)
		• Compound A formed by sevoflurane and soda lime at low flows
		• Carbon monoxide formed with desiccated absorbent (greatest with desflurane and Baralyme)
		• Case reports of fires created by desiccated Baralyme and sevoflurane
		• Unrecognized desiccation or failure of indicator dye to change can lead to rebreathing
		
		$CO_2 + H_2O \rightarrow H_2CO_3$
		$H_2CO_3 + 2NaOH \ (KOH) \rightarrow Na_2CO_3 \ (K_2CO_3) + 2H_2O + heat$
		$Na_2CO_3 \ (K_2CO_3) + Ca(OH)_2 \rightarrow CaCO_3 + 2NaOH \ (KOH)$
		
		• Chemical reaction with CO$_2$ and soda lime

Scavenger systems	• Waste-gas scavengers dispose of gases that have been vented from the breathing circuit by the APL valve and ventilator spill valve
	• Different types of scavenging systems
	  ▸ Charcoal
	  ▸ Passive systems: hose vents waste outside building without vacuum
	  ▸ "Closed" interface with positive/negative pressure relief valves
	  ▸ Higher occupational exposure risk
	  ▸ Active systems: hose vents waste outside building with vacuum
	  ▸ "Open" interface
	• National Institute for Occupational Safety and Health (NIOSH) recommends limiting the room concentration of nitrous oxide to 25 ppm and halogenated agents to 2 ppm (0.5 ppm if nitrous oxide is also being used)
		• Improper function of valves with "closed" interface can expose the patient to negative pressure (i.e., from vacuum) or positive pressure/barotrauma
		• Occupational exposure (i.e., from obstruction/occlusion of scavenging tubing)

FIGURE 48-1. Basic circle circuit configuration

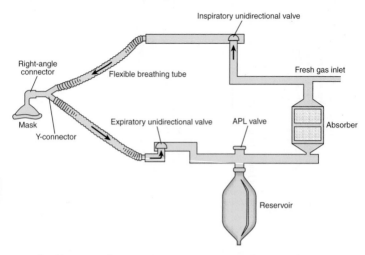

APL: adjustable pressure limiting (valve). Reproduced from Morgan GE, Mikhail MS, Murray MJ. *Clinical Anesthesiology*. 4th ed. Figure 3-10. Available at: http://www.accessmedicine.com. Copyright © The McGraw-Hill Companies, Inc. All rights reserved.

REFERENCES

For references, please visit **www.TheAnesthesiaGuide.com**.

CHAPTER 49
Mechanical Ventilation in the Operating Room

Sauman Rafii, MD and J. David Roccaforte, MD

BASICS

- Involves intermittent administration of positive pressure:
  - Expiratory phase is passive:
    - Flow out of patient is determined by airway resistance and lung elastance (1/compliance)
- In general, ventilators in anesthesia machines are simpler than ventilators seen in an ICU setting; however, the distinction between the two is increasingly blurred

MODES OF MECHANICAL VENTILATION

- Controlled mechanical ventilation:
  - ▸ Designed for anesthetized, and often paralyzed, patients
  - ▸ Volume controlled and pressure controlled:
    - Volume controlled (Figure 49-1):
      - ◆ A tidal volume and a respiratory rate are programmed
      - ◆ Tidal volumes are constant, but airway pressures vary with airway resistance and lung and chest wall compliances
    - Pressure controlled (Figure 49-2):
      - ◆ Inspiratory pressure, inspiratory time, and respiratory rate are programmed
      - ◆ The ventilator delivers a constant pressure during inspiration
      - ◆ The inspired pressure with each breath is constant, but tidal volumes may change with any changes in airway resistance and lung and chest wall compliances (i.e., abdomen insufflation, bronchospasm, ETT kinking, secretions in ETT)
      - ◆ Need to closely monitor actually delivered Vt
      - ◆ May be useful in conditions under which high peak pressures are generated under volume-controlled ventilation, for example, ALI/ARDS, morbidly obese patients, laparoscopic surgery in patients in steep Trendelenburg position
      - ◆ No evidence that "protective ventilation" used for ARDS patients improves outcome in patients with healthy lungs
- Partially controlled mechanical ventilation:
  - ▸ Designed for spontaneously breathing patients. Not all OR ventilators have these modes

FIGURE 49-1. Volume-targeted square wave flow controlled-mode ventilation

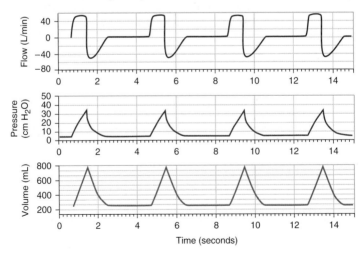

Note that inspiratory flow is constant while pressure increases until the start of expiration. Also, there is no negative deflection before each breath, as the breaths are not initiated by the patient. Vt 700 mL, RR 15, I:E 1:2, PEEP 5 cm H₂O. Reproduced with permission from Hess DR, MacIntyre NR, Mishoe SC, et al, eds. *Respiratory Care: Principles and Practice.* Philadelphia: WB Saunders; 2002:786–791. © Elsevier.

FIGURE 49-2. Pressure-targeted controlled-mode ventilation (PCV)

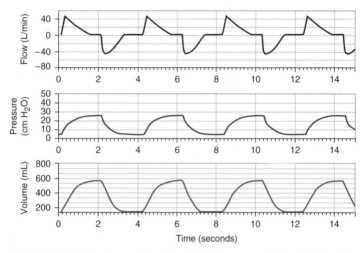

Note that inspiratory flow increases to achieve the target pressure, and then decreases as the lungs fill. $P_{inspired}$ 25 cm H_2O, RR 15, I:E 1:1, PEEP 5 cm H_2O. Reproduced with permission from Hess DR, MacIntyre NR, Mishoe SC, et al, eds. *Respiratory Care: Principles and Practice.* Philadelphia: WB Saunders; 2002:786–791. © Elsevier.

- Modes:
  - Synchronized intermittent mandatory ventilation (SIMV; Figure 49-3):
    - A tidal volume and a respiratory rate are programmed
    - The patient may spontaneously breathe at a rate higher than that which is programmed
    - The ventilator will allow this, but will not assist the patient's spontaneous breaths
  - Pressure support ventilation (PSV; Figure 49-4):
    - The patient breathes spontaneously
    - With each breath, the ventilator adds a programmed amount of pressure to assist the patient
    - Typically 5 cm H_2O will eliminate the extra work of breathing due to the resistance of the circuit and the ETT. Beyond that, the machine assists the patient's breathing
  - SIMV + PSV combines the two previous modes:
    - Mechanical breaths are delivered
    - Spontaneous breaths are assisted

OTHER SETTINGS

- Positive end-expiratory pressure (PEEP):
  - A constant amount of pressure is maintained in the airways throughout the expiratory cycle
  - Improves oxygenation by preventing collapse of alveoli
  - Might prevent atelectasis:
    - Atelectasis is constant during mechanical ventilation and is multifactorial (compression, absorption, loss of surfactant)
    - Intermittent vital capacity (recruitment) maneuvers, inflating lungs to 40 cm H_2O, lasting for only 7–8 seconds, can reinflate collapsed alveoli

FIGURE 49-3. Volume-targeted synchronized intermittent mandatory ventilation (SIMV)

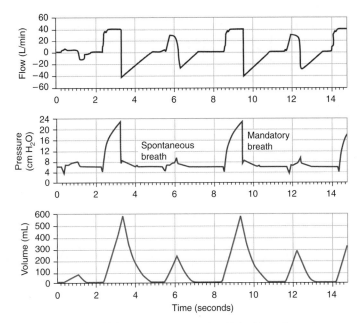

Pressure support can be added to support spontaneous breaths, but it is not the case here; spontaneous breaths are not assisted. SIMV RR 10, Vt 600 mL, PS 0, PEEP 5 cm H_2O. Reproduced with permission from Hess DR, MacIntyre NR, Mishoe SC, et al, eds. *Respiratory Care: Principles and Practice.* Philadelphia: WB Saunders; 2002:786–791. © Elsevier.

- Fraction of inspired oxygen (FiO_2):
  ‣ This is measured by the machine after the mixture of the fresh gas flows and recirculated breath:
    ▪ An oxygen analyzer utilizes electrochemical sensors to determine the partial pressure. It may be located in the inspiratory or expiratory limb of the circuit
- I:E ratio:
  ‣ Ratio of the amount of time spent in inspiration and exhalation
  ‣ Example: an I:E ratio of 1:2 with a programmed respiratory rate of 10 breaths/min (6 seconds per cycle), 2 seconds would be spent in inspiration and 4 seconds would be spent in exhalation
  ‣ The I:E ratio should be lower (e.g., 1:4) in patients with COPD or bronchospasm, in order to allow enough time for full exhalation and prevent breath stacking
  ‣ On the other hand, inverse ratio ventilation (i.e., I:E of 1:1, or even 1:0.5) can be used in patients with stiff lungs (ARDS, morbid obesity) in order to increase the time spent in inspiration and improve oxygenation. However, this technique is somewhat falling out of favor

FIGURE 49-4. Pressure support mode ventilation (PSV)

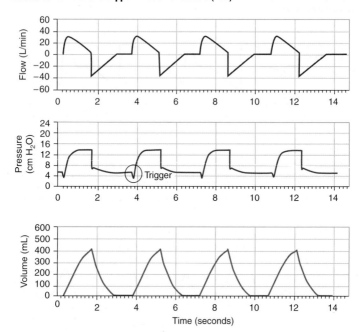

Note the negative deflection in the pressure curve. This indicates that the patient is taking a spontaneous breath, and, thus, triggering the ventilator to deliver the predetermined amount of pressure support. As with PCV, inspiratory flow increases to achieve the target pressure, and then decreases as the lungs fill. Pressure support (PS) 14 cm H_2O, PEEP 5 cm H_2O. Reproduced with permission from Hess DR, MacIntyre NR, Mishoe SC, et al, eds. *Respiratory Care: Principles and Practice.* Philadelphia: WB Saunders; 2002:786–791. © Elsevier.

REFERENCES

For references, please visit **www.TheAnesthesiaGuide.com**.

CHAPTER 50
Full Stomach

Elisabeth Falzone, MD and Jean-Pierre Tourtier, MD

MAIN RISK

Aspiration of gastric contents with subsequent severe chemical pneumonitis (Mendelson syndrome) and/or pneumonia.

Aspiration occurs in the presence of a triad:
- Fluid or solids in the stomach
- Vomiting or passive regurgitation
- Depression of the airway protective reflexes

PATIENTS AT RISK FOR ASPIRATION OF GASTRIC CONTENTS

- Breach of NPO guidelines or emergent (nonelective) surgical procedure
- Acute or chronic, upper or lower, GI pathology (e.g., intestinal obstruction, Barrett esophagus, GERD)
- Obesity; increased risk if bariatric surgery
- Opioid administration, sedation, impaired level of consciousness
- Increased ICP, neurological disease affecting gastric emptying, esophageal sphincter tone, or upper airway reflexes; diabetes with autonomic dysfunction leading to gastroparesis
- ESRD
- Difficult intubation/airway
- Pregnancy beyond 18–20 weeks of gestation

DIAGNOSIS OF FULL STOMACH

- History
- Preanesthetic ultrasonographic measurement of the antral cross-sectional area (not performed routinely):
  ‣ Upright 45°, low-frequency (2–5 MHz) probe
  ‣ Antrum imaged in a parasagittal plane in the epigastric area using the left lobe of the liver, the inferior vena cava, and the superior mesenteric vein as internal landmarks
  ‣ Anteroposterior and craniocaudal diameters measured
  ‣ $CSA = (AP \times CC \times \pi)/4$
  ‣ "At-risk" stomach if CSA $\geq$340 mm^2

PREMEDICATION

- H$_2$ antagonist: two oral doses of ranitidine (150 mg)—one the night before surgery and one on the morning of surgery (to decrease gastric acidity)
- Alternatively, nonparticulate antacid (sodium citrate) 30 mL PO before bringing patient to the OR

PROCEDURE

- It is best to use GA and protect the airway by a cuffed endotracheal tube. Regional anesthesia with minimal sedation can be considered in selected cases, after carefully weighing risks and benefits
- Empty the stomach with a nasogastric tube (if not contraindicated), although this by no means guarantees that there will not be regurgitation of gastric contents. If NGT in place, put in suction and do not remove before induction

- Preoxygenate well (3 minutes or several FVC breaths) until FeO_2 above 80%
- Rapid sequence intubation:
  - *Hypnotic*: propofol 2.5 mg/kg (or etomidate 0.3 mg/kg or ketamine 3–4 mg/kg if concern about hemodynamic stability)
  - *NMB*:
    - Succinylcholine 1 mg/kg (do not "precurarize" with a nondepolarizing agent to avoid fasciculations, as this will delay onset of NMB)
    - Rocuronium if contraindication to succinylcholine (hyperkalemia, allergy, myopathy, paraplegia/tetraplegia, absent/abnormal plasma pseudocholinesterase) in patient not at risk for difficult intubation: 0.6–0.9 mg/kg
  - Sellick maneuver: probably not very effective but little potential to harm:
    - The cricoid cartilage is pushed against the body of the sixth cervical vertebra, compressing the esophagus to prevent passive regurgitation
    - The cricoid cartilage can be located inferior to the thyroid prominence and cricothyroid membrane
    - Cricoid pressure is applied before intubation, immediately after injection of induction medications, and **should not be released** until ETT position is confirmed by $EtCO_2$ and auscultation
    - The cricoid cartilage should be fixed between digits and then pressed backwards at a force of 20–30 N (training with a sealed 50 mL syringe: compression of the syringe to 34 mL approximates 30 N of pressure)
    - Cricoid pressure must be released if active vomiting supervenes, to reduce the risk of esophageal rupture
  - No mask ventilation to avoid stomach insufflation
  - Intubation after 45–60 seconds with succinylcholine (end of fasciculations) or 60–90 seconds with rocuronium
- Extubate only when patient fully alert, responding to commands, and NMB fully reversed

REFERENCES

For references, please visit **www.TheAnesthesiaGuide.com**.

CHAPTER 51
Difficult Intubation and Various Tools

Samir Kendale, MD

DIFFICULT AIRWAY ALGORITHM

See figure 51-1 on the following page.

FIGURE 51-1. Difficult airway algorithm

DIFFICULT AIRWAY INTUBATION

1. Assess the likelihood and clinical impact of basic management problems:
   A. Difficult ventilation
   B. Difficult intubation
   C. Difficulty with patient cooperation or consent
   D. Difficult tracheostomy

2. Actively pursue opportunities to deliver supplemental oxygen throughout the process of difficult airway management.

3. Consider the relative merits and feasibility of basic management choices:

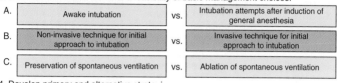

A. Awake intubation vs. Intubation attempts after induction of general anesthesia

B. Non-invasive technique for initial approach to intubation vs. Invasive technique for initial approach to intubation

C. Preservation of spontaneous ventilation vs. Ablation of spontaneous ventilation

4. Develop primary and alternative strategies:

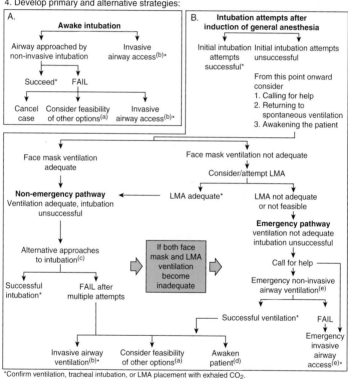

*Confirm ventilation, tracheal intubation, or LMA placement with exhaled CO_2.

a. Other options include (but are not limited to): surgery utilizing face mask or LMA anesthesia, local anesthesia infiltration or regional nerve blockade. Pursuit of these options usually implies that mask ventilation will not be problematic. Therefore, these options may be of limited value if this step in the algorithm has been reached via the Emergency Pathway.

b. Invasive airway access includes surgical or percutaneous tracheostomy or cricothyrotomy.

c. Alternative non-invasive approaches to difficult intubation include (but are not limited to): use of different laryngoscopic blades, LMA as an intubation conduit (with or without fiberoptic guidance), fiberoptic intubation, intubating stylet or tube changer, light wand, retrograde intubation, and blind oral or nasal intubation.

d. Consider re-preparation of the patient for awake intubation or canceling surgery.

e. Options for emergency non-invasive airway ventilation include (but are not limited to): rigid bronchoscope, esophageal-bracheal combitube ventilation, or transtracheal jet ventilation.

Reproduced with permission from Practice guidelines for management of the difficult airway: an updated report by the American Society of Anesthesiologists Task Force on Management of the Difficult Airway. *Anesthesiology.* 2003;98:1269.

TECHNIQUES FOR DIFFICULT AIRWAYS

Characteristics of Various Tools Used to Secure Difficult Airways		
Device	Pros	Cons
Bougie	Useful for grade 2 or 3 view, inexpensive	No visualization of cords, blind insertion may cause trauma
Fiber-optic	Confirmation of tube depth, avoidance of neck mobilization, can be performed awake, high chance of success with skilled operator	Time consuming, no rapid sequence, cost of equipment, success rate operator dependent
Laryngeal mask airway (LMA)	Ease of use, lower resistance airway, less chance of dental injury, reduced sore throat, reduced hemodynamic and IOP changes	May be unsafe in procedures requiring head movement or position other than supine, does not prevent aspiration, not protective against laryngospasm
Intubating LMA (i.e., Fastrach, AirQ)	Ease of use, ability to ventilate allows time to intubate	Success not guaranteed, no visualization of vocal cords, potential esophageal, pharyngeal, or laryngeal trauma due to blind insertion, more minor complications than standard LMA (sore throat, difficulty swallowing), no rapid sequence
Video laryngoscope (i.e., Glidescope, McGrath)	May help minimize neck movement, ease of obtaining view of cords, may be used for rapid sequence, useful for teaching	ETT may be difficult to pass, risk of failure in patients with cervical deformity
Airtraq	Ease of use, ability to visualize cords, reduced hemodynamic changes, reduced cervical spine motion, disposable	Cost, requires good mouth opening, single blade size
Retrograde intubation	Inexpensive Portable	Invasive procedure requiring multiple items Time consuming
Cricothyrotomy	Inexpensive Portable	Invasive procedure

BOUGIE

The gum elastic bougie is a ~25″ long flexible stylet with angled tip.

Indications: poor grade laryngoscopy, suspected cervical spine injury.

Contraindications: contraindication to laryngoscopy, inaccessible oral cavity.
• Perform standard laryngoscopy, attempting to identify arytenoids
• Lubricate bougie
• Insert angled end of bougie blindly under epiglottis, probing for opening
• Insert until clicks felt along tracheal rings
• If no clicks, continue insertion until resistance felt against smaller airways
• Retract bougie from area of resistance

- Advance endotracheal tube over bougie into trachea without advancing bougie
- Remove bougie and confirm endotracheal tube placement

FIBER-OPTIC INTUBATION

Indications: difficult airway, avoiding neck extension or mandibular distraction, awake intubation.

Contraindications: bleeding in airway, lack of time, lack of patient cooperation if awake.

(See chapter 53.)

A. Laryngeal mask airway (LMA)

Supraglottic ventilatory device consisting of anatomically shaped silicone cuff attached to tube for connection to circuit.

Contraindications: risk of aspiration (GERD, obesity, pregnancy, full stomach, upper abdominal surgery, etc.), facial trauma, pharyngeal obstruction, patients requiring high insufflation pressures, restricted access to airway.

- Choose appropriate size, typically based on patient weight and/or mouth opening
- Deflate cuff

LMA Size Based on Weight			
1	Up to 5 kg	3	30–50 kg
1.5	5–10 kg	4	50–70 kg
2	10–20 kg	5	70–100 kg
2.5	20–30 kg	6	>100 kg

- Lubricate posterior (convex) area of LMA, avoiding excessive lubricant
- Ensure adequate anesthesia prior to insertion
- Extend head and flex neck
- Holding LMA with thumb and index finger, press tip against hard palate (see Figure 51-2)
- Press mask into posterior pharyngeal wall. Position into place using index finger (see Figure 51-3)
- Confirm LMA is midline
- Inflate cuff; the LMA will typically "pop out" slightly
- Confirm placement by bilateral breath sounds and positive $EtCO_2$
- Monitor cuff inflation pressure (<25 cm H_2O) if prolonged case and/or N_2O used

B. Intubating LMA (i.e., Fastrach, AirQ)

Supraglottic airway curved to align opening with glottis and enlarged mask to allow passage of endotracheal tube.

- Choose appropriate size as above
- Ensure adequate anesthesia and/or paralysis for endotracheal intubation
- Lubricate endotracheal tube
- Introduce endotracheal tube through LMA; a slight upward pull on the handle of the Fastrach might facilitate ETT passage. The Fastrach requires use of a special ETT, while the AirQ can accommodate a regular ETT (see Figure 51-4)
- Confirm placement of endotracheal tube (auscultation, chest rising, $EtCO_2$)
- Slide LMA out of pharynx, maintaining counterpressure on the ETT, using the stabilizing rod provided with the Fastrach or a stylet provided with the AirQ (see Figure 51-5). Remove rod prior to complete LMA extraction to avoid tearing off the ETT pilot balloon
- Reconnect circuit to endotracheal tube

FIGURE 51-2. Insertion of LMA

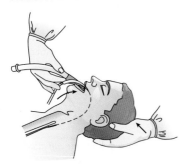

Reproduced with permission from LMA North America, Inc.

FIGURE 51-3. Positioning of LMA using index finger

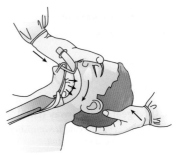

Reproduced with permission from LMA North America, Inc.

FIGURE 51-4. Insertion of ETT through intubating LMA

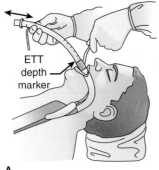
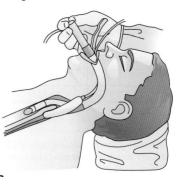

A   **B**

(A and B) Reproduced with permission from LMA North America, Inc.

FIGURE 51-5. Removal of intubating LMA once ETT inserted

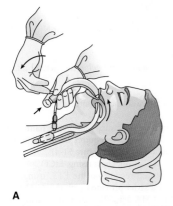
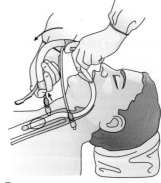

A   **B**

(A and B) Remove rod prior to complete LMA extraction to avoid tearing off the ETT pilot balloon. Reproduced with permission from LMA North America, Inc.

C. Video laryngoscope (i.e., GlideScope, McGrath)

Blade with incorporated camera transmitting to view on separate screen (GlideScope) or integrated display (McGrath).
- Introduce laryngoscope in midline position

FIGURE 51-6. Insertion of GlideScope

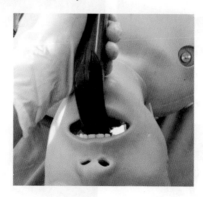

- Visualize uvula, and then epiglottis on screen
- Insert tip of blade into vallecula and lift laryngoscope to obtain view of cords on screen
- Advance styletted tube through vocal cords under video guidance; *NB*: difficulty inserting the ETT is often due to a position of the video laryngoscope that is **too deep**, too close to the vocal cords
- Withdraw stylet once ETT tip is through cords and complete advancement of tube

FIGURE 51-7. Visualization of the uvula, then the epiglottis

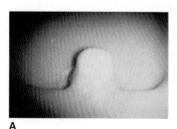

A   B

FIGURE 51-8. Visualization of the vocal cords

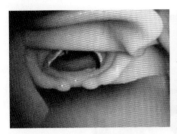

FIGURE 51-9. Insertion of the styletted ETT under vision

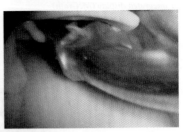

FIGURE 51-10. Insertion of the Airtraq with ETT loaded into channel

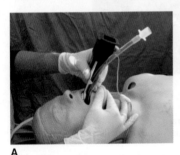

A

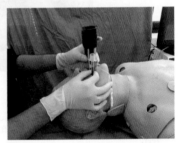

B

D. Airtraq

Optical laryngoscope that provides view of glottis without alignment of axes and includes channel for holding and advancing endotracheal tube.

- Turn on LED at least 30 seconds prior to intubation
- Load lubricated endotracheal tube into channel
- Introduce laryngoscope in midline position
- Advance over tongue and visualize epiglottis
- Place tip into vallecula and lift up to visualize cords
- Center cords in visual field by gently maneuvering device back and up
- Advance tube through cords under visualization through eyepiece
- Pull device laterally and rotate to remove device while securing tube in place

RETROGRADE INTUBATION

Indications: facial trauma, blood in oropharynx, failure of other methods.

Contraindications: lack of familiarity, laryngeal trauma or stenosis, distorted neck anatomy.

(See chapter 54.)

FIGURE 51-11. Advance ETT into visualized vocal cords

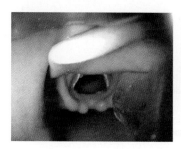

FIGURE 51-12. Removal of Airtraq after the ETT is disengaged from channel

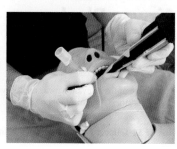

CRICOTHYROTOMY

Indications: trauma in which other methods are impossible, failure to intubate or ventilate, severe obstruction of upper airway.

Contraindications: distorted neck anatomy, laryngeal pathology or trauma, lack of familiarity.

- Locate and palpate cricothyroid membrane
- Prep area
- Grip thyroid cartilage and palpate cricothyroid membrane
- With opposite hand, make incision vertically from thyroid cartilage to inferior cricoid cartilage (~2–3 cm)
- Retract skin and subcutaneous tissue
- Palpate cricothyroid membrane again
- Make incision horizontally through lower part of cricothyroid membrane (~1–1.5 cm)
- Spread apart the cricothyroid membrane to allow insertion of dilator
- Insert dilator, superiorly to inferiorly
- Insert endotracheal or tracheostomy tube while dilator is in place
- Inflate cuff and confirm position
- Secure into place

REFERENCES

For references, please visit **www.TheAnesthesiaGuide.com**.

CHAPTER 52
Airway Blocks

Edward C. Lin, MD

Knowledge of the relevant airway anatomy and innervation is essential to successful airway anesthesia (Figures 52-1 and 52-2).

FIGURE 52-1. Upper airway anatomy and innervation

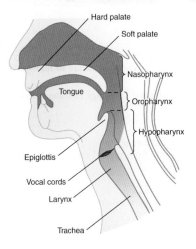

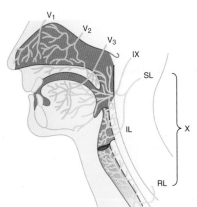

V₁   Ophthalmic division of trigeminal nerve (anterior ethmoidal nerve)

V₂   Maxillary division of trigeminal nerve (sphenopalatine nerves)

V₃   Mandibular division of trigeminal nerve (lingual nerve)

IX   Glossopharyngeal nerve

X   Vagus nerve
     SL   Superior laryngeal nerve
     IL   Internal laryngeal nerve
     RL   Recurrent laryngeal nerve

FIGURE 52-2. Innervation of the larynx

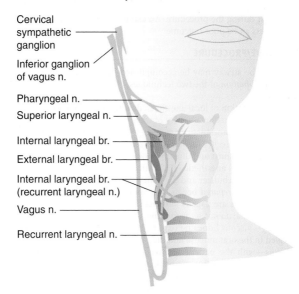

- Cervical sympathetic ganglion
- Inferior ganglion of vagus n.
- Pharyngeal n.
- Superior laryngeal n.
- Internal laryngeal br.
- External laryngeal br.
- Internal laryngeal br. (recurrent laryngeal n.)
- Vagus n.
- Recurrent laryngeal n.

Reproduced with permission from Brown DL. *Atlas of Regional Anesthesia.* 4th ed. Philadelphia: Saunders; 2010:193. © Elsevier.

Nerves of the Airway with Area of Innervation	
Nerve	Relevant sensory innervation
Trigeminal	Mucus membranes of the nose, superior and inferior surfaces of the hard and soft palate, anterior two thirds of tongue
Glossopharyngeal	Posterior one third of tongue, vallecula, anterior surface of the epiglottis, walls of pharynx, tonsils
Superior laryngeal	Base of the tongue, epiglottis, aryepiglottic folds, arytenoids
Recurrent laryngeal	Larynx below the vocal cords, trachea

PREOPERATIVE/PREPROCEDURAL

- **Consent** the patient for the procedure, taking care to **explain** in simple language what will happen and answering any questions. A calm and informed patient is more likely to cooperate than one who is confused and frightened
- **Sedation** for patient comfort is often critical, but take care to carefully titrate medications such as midazolam (1–3 mg IV) or fentanyl (25–50 μg IV) that may cause respiratory depression. **Dexmedetomidine**, an alpha 2 agonist with sedative but not respiratory depressive properties, may be considered (may start IV at 4 μg/kg/h, and then decrease to 1.5–2 μg/kg/h once patient becomes visibly sedated)
- **Antisialagogues** (e.g., glycopyrrolate 0.2–0.4 mg IV, caution in tachycardic patients) to decrease oral secretions may be useful to improve the effectiveness of topicalization and to improve fiber-optic visualization

- **Alert** the OR staff to the possibility of a difficult intubation. Be sure to discuss with the surgeon the possibility of needing a **surgical airway**. Consider asking a colleague to assist during the procedure. An extra pair of hands can be the difference between success and a poor outcome

INTRAOPERATIVE/PROCEDURE

- Anesthetizing the airway may be accomplished by *topicalization*, *invasive airway blocks*, or a *combination* of the two techniques
  - ‣ *Topicalization*:
    - Involves application of local anesthetic directly to the mucosa
    - May be accomplished in a variety of ways:
      - ◆ *Atomizer*—local anesthetic (e.g., 5–10 mL of 2% lidocaine) is dispersed via an atomizer device (e.g., Mucosal Atomizer Device [MAD], Wolfe Troy Medical, Inc.) into a fine mist and directly sprayed onto the desired mucosa
      - ◆ *Nebulizer*—local anesthetic (e.g. 8 mL of 2% lidocaine) is placed into breathing treatment nebulizer and the patient inhales the resultant mist
      - ◆ *Commercially prepared* benzocaine sprays such as Hurricaine®—three brief 1-second sprays are usually sufficient. (*Note*: Benzocaine may cause methemoglobinemia; *do not spray for more than 3 seconds!*)
      - ◆ *Gargling*—viscous lidocaine (e.g., 5–10 mL of 2% viscous lidocaine) may be gargled in the oral mucosa and then spit out
      - ◆ *Melting*—with the patient semirecumbent, 2% lidocaine ointment can be placed on a wooden tongue blade and given to the patient to place on the tongue, as far as possible without gagging. The patient is instructed to let the ointment melt without swallowing. Alternatively, for a nasal intubation, the ointment can be injected into both nares using a syringe (5 mL in each naris). With both techniques, after a few minutes, the ointment will melt and drip down the airway, and the patient will start coughing, signaling some degree of aspiration, and adequate topicalization above the vocal cords
  - ‣ Airway blocks:
    - Airway blocks are more invasive than topicalization, but provide excellent anesthesia to the airway

Technique of Different Airway Blocks with Location of Anesthetized Area		
Block	Technique	Area blocked
Glossopharyngeal nerve block 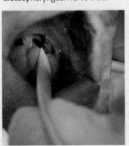 Reproduced with permission from Hadzic A. *The New York School of Regional Anesthesia Textbook of Regional Anesthesia and Acute Pain Management.* New York: McGraw-Hill; 2006. Figure 19-5. Copyright © The McGraw-Hill Companies, Inc. All rights reserved.	The patient's mouth is first opened. While retracting the tongue, the tip of a 22–25 G spinal needle is inserted into the base of one posterior tonsillar pillar and local anesthetic (e.g., 1–2 mL of 2% lidocaine) is injected after negative aspiration. The procedure is then repeated on the other side. Alternatively, a pledget soaked in 4% lidocaine can be placed in the appropriate location and kept in place for 5 minutes	Posterior one third of tongue, vallecula, anterior surface of the epiglottis, walls of pharynx, tonsils

(continued)

Technique of Different Airway Blocks with Location of Anesthetized Area (*continued*)		
Block	Technique	Area blocked
Superior laryngeal nerve 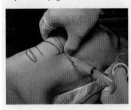 Reproduced with permission from Hadzic A. *The New York School of Regional Anesthesia Textbook of Regional Anesthesia and Acute Pain Management*. New York: McGraw-Hill; 2006; Figure 19-7. Copyright © The McGraw-Hill Companies, Inc. All rights reserved.	The hyoid bone is first identified and then displaced toward the side to be blocked. A 25 G needle is inserted, contacts the greater cornu of the hyoid bone and then walked off inferiorly and advanced 1–2 mm. Local anesthetic (e.g., 1–2 mL of 2% lidocaine) is then injected after negative aspiration. The procedure is then repeated on the other side	Base of the tongue, epiglottis, aryepiglottic folds, arytenoids
Transtracheal nerve block 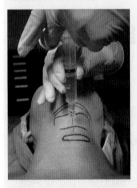 Reproduced with permission from Hadzic A. *The New York School of Regional Anesthesia Textbook of Regional Anesthesia and Acute Pain Management*. New York: McGraw-Hill; 2006. Figure 19-9. Copyright © The McGraw-Hill Companies, Inc. All rights reserved.	The cricothyroid membrane is first identified inferior to the thyroid cartilage and superior to the cricoid cartilage A 20–22 G angiocath is threaded over the needle through the cricothyroid membrane (a soft catheter avoids injuring the back wall when the patient coughs) After air is aspirated (to confirm placement of catheter tip into the airway), local anesthetic (e.g., 2–3 mL of 2% lidocaine) is injected rapidly The patient will cough, which will spread the local anesthetic	Larynx below the vocal cords, trachea *NB*: This block is actually a form of topicalization, but is usually classified with airway blocks as it involves a needle puncture

- Anesthetizing the nasopharynx:
  - Although direct nerve block of the nerves innervating the nasal mucosa is possible (by blocking the sphenopalatine ganglion), it is not commonly performed and will not be discussed here
  - Common techniques for nasal topicalization are:
    - *Soaked cotton swabs*—cotton swabs are soaked in local anesthetic (e.g., lidocaine or cocaine), and then placed through the nares against the mucosa for several minutes
    - *Nasal airways*—nasal airways of varying sizes are first coated with viscous lidocaine and the smallest airway is then inserted through the nares. After the airway is allowed to sit for 1 minute, a progressively larger airway is inserted and allowed to sit. This process is repeated until the largest airway has been placed. This allows topicalization and dilation of the nasal passage

- Consider use of vasoconstrictors to reduce nasal bleeding:
  - Cocaine 4%—maximum dose 200 mg, potential for abuse, concern for tachycardia and dysrhythmia
  - Phenylephrine—may be added to local anesthetic solutions (e.g., 1 mL of 1% Neosynephrine may be added to 3 mL of 2% lidocaine to make a 0.25%/1.5% solution, respectively)
  - Vasoconstrictor sprays such as oxymetazoline (Afrin®): two puffs in each nostril prior to bringing patient to OR, and two puffs again after 5–10 minutes
    All vasoconstrictors have a potential for systemic absorption and severe hypertension. **DO NOT USE BETA-BLOCKERS** to treat vasoconstrictor-induced hypertension: risk of heart failure, pulmonary edema, and death!
- Most practitioners use a combination of topicalization and transtracheal block. Glossopharyngeal and superior laryngeal nerve blocks are rarely used nowadays

REFERENCES

For references, please visit **www.TheAnesthesiaGuide.com**.

CHAPTER 53
Awake Fiber-Optic Intubation

Arthur Atchabahian, MD

NASAL VERSUS ORAL INTUBATION

Advantages of nasal intubation	Disadvantages of nasal intubation
• Easier, as the path is straighter from nasopharynx to glottis • Less gagging as minimal contact with tongue base • Patient cannot bite tube/bronchoscope	• Potential for epistaxis (avoid, e.g., in pregnant patients) • Risk of sinusitis if kept in place for >48 h

PREPARATION

- Patient must be given a complete explanation of the entire procedure, to enhance cooperation, and to allay anxiety
- Adequate IV access
- Check equipment; all medications, including emergency medications, immediately available
- Backup airway access devices (LMAs, cricothyrotomy kits) should be immediately available
- Obtain knowledgeable help if available
- Surgeon informed, available for surgical airway if needed:
  - In some especially difficult cases, the neck might be prepped, and the surgeon gowned, ready to secure a surgical airway if needed

SEDATION

- Adequate sedation is important to minimize anxiety and hemodynamic swings
- However, avoid excessive sedation leading to airway obstruction and hypoventilation, which could be catastrophic in patients with difficult/impossible mask/airway
- Use small amounts of midazolam (1–2 mg) to provide amnesia
- A dexmedetomidine infusion, starting at 4 µg/kg/h, until eye closure and visible relaxation, and then decreased to 1.5–2 µg/kg/h, provides adequate sedation with little or no respiratory depression or obstruction:
  ‣ Monitor for bradycardia; reduce infusion rate if needed

AIRWAY PREPARATION TECHNIQUES

- 100% O_2 by non-rebreather mask for at least 5 minutes
- Unless rate-dependent angina, antisialagogue (glycopyrrolate 0.2–0.4 mg IV), and, if indicated, metoclopramide (10 mg IV)
- Airway blocks (see Chapter 52) can be used depending on personal preferences:
  ‣ Transtracheal block useful as other techniques do not topicalize trachea (below the cords)
  ‣ Glossopharyngeal and superior laryngeal blocks less widely used currently; adequate topicalization and dexmedetomidine is usually sufficient
- For anticipated oral approach:
  ‣ Patient is asked to swish, gargle, and spit out 3–4 mL lidocaine 4% several times, *or*
  ‣ The oropharynx is sprayed with topical benzocaine/tetracaine preparations (e.g., Hurricane; do not exceed 3 seconds of spraying: risk of methemoglobinemia with benzocaine)
  ‣ 6 mL lidocaine 4% is nebulized using a handheld nebulizer
- For anticipated nasal approach:
  ‣ Patient self-administers three puffs of a nasal vasoconstrictor (oxymetazoline 0.05% [Afrin®]) into each nostril
  ‣ 5 mL of viscous lidocaine 2% is administered into each nostril; patient is asked to retain volume in nostrils as long as possible, and then asked to inhale and swallow the volume; this procedure is repeated for a second dose
  ‣ 6 mL lidocaine 4% is nebulized using a handheld nebulizer

TECHNIQUE FOR ORAL APPROACH

- Patient positioned to maximize access to mouth, and to align the oral, pharyngeal, and laryngeal axes, thus placing the patient in a "sniffing" position:
  ‣ Typically, the patient is positioned supine or semirecumbent, with the operator standing behind the head
  ‣ Occasionally, for example, in the morbidly obese or for patients with neck masses, having the patient sitting up, with the operator standing in front of the patient, can facilitate the procedure and reduce airway obstruction
- Generously lubricate appropriately sized endotracheal tube (ETT), and position tube into a Berman oral airway, ensuring that the tube slides easily within the lumen of the airway:
  ‣ An Ovassapian airway (see Figure 53-1) can also be used and has the advantage of being easier to extract from the ETT
  ‣ With a Berman airway, the ETT connector will have to be disconnected in order to remove the airway
- Advance the ETT beyond the edge of the Berman airway and test the cuff, to ensure that placement of the tube into the airway did not disrupt integrity of the cuff, and then retract the tube into the airway until both tips are aligned
- Place Berman/ETT into midline of the mouth so that it fits comfortably and is well tolerated by the patient; supplemental oxygen may be administered via a nasal cannula. Suction oropharynx
- Advance the fiber-optic bronchoscope (FOB) through the lumen of the ETT, visualizing structures as it exits the tube. Additional lidocaine may be sprayed onto the mucosal surfaces as needed

FIGURE 53-1. Ovassapian (A) and Berman (B) airways

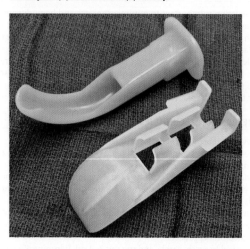

FIGURE 53-2. Initial position for fiberoptic intubation: ETT inside airway

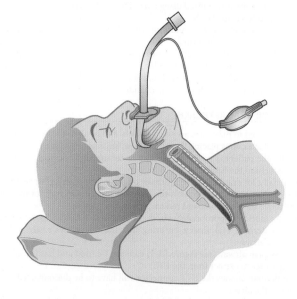

Reproduced with permission from Ovassapian A. *Fiberoptic Endoscopy and the Difficult Airway.* 2nd ed. Philadelphia: Lippincott-Raven; 1996:77.

FIGURE 53-3. View of epiglottis

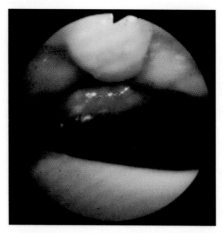

- The FOB has to first go up (anterior) about 45° after exiting the airway, going under the epiglottis (see Figure 53-3) toward the vocal cords
- Identify glottic opening (Figure 53-4), and advance the tip of the FOB beyond the vocal cords into the trachea, identifying tracheal rings and carina (Figure 53-5) to confirm location
- The FOB has then to go down (posterior) about 45°, as the trachea has an anterior-to-posterior slope (Figures 53-6 and 53-7)

FIGURE 53-4. View of glottic opening

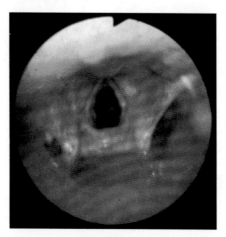

FIGURE 53-5. View of tracheal rings and carina

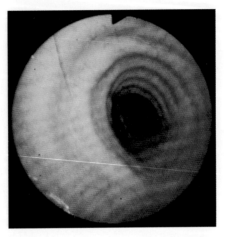

FIGURE 53-6. Orienting FOB downward (posterior)

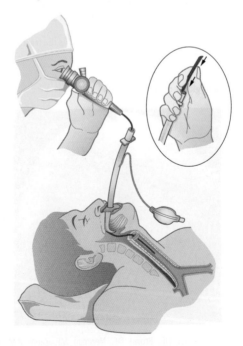

FIGURE 53-7. FOB direction changes for oral intubation

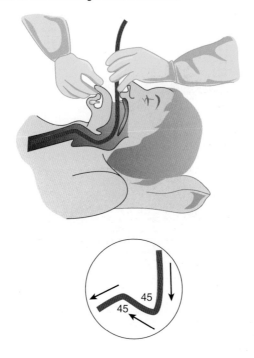

- Using the FOB as a guide, slowly advance the ETT through the airway over the scope and into the trachea (Figure 53-8)
- The ETT is advanced blindly and the bevel can on occasion be caught on the larynx (arytenoid cartilages, vocal cords, etc)
  ► In order to minimize that risk, the ETT should be rotated 90° counterclockwise (Murphy eye on top) so the bevel remains close to the scope
  ► Alternatively, an ETT with a soft tip (ETT of the LMA Fastrach®) or a tapered tip (several models) can be used
- Position the ETT so that the carina can be visualized with the FOB through the ETT; confirm by lung auscultation and presence of CO_2. Ideally, the ETT should be 3–6 cm from the carina
- When the endotracheal position of the ETT is confirmed, induce GA with IV drugs and connect ETT to circuit

FIGURE 53-8. Advancing ETT over FOB into trachea

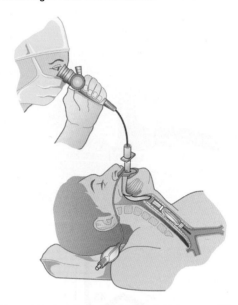

Reproduced with permission from Ovassapian A. *Fiberoptic Endoscopy and the Difficult Airway.* 2nd ed. Philadelphia: Lippincott-Raven; 1996:77.

FIGURE 53-9. ETT bevel over FOB without (A; bevel at risk of getting caught on laryngeal structures) and with 90° counterclockwise rotation (B; bevel "railroading" on the scope)

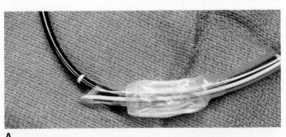

A

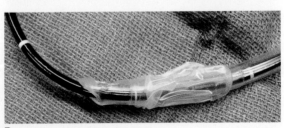

B

FIGURE 53-10. Soft tip versus tapered tip

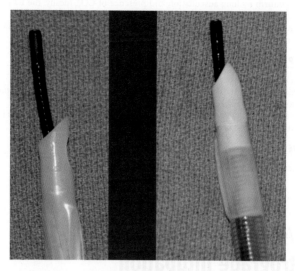

Endotracheal tubes over a 4.0-mm flexible bronchoscope. The tube designed for intubation through the LMA Fastrach (right) has a curved tip, which eases passage of the tube into the trachea. Reproduced from Longnecker DE, Brown DL, Newman MF, Zapol WM. *Anesthesiology*. Figure 35-26. Available at: http://www.accessanesthiology.com. Copyright © The McGraw-Hill Companies, Inc. All rights reserved.

TECHNIQUE FOR NASAL APPROACH

- Patient is positioned such that the head is in midline and in slight extension, and access to nostrils is unimpeded
- Generously lubricate two nasal airways (as large as the nostrils can accommodate) with viscous lidocaine, and place one airway into each nostril
- Select an appropriately sized ETT (conventional or nasal RAE preformed tube), preferably slightly smaller than the size of the nasotracheal airway placed earlier, and lubricate generously
- Remove the nasal airway from the side that provided the least resistance in placement, and provide supplemental oxygen through the other airway by nasal cannula
- Place ETT into nostril and slowly advance tube directing it posteriorly until a slight "give" is felt, indicating passage of the tube past the nasal turbinates
- Advance the FOB through the lumen of the ETT into the nasopharynx, and advance slowly, identifying structures leading to the glottic opening
- Identify glottic opening, and advance the tip of the FOB beyond the vocal cords into the trachea, identifying tracheal rings and carina to confirm location
- Using the FOB as a guide, slowly advance the ETT over the scope and into the trachea:
  ▸ The ETT is advanced blindly and the bevel can on occasion be caught on the larynx (arytenoid cartilages, vocal cords, etc)
  ▸ In order to minimize that risk, the ETT should be rotated 90° counterclockwise (Murphy eye on top) so the bevel remains close to the scope. Some authors, however, advocate rotating the ETT clockwise for nasotracheal intubation
  ▸ Alternatively, an ETT with a soft tip (ETT of the LMA Fastrach®) or a tapered tip (several models) can be used

- Position the tube so that the carina can be visualized with the FOB through the ETT; confirm by lung auscultation and presence of CO_2. Ideally, the ETT should be 3–6 cm from the carina
- When the endotracheal position of the tube is confirmed, induce GA with IV drugs and connect ETT to circuit

ASLEEP INTUBATION

- For a nasal approach, prepare nares as described above prior to induction
- Similar technique (nasal or oral) following preoxygenation and IV induction
- Suction pharynx before inserting FOB
- Have an assistant provide adequate jaw lift, as the tongue will fall back with the loss of muscle tone and occlude the pharynx

REFERENCES

For references, please visit **www.TheAnesthesiaGuide.com**.

CHAPTER 54
Retrograde Intubation
Arthur Atchabahian, MD

INDICATIONS

- Any difficult intubation in patients whose cricothyroid membrane can be located
- Especially suited for facial trauma (nasal intubation contraindicated)

PATIENT PREPARATION IS KEY!

- If possible, discuss all aspects of procedure with patient to enhance cooperation and to minimize anxiety
- However, often performed as an emergency procedure
- Use of an antisialagogue (glycopyrrolate) is strongly recommended
- Use of anxiolytics (midazolam, dexmedetomidine) is urged but not required
- Adequate topicalization of mucous membranes is also strongly recommended

EQUIPMENT (SEE FIGURE 54-1)

- 5 mL of 2% lidocaine in 10 mL syringe with 25 G needle
- Retrograde intubation access kit (if not available, this technique has been performed using a Tuohy needle and an epidural catheter):
  - ▸ *NB*: Some kits have a tube exchanger that allows insufflating oxygen; these exchangers have only one tapered end
- Magill forceps
- Appropriately sized endotracheal tube
- Viscous lidocaine for topicalization of mucous membranes and for lubrication

FIGURE 54-1. Contents of retrograde intubation kit

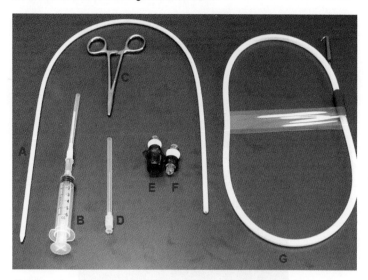

(A) Hollow tube exchanger (note tapered end on the left); (B) syringe with Angiocath; (C) clamp; (D) needle; (E) standard 15-mm adapter connector for oxygen administration through tube exchanger using an Ambu-type bag or an anesthesia machine circuit; (F) Luer Lock adapter and connector for oxygen administration through tube exchanger using a jet ventilation device; (G) guidewire with J-tip visible.

TECHNIQUE

- IV access secured
- Oxygen by nasal cannula
- If possible, topicalization performed by gargling and swishing of viscous lidocaine
- Patient supine with head extended to expose neck, cricothyroid membrane identified by palpation and marked
- Skin wheal using lidocaine 2% is made over the cricothyroid membrane. Stabilize larynx between thumb and index. The needle is advanced through the cricothyroid membrane until air is aspirated into the syringe. 3 to 4 mL of lidocaine 2% is injected into the trachea for topicalization of subglottic structures. The patient will cough. Have assistants maintain patient to avoid movement that could cause the needle to injure the back wall of the trachea
- Once topicalization of the airway is complete, connect the introducer needle of the retrograde intubation kit to a 10 mL syringe with 5 mL of saline. Stabilize larynx as above. Insert needle through the cricothyroid membrane with the bevel facing upward and the needle directed cephalad at a 45° angle to the skin. A distinct pop is felt as the cricothyroid membrane is pierced, and air can be aspirated into the syringe (see Figure 54-2)

FIGURE 54-2. Insertion of needle though cricothyroid membrane

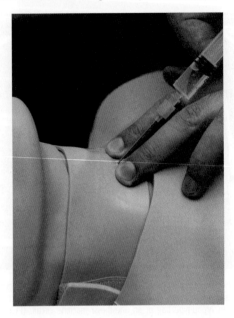

- The needle in the airway is maintained in place with one hand while the syringe is removed from the hub. The guidewire supplied in the retrograde intubation kit is slowly advanced through the needle (see Figure 54-3), directed cephalad, while an assistant observes the oropharynx for the tip of the guidewire (this may require several passes)

FIGURE 54-3. Insertion of the guidewire

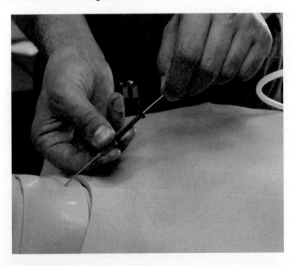

- The guidewire has a J-tip and a straight tip. It also has two marks, which correspond to the length of wire that has to be at the skin by the cricothyroid membrane, depending on which tip is inserted

FIGURE 54-4. Retrieving the guidewire

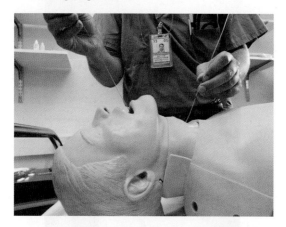

- Once the tip is visualized in the oropharynx, it may be retrieved with a Magill forceps and pulled *slowly* to exit the mouth, so as not to pull the proximal end of the guidewire into the trachea (see Figure 54-4)

FIGURE 54-5. Placement of Kelly clamp on the black mark

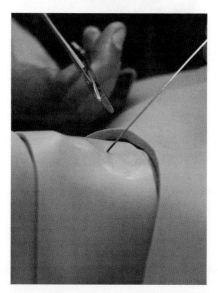

- Once the distal mark is by the skin, the needle in the cricothyroid membrane is removed and a Kelly clamp is placed on the mark to prevent the wire from being pulled any further in the trachea (see Figure 54-5)

FIGURE 54-6. Placement of tube exchanger

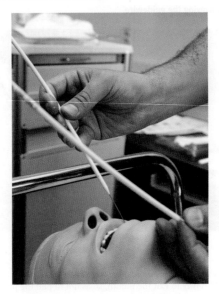

FIGURE 54-7. Proximal black mark

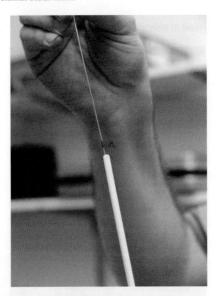

Proximal black mark (A) seen, indicating that the tube exchanger is against the cricothyroid membrane.

- After lubricating the endotracheal tube exchanger, it is advanced, *tapered side first*, over the guidewire into the trachea until resistance is felt. The proximal black mark should then be visible beyond the tube exchanger (see Figures 54-6 and 54-7)
- The appropriately sized endotracheal tube can now be railroaded over the tube exchanger (rotate 90° counterclockwise as for fiber-optic intubation) until it is seated in the trachea (see Figures 54-8 and 54-9). Ensure that depth markings on the tube exchanger match markings on the ETT to ensure that the ETT is not caught on the larynx. The ETT is then barely past the vocal cords, as its tip is at the level of the cricothyroid membrane

FIGURE 54-8. Insertion of ETT; remember to rotate 90° counterclockwise

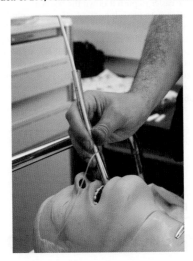

FIGURE 54-9. Ensure that depth markings on ETT and tube exchanger match

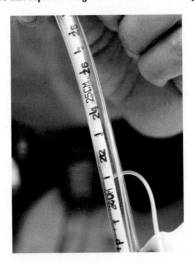

- The tube exchanger and wire are then removed together, and the ETT is pushed down into the trachea. Confirm ETT placement by end-tidal CO_2
- A small occlusive dressing may be placed over the neck at the needle entry site

VARIATIONS

- The guidewire can be retrieved through the nose for a nasal intubation. This technique is contraindicated in case of facial trauma, as a fracture of the cribriform plate can cause the guidewire to enter the cranium
- An alternative technique is to insert the ETT directly over the guidewire without using the tube exchanger. This might make it more difficult to insert the ETT past the vocal cords, as the bevel might get caught. However, if the guidewire is passed through the Murphy eye rather than the tip of the ETT, the tip will be inserted more distally and it will be easier to push it down the trachea
- Yet another alternative is to use a long guidewire (typically borrowed from urological or vascular surgical supplies). The guidewire is inserted as described above. Its tip is then threaded into the instrument port of a fiber-optic bronchoscope. Do not forget to position the ETT over the FOB *before* threading the wire. The FOB is then inserted, guided by the guidewire, until it reaches the cricothyroid membrane. The guidewire is removed, and the FOB is then pushed down the trachea to visualize the carina. The ETT is threaded over the FOB as in a classic FOB-assisted intubation

REFERENCES

For references, please visit **www.TheAnesthesiaGuide.com**.

CHAPTER 55
High-Frequency Jet Ventilation (HFJV)

Brooke Albright, MD

DESCRIPTION

- Open mechanical ventilation system that may improve gas exchange at lower peak and mean airway pressures than conventional ventilation
- Pulsed cycles of small tidal volumes (2–5 mL/kg) at high frequencies (50–150 breaths/min)
- Inspiration: via a small cannula that delivers a jet stream of pulsed breaths to the lungs. The jet stream cannula should be small enough to avoid "sealing" the airway. Typically the cannula is placed through the vocal cords in the trachea, but in an emergency setting, a cannula or a large-bore Angiocath can be introduced through the cricothyroid membrane
- Expiration: passive around jet nozzle
- High-frequency jet ventilation (HFJV) parameters and settings:
  ▸ Driving pressure: major determinant of tidal volume. Driving pressure settings are usually 20–25 psi in adults, with a maximum of 50 psi
  ▸ Inspiration time and respiratory frequency: the major determinants of "auto-PEEP" (air trapping). Inspiration time is usually set at 30–40% and respiratory frequency is between 50 and 150 bpm. By increasing either value, auto-PEEP is increased, which allows recruitment of alveoli, optimization of V/Q matching, and improvement in oxygenation. Auto-PEEP may also be beneficial when a "still" surgical field is desired because chest wall excursions are reduced

- ▸ FiO_2: always set at 100%. It is the oxygen concentration at the jet nozzle. However, the actual FiO_2 in the alveoli is significantly lower due to the Venturi effect (negative pressure around gas flow that drags air from the environment into the airway) and the use of an open system
- ▸ Humidification: used when prolonged jet ventilation anticipated in order to avoid mucus membrane damage or formation of mucus clot leading to airway obstruction
- The mechanism of gas exchange is unlike that in conventional ventilation: CO_2 elimination is possible because of a combination of bulk convection, molecular diffusion, and turbulence of convective flow
- Due to the lower peak and mean airway pressures in HFJV, intrathoracic pressures are decreased leading to increased venous return and improved cardiac function

INDICATIONS

- Certain procedures requiring a shared or still operative field:
  - ▸ Bronchosopy
  - ▸ Laryngoscopy
  - ▸ Tracheal reconstruction
  - ▸ Laryngeal resection
  - ▸ One-lung ventilation
- Respiratory failure in patients with:
  - ▸ Bronchopleural and tracheoesophageal fistulas
  - ▸ Laryngeal neoplasms
  - ▸ Barotrauma
  - ▸ Pulmonary fibrosis
  - ▸ Severe ARDS
  - ▸ Pulmonary hemorrhage
  - ▸ Persistent fetal circulation in the neonate to enhance CO_2 elimination
  - ▸ Infants with congenital diaphragmatic herniation
- Difficult airways: the "cannot ventilate, cannot intubate" patient (through crico-thyrotomy)

COMPLICATIONS/SIDE EFFECTS

- Barotrauma (high pressure buildup in a closed tissue pocket):
  - ▸ May lead to pneumothorax, pneumomediastinum, and subcutaneous emphysema
  - ▸ Avoid by allowing adequate expiratory time and keeping the airway system open (avoid use in upper airway obstruction; if needed, place oral/nasal airway to maintain patency)
  - ▸ Assure automatic shutoff mechanisms are properly functioning to allow termination of ventilation in overpressure situations
- Tracheal injury:
  - ▸ Always use adequate humidification
- Excessive auto-PEEP and dynamic hyperinflation:
  - ▸ Usually occurs at frequencies above 150 bpm
  - ▸ Avoid malposition of the jet ventilator catheter tip in the proximal conducting airways—should be at level of carina
  - ▸ Auto-PEEP is usually a desired feature but can result in worsening ventilation and compromise systemic circulation
- Hypercapnia:
  - ▸ More common when high respiratory frequencies used
  - ▸ Avoid in patients with obesity, reduced chest wall compliance, COPD, or increased baseline CO_2 levels:
    - ▪ However, some clinical trials show HFJV can be used safely even in COPD and bullous emphysema
  - ▸ Consider switching to CMV periodically to check $PetCO_2$. Can check ABG if arterial line is available. May be treated by increasing tidal volumes (increase driving pressure or inspiratory time, or decrease respiratory rate)

PEARLS

- Ventilator settings must be individualized for each patient according to his or her lung compliance and physiologic needs:
  - ‣ Adjustable HFJV parameters include driving pressure, frequency, and inspiratory time
- Auto-PEEP is a desired feature of HFJV
- Inhalational anesthetics cannot be used with HFJV; use TIVA
- Ability to monitor FiO_2, $PetCO_2$, Paw, and VT is limited due to its open airway system and greater dead space ventilation
- HFJV can be used in situations where a "still" surgical field is required, or in the management of the difficult airway

REFERENCES

For references, please visit **www.TheAnesthesiaGuide.com**.

CHAPTER 56
Antidotes

Clement Hoffmann, MD and Jean-Pierre Tourtier, MD

NEOSTIGMINE

- *Indication*: reversal of nondepolarizing muscle relaxants for patients with residual neuromuscular block (TOF ratio <0.9)
- Mechanism of action: reversibly inhibits acetylcholinesterase and thus potentiates the nicotinic and muscarinic effects of acetylcholine
- Only use if ≥1 response on TOF
- *Dose*: 50–70 µg/kg
- Glycopyrrolate 10–15 µg/kg associated to prevent adverse parasympathetic side effects of neostigmine (muscarinic effects: bradycardia, bronchospasm, increased secretions, etc)
- Atropine possible too (20 µg/kg), but more tachycardia and less antisialagogue action than glycopyrrolate. Also, atropine crosses the BBB and can cause CNS side effects
- Onset time: 10 minutes
- Goal: TOF ratio >0.9
- Contraindications: unstable asthma, Parkinson disease, deep NMB with no response on TOF, succinylcholine
- In children, edrophonium 500 µg/kg paired with atropine 20 µg/kg is often used instead of neostigmine. The onset time is shorter, although the difference is probably not clinically significant

SUGAMMADEX

- *Currently not approved by the FDA, not available in the United States*
- Indication: reversal of NMB by selective biding of nondepolarizing steroidal muscle relaxants (aminosteroids)—rocuronium, vecuronium, and pancuronium
- Dose: reversal of rocuronium or vecuronium:
  - ‣ With 4/4 on TOF: 2 mg/kg (onset time: 1 minute)
  - ‣ With 2/4 on TOF: 4 mg/kg (onset time: 2 minutes)
  - ‣ No response on TOF: 16 mg/kg (onset time: 2 minutes)

NALOXONE

- Morphine antagonist (mu-opioid receptor competitive antagonist)
- *Indicated for*:
  - ▸ Opioid overdose
  - ▸ Treatment for side effects of IV or neuraxial morphine: respiratory depression, CNS depression, urinary retention
- *Contraindications*: allergy, caution in patients at risk for myocardial ischemia because it can result in increased sympathetic activity
- *Dose*: one vial IV (400 μg in 1 mL) diluted in 9 mL normal saline, titration milliliter per milliliter until respiratory rate >12/min. Avoid giving more than needed because of severe pain, difficult to treat, and agitation
- Onset time: 1 minute, and effects may last up to 45 minutes (shorter than duration of action of most opioids)—risk of "remorphinization"
- Maintain by continuous infusion, adjusted to clinical response (e.g., two vials [800 μg] over 3 hours)

FLUMAZENIL

- *Indicated for*: reversal of sedative and hypnotic effects of benzodiazepines
- *Contraindications*: allergy to benzodiazepines, chronic treatment with benzodiazepines (withdrawal syndrome with risk of seizure), intoxication with medications that can cause seizures (e.g., tricyclic antidepressants), inability to monitor (duration of action of flumazenil is shorter than that of most benzodiazepines)
- *Dose*: bolus 0.3 mg, and then titration 0.2 mg/min (maximum 2 mg); maintain by IV infusion 0.1–0.4 mg/h

INTRALIPID (SEE CHAPTER 119)

- Indication: rescue for cardiac toxicity associated with local anesthetics, especially bupivacaine and ropivacaine—arrhythmia, severe hypotension, or asystole
- Contraindications of Intralipid administration for nutrition: severe disorders of fat metabolism such as severe liver damage, acute myocardial infarction, shock, dyslipidemia, hemostatic abnormalities, hypersensitivity to Intralipid; none of these contraindications apply when used for LA toxicity
- Recommended dose: 1.5 mL/kg of 20% Intralipid IV bolus (can be repeated once if persistent asystole) followed by a continuous infusion of 0.25 mL/(kg min) for 30 minutes (the rate of the infusion should be increased to 0.5 mL/(kg min) for 60 minutes if blood pressure decreases)
- See www.lipidrescue.org

METHYLENE BLUE

- Indication: treatment for methemoglobinemia (caused by prilocaine, benzocaine) above 20% or associated with hypoxemia signs
- Conversion of methemoglobin to hemoglobin by acceleration of the enzymatic reduction of methemoglobin by NADPH methemoglobin reductase
- Warning: can cause methemoglobinemia at high concentrations!
- Dose: initial 1–2 mg/kg over 5 minutes; effects are seen in 20 minutes to 1 hour, may be repeated in 1 hour if necessary with a dose of 1 mg/kg (maximal dose 7 mg/kg)
- Contraindications: renal failure, hypersensitivity to methylene blue or any component; use with caution when G6PD deficiency
- Treatment failure: ongoing exposure, patient with deficient NADPH methemoglobin reductase

REFERENCES

For references, please visit **www.TheAnesthesiaGuide.com**.

CHAPTER 57
Ambulatory Anesthesia

Jennifer Wu, MD, MBA

BASICS

- Patients come from home on the day of surgery and are discharged home shortly after surgery
- Ambulatory surgery centers are often separate from hospitals, and so do not have the resources to:
  ‣ Admit patients postoperatively
  ‣ Mechanically ventilate postoperatively
  ‣ Transfuse blood
  ‣ Insert invasive monitors (arterial line, central line)
- Procedure selection is important to *avoid*:
  ‣ Lengthy procedures
  ‣ Large fluid shifts and/or blood loss
  ‣ Postoperative pain management requiring IV agents
  ‣ Prolonged mechanical ventilation
- If a patient needs to be stabilized or admitted from a surgery center, he or she must be transferred to an admitting hospital by ambulance

PREOPERATIVE

- Patients may have their initial preanesthesia evaluation on the day of surgery, or in the week prior at an anesthesia clinic or by telephone
- Anesthetic information may be administered by handout, telephone, or video
- Patient selection:
  ‣ ASA 1 and 2 patients
  ‣ ASA 3 patients who are optimized
- Identify risk factors for unanticipated admission and consider canceling/performing in hospital:
  ‣ Respiratory issues:
    ▪ Requires home oxygen; Sleep apnea, especially if home CPAP
    ▪ History of difficult airway
    ▪ History of prolonged ventilation
  ‣ Severe postoperative nausea and vomiting
  ‣ History of chronic pain or substance abuse
  ‣ Psychiatric disorders
  ‣ Postoperative delirium
- Consider regional anesthesia to reduce postoperative opioid use

INDUCTION

- Use short-acting agents with strong safety profile:
  ‣ Propofol:
    ▪ Rapid induction and recovery
    ▪ Decreases incidence of PONV
  ‣ Avoid etomidate, which is associated with PONV
  ‣ Succinylcholine is short-acting but can cause myalgia
- Consider LMA to eliminate the need for muscle relaxation and reversal
- Consider monitored anesthesia care and regional anesthesia

MAINTENANCE

- Use short-acting agents
- Consider TIVA to reduce postoperative nausea and vomiting
- Administer prophylactic antiemetics (see chapter 69):
  ‣ Dexamethasone 8 mg IV after induction
  ‣ Ondansetron 4 mg IV 30 minutes before end of surgery
  ‣ Droperidol 0.625 mg IV for high-risk patients; black box warning mandates EKG monitoring postoperatively

POSTOPERATIVE

- Seek to eliminate time in the PACU by aggressively avoiding nausea, using nonopioid methods to treat pain
- Patients may or may not need to void postoperatively, depending on the type of surgery and institutional guidelines
- Aldrete-based criteria for discharge home (see chapter 69)
- Patients must be provided with instructions for routine care and possible emergencies
- Patients must have a reliable adult escort home

PEARLS AND TIPS

- The most common anesthetic cause of postoperative unanticipated admission is nausea and vomiting. The second most common cause is pain
- A well-organized system for administering regional anesthesia does not delay surgery and results in better postoperative pain control and faster discharge home
- An ambulatory surgery center should have standard anesthesia equipment, suction, oxygen, emergency resuscitative equipment, treatment for MH (if general anesthesia is performed), and treatment for local anesthetic toxicity (if regional anesthesia is performed)

REFERENCES

For references, please visit **www.TheAnesthesiaGuide.com**.

CHAPTER 58
Opioids, Induction Agents, Neuromuscular Blockers

Brian J. Egan, MD, MPH

Opioids			
Medication	**Pharmacology**		**Clinical pearls**
Morphine	Class	Phenanthrene	• IV/IM dosing equipotent
	Dose	1–3 mg	• IV dosing may produce less nausea/vomiting
	Relative potency	1	• Active metabolite (morphine 6-glucuronide) accumulates with renal insufficiency/failure
	Onset/peak	5/20 min	• Intrathecal/epidural use: hydrophilic nature allows for single dose to have prolonged effect at the mu receptors within the substantia gelatinosa (12–24 h). Migration to brain stem can produce delayed respiratory depression
	Metabolism	Hepatic	
	Side effects	Causes common opioid side effects[1] as well as histamine release	
Hydromorphone (Dilaudid)	Class	Phenanthrene	• Good alternative to morphine in renal insufficiency
	Dose	0.1–0.4 mg	• Purported to have less emetogenic effect compared with morphine
	Relative potency	7.5	
	Onset/peak	5/20 min	
	Metabolism	Hepatic	
	Side effects	Common opioid side effects[1]	
Meperidine (Demerol)	Class	Phenylpiperidine	• Most effective opioid at decreasing postoperative shivering
	Dose	12.5–100 mg	• Use in renal insufficiency can lead to accumulation of the metabolite, normeperidine, which can cause seizures
	Relative potency	0.1	
	Onset/peak	5/20 min	
	Metabolism	Hepatic	• Atropine-like structure can increase HR; does not cause miosis
	Side effects	Interaction with MAOIs can cause fatal hypermetabolic reaction	

(continued)

Opioids (*continued*)			
Medication	Pharmacology		Clinical pearls
Fentanyl (Sublimaze)	Class	Phenylpiperidine	• Use as analgesic component of TIVA at 0.2–1.5 µg/kg/h • Context-sensitive half-time (CSHT) leads to prolonged elimination with infusions greater than 2 h • Terminate infusion 30 min prior to expected emergence to allow drug accumulated in other compartments to be eliminated
	Dose	25–50 µg	
	Relative potency	100	
	Onset/peak	1/5 min	
	Metabolism	Hepatic	
	Side effects	Common opioid side effects[1] and chest wall rigidity	
Sufentanil (Sufenta)	Class	Phenylpiperidine	• As component of TIVA has more favorable CSHT but will accumulate with longer infusions • Very rapid onset
	Dose	5–10 µg	
	Relative potency	1,000	
	Onset/peak	30 s/1 min	
	Metabolism	Hepatic	
	Side effects	Common opioid side effects[1]	
Alfentanil (Alfenta)	Class	Phenylpiperidine	• Good alternative to remifentanil as bolus agent for brief periods of more intense stimulation • Good choice of analgesic component of TIVA (0.5–3 µg/(kg min)) when duration anticipated to be longer than 8 h (although remifentanil still superior in terms of recovery)
	Dose	100–300 µg	
	Relative potency	15	
	Onset/peak	30 s/1 min	
	Metabolism	Hepatic	
	Side effects	Common opioid side effects[1] Chest wall rigidity at high doses or with rapid administration	
Remifentanil (Ultiva)	Class	Phenylpiperidine	• With a flat CSHT with infusion of any duration, excellent TIVA component • Rapid onset and offset makes it good for blunting sympathetic effects of brief periods of increased stimulation • Very-low-dose infusions can be used for sedation; however, works synergistically with propofol to cause respiratory depression and apnea
	Dose	5–50 µg IV	
	Relative potency	100	
	Onset/peak	30 s/1 min	
	Metabolism	Tissue esterases	
	Side effects	Common opioid side effects.[1] Acute opioid desensitization, hyperalgesia	

[1]Common opioid side effects include nausea/vomiting, respiratory depression, urinary retention, pruritus, constipation, sedation, and miosis. Doses given are typical one-time bolus doses, not total doses for a given procedure.

FIGURE 58-1. Context-sensitive half-time of opioids

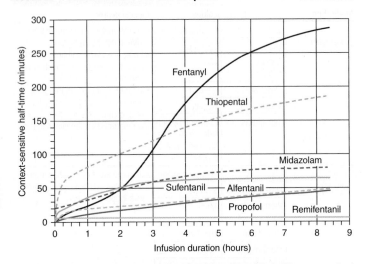

Curves are based on simulated pharmacokinetic models. Solid and dashed lines are used only to distinguish overlapping curves. Propofol and thiopental added for comparison purposes. Reproduced from Longnecker DE, Brown DL, Newman MF, Zapol WM. *Anesthesiology*. Figure 68-6. Available at: http://www.accessanesthiology.com. Copyright © The McGraw-Hill Companies, Inc. All rights reserved.

INDUCTION AGENTS

See table on following page.

Induction Agents			
Medication	Pharmacology		Clinical pearls
Propofol	Class	Alkylphenol	• Does not possess analgesic properties • 70% of patients experience pain with injection • Use within 6 h after opening • Favorable CSHT allows use as component of TIVA (75–150 µg/kg/min) • Rapid offset allows use as sedation in ICU or component of MAC (25–75 µg/kg/min) • Antiemetic at low doses (e.g., 10 mg IV or 10 µg/kg/min) • Prolonged infusions have caused "propofol infusion syndrome" (metabolic acidosis with bradycardia, hyperlipidemia, hepatomegaly, rhabdomyolysis, and green urine)
	Induction dose	1–2.5 mg/kg (age dependent)	
	Onset/duration	30 s/8 min	
	Metabolism	Hepatic and extrahepatic mechanisms	
	Side effects	Hypotension	
Thiopental	Class	Barbiturate	• No longer available for use in the United States • Infiltration causes severe pain and tissue injury • Contraindicated with porphyria • Possible histamine release and bronchospasm • If BP maintained, useful as neuroprotective agent as decreases $CMRO_2$ (maximum at burst suppression on EEG) and decreases ICP due to decreased CBF • Not useful as continuous infusion due to prolonged CSHT
	Induction dose	3–5 mg/kg	
	Onset/duration	30 s/6–10 min	
	Metabolism	Hepatic	
	Side effects	Hypotension in debilitated or hypovolemic patient	
Midazolam	Class	Benzodiazepine	• More commonly used as a premedication or hypnotic–sedative component of MAC (causes both anxiolysis and anterograde amnesia) • When used alone, minimal effect on ventilation and blood pressure • Also has anticonvulsant effects that are useful in conjunction with local anesthetic administration • Can be given PO, 0.5 mg/kg, to facilitate pediatric induction
	Induction dose	0.2–0.3 mg/kg	
	Onset/duration	1–3 min/peaks 5 min; can result in prolonged sedation	
	Metabolism	Hepatic Decreases with age	
	Side effects	Synergistic respiratory depression with opioids and propofol	

(continued)

Induction Agents (*continued*)

Medication	Pharmacology		Clinical pearls
Ketamine	Class	PCP derivative	• Unique in its analgesic properties (NMDA antagonist) • Increases salivation/lacrimation (can attenuate with anticholinergic) • Produces bronchodilation and a centrally mediated sympathetic stimulation (increased BP, HR, and CO); however, will still produce hypotension in hypovolemic patient • Minimal suppression of ventilation when used alone • Can be used to supplement failed regional (0.2–0.8 mg/kg IV) • Resurgence in use related to opioid-sparing effect and ability to decrease opioid tolerance at subanesthetic doses (1–3 μg/kg/min)[2]
	Induction dose	1–2 mg/kg IV and 4–6 mg/kg IM	
	Onset/duration	30 s/3 min	
	Metabolism	Hepatic	
	Side effects	Psychotomimetic effects	
Etomidate	Class	Imidazole	• Minimal decrease in BP with induction doses; however, will still produce hypotension in hypovolemic patient • Has no analgesic effect • Adrenal suppression for 4–6 h after injection; therefore, infusion or repeat dosing best avoided, avoid in septic patient • Pain and myoclonic movements with induction are common (>50%) • May be associated with increased risk of PONV
	Induction dose	0.2–0.3 mg/kg	
	Onset/duration	30/100 s for every 0.1 mg/kg	
	Metabolism	Ester hydrolysis	
	Side effects	Adrenal suppression (for 4–8 h after induction dose)	

NEUROMUSCULAR BLOCKING AGENTS

See table on following page.

Neuromuscular Blocking Agents

Muscle relaxant	Class	Intubating dose (mg/kg)	Infusion dose	Onset	Duration (min)	Metabolism
Pancuronium	Aminosteroid	0.1	NA	3–5 min	60–90	Renal >> hepatic
Vecuronium	Aminosteroid	0.08–0.1	1.0 µg/kg/min	3–5 min	20–35	Hepatic ≅ renal
Rocuronium	Aminosteroid	0.6–1.2	0.01–0.012 mg/kg/min	1–2 min	20–35	Hepatic > renal
Mivacurium[1]	Benzylisoquinoline	0.25	5–6 mg/kg/min	2–3 min	12–20	Enzymatic hydrolysis
Cisatracurium	Benzylisoquinoline	0.15–0.2	1–1.5 mg/kg/min	3–5 min	20–35	Hoffman elimination
Atracurium[1]	Benzylisoquinoline	0.4–0.5	9–10 µg/kg/min	3–5 min	20–35	Hoffman elimination
Succinylcholine	Depolarizing	1–2	2.5 mg/min titrated to twitch response	30–60 s	6–9	Pseudocholinesterase

[1]No longer available in the United States.

NMB REVERSAL

- Qualitative measures of residual weakness poor:
  - *Tactile* absence of fade on train-of-four (TOF) 4/4 still compatible with clinically significant blockade
  - Sustained tetany at 100 Hz for 5 seconds suggests TOFR ≥0.85
  - Respiratory parameters (Vt, FVC, NIF, $EtCO_2$) are inadequate to determine residual weakness
  - The application of tetanus produces facilitated (enhanced) results of TOF or tetany for 5–10 minutes
- Residual paralysis leads to increased risk of perioperative mortality and morbidity:
  - Weakened upper airway may be less able to prevent aspiration
  - Increased risk of severe hypoxemia (SpO_2 <93%) in PACU
  - May be risk factor for atelectasis
- Do not assume a single intubating dose of NMB has worn off by case end. Rocuronium capable of producing clinically significant residual blockade at 3 hours
- Anticholinesterase reversal has risks:
  - Overdosing may exacerbate weakness
  - Ceiling effect reached at between 0.04 and 0.07 mg/kg due to nearly 100% inhibition of enzyme. May not be adequate to overcome NMB
  - Increased secretions and bradycardia have to be offset with anticholinergics; arrhythmias common
  - May increase risk of PONV (unclear)
- Too dense a block (0 twitches) not reversible but 4/4 twitches may still have TOFR <0.4 and still require reversal:
  - Never reverse 0 twitches. Patient will be weak
  - Reverse two to three twitches with 0.05 mg/kg neostigmine
  - May reverse one twitch but, remember, it may take up to 30 minutes to achieve sustained tetanus
  - Reverse TOF of 4 with fade with 0.03 mg/kg
  - TOF of 4 without fade may require as little as 0.02 mg/kg of neostigmine
- Succinycholine infusion can also be guided by use of nerve stimulator. Avoid stage 2 blockade by monitoring for development of fade

NMB MONITORING (FIGURES 58-2 AND 58-3)

NB: Ensure to place black (negative) electrode distally for optimal response.

A. TOF

- Twitches progressively fade as relaxation increases
- Ratio (difficult to estimate) of the responses to the first and fourth twitches is a sensitive indicator of nondepolarizing muscle paralysis
- More convenient to visually observe the sequential disappearance of the twitches:
  - Disappearance of the fourth twitch represents a 75% block
  - The third twitch an 80% block
  - The second twitch a 90% block
- Clinical relaxation usually requires 75–95% neuromuscular blockade

B. Tetany at 50 or 100 Hz

- Sensitive test of neuromuscular function
- Sustained contraction for 5 seconds indicates adequate—but not necessarily complete—reversal from neuromuscular blockade
- Painful in conscious patient

C. Double burst stimulation (DBS)

- Two variations of tetany that are less painful to the patient
- DBS is more sensitive than TOF stimulation for the clinical (i.e., visual or tactile) evaluation of fade

Diaphragm, rectus abdominis, laryngeal adductors, and orbicularis oculi muscles recover from NMB earlier than the adductor pollicis.

Other, less reliable indicators of adequate recovery include:
- Sustained (5 seconds) head lift
- Ability to generate an inspiratory pressure of at least −25 cm H$_2$O
- Forceful handgrip

FIGURE 58-2. Sites suitable for nerve stimulation

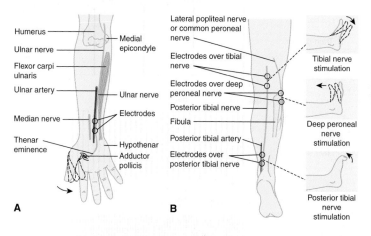

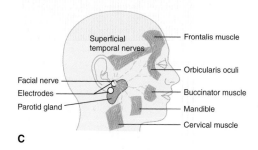

(A) Ulnar nerve; (B) tibial, deep peroneal, and posterior tibial nerves; (C) facial nerve. Reproduced with permission from Ali HH. Monitoring neuromuscular function. *Semin Anesth.* 1989;8:158. © Elsevier.

FIGURE 58-3. Patterns of electrical impulses for monitoring of NMB

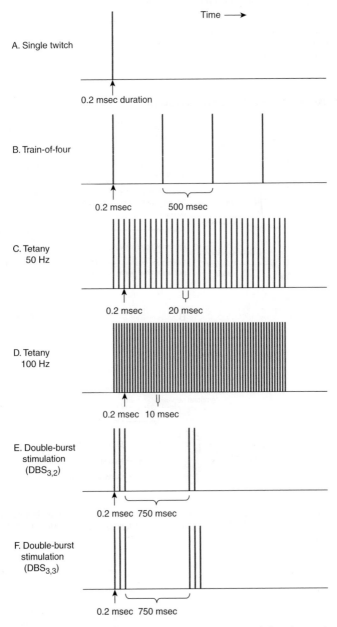

All stimuli are 200 microseconds in duration, of square-wave pattern, and of equal current intensity. (A) Single twitch; (B) train-of-four; (C) tetany 50 Hz; (D) tetany 100 Hz; (E) double-burst stimulation (DBS₃,₂); (F) double-burst stimulation (DBS₃,₃). Reproduced from Morgan GE, Mikhail MS, Murray MJ. *Clinical Anesthesiology.* 4th ed. Figure 6-32. Available at: http://www.accessmedicine. com.

REFERENCES

For references, please visit **www.TheAnesthesiaGuide.com**.

CHAPTER 59
Common Drugs Encountered in the OR

Ruchir Gupta, MD

All dosages are for adults unless otherwise specified. For details on pediatric dosages, please refer to Chapter 167.
• Abciximab (ReoPro): see table on antiplatelet agents
• Acetazolamide (Diamox): see table on diuretics
• (Aldactone) Spironolactone: see table on diuretics
• Alfentanil (Alfenta): see table on opioids
• Aminocaproic acid (Amicar): see table on antifibrinolytics
• (Anectine) Succinylcholine: see table on neuromuscular blocking agents

Anticholinergics				
	Tachycardia	Bronchodilation	Sedation	Antisialagogue
Atropine	+++	++	+	++
Scopolamine	+	+	+++	++
Glycopyrrolate (Robinul) (does not cross BBB)	++	++	0	+++

ANTICOAGULANTS AND REVERSAL

See table on following page.

Anticoagulants and Reversal

Drug

Argatroban	Direct thrombin inhibitor	2 μg/kg/min infusion up to 10 μg/kg/min (HIT), 350 μg/kg IV over 2–5 min with 25 μg/kg/min infusion (PCI in patients with HIT)
Antithrombin III (ATIII, Thrombate III)	Binds coagulation factors, preventing formation of clot	Determine preinfusion (baseline) antithrombin III concentration and calculate initial (loading) dosage using following formula:

Initial dose (U) =
$$\frac{(\text{desired ATIII concentration} - \text{baseline AT III concentration [\% of normal]}) \times \text{weight (kg)}}{1.4}$$

Administer dose to increase antithrombin III concentration to a suggested level of 120% of normal using formula

Enoxaparin (Lovenox)	Accelerates activity of antithrombin III	30–40 mg SC bid (DVT prophylaxis), 1 mg/kg SC q12 h or 1.5 mg/kg SC q day (Tx of DVT), 1.5 mg/kg/dose SC q12 h (ACS)
Protamine	Combines with heparin (strong acid) to form a stable complex (salt)	1 mg protamine per mg of active heparin
Warfarin (Coumadin)	Inhibits factors 2, 7, 9, 10 and proteins C and S	5 mg PO, and then maintenance of 2–10 mg PO for goal INR of 2–3

Antiemetics

Drug	Dose (IV)	Mechanism	Anesthetic considerations
Ondansetron (Zofran)	4 mg (adults), 0.1 mg/kg (pediatrics) up to 4 mg	5-HT3 receptor antagonist	Prolongs QT interval Hepatic clearance
Granisetron (Kytril)	1 mg (adults), 10 μg/kg (pediatrics)	5-HT3 receptor antagonist	
Dolasetron (Anzemet)	12.5 mg (adults), 0.35 mg/kg	5-HT3 receptor antagonist	
Droperidol (Inapsine)	1–2 μg/kg (adults), 0.1 mg/kg (pediatrics)	DA antagonist, blocks release of NE, 5-HT, GABA	Prolongs QT interval (black box warning), hypotension, extrapyramidal effects, avoid in pheochromocytoma, avoid in patients receiving L-dopa therapy
Dexamethasone (Decadron)	4–12 mg	Antiemetic mechanism unclear	Administer with caution in patients with DM Useful if airway trauma during repeated intubations Useful as antiemetic (4 mg)
Metoclopramide (Reglan)	0.25 mg/kg	DA antagonist centrally, peripheral cholinomimetic	Avoid in patients with pheochromocytoma Can cause extrapyramidal side effects, neuroleptic malignant syndrome Does not affect gastric pH
Promethazine (Phenergan)	12.5–25 mg	H1 receptor antagonist DA blocker Partial alpha-blocker	Respiratory depression CNS depression Rare neuroleptic malignant syndrome

Antifibrinolytics

Drug	Dosage	Mechanism of action
Aminocaproic acid (Amicar)	Acute bleeding: 4–5 g during the first hour, followed by 1 g/h for 8 h or until bleeding controlled (maximum daily dose: 30 g) Thrombocytopenia: 0.1 g/kg over 30–60 min	Blocks activation of plasminogen to plasmin
Aprotinin (Trasylol)	2 million KIU (280 mg; 200 mL) loading dose IV over 25–30 min 2 million KIU (280 mg; 200 mL) into the pump prime volume 500,000 KIU/h (70 mg/h; 50 mL/h) IV during procedure	Serine protease inhibitor that decreases fibrinolysis and the inflammatory pathway by interfering with the chemical mediators (thrombin, plasmin, kallikrein)

Antiplatelet Agents

Drug	Mechanism of action	Dose
Abciximab (ReoPro)	Inhibits platelet aggregation by inhibiting glycoprotein IIB/IIIA surface antigen	Bolus 0.25 mg/kg administered over 10–60 min prior to PCI, and then as an infusion at 10 µg/min
Clopidogrel (Plavix)	Inhibits platelets by binding ADP	Load 300 mg PO, maintenance 75 mg PO q day
Eptifibatide (Integrilin)	Inhibits platelet aggregation by inhibiting glycoprotein IIB/IIIA surface antigen	Bolus 180 µg/kg, and then 2 µg/kg/min infusion
Ticlopidine (Ticlid)	Inhibits platelets by binding ADP	250 mg PO BID

- Antithrombin III (Thrombate III): see table on anticoagulants and reversal

Anxiolytics

Midazolam (Versed)	0.01–0.1 mg/kg
Diazepam (Valium)	0.04–0.2 mg/kg

- (Anzemet) Dolasetron: see table on antiemetics
- Aprotinin (Trasylol): see table on antifibrinolytics
- Argatroban: see table on anticoagulants and reversal
- Atracurium (Tracrium): see table on neuromuscular blocking agents
- Atropine: see table on anticholinergics/see table on reversal agents
- (Benadryl) Diphenhydramine: see table on common drugs
- Cisatracurium (Nimbex): see table on neuromuscular blocking agents
- Clopidogrel (Plavix): see table on antiplatelet agents

Common Drugs Seen in the OR Setting

Drug	Dose IV (indication)	Comments
Indigotindisulfonate (Indigo Carmine)	40 mg slowly	Used for evaluation of urine output. May cause transient decrease in pulse oximeter reading and elevated BP for 15–30 min
Methylene blue	1–2 mg/kg over 10 min (methemoglobinemia) 100 mg (marker for GU surgery)	Causes transient decrease in measured pulse oximeter reading, hemolysis in patients with G6PD deficiency, HTN
Glucagon (GlucaGen)	0.25–0.5 mg (duodenal relaxation) 5 mg bolus (refractory beta-blocker toxicity) 0.5–1 mg (hypoglycemia)	Associated with anaphylaxis, hyperglycemia, nausea, vomiting
Diphenhydramine (Benadryl)	10–50 mg (acute mild allergic reaction)	Sedative properties, may cause decrease in BP
Haloperidol (Haldol)	0.5–5 mg (mild–moderate agitation) 10–20 mg (severe agitation) 1 mg (PONV)	May cause extrapyramidal symptoms, prolonged QT (torsades de pointes), NMS
Famotidine (Pepcid)	20 mg	H_2 receptor antagonist

Corticosteroids

Drugs	Indications with dosage	Comments
Dexamethasone (Decadron)	Cerebral edema (10 mg, 4 mg q6 h), airway edema (4–6 mg)	Immunosuppressant, delayed wound healing
Hydrocortisone (Solu-Cortef)	Acute adrenal insufficiency (100 mg, and then 300 mg q8 h), shock (1.5–4 mg/kg per day from surgical start to 24 h), physiologic replacement (500–2,000 mg), stress dosing (1–2 mg/kg, and then 0.5–1 mg/kg q6 h)	Abrupt withdrawal can cause adrenocortical insufficiency
Methylprednisolone (Solu-Medrol)	Spinal cord injury (30 mg/kg IV over 15 min, after 45 min 5.4 mg/kg/h × 23 h) Status asthmaticus (2 mg/kg)	Very potent. Almost no mineralocorticoid properties

- (Coumadin) Warfarin: see table on anticoagulants and reversal
- Dexamethasone (Decadron): see table on corticosteroids
- (Diamox) Acetazolamide: see table on diuretics
- Diazepam (Valium): see table on anxiolytics
- (Dibenzyline) Phenoxybenzamine: see Chapter 47
- (Dilantin) Phenytoin: see Chapter 106
- Diphenhydramine (Benadryl): see table on common drugs
- (Diprivan) Propofol: see table on induction agent

Diuretics

Drug	Dosage (indications)	Precautions/side effects	Serum pH	Na	Cl⁻	K⁺	Glucose	Uric acid	Ca²⁺	Mg
Carbonic anhydrase inhibitor: acetazolamide (Diamox)	250–500 mg IV q day (CHF), 250–375 mg IV q day (glaucoma), 125–250 mg PO q6–12 h (mountain sickness), 8–30 mg/kg PO per day in divided doses (seizure prophylaxis)	Ototoxicity, Stevens–Johnson syndrome, seizures, GI irritation, hyperchloremic metabolic acidosis, BM depression	↓		←	↓				
Loop diuretics: furosemide (Lasix)	10–20 mg IV over 1–2 min, may repeat, not to exceed 200 mg (CHF, edema, HTN, nonobstructive oliguria)	Hepatic encephalopathy (with hepatic failure) Pancreatitis Gastric irritation Tinnitus Paresthesias Vertigo Aplastic anemia (rare) Erythema multiforme Purpura Photosensitivity Stevens–Johnson syndrome Orthostatic hypotension Increased cholesterol/TG	←	↓	←	↓	←–	←–	↓	↓

(continued)

Diuretics (continued)

Drug	Dosage (indications)	Precautions/side effects	Serum pH	Na	Cl⁻	K⁺	Glucose	Uric acid	Ca²⁺	Mg
Thiazide diuretics: hydrochlorothiazide (Aquazide)	25 mg PO q day, may increase to 50 mg (HTN, nephrocalcinosis, osteoporosis, DI)	Gout	↑	↓	↓	↓	↑	↑	↑	
Aldosterone antagonist: spironolactone (Aldactone)	50–100 mg PO q day, given in either single or divided doses (HTN); 25–100 mg PO q day (hypokalemia); 100 mg PO q day, given in either single or divided doses (edema). Initially, 400 mg PO for 4 days or 400 mg PO for 3–4 weeks to diagnose the condition (hyperaldosteronism, nephrotic syndrome)	Abdominal pain Agranulocytosis Amenorrhea Drowsiness Erythema Gastritis Gynecomastia Hirsutism Impotence (erectile dysfunction) Infertility Maculopapular rash Mastalgia Menstrual irregularity		↓	↑	↑	–			
K⁺-sparing diuretics: triamterene (Dyrenium)	100 mg PO (edema, ascites)	Diarrhea; dizziness or light-headedness when standing or sitting up; headache; loss of appetite; nausea		↓		↑–	↑–	↑	↑	

- Dolasetron (Anzemet): see table on antiemetics
- Droperidol (Inapsine): see table on antiemetics
- Edrophonium (Tensilon): see table on reversal agents
- Enoxaparin (Lovenox): see table on anticoagulants and reversal
- Eptifibatide (Integrilin): see table on antiplatelet agents
- Etomidate (Amidate): see table on induction agents
- Famotidine (Pepcid): see table on common drugs
- Fentanyl (Sublimaze): see table on opioids
- Furosemide (Lasix): see table on diuretics
- Glucagon (GlucaGen): see table on common drugs
- Glycopyrrolate (Robinul): see tables on anticholinergics and on reversal agents
- Granisetron (Kytril): see table on antiemetics
- Haloperidol (Haldol): see table on common drugs
- Heparin: see chapter 12
- Hydrocortisone (Solu-Cortef): see table on corticosteroids
- Indigotindisulfonate (Indigo Carmine): see table on common drugs

Induction Agents	
Etomidate (Amidate)	0.2–0.4 mg/kg
Ketamine (Ketalar)	1–2 mg/kg
Propofol (Diprivan)	1.5–2.5 mg/kg
Thiopental (Pentothal)	3–5 mg/kg

- (Integrilin) Eptifibatide: see table on antiplatelet agents
- Ketamine (Ketalar): see table on induction agents
- (Kytril) Granisetron: see table on antiemetics
- (Lasix) Furosemide: see table on diuretics
- (Lovenox) Enoxaparin: see table on anticoagulants and reversal
- Midazolam (Versed): see table on anxiolytics
- Methylene blue: see table on common drugs
- Methylprednisolone (Solu-Medrol): see table on corticosteroids
- Metoclopramide (Reglan): see table on antiemetics
- Neostigmine (Prostigmine): see table on reversal agents

Neuromuscular Blocking Agents		
Atracurium (Tracrium)	0.4–0.5 mg/kg	Infusion: initially 0.4–0.5 mg IV bolus, followed by 9–10 µg/kg/min
Cisatracurium (Nimbex)	0.15–0.2 mg/kg	Infusion: 0.15–0.2 mg/kg IV bolus followed by 1–3 µg/kg/min
Rocuronium (Zemuron)	0.6–1.2 mg/kg	Infusion: 0.01–0.012 mg/kg/min
Vecuronium (Norcuron)	0.08–0.1 mg/kg	Infusion: initial IV bolus (0.08–0.3 mg/kg), followed by (after 20–40 min) 1 µg/kg/min infusion (usual range: 0.8–1.2 µg/kg/min)
Succinylcholine (intubating dose) (Anectine)	1 mg/kg 4 mg/kg IM	Infusion: 2.5 mg/min (0.5–10 mg/min)

- (Norcuron) Vecuronium: see table on neuromuscular blocking agents
- Ondansetron (Zofran): see table on antiemetics

Opioids	
Fentanyl (Sublimaze)	0.5–2.5 µg/kg
Sufentanil (Sufenta)	0.1–1 µg/kg
Alfentanil (Alfenta)	50–70 µg/kg
Remifentanil (Ultiva)	0.5–1.0 µg/kg/min

- (Phenergan) Promethazine: see table on antiemetics
- Phenoxybenzamine (Dibenzyline): see chapter 47
- Phentolamine (Regitine): see chapter 47
- Phenytoin (Dilantin): see chapter 106
- Physostigmine: see table on reversal agents
- (Plavix) Clopidogrel: see table on antiplatelet agents
- Propofol (Diprivan): see table on induction agents
- (Prostigmine) Neostigmine: see table on reversal agents
- Protamine: see table on anticoagulants and reversal
- (Regitine) Phentolamine: see chapter 47
- Remifentanil (Ultiva): see table on opioids
- (ReoPro) Abciximab: see table on antiplatelet agents

Reversal Agents	
Neostigmine (Prostigmine)	0.05–0.08 mg/kg
Physostigmine	0.01–0.03 mg/kg
Edrophonium (Tensilon)	0.5–1 mg/kg
Atropine	0.007–0.014 mg/kg
Glycopyrrolate (Robinul)	0.008–0.016 mg/kg

- Rocuronium (Zemuron): see table on neuromuscular blocking agents
- Scopolamine: see table on anticholinergics
- (Solu-Cortef) Hydrocortisone: see table on corticosteroids
- (Solu-Medrol) Methylprednisolone: see table on corticosteroids
- Spironolactone (Aldactone): see table on diuretics
- (Sublimaze) Fentanyl: see table on opioids
- Succinylcholine (Anectine): see table on neuromuscular blocking agents
- Sufentanil (Sufenta): see table on opioids
- (Tensilon) Edrophonium: see table on reversal agents
- Thiopental (Pentothal): see table on induction agents
- (Thrombate III) Antithrombin III: see table on anticoagulants and reversal
- Ticlopidine (Ticlid): see table on antiplatelet agents
- (Trasylol) Aprotinin: see table on antifibrinolytics
- Triamterene (Dyrenium): see table on diuretics
- (Ultiva) Remifentanil: see table on opioids
- (Valium) Diazepam: see table on anxiolytics
- Vecuronium (Norcuron): see table on neuromuscular blocking agents
- (Versed) Midazolam: see table on anxiolytics
- Warfarin (Coumadin): see table on anticoagulants and reversal
- (Zofran) Ondansetron: see table on antiemetics

CHAPTER 60
Inhalation Agents

Jennifer Wu, MD, MBA

BASICS

- Potent (halogenated) agents currently in use: isoflurane, sevoflurane, desflurane; older agents: halothane, enflurane, methoxyflurane
- Nitrous oxide chemically unrelated
- Blood gas partition coefficient is a measure of solubility of the inhalation agents. The less soluble the agent, the more rapid the onset and offset:
  - ▸ Liposolubility: halothane > isoflurane > sevoflurane > desflurane

Anesthetic Effect of Various MAC Values	
MAC value	Effect
1 MAC	Alveolar concentration of anesthetic agent necessary to prevent movement in response to surgical incision in 50% of patients
1.5 MAC	90% will not move
0.3 MAC	MAC awake: patients will become conscious if no other agent used

Factors Affecting MAC				
	Age	Temperature	Substances	Other
Increased MAC	Young (maximum at age 6 months)	Hyperthermia	• Acute amphetamines • Chronic alcohol	
Decreased MAC	Old	Hypothermia	• Acute alcohol • Concurrent opioids	Pregnancy Regional anesthesia

PROPERTIES OF VOLATILE ANESTHETICS

See table on following page.

Properties of Volatile Anesthetics

	Desflurane	Sevoflurane	Isoflurane	Nitrous oxide
MAC (%)	6.0	1.7	1.2	105
B:G partition coefficient	0.45	0.65	1.4	0.47
Pungent	Yes	No	Yes	No
SVR	Decrease	Decrease	Decrease	Increase
Heart rate	Increase secondary to sympathetic stimulation	No change	Increase secondary to baroreceptor reflex from decreased MAP	Moderate increase secondary to sympathetic stimulation
MAP	Transient increase with rapid rise in concentration, and then decrease	Decrease	Decrease	Variable
Contractility	Decrease	Decrease	Decrease	Decrease
Metabolism	Minimal	Moderate	Minimal	No
Other properties	• Agent that is most likely to form carbon monoxide when in contact with dry CO_2 absorbent	• Breakdown product compound A is nephrotoxic in animals (unclear clinical significance) • Avoid flows <2 L/min		• Expands air spaces (bowel, lung blebs) • Increases pulmonary vascular resistance
Clinical considerations	• Faster emergence than sevoflurane and isoflurane	• Good for inhalation induction	• Inexpensive	• May increase nausea • Second gas effect speeds induction and emergence

CARDIOVASCULAR EFFECTS

- All halogenated agents are vasodilators; hypotension can result with high inhaled concentrations
- Desflurane has a sympathomimetic effect, especially during rapid increase in concentration, with tachycardia and possibly hypertension. This usually resolves after a few minutes
- Halothane also depresses myocardium (useful in tetralogy of Fallot)
- N_2O has a mild sympathomimetic effect, usually not clinically significant

Effect of Intracardiac Shunts on Speed of Inhalation Induction

Shunt	Speed of inhalation induction
L → R	Faster
R → L	Slower

Respiratory Effects	
Increase	Decrease
Bronchodilation	Ventilatory response to hypercarbia
Respiratory rate	Ventilatory response to hypoxia
	Hypoxic pulmonary vasoconstriction
	Tidal volume
	Minute ventilation

Neurologic Effects		
	Cerebral blood flow	Cerebral metabolic rate
Desflurane	Vasodilation	Decrease
Sevoflurane		
Isoflurane		
Nitrous oxide	Vasodilation	Increase

- All inhalation agents interfere with somatosensory-evoked potential monitoring: See chapter 105
  - ▸ Decrease in amplitude
  - ▸ Increase in latency
  - ▸ Maintenance of general anesthesia at a half MAC or less is usually acceptable (+IV propofol infusion)
  - ▸ Avoid rapid changes in concentration

OBSTETRICS

- Pregnancy decreases the MAC
- Desflurane, sevoflurane, and isoflurane relax the uterus

NEUROMUSCULAR EFFECTS

- Desflurane, sevoflurane, and isoflurane cause muscle relaxation and potentiate nondepolarizing muscle relaxants
- Desflurane, sevoflurane, and isoflurane can trigger malignant hyperthermia in genetically susceptible patients

Toxicity				
	Desflurane	Sevoflurane	Isoflurane	Nitrous oxide
Liver		Metabolized to inorganic fluoride	Rarely causes hepatitis	
Renal		Nephrotoxicity in animals		
Soda lime interaction	CO production associated with dry soda lime	Compound A produced when flows are low for prolonged time		
Malignant hyperthermia	May trigger	May trigger	May trigger	Safe to use in MH-susceptible patient

REFERENCES

For references, please visit **www.TheAnesthesiaGuide.com**.

CHAPTER 61
Intraoperative Events

Tanuj P. Palvia, MD and Jason Lau, MD

BRADYCARDIA

- Stable or unstable?
  - ‣ Is the patient in cardiopulmonary arrest? Initiate ACLS Protocol
  - ‣ Assess the airway. Ensure the adequacy of oxygenation and ventilation
  - ‣ Assess for hypotension. If patient is hypotensive, immediately communicate with the surgeon and examine the surgical field for possible causes. Then the following steps should be undertaken as necessary:
    - Turn off the anesthetic vaporizer
    - Administer crystalloid bolus as appropriate
    - Administer atropine 0.01 mg/kg
    - Consider epinephrine 10–50 µg IV bolus
    - If necessary, start epinephrine infusion at 2 µg/min and titrate as necessary
  - ‣ Consider intraoperative EKG, A-line, CVP monitoring
  - ‣ Consider use of external pacemaker (transvenous or transcutaneous)
- Once patient is stabilized, or if stable, identify cause and treat: identify P waves and QRS complexes (see chapter 5):
  - ‣ Each QRS is preceded by a P wave:
    - Sinus bradycardia, sinus pause
  - ‣ No P waves are visible:
    - Irregular QRS rate: A-Fib with slow ventricular response
    - Wide QRS: sinoatrial block
  - ‣ There are more P waves than QRS complexes:
    - PR getting longer, and then P without QRS: second-degree AV block Mobitz 1 (Wenckebach)
    - PR constant, occasional P without QRS: second-degree AV block Mobitz 2
    - No relation between P and QRS: third-degree AV block
- Possible causes:
  - ‣ Airway issues:
    - Hypoventilation? Increase respiratory rate and/or tidal volume
    - Hypoxia? Increase FiO_2 and/or PEEP
  - ‣ Hypotension:
    - See Event below
  - ‣ Consider a cardiopulmonary event:
    - Tension pneumothorax
    - Hemothorax
    - Tamponade
    - Embolism—gas, amniotic, thrombus, fat
    - Sepsis
    - Myocardial depression—drugs, ischemia, electrolytes, trauma
  - ‣ Pharmacological cause:
    - Volatile agent overdose (or adequate dosing in susceptible patient), induction drugs, succinylcholine (especially if redosing), neostigmine, opioids. Identify drugs given by surgeon (e.g., vasoconstrictors)
  - ‣ Vagal reflex:
    - Discontinue stimulation; atropine if needed
  - ‣ Undetected blood loss:
    - Obtain additional IV access and replace fluids. Ensure cross-matched blood is available; transfuse as needed

- ‣ Consider other causes:
  - ▪ Regional/neuraxial anesthetics: Bezold–Jarisch reflex causing vasodilation + bradycardia up to arrest. Ensure normovolemia; administer epinephrine IV boluses (start 10–50 µg, increase if needed)
  - ▪ Surgical factors: IVC compression, retractor placement, pneumoperitoneum

TACHYCARDIA

- Stable or unstable?
  - ‣ Is the patient in cardiopulmonary arrest (e.g., ventricular fibrillation, pulseless ventricular tachycardia)? Initiate ACLS Protocol immediately
  - ‣ What is the blood pressure?
    - ▪ Hypertensive? (Consider hypertensive causes discussed in the section "Hypertension.")
    - ▪ Hypotensive?
      - ◆ Reconfirm blood pressure
      - ◆ Turn off vaporizers
      - ◆ Administer crystalloids appropriately
- Diagnose rhythm: See chapters 5 and 16
  - ‣ QRS duration <0.08 seconds:
    - ▪ Regular: attempt vagal stimulus (carotid massage, ocular pressure, Valsalva, unless contraindicated):
      - ◆ Each QRS is preceded by a P wave: SVT
      - ◆ There are more P waves than QRS complexes: atrial flutter or reentrant tachycardia
    - ▪ Irregular:
      - ◆ There are no P waves: A-Fib
      - ◆ Each QRS is preceded by a P wave: reentrant tachycardia
  - ‣ QRS duration >0.12 seconds:
    - ▪ Regular:
      - ◆ P not visible, or dissociated from QRS: ventricular tachycardia
      - ◆ Each QRS is preceded by a P wave: SVT + BBB
      - ◆ There are more P waves than QRS complexes: atrial flutter + BBB or reentrant tachycardia + BBB
    - ▪ Irregular:
      - ◆ No P waves: A-Fib + BBB
      - ◆ There are more P waves than QRS complexes: reentrant tachycardia + BBB
- Treat:
  - ‣ Poorly tolerated tachycardia (altered mental status, shock, chest pain), sinus or otherwise?
  - ‣ Sinus tachycardia? Identify cause (see below) and treat. If no cause identified, consider beta-blockade
  - ‣ Arrhythmia?
    - ▪ Ventricular tachycardia: lidocaine 1 mg/kg IV; DC cardioversion if poorly tolerated
    - ▪ A-Fib: titrate beta-blocker/Ca channel blocker
    - ▪ SVT: adenosine 6–12 mg IV
  - ‣ Use synchronized cardioversion (start at 100 J, and then 200 J)
- Once patient is stabilized, identify cause and treat:
  - ‣ Reflex stimulation:
    - ▪ Surgical stimulation, laryngoscopy? Ensure adequate anesthesia/analgesia
  - ‣ Hypovolemia? Review fluid status:
    - ▪ Blood loss—check Hct, cross-match, and transfuse blood products
    - ▪ Dehydration—improve IV access and begin fluid replacement
    - ▪ Consider excessive diuresis, sepsis
  - ‣ Pharmacological cause:
    - ▪ Consider induction/inhalation agent, atropine/glycopyrrolate, local anesthetic toxicity, epinephrine, vasopressors
    - ▪ Consider patient history of cocaine/methamphetamine use

- Airway:
  - Hypoventilation? Increase tidal volume and/or respiratory rate
  - Hypoxemia? Increase FiO_2 and/or PEEP
- Other causes:
  - Cardiopulmonary problems: HTX, PTX, tamponade, embolism, myocardial irritability (from drugs, ischemia, electrolytes, trauma), pulmonary edema
  - Anaphylaxis
  - Malignant hyperthermia

HYPOTENSION

Fall in BP by >20% from baseline, or below predetermined limits (e.g., SBP 90 mm Hg, MAP 60 mm Hg).

- For an unstable patient:
  - Ensure adequate oxygenation/ventilation
  - Confirm BP measurement; palpate pulse (if strong, hypotension unlikely); if severe vasoconstriction, consider A-line into large (femoral) artery, as radial measurement might be unreliable
  - Is the patient in cardiopulmonary arrest? Initiate ACLS Protocol
  - Turn off vaporizer; d/c all vasodilating drugs
  - Improve blood return: lie flat; elevate legs
  - Administer crystalloid bolus 10 mL/kg; repeat as appropriate
  - Give phenylephrine (1 µg/kg) (or if HR low, ephedrine [5–10 mg]). If no effect, consider epinephrine (10–50 µg) bolus
  - If necessary, epinephrine infusion starting at 2 µg/min
  - Consider EKG, A-line, CVP monitoring, PAC insertion, TTE/TEE for cardiac assessment
  - Also consider anaphylaxis, bradycardia, hypoxemia
- Once patient is stabilized, identify cause and treat:
  - Hypovolemia? Review fluid status, U/O, Hct:
    - Blood loss—check Hct, cross-match, and transfuse blood products
    - Dehydration—place additional IV access as needed; begin fluid replacement
    - Consider excessive diuresis, sepsis
  - Pharmacological cause:
    - Induction/inhalation agent, opioids, succinylcholine, anticholinesterases, local anesthetic toxicity, vancomycin, protamine
    - Administration error: infusion pump malfunction, medication error, drugs administered by surgeon
  - Other causes:
    - Cardiopulmonary problems: ischemia/MI, HTX, PTX, tamponade, embolism, myocardial depression (from drugs, ischemia, electrolytes, trauma), sepsis
    - Regional/neuraxial anesthesia: sympathectomy, vasodilation, bradycardia, respiratory failure. Tx: volume loading, vasopressors, airway support, left lateral displacement in parturients
    - Surgical factors: vagal reflexes, IVC compression/obstructed venous return, retractor placement, pneumoperitoneum, positioning

HYPERTENSION

BP >20% above baseline, or above predetermined limits.

- Immediate treatment:
  - Ensure adequate oxygenation and ventilation
  - Confirm blood pressure measurement (NIBP on different site, transducer level/calibration, etc.)
  - Discontinue ongoing vasopressor infusions
  - Assess depth of anesthesia and increase as necessary:
    - Check for errors in delivery of anesthesia

- Identify precipitating factors:
  ‣ Depth of anesthesia:
    ▪ Titrate anesthetic appropriately
  ‣ Reflex stimulation:
    ▪ Consider surgical stimulation, laryngoscopy? Discuss with surgeon; cease stimulation. Administer appropriate dose of opioids
  ‣ Airway problems—is hypertension related to hypercarbia?
  ‣ Consider medication errors, drugs administered by surgeon
  ‣ Consider underlying conditions:
    ▪ Preexisting hypertension
    ▪ Pheochromocytoma
    ▪ Hyperthyroidism
    ▪ Malignant hyperthermia
    ▪ Raised intracranial pressure
    ▪ Fluid overload
- Consider antihypertensive therapy—titrate drugs to effect:
  ‣ If normal heart rate, give labetalol 0.1–0.25 mg/kg, or initiate nicardipine infusion at 5 mg/h
  ‣ If tachycardic, give metoprolol 0.01–0.3 mg/kg or esmolol 0.25–1 mg/kg

HYPOCARBIA

- Is the patient stable or unstable?
  ‣ Is the patient in cardiopulmonary arrest? If so, initiate ACLS Protocols immediately
  ‣ Consider a cardiopulmonary event:
    ▪ Tension pneumothorax
    ▪ Hemothorax
    ▪ Tamponade
    ▪ Embolism—gas, amniotic, thrombus
    ▪ Sepsis
    ▪ Myocardial depression—from drugs, ischemia, electrolytes, trauma
  ‣ Having excluded cardiopulmonary etiologies, the next step should be to assess the airway:
    ▪ Ensure the adequacy of oxygenation and ventilation
    ▪ Ventilate by hand
    ▪ Check circuit, scavenging, valves, vaporizers, monitors, **capnograph**
    ▪ Check endotracheal tube/LMA
  ‣ Assess breathing/circulation
- Once stabilized, determine cause: metabolic versus respiratory alkalosis:
  ‣ Metabolic:
    ▪ Diuretics, vomiting, ileus, diarrhea, polyuric states
    ▪ Steroids, bronchodilators, catecholamines, TPN, insulin
    ▪ Hypovolemia
    ▪ Post massive blood transfusion
  ‣ Respiratory:
    ▪ Hyperventilation
- Treatment:
  ‣ Address underlying cause
  ‣ Ensure adequate ventilation:
    ▪ If controlled ventilation:
      ◆ Adjust respiratory rate and/or tidal volume
      ◆ Give muscle relaxant/analgesic if breathing over ventilator
    ▪ If spontaneous ventilation (LMA/MAC):
      ◆ Give analgesic
      ◆ Deepen anesthetic
  ‣ Fluid replacement—consider colloids
  ‣ Check ABG with electrolytes hourly

- Consider $MgSO_4$ 0.1–0.2 mmol/kg IV
- Consider IV KCl, phosphate

HYPERCARBIA

- Assess the airway:
  - Ensure the adequacy of oxygenation and ventilation
  - Ventilate by hand
  - Check circuit, scavenging, valves, vaporizers, monitors, **capnograph**
  - Check endotracheal tube/LMA
- Determine cause: metabolic versus respiratory:
  - Metabolic:
    - Shock state: cardiogenic, hypovolemic, septic, distributive
    - Sepsis
    - Trauma
    - Diabetic emergencies
    - Ischemia
    - Hepatic/renal failure
    - Acetazolamide
    - Epinephrine infusion
    - Methanol/alcohol/ethylene glycol ingestion
  - Respiratory:
    - CO_2 absorption from laparoscopy
    - Hypoventilation:
      - Anatomical: distended abdomen, loss of integrity of chest wall/diaphragm
      - Lithotomy/Trendelenburg position
      - CNS depression
      - Muscle weakness
      - Preexisting conditions
      - Pharmacological: NMB, high spinal
    - Coughing/breath holding/light anesthesia:
      - Rapidly deepen anesthesia
    - Airway obstruction—laryngospasm, bronchospasm:
      - Laryngospasm: hold positive pressure, IV propofol 20–40 mg, succinylcholine 20–30 mg IV
      - Bronchospasm: see section "Bronchospasm." Deepen anesthesia, inhaled beta-2 agonists, steroids
- Treatment:
  - Address underlying cause
  - Ensure adequate ventilation (if hypoventilation):
    - Controlled ventilation:
      - Adjust tidal volume and/or respiratory rate
    - Spontaneous ventilation (LMA/MAC):
      - Assess for obstruction: chin lift, nasal trumpet, oral airway
      - Lighten anesthetic
  - Support circulation with volume and inotropes
  - Draw ABG and measure anion/osmolal gaps
  - IV $NaHCO_3$ indicated in bicarbonate losing states with normal anion gap (e.g., renal tubular acidosis)

INCREASED PEAK AIRWAY PRESSURES

Definition: An increase in PIP 5 cm H_2O or greater during PPV or a PIP greater than 40 cm H_2O.

Causes: Obstruction/increased resistance in the breathing circuit, ETT, or patient.

- *Circuit*: Kinked hose, failure of pressure check valves, closed inspiratory, expiratory or pop-off valve
- *ETT*: Kinked ETT, endobronchial intubation, foreign body, secretions or mucus plugging in ETT, herniated ETT cuff obstructing ETT outlet

- *Patient*: Raised intra-abdominal pressure, pulmonary aspiration of gastric contents, bronchospasm, atelectasis, decreased chest wall or diaphragmatic compliance, unusual patient position or abnormal anatomy (scoliosis), pulmonary edema, pneumothorax
- *Drug induced*: Opioid-induced chest wall rigidity, inadequate muscle relaxation, malignant hyperthermia

A. Management

- Increase FiO_2 to 100%
- Switch to manual ventilation and rule out causes of obstruction

Circuit obstruction:

- Disconnect Y piece from ETT and compress reservoir bag:
  - ▸ If airway pressure is high, obstruction is present in the breathing circuit
  - ▸ Ventilate using a backup system until the ventilator is fixed

ETT obstruction:

- Increase in plateau pressure → possibly kinked tube
- Pass a suction catheter down the ETT to evaluate for obstruction and suction while removing catheter
- If the ETT is obstructed, remove the ETT, and replace with a new ETT; use FOB or ETT exchanger if difficult intubation

Patient related:

- Usually no change in plateau pressure
- Auscultate both sides of the patient's chest for equal BS B/L, wheezes, or crackles:
  - ▸ If breath sounds are unequal, consider endobronchial intubation, check taping of tube
  - ▸ If wheezes present, consider bronchospasm
  - ▸ If crackles are present, consider pulmonary edema
- Check BP and heart rate; perform chest percussion; consider pneumothorax

Miscellaneous:

- Malignant hyperthermia
- Ensure depth of anesthesia is sufficient
- Administer NMB for possible chest wall rigidity from opiates, or insufficient muscle relaxation
- Surgical position/retraction, abnormal anatomy

OLIGURIA

Definition: Urine output below 0.5 mL/kg/h.

Causes:

- Decreased renal perfusion from volume status or cardiac output
- Increased vasopressin (stress response to surgery)
- Renal failure
- Physical obstruction of urinary flow

A. Management

Mechanical:

- Irrigate Foley to rule out kinked, clotted, or poorly positioned Foley catheter (above bladder level, etc.)
- Communicate with surgeon: aortic cross-clamping, compression/ligature of the ureters?
- Inject IV methylene blue/indigo carmine to r/o severed ureter

Hypovolemia:

- May be accompanied by tachycardia, hypotension
- Test bolus 300–500 mL colloid or crystalloid; if no response, may bolus again if no sign of overload
- Consider TTE/TEE or invasive monitoring to assess volume status

Cardiac:

If patient has cardiac history (CHF) or there is concern for cardiac cause of oliguria, consider:

- PA catheter or TEE
- Optimize volume status
- Inotropic support if CO continues to be low: dobutamine, dopamine 2–10 µg/kg min
- Keep MAP above 80 mm Hg as renal function may be pressure dependent, particularly in patients with chronic HTN

Miscellaneous:

- Acute renal failure: r/o shock or hypotension, crush syndrome (myoglobinuria), or transfusion reaction (hemoglobinuria)
- Check Hgb/Hct and transfuse for significant anemia
- If other causes excluded, consider diuretic (furosemide 5 mg IV, or mannitol). Chronic diuretic users may need this to maintain normal UOP
- Restrict K^+ until renal failure has been ruled out

HYPOXEMIA

Definition: SaO_2 <90% or Pao_2 <60 mm Hg.

Causes:

- Hypoventilation
- Low inspired FiO_2
- V/Q mismatch e.g., PE
- Increased shunt
- Poor oxygen delivery (e.g., low CO) might lead to lower displayed SpO_2 despite normal SaO_2 check ABG if in doubt

A. Management

- Increase FiO_2 to 100%
- Consider ABG
- If shortly after intubation, esophageal intubation until proven otherwise

Hypoventilation:

- Measure $EtCO_2$
- Evaluate for adequate ventilation (B/L BS); monitor for circuit leak

Shunting:

- Atelectasis: recruitment maneuvers, add PEEP
- Bronchospasm: manually ventilate to evaluate pulmonary compliance; large gradient between peak and plateau airway pressure
- Collapsed lung (secretion/pneumonia/mainstem intubation):
  ‣ Auscultate for equal BS B/L; watch chest movement
  ‣ Check position of ETT and reposition if necessary
  ‣ Suction obstructive secretions/possibly bronchoscopy assisted
  ‣ Add PEEP
  ‣ Intermittent sighs (large breaths in between normal Vt)

Miscellaneous:

- Adjust SpO_2 probe if poor waveform
- Poor cardiac output:
  ‣ Restore adequate circulating blood volume
  ‣ Transfuse for low Hct
  ‣ Consider inotropes
- Evaluate for methemoglobinemia or carboxyhemoglobin
- Decrease volatile anesthetics to decrease inhibition of hypoxic pulmonary vasoconstriction

BRONCHOSPASM (SEE ALSO CHAPTER 205)

Definition: Partially reversible bronchiolar constriction initiated by noxious stimuli, asthma, COPD.

Symptoms:
- Wheezing
- Increased peak pressures with unchanged plateau pressures
- Decreasing exhaled tidal volumes
- Slowly rising waveform on capnograph

A. Management

- Increase FiO_2 to 100%
- If prior to/during induction, use propofol over thiopental
- Manual ventilation to evaluate compliance
- Auscultate for wheezing or diminished breath sounds
- Check ETT position using direct laryngoscopy or fiber-optic (ensure that it is not mainstem or against the carina)
- Pass a suction catheter down ETT to r/o kinking, obstruction by secretions

Mild bronchospasm:
- Increase anesthetic depth
- Administer a beta-2 agonist by metered dose inhaler (four to eight puffs); repeat after 5 minutes if needed

Severe bronchospasm:
- Beta-2 agonist MDI or nebulizer; if unsuccessful, use SQ epinephrine
- Administer IV corticosteroids (give early as peak effect delayed by 3–4 hours): methylprednisolone IV 100 mg bolus
- Discontinue drugs that cause histamine release (e.g., morphine, thiopental, meperidine)

REGURGITATION/ASPIRATION

Definition: Aspiration of gastric contents in patients who are unable to protect their airway.

A. Prevention

- Nonemergent surgery $\rightarrow$ light meals >6 hours prior, clear liquids >2 hours prior
- Decrease pH and gastric volume prior to administration of anesthesia:
  - Nonparticulate antacids: will increase gastric volume
  - H2 antagonists
  - Proton pump inhibitors
  - Prokinetic agents
  - Consider gastric suctioning prior to induction of anesthesia
- Apply cricoid pressure until the ETT position is confirmed (effectiveness unclear)
- Intubate the trachea and inflate the ETT cuff quickly
- Gastric suctioning prior to extubation
- Extubate the patient only after recovery of protective laryngeal reflexes

B. Management

- If the ETT is not in place, tilt head down, turn head to side, suction upper airway, and then place ETT and suction through the ETT
- Perform **suctioning prior to positive pressure ventilation** to avoid forcing particulate matter down to distal airways
- FiO_2 to 100%
- Consider PEEP for improved oxygenation
- If risk of particulate aspiration, perform bronchoscopy, possible lavage and suctioning

- Consider antibiotics if known aspiration of feculent material
- If low likelihood in ambulatory outpatient with no signs of hypoxemia, cough, wheeze, or radiographic abnormalities within 6 hours, outpatient follow-up is a possibility
- Monitor ×24–48 hours if high likelihood of aspiration
- Serial temperature checks, WBC counts, CXR (fluffy infiltrates), and ABG
- Provide supportive care; consider ARDS therapy
- No steroids
- Do not treat pulmonary edema unless hypervolemia present

REFERENCE

For references, please visit **www.TheAnesthesiaGuide.com**.

CHAPTER 62
Postoperative Complications

Teresa A. Mulaikal, MD and Sansan S. Lo, MD

PERIOPERATIVE VISUAL LOSS IN NONOCULAR SURGERY

Incidence of perioperative ocular injury ranges from 0.002% to 0.2%, highest in cardiac and spine surgery.

Most common ocular injury in nonophthalmologic surgery is corneal abrasion.

Most common cause of permanent perioperative visual loss is ischemic optic neuropathy.

Most Common Causes of Perioperative Visual Loss			
	Corneal abrasion	Retinal ischemia	Ischemic optic neuropathy
Symptoms	Painful foreign body sensation, visual acuity may be intact	Painless loss of vision Unilateral Periorbital edema Proptosis Chemosis Extraocular muscle injury Ecchymosis	Painless loss of vision Bilateral
Etiology	Corneal epithelial defect in anterior segment	Central retinal artery occlusion Branch retinal artery occlusion (retinal microemboli or vasospasm) Elevated intraocular pressure	Unknown, perhaps related to optic nerve ischemia, vascular insufficiency, although often no other clinically significant end-organ damage

(continued)

	Corneal abrasion	Retinal ischemia	Ischemic optic neuropathy
Most Common Causes of Perioperative Visual Loss (*continued*)			
Risk factors	Unprotected, exposed eyes Intraoperative contact lens use	Prone positioning Spine surgery Cardiac surgery, bypass External orbital pressure	Prone positioning Spine surgery (PION) Cardiac surgery (AION) Prolonged surgery ?Deliberate hypotension ?Hypoxia ?Hemodilution ?Vasoconstrictors ?Anemia ?Elevated venous pressure (e.g., Trendelenburg)
Diagnosis	Slit lamp examination with fluorescein	Afferent pupillary defect Pale swollen optic disc Cherry red retina Ground glass retina	Afferent pupillary defect or nonreactive pupil (CNII) AION: optic disc edema PION: normal optic disc Abnormal visual-evoked potentials
Treatment	Antibiotic drops	IV acetazolamide 5% CO_2 + O_2 inhalation Ocular massage ?Ophthalmic artery fibrinolysis	Attempt to optimize oxygenation and orbital perfusion pressure, although no definitive treatment
Prognosis	Good prognosis Expect recovery	Poor prognosis Permanent visual loss	Poor prognosis Permanent visual loss
Prevention	Tape eyes securely No benefit to lubricant Remove contact lenses	Avoid external orbital pressure Frequently examine eyes during prone cases	Stage long spine procedures Nadir hematocrit does not differ in patients with ION and those unaffected in noncardiac surgery Massive fluid replacement may be a risk factor for ION (no clear evidence)

PION, posterior ischemic optic neuropathy; AION, anterior ischemic optic neuropathy; CNII, optic nerve; ?, possible, unproven.

COMMON PERIOPERATIVE NEUROPATHIES DURING GENERAL ANESTHESIA

Mechanism of nerve injury: stretch, compression, transection, ischemia, metabolic, neoplastic, radiation.

Double crush hypothesis: preexisting neuropathies increase the incidence of subsequent nerve injury.

Prognosis: best with sensory loss, worst with motor weakness and atrophy, poor prognosis with nerve transection.

Common Neuropathies During General Anesthesia

	Ulnar, C8–T1	Radial, C5–C8 and T1	Brachial plexus, C5–T1	Sciatic, L4–S3	Femoral, L2–L4	Obturator, L2–L4 (ventral rami)
Symptoms	Paresthesias of fourth and fifth digits Hypothenar atrophy, weakness of wrist flexion	Paresthesias on the dorsum of the hand or posterior arm Wrist drop Limited extension at elbow	Paresthesias, weakness, and atrophy in distribution of specific nerve roots	Loss of hip extension, knee flexion *Common peroneal:* loss of dorsiflexion, eversion, paresthesias in dorsum of foot *Tibial:* loss of plantar flexion and inversion, paresthesias on plantar aspect of foot	Loss of hip flexion, adduction, knee extension Paresthesias in anterior and medial thigh, medial calf Lateral femoral cutaneous nerve: L2–L3, isolated sensory nerve, paresthesias in lateral aspect of thigh, *meralgia paresthetica*	Loss of hip adduction Paresthesias of medial, distal two thirds of thigh, including posterior region
Etiology	External pressure as nerve courses posterior to medial epicondyle of humerus and posteriomedially to tubercle of ulna coronoid process	Pressure in the spiral groove of humerus Possibly frequent inflation of blood pressure cuff Overextension of forearm at elbow	Hyperabduction of arms more than 90° from table, "stretch injury" Median sternotomy during dissection of IMA Steep Trendelenburg + shoulder brace Axillary cannulation	Lithotomy: sciatic nerve stretch with complete leg extension, or excessive external hip rotation Compression of common peroneal nerve on lateral head of fibula Total knee arthroplasty Total knee arthroplasty: tourniquet, realignment of valgus knee	Abdominal retraction Lithotomy: femoral nerve compression under inguinal ligament with extreme hip flexion, abduction, external rotation Retroperitoneal hematoma Total hip arthroplasty	Lithotomy

Diagnosis	Physical exam EMG NCS					
Treatment	Physical therapy Nerve transposition	Tendon transfer		Physical therapy		
Prevention	Pressure point padding Neurophysiologic monitoring Supination or neutral forearm positioning	Pressure point padding Neurophysiologic monitoring	Avoid arm hyperextension Avoid asymmetric sternal retraction Shoulder brace on acromioclavicular joint	In lithotomy, limit hip flexion and abduction of thighs, minimal external hip rotation Limit duration of lithotomy to <2 h	In lithotomy, limit hip flexion and abduction of thighs, minimal external hip rotation Limit duration of lithotomy to <2 h Use of short lateral retractor blades	Limit duration of lithotomy to <2 h
Risk factors	Preexisting neuropathy Male Obesity Prolonged surgery	Preexisting neuropathy			Preexisting neuropathy Thin body habitus	Preexisting neuropathy

EMG: electromyography; NCS: nerve conduction studies; IMA: internal mammary artery.

Perioperative Dental Injury	
Etiology and timing of injury	Laryngoscopy (50–70%) Emergence and extubation (9–20%)
Risk factors	Mallampati III and IV Emergency surgery General anesthesia with endotracheal intubation Prominent maxillary incisors (most vulnerable to injury) Oropharyngeal airway placement Aggressive suctioning Poor dentition

Prevention	Secure loose tooth with suture, wrap suture around adjacent
	    stable teeth, tape to ipsilateral cheek
	Remove loose teeth prior to induction
	Placement of soft bite block between mandibular and
	    maxillary molars

Treatment	Store dislodged teeth in saline or cold milk Reimplantation by dental surgery
Prognosis	Best if reimplantation occurs within 30 min of injury

Iatrogenic Airway Trauma	
Adverse outcomes	Laryngitis Vocal cord injury Arytenoid dislocation Tracheobronchial rupture Mucosal necrosis Hematoma formation Esophageal perforation Creation of false lumen in membranous trachea (e.g., by bougie)
Risk factors	Double-lumen endotracheal tube placement Cuff overinflation Inappropriately large endotracheal tubes Red rubber endotracheal tubes
Diagnosis	Physical exam: hoarseness, stridor, crepitus Fiber-optic bronchoscopy Imaging
Prevention	Use of age-appropriate and size-appropriate endotracheal tubes Avoid cuff overinflation Ensure adequate leak pressures around endotracheal tube in pediatric cases
Treatment	Thoracic surgery consultation ENT consultation

AWARENESS DURING ANESTHESIA

Definition: explicit recall during general anesthesia.

Incidence of anesthesia awareness is 0.1–0.2% and most patients report awareness well after PACU discharge.

Majority of cases occur during maintenance of anesthesia, with less frequent use of benzodiazepines, opioids, volatile agents, and intravenous agents in reported cases.

The use of processed EEG monitoring (e.g., BIS, Entropy) to decrease the incidence of awareness is controversial.

Signs and Treatment of Anesthesia Awareness	
Intraoperative signs	Hypertension Tachycardia Patient movement
Etiology	Light anesthesia Machine malfunction
Patient symptoms	Inability to move Sensation of weakness, paralysis Hearing voices, noises, words Feelings of anxiety or impending doom
Diagnosis	Modified Brice questionnaire
Risk factors	History of awareness Light anesthesia Neuromuscular blocking agents Female gender Chronic opioids, alcohol, benzodiazepine, or other CNS depressants Acute amphetamine use Cardiac surgery Cesarean section under general anesthesia Trauma surgery Rigid bronchoscopy or microlaryngeal endoscopic surgery Difficult intubation
Prevention	No paralysis unless surgically indicated Processed EEG monitoring of controversial value
Treatment	Referral to psychiatry Psychotherapy for management of posttraumatic stress disorder

Modified Brice Questionnaire
• What was the last thing you remember before you went to sleep for your operation? • What was the first thing you remember after your operation? • Can you remember anything in between these two periods? • Did you dream during your operation? • What was the most unpleasant thing you remember about your operation?

REFERENCES

For references, please visit **www.TheAnesthesiaGuide.com**.

CHAPTER 63
OR Fires

Jean Charchaflieh, MD, DrPH, FCCM, FCCP

OCCURRENCE

- Most recent (2010) estimates: 550–650 occurrences per year in the United States
- Oxygen-enriched atmosphere (OEA) involved in 72–74% of fires; alcohol prep solutions and drapes are most common fuels
- Most fire-related burn claims involved plastic surgery performed on the face under MAC with supplemental O_2 where electrosurgical unit (ESU) comes in contact with drapes/gauze wet with alcohol prep solution

RISK FACTORS

Three elements must exist for fire to occur: ignition source, fuel and oxidizer.

The APSF Fire Prevention Algorithm recommends securing the airway with ET tube or LMA if >30% oxygen is required to maintain oxygen saturation.

TABLE 63-1	Examples of Elements of Fire Triad in an OR Setting	
Ignition source (heat)	Fuel	Oxidizer
Electrosurgical units (ESU)	Prep solutions: alcohol, chlorhexidine, benzoin, Mastisol, acetone, petrolatum products	O_2
Fiber-optic light source	Surgical drapes, gowns, sponges, packs, sutures, mesh	N_2O
Laser beams	Plastic/PVC/latex products (ETT, masks, nasal cannulas, tubings)	Air
Drills	Intestinal gases (CH_4, H_2)	
External defibrillation	Hair, other bodily tissues	

MECHANISMS AND PREVENTION

TABLE 63-2	Elements of Fire in the OR: Mechanisms and Prevention
Mechanism	Prevention
Oxygen: • $FiO_2 \geq 21\% \rightarrow \Uparrow$ ignition, temperature, combustion • O_2 heavier than air $\rightarrow$ collects under drapes • O_2 at 3 L/min via NC $\rightarrow FiO_2$ 70–80% under drapes • D/C NC $O_2 \rightarrow FiO_2 \Downarrow$ to 30% in 30 s	**Oxygen:** • Provide lowest FiO_2 consistent with adequate SaO_2 • Use O_2 "for rescue only" • Tape NC in place to avoid blowing O_2 into surgical field • Discontinue O_2 60 s before use of ESU
N_2O: • FiO_2 25% + N_2O 75% $\approx FiO_2$ 100% in ability to support combustion • $N_2O \Uparrow$ risk of fire when combined with intestinal gases ($CH_4 + H_2$), which act as fuels	**N_2O:** • Avoid N_2O during cases where ESU is used on gas-filled intestines (GI obstruction)
Volatile anesthetics: • Sevoflurane + desiccated Baralyme may $\rightarrow$ fire	**Volatile anesthetics:** • Replace Baralyme regularly, especially on Monday morning

(continued)

TABLE 63-2 Elements of Fire in the OR: Mechanisms and Prevention (*continued*)	
Mechanism	Prevention
Hair: • Retains prep solutions longer, ignites easily	**Hair:** • Clip hair in operative site or render it nonflammable by heavy coating with water-soluble lubricant jelly • Instruct patients not to use petroleum-based facial creams and hair products
Drapes and towels: • Absorb O_2 and alcohol → facilitate ignition • Fire-resistant cotton towels → "surface fiber flame propagation," that is, fire underneath drapes without drapes being on fire → ignition of materials at some distance from operative site with no intermediate fire ("mysterious spark")	**Drapes and towels:** • Thoroughly moistened gauze in operative field • Minimize drape tenting to prevent entrapment of O_2 and alcohol vapors
Skin prep solutions: • Alcohol-based solutions extremely flammable (ChloraPrep: 2% chlorhexidine gluconate + 70% isopropyl alcohol)	**Skin prep solutions:** • Do not drape or use ignition source until skin is completely dry (minimum 3 min on hairless skin and up to 1 h in hair) • When prepping the neck area, place towels under each side to absorb excess solution • Remove any soaked materials before using ignition source • Wipe away excess prep solution before draping to prevent vapor collection under tented drapes
ESU: • Unipolar ESU → higher temperatures than bipolar ESU • Both are ignition sources at the tip with as little as 20% alcohol (ChloraPrep has 70% alcohol)	**ESU:** • Avoid using ESU with flammable materials in OEA • Use bipolar ESU at lowest temperature possible • Holster ESU when not in use • Deactivate ESU before the tip leaves surgical site • Frequently clean ESU tip to prevent carbon accumulation, which leads to heat buildup
ETT: • Ease of flammability: polyvinyl chloride (PVC) > red rubber > silicone > metal tube (metal wrapping of tubes not FDA approved) • PVC produces most toxic products • Silicone produces silica ash → late silicosis • Thin ETT cuff highly susceptible to puncture by laser, which leads to OEA at surgical site	**ETT:** • Fill cuff with colored saline to signal puncture • Use moistened gauze over visible cuff • Place cuff as far down in trachea as possible • Consider jet ventilation through ventilating bronchoscope (risks include barotrauma, pneumothorax, distal bronchial seeding of virus) • Helium reduces index of flammability by only 1–2%

IMMEDIATE INTERVENTIONS IN AN OR FIRE/AIRWAY FIRE

- Remove ignition source immediately (surgeon)
- Stop ventilation and disconnect circuit (anesthesiologist)
- Place flaming material in water
- Use saline/water to quench fire
- Use RACE acronym to stop fire: rescue, alarm, confine, extinguish
- Use PASS acronym to operate extinguisher: pull, aim, squeeze, sweep
- Ventilate via FM with O_2 100% and continue anesthesia
- Perform DL and bronchoscopy to survey damage and remove debris
- Perform bronchial lavage in blowtorch-type fire (fire interior to ETT) with fiber-optic assessment of distal airway
- Reintubate if airway damage
- Consider low tracheotomy for severe airway damage
- Obtain CXR
- Consider prolonged intubation and mechanical ventilation for pulmonary damage from heat/smoke inhalation
- Assess oropharynx and face and any burned area for size and depth
- See chapter 218 for further care

REFERENCES

For references, please visit **www.TheAnesthesiaGuide.com**.

CHAPTER 64
Blood Products and Transfusion

Ruchir Gupta, MD and Gebhard Wagener, MD

NB: Hb (g/dL) ~ Hct (%)/3.

BLOOD PRODUCTS

See table on following page.

Blood Products

Product	Definition	Indication	Benefits	Risks
RBC		Indication for transfusion varies • Hct <21 for ASA 1 or 2, Hct <31 for anyone with documented or suspected cardiac pathology (e.g., elderly) (controversial) • In OR, often clinical judgment (labs take time, and Hct will not drop right away with acute bleeding) Allowable blood loss (ABL): weight (kg) × EBV (70 mL/kg for males, 65 mL/kg for females) × $(H_{initial} - H_{final})$	250 mL with 70% Hct Each unit will increase Hct by ~4%	• Hypocalcemia (citrate) • Hyperkalemia • Thrombocytopenia • Hepatitis C • ABO incompatibility • Bacterial contamination, or endotoxin if donor septic
Platelets		Platelet count should be >100,000 with minimum required for surgery at 50,000	Each "large" unit (6 individual units) increases platelets by 10,000	Stored at 20–24°. Thus, greater risk of bacterial contamination. Any fever in 6 h of transfusion is platelet-induced sepsis unless proven otherwise
FFP	Fluid portion obtained from a single unit of whole blood that is frozen within 6 h of collection Contains all plasma proteins including all clotting factors except platelets	• Isolated factor deficiencies • Reversal of warfarin therapy • Correction of coagulopathy associated with liver disease • Massive blood transfusions and continued bleeding following platelet transfusion • Antithrombin III deficiency or thrombotic thrombocytopenic purpura (TTP) • Management of heparin resistance	Each unit increases level of clotting factors by 2–3% in adults Initial therapeutic dose → 10–15 mL/kg Goal = 30% of normal coagulation factor concentration	Same infectious risk as unit of whole blood Sensitization to plasma proteins ABO-compatible units should generally be given, but not mandatory Warm to 37°C prior to transfusion
Cryoprecipitate	Portion of plasma that precipitates when FFP is thawed at 4°C	• Hemophilia • vWF deficiency • Hypofibrinogenemia	80–100 U of factor VIII, 100–250 mg of fibrinogen, 50–60 mg of fibronectin, 40–70% of normal vWF levels, and anti-A and anti-B antibodies	Infections Allergic reactions

Blood Products Pretreatment and Indications

Type	Definition	Products	Indications
Leukocyte-reduced Most blood products are leukocyte-reduced since the 1990s	Filtering to reduce WBC from 1–2 billions to ~5 millions in a unit of RBCs	RBC, platelets	Prevention of • HLA immunization • Febrile nonhemolytic reactions • Immunosuppression Decrease CMV transmission
Phenotyped	Cross-matched for antigens other than ABO and Rhesus	RBC, platelets	Patients on chronic transfusion therapy (sickle cell disease, thalassemia, etc.)
Irradiated	Gamma irradiation of cellular components (lymphocytes) that reduce their ability to cause GVHD in immunocompromised recipients	RBC, platelets (decreases survival of viable platelets)	High-risk patients: • Bone marrow transplant recipient • Severe congenital immunodeficiency syndromes Intermediate-risk patients: • Premature infants undergoing exchange transfusions • Leukemia/lymphoma • Chemotherapy-induced bone marrow suppression
CMV-screened	Blood from donors who have been screened for CMV antibodies	RBC, platelets	• Pregnant women • Premature infants born to CMV-seronegative mothers • CMV-seronegative recipients of allogeneic bone marrow transplants from CMV-seronegative donors • CMV-seronegative patients with acquired immunodeficiency syndrome

Blood Product Compatibility by ABO Type

Recipient's blood type	Compatible RBCs	Compatible plasma products	Compatible platelets	
			Primary choice	Secondary choice
A	A, O	A, AB	A, AB	B, O
B	B, O	B, AB	B, AB	A, O
O	O	O, A, B, AB	O	A, B, AB
AB	O, A, B, AB	AB	AB	A, B, O

Transfusion Reactions

Reaction	Causes	Signs	Treatment
Urticarial-pruritic	Allergenic substances in donor plasma react with preexisting IgE antibodies in recipient	Pruritus and urticaria	Slow or stop transfusion
Febrile nonhemolytic reaction	Interaction between recipient antibodies and antigens present on leukocytes and platelets of the donor	↑ temperature, rarely >38°C Chills and shivering sometimes → requiring discontinuation of transfusion	Administer antipyretics Support oxygenation and circulation; maintain urine output (consider diuretics) Send blood samples for free hemoglobin and recross-match Use only O negative blood if blood necessary in interim Send for PT, PTT, platelets, fibrinogen If history of repeated febrile reactions, transfuse WBC-depleted red cells made by centrifugation, filtration, freeze–thaw technique
Febrile hemolytic reaction	Interaction between recipient antibodies and antigens present on RBCs of the donor	Increased temperature, hypotension, hemoglobinuria, and DIC	Support oxygenation and circulation; maintain urine output (consider diuretics) Send blood samples for detection of free hemoglobin and recross-match Use only O negative blood if blood necessary in interim Send for PT, PTT, platelets, fibrinogen
Anaphylactic	Antigen–antibody reaction resulting in massive degranulation of mast cells and basophils	Wheezing and hypotension	Stop transfusion; maintain oxygenation, ventilation, and inotropic support with aid of vasopressors (epinephrine 10–100 μg IV) if necessary; corticosteroids also helpful Send blood samples for detection of free hemoglobin and recross-match Use only O negative blood if blood necessary in interim Send for PT, PTT, platelets, fibrinogen
Transfusion-related acute lung injury (TRALI)	Etiology not fully understood but antibodies to human leukocyte antigens have been implicated	Noncardiogenic pulmonary edema following transfusion	Primarily supportive with mechanical ventilation. Diuretics are best avoided

(continued)

Transfusion Reactions (*continued*)

Reaction	Causes	Signs	Treatment
Bacterial contamination	Usually skin-associated bacteria (i.e., gram + cocci). Most commonly in platelets	Fever and chills, hypotension, nausea, vomiting, diarrhea, oliguria, and shock. Dyspnea, wheezing, bleeding due to DIC	Antibiotics, supportive, best treatment is prevention
Delayed hemolytic transfusion reaction (DHTR)	Occurs after previous alloimmunization to antigen. Over time, antibodies drop below a level, and reexposure to antigen triggers immune response	Sudden drop in Hb 3–14 days after transfusion below pretransfusion level (profound anemia), profound hyperbilirubinemia (jaundice), fever	Supportive treatment
Posttransfusion purpura	Alloantibodies to donor platelets, leading to thrombocytopenia	Severe thrombocytopenia, mucous membrane bleeding, fever, chills	Steroids, IVIG For patients refractory to IVIG therapy, plasma exchange

Risks of Blood Transfusion

Type	Occurrence per number of RBC units transfused
Infectious	
Human immunodeficiency virus	1 in 1.4–2.4×10^6
Hepatitis B	1 in 58,000–149,000
Hepatitis C	1 in 872,000–1.7×10^6
Bacterial infection	1 in 2,000
Immunologic reactions	
Febrile nonhemolytic transfusion reactions	1 in 100
Anaphylactic transfusion reactions	1 in 20,000–50,000
ABO mismatch	
Hemolysis	1 in 60,000
Death	1 in 600,000
Leukocyte-related target organ injury	1 in 20 to 1 in 50
Transfusion-related acute lung injury	1 in 2000
Posttransfusion purpura	Rare
Transfusion services error	
Donor screening error	1 in 4×10^6
Transfusion services error	1 in 14,000

American Society of Anesthesiology Guidelines for Transfusion of Red Blood Cells in Adults
• Transfusion for patients on cardiopulmonary bypass with hemoglobin level ≤6.0 g/dL is indicated
• Hemoglobin level ≤7.0 g/dL in patients older than 65 years and patients with chronic cardiovascular or respiratory diseases justifies transfusion
• For stable patients with hemoglobin level between 7 and 10 g/dL, the benefit of transfusion is unclear
• Transfusion is recommended for patients with acute blood loss more than 1,500 mL or >30% of blood volume
• Evidence of rapid blood loss without immediate control warrants blood transfusion

Reproduced with permission from Ferraris VA, et al. Perioperative blood transfusion and blood conservation in cardiac surgery: the Society of Thoracic Surgeons and The Society of Cardiovascular Anesthesiologists clinical practice guideline. *Ann Thorac Surg*. 2007;83 (5 Suppl):S27.

Electrolyte Composition of Crystalloid IV Fluids							
Solution	Na (mmol/L)	Cl (mmol/L)	K⁺ (mmol/L)	Ca²⁺ (mmol/L)	Mg (mmol/L)	HCO₃ (mmol/L)	Lactate (mmol/L)	Glucose (mg/dL)
Lactated Ringer's	130	109	4	3	–	–	28	–
Normal saline	154	154	–	–	–	–	–	–
D5W	–	–	–	–	–	–	–	5,000
Plasma-Lyte	141	103	4	5	2	26	–	–

REFERENCES

For references, please visit **www.TheAnesthesiaGuide.com**.

CHAPTER 65
Massive Transfusion, Factor VII (Including von Willebrand Disease)

Gebhard Wagener, MD and Ruchir Gupta, MD

MANAGEMENT OF BLEEDING AND MASSIVE TRANSFUSION

A. Massive blood loss and transfusion

• Definition: replacement by transfusion of more than 50% of a patient's blood volume in 12–24 hours
• Contact blood bank and activate rapid transfusion protocol if available: the blood bank will then always keep a certain number of blood products on hold for this patient

B. Management

Avoid acidosis:
• Acidosis affects coagulation factor involving calcium and phospholipids

Avoid hypothermia:
- Hypothermia slows any enzymatic activity including coagulation factors and activation of platelets by von Willebrand factor (vWF)
- Not detected by laboratory tests: samples are warmed to 37°C
- Not correctable with plasma and factor concentrates

Check coagulation profiles (including fibrinogen levels) frequently.

Avoid citrate toxicity:
- Metabolic alkalosis:
  ‣ pH of PRBC at 37°C = 7.10 due to citric acid and production of lactate by red cells during storage; however, metabolism of 1 mmol of citrate generates 3 mEq of bicarbonate (23 mEq of bicarbonate/1 U PRBC)
- Hypocalcemia:
  ‣ Citrate binds ionized calcium: measure calcium frequently and replace generously

Avoid hyperkalemia:
- Potassium levels in stored PRBC increase by 1 mEq/L
- Peak K concentration: 90 mEq/L in PRBC
- Measure K concentration frequently
- Treat hyperkalemia aggressively: insulin/glucose, calcium, furosemide, dialysis (continuous venovenous hemodialysis [CVVHD])
- Consider washing PRBC in Cell Saver if plasma K >5 mmol/mL or rapidly rising
- Consider storing 2–3 U washed PRBC prior to surgery in case of massive bleeding and worsening hyperkalemia
- Replace calcium generously

C. Transfusion

Consider 1:1:1 resuscitation: 1 U PRBC combined with 1 U plasma and 1 U platelets.

Recent studies have shown a survival benefit of 1:1:1 transfusion in combat and civilian trauma.

Plasma

Dilutional coagulopathy: 500 mL blood loss causes a 10% decrease in clotting factors.

Coagulopathy can occur with a 25% decrease of clotting factors (usually 8–10 U packed red blood cells).

Dose for reversal of anticoagulants:
- Determine current and target INR
- Convert INR to approximate percentage of prothrombin complex:
  ‣ INR 1 = 100 (%)
  ‣ INR 1.4–1.6 = 40
  ‣ INR 1.7–1.8 = 30
  ‣ INR 1.9–2.1 = 25
  ‣ INR 2.2–2.5 = 20
  ‣ INR 2.6–3.2 = 15
  ‣ INR 4.0–4.9 = 10
  ‣ INR > 5 = 5 (%)
- Amount of FFP (mL) = (target level [%] − current level [%]) × weight (kg)

Platelets

Fifty percent decrease in platelets with 10–12 U of packed red blood cells.

Transfuse if platelets <50,000 and bleeding or <20,000 without bleeding.

Six units of platelets (=1 "large" unit) increases platelet count by 5–10,000.

Avoid and treat disseminated intravascular coagulation (DIC)
- Depletion of coagulation factors and release of tissue factor from injured tissue
- Consumptive coagulopathy causes widespread coagulopathy and thrombosis

- Fragmentation of erythrocytes generates schistocytes and hemolysis
- Common after head trauma, obstetrical bleeding, sepsis, and malignancy
- Consider DIC if hemorrhage persists despite adequate transfusion
- Observe IV and central line insertion sites for bleeding
- Always check fibrinogen level when sending coagulation profiles
- Test: elevated D-dimers, thrombocytopenia, prolonged PT, PTT, INR, decreased fibrinogen

Disseminated Intravascular Coagulation (DIC) Score			
Platelet count	>100,000 = 0	50,000–100,000 = 1	<50,000 = 2
Elevated fibrin degradation products	Normal = 0	Moderate elevation = 2	Strong elevation = 3
PT above upper limit of reference range	<3 s = 0	3–6 s = 1	>6 s = 2
Fibrinogen	>100 mg/dL = 0	<100 mg/dL = 1	

Score ≥5: compatible with overt DIC.

Cryoprecipitate:
- After thawing of plasma a precipitate can be separated by centrifuging and then frozen to produce cryoprecipitate
- One unit cryoprecipitate (=10–15 mL) contains high concentrations of factor VIII (80–110 IU), 200 mg of fibrinogen, fibronectin, factor XIII, and vWF
- Ten units cryoprecipitate will increase the fibrinogen level by about 70 mg/dL
- Indicated for DIC, low fibrinogen levels, and if large volume plasma transfusion cannot be tolerated

Desmopressin (DDAVP):
- Synthetic vasopressin that causes release of vWF from endothelium
- Treatment of vWF deficiency, qualitative platelet disorders, and mild hemophilia
- Uremic coagulopathy
- Mild–moderate von Willebrand disease with factor VIII coagulant activity levels >5%
- Hemophilia A (factor VIII activity levels >5%)
- Dose: 0.3 μg/kg slowly intravenous

Prothrombin complex concentrate:
- Contains factors II, VII, IX, and X, proteins C and S
- Superior to plasma for reversing oral anticoagulant toxicity: more effective while avoiding large volume transfusion
- Benefit in trauma and massive bleeding remains to be subject of further studies

Recombinant factor VIIa:
- High levels of activated factor VII activate factor X cascade even with low levels of factors VII and IX and trigger coagulation
- Needs exposure to tissue factor: spontaneous thrombosis unlikely unless tissue factor is exposed (vascular anastomosis)
- Approved as prophylaxis and treatment for bleeding in patients with hemophilia with inhibitors against factor VIII or IX
- Frequently used in desperate situations of massive hemorrhage
- Randomized trials:
  ‣ *Intracranial hemorrhage*: Decreases hematoma expansion but no survival benefit
  ‣ *Liver transplantation*: No benefit of single or repeated doses of recombinant factor VIIa
  ‣ *Trauma*: Reduction in transfusion requirements but no difference in mortality in blunt and penetrating trauma
- Dose and treatment algorithm

FIGURE 65-1. Algorithm for the treatment of massive bleeding with factor VII

1.	Is the patient a candidate for Factor VII?

a. *Patient Location: ICU, OR or ED?*
   • No: Do not give Factor VII
   • Yes: proceed to b

b. *All available warming strategies, surgical interventions, liquid sealants and/or other conventional methods of hemostasis utilized?*
   • No: Do not give Factor VII
   • Yes: proceed to c

c. *Transfusion requirements: >10 units of FFP in <6 hours and >10 units of pRBC in <6 hours?*
   • No: Do not give Factor VII
   • Yes: proceed to d

d. *Fibrinogen level?*
   • Less than 100 mg/dl: Give more Cryoprecipitate
   • Greater than 100 mg/dl. Proceed to "e"

e. *Platelet count?*
   • Less than 70,000/mm^3: Give more Platelets
   • Greater than 70,000/mm^3. Proceed to "f"

f. *Fibrin Split Products (FSP)?*
   • Greater than 160 mcg/ml. Do not give Factor VIIa
   • Less than 160 mcg/ml. Start Factor VIIa

2.	Factor VIIa Dosing Guidelines:

a. Start with 90 mcg/kg IV Bolus X 1 (Round off to 1200 mcg increments).

b. Repeat with 120 mcg/kg IV Bolus X 1 (Round off to 1200 mcg increments).

c. Repeat same dose after 2 hours.

d. Re-evaluate patient after 2 doses.
   • At every cycle, reexamine patients for other surgical sources of bleeding
   • If no sign of hemostasis is seen after 2 doses, stop here and do not continue further with Factor VIIa

This algorithm is only a suggestion and modifications may be required depending on institution, location, and patient.

REFERENCES

For references, please visit **www.TheAnesthesiaGuide.com**.

CHAPTER 66
Autologous Transfusion

Rita Parikh, MD

- Donation is made by intended recipient
- Safest blood—no exposure to foreign alloantigens or transfusion-transmissible viral infections
- Can avoid the formation of red cell, white cell, or HLA antibodies
- Useful especially if patient has rare blood type or multiple alloantibodies
- Four broad classifications of autologous donation:
  ‣ Preoperative donation
  ‣ Perioperative hemodilution (acute normovolemic hemodilution [ANH])
  ‣ Intraoperative collection (AKA Cell Saver)
  ‣ Postoperative salvage

Factors to determine whether a patient should undergo preoperative autologous donation (PAD):
- Date of surgery:
  ‣ Generally the patient donates 1 U per week, as long as predonation Hgb and Hct remain >11 g/dL and ≥33%, respectively
  ‣ Minimum of 3 days between collections
  ‣ Minimal allowable time between the last donation and surgery is 72 hours to allow for volume repletion
- Expected surgical blood loss
- Patient's hemoglobin and hematocrit
- Availability of blood supply (rare groups, antibodies)
- Religious beliefs (some Jehovah's Witnesses will accept autologous blood; others will accept hemodilution only if continuity maintained with the IV collection bag)
- Acceptable peripheral venous access
- Existence of underlying conditions that could be worsened by donating or that would preclude donation

The technique that should be used in order to avoid or decrease the chance of receiving allogeneic blood should be discussed in advance with the patient, and the risks and benefits of each addressed.

PREOPERATIVE AUTOLOGOUS DONATION

A. Indication
- Often ordered for use in elective surgeries such as orthopedic, selected gynecologic, and cardiovascular or prostate surgeries
- Major indication—anticipation that at least 1 U of blood will be needed intraoperatively or postoperatively

B. Method
- Hemoglobin ≥11 g/dL
- Give PO iron for 3 weeks, can also be supplemented with recombinant EPO 40,000 U SQ q7 days
- PAD accomplished by whole blood phlebotomy or red cell apheresis
- Frequency of donation—no more than q3 days and not less than 72 hours before scheduled surgery
- Administer units in chronological order

C. Risks
- Iatrogenic anemia resulting after donation
- Iatrogenic hypovolemia after donation

- Some underlying medical conditions may be worsened by donating blood
- Same adverse reactions that can occur with allogeneic whole blood or apheresis donation
- Risk of bacterial contamination if inadequate skin prep or if patient is bacteremic
- Clerical error leading to transfusion of another unit of blood

D. Benefits

- Age: no upper or lower limit
- Parental/guardian consent for patients under 17 years of age
- Weight—no minimum weight
- If <50 kg, adjust amount of blood removed
- If <300 mL, adjust amount of anticoagulant
- Conserve nontransfused units for postoperative period
- Patients with chronic viral infections or risks associated with nonbacterial infections (hepatitis or HIV) are eligible to donate in many situations

E. Contraindications

- Preexisting conditions: symptomatic CAD, CHF, MI within past 6 months, and/or medication(s) for cardiovascular disease emphysema, or COPD
- Uncontrolled HTN, known cerebrovascular disease (including CVA within 6 months), and AS
- Presence or evidence of bacterial infection

Relative contraindications:
- Low initial hematocrit and blood volume (body weight <110 lb)
- Inadequate peripheral venous access

ACUTE NORMOVOLEMIC HEMODILUTION

A. Indication

Most notably cardiopulmonary bypass.

B. Method

- Surgical or anesthesiology team withdraws blood preoperatively and replaces it with crystalloid or colloid solutions
- Blood is reinfused during or after the surgical procedure
- Blood is collected in standard blood bags containing anticoagulant/preservative and is stored at room temperature
- Technique used must ensure sterility
- Units may be stored in OR at room temperature for <8 hours or at 1–6°C for 24 hours (to preserve platelets and coagulation factors)
- Blood units for ANH are reinfused in the reverse order of collection so that the last unit reinfused carries the highest hematocrit level (last unit collected infused first)

C. Benefits

- Produce normovolemic hemodiluted state
- Blood stored at room temperature <8 hours that is not infused at the end of procedure can be stored in a monitored refrigerator
- Units may not be stored for >24 hours if the arm was not adequately prepared before phlebotomy or if the information is unknown

D. Contraindications

- Perioperative blood may not be used for transfusion for other patients

INTRAOPERATIVE BLOOD SALVAGE (IBS; ALSO KNOWN AS "CELL SAVER")

A. Indication

Used commonly during cardiovascular surgical procedures, aortic reconstruction, spinal instrumentation, joint arthroplasty, liver transplantation, resection of AVMs, and occasionally in trauma cases.

B. Method

- Blood-containing fluid (typically NS or RL) is aspirated from the operative site, centrifuged or washed, and reinfused through a filter during the operative or postoperative period
- IBS is most effective during surgical procedures in which relatively large amounts of blood (e.g., vascular procedures) pool in body cavities. This makes it relatively easy to aspirate the blood without introducing significant amounts of air, which can produce frothing and subsequent hemolysis
- Washing the blood before reinfusion removes fibrin, activated clotting factors, cellular debris, and other metabolites
- Most devices can concentrate the RBCs to hematocrit in the range of 45–65%

C. Risks

- Hemolysis, DIC, sepsis, and air embolism
- Potential complications of IBS are reinfusion of fat, microaggregates (platelets and leukocytes), air, red cell stroma, free Hb, heparin, bacteria, and debris. Most of these are removed by cell salvage equipment and via use of filters
- Salvaged blood is deficient in platelets and coagulation factors

D. Benefits

- Intraoperative blood units collected and processed under sterile conditions by a collection device that washes with 0.9% saline can be transfused immediately or stored at room temperature for 6 hours or at 1–6°C for 24 hours provided that the refrigerated storage begins within 4 hours after the end of collection
- Posttransfusion survival of perioperatively salvaged red cells has shown to be comparable to that of allogeneic cells

E. Contraindications

- Infection
- Malignant cells
- Bowel contents, amniotic fluid, and procoagulants in the operative field

POSTOPERATIVE BLOOD SALVAGE (PBS)

A. Indication

- Cardiopulmonary bypass
- Cardiovascular and thoracic procedures
- Arthroplasty

B. Method

- Recovery of blood from a surgical site that may be reinfused into the patient with or without processing, usually of value only within the first 24 or 48 hours after surgery in patients actively bleeding into a closed site (e.g., chest cavity after CPB, joint cavity drainage)
- Blood contained in a plastic container must be filtered (washing is optional) before it is returned to the patient

C. Risks

- Risk of introducing cellular debris and platelet aggregates if blood is not filtered prior to administration

- Risk of proliferation of bacteria if blood is not reinfused within 6 hours after collection
- Unwashed salvaged blood shown to contain thromboplastic material, interleukins, complement, fibrin degradation products, and factors from activated leukocytes and platelets that activate the coagulation process in recipients

D. Benefits

- Blood is usually defibrinated; does not require anticoagulation before transfusion
- Although dilute, the blood is sterile and contains viable red cells

E. Contraindications

- Infection or malignant tumor cells in the site from which the blood is being salvaged or when the rate of blood loss is <50 mL/h

Medications Used to Prevent Anemia in the Context of Autologous Transfusion			
Medication	Indications	Dosing	Contraindications
Iron	Systematic if donation	200 mg iron PO q day (i.e., 300 mg Fe fumarate PO BID, or 325 mg Fe sulfate PO TID)	Side effects: GI intolerance, black stools
Folate	Systematic if donation	1 mg PO q day	Pernicious/aplastic anemia (unless vit B12 also administered)
Erythropoietin (EPO)	Donation or preoperative anemia Patient can donate an additional 1–2 U Weigh indication as very expensive; mostly valuable for large blood loss and rare blood group and/or antibodies	600 IU/kg once a week (D21, 14, 7 preoperatively, and then day of surgery) • Systematic if donation • Only if Hb <13 g/dL if no donation; usually two doses are enough	• Uncontrolled HTN • Hypersensitivity • Post-EPO erythroblastopenia • Contraindication to thromboprophylaxis

REFERENCES

For references, please visit **www.TheAnesthesiaGuide.com**.

CHAPTER 67
Prevention of Venous Thromboembolism (VTE)

Jessica Spellman, MD

- Venous thromboembolism (VTE) represents a major preventable cause of perioperative morbidity (postphlebitic syndrome) and mortality (fatal pulmonary embolism [PE])
- Cost-effectiveness of thromboprophylaxis as well as little or no increase in clinically important bleeding with prophylactic doses has been demonstrated

Risk Factors for VTE	
• Surgery	• High estrogen states (pregnancy and postpartum, OCPs, HRT, estrogen receptor modulators)
• Major trauma or lower extremity injury	• Erythropoiesis-stimulating agents
• Immobility	• Myeloproliferative disorders
• Cancer and cancer therapy	• Acute medical illness
• Venous compression	• Inflammatory bowel disease
• Prior VTE	• Nephrotic syndrome
• Age >60 years	• Paroxysmal nocturnal hemoglobinuria
• Obesity	• Thrombophilia (inherited or acquired)
• Central venous catheterization	

Surgical patients can be generalized into groups based on level of risk for VTE.

Risk Level for VTE Based on Surgery		
Risk level	Patient group	Risk of DVT without prophylaxis (%)
Low	Minor surgery in mobile patients	<10
Moderate	Most general, open gynecologic or urologic surgery patients	10–40
High	Hip or knee arthroplasty Hip fracture surgery Major trauma Spinal cord injury	40–80

Thromboembolism Prophylaxis Recommendations for Level of Risk of VTE from the American College of Chest Physicians (ACCP), 2008	
Risk level	Suggested thromboprophylaxis options
Low	No specific thromboprophylaxis Early and "aggressive" ambulation
Moderate	LMWH LDUH bid or tid Fondaparinux
Moderate with high bleeding risk	Mechanical thromboprophylaxis Consider anticoagulant thromboprophylaxis when high bleeding risk decreases
High	LMWH Fondaparinux Oral vitamin K antagonist (INR 2–3)
High with high bleeding risk	Mechanical thromboprophylaxis Consider anticoagulant thromboprophylaxis when high bleeding risk decreases

LMWH, low-molecular-weight heparin; LDUH, low-dose unfractionated heparin.

If additional risk factors are present (see Table of Risk Factors for VTE), consideration should be given to increasing the intensity or duration of prophylaxis.

MECHANICAL THROMBOPROPHYLAXIS

TABLE 67-1 Mechanical Thromboprophylaxis Strategies
Early and frequent ambulation
Graduated compression stockings (GCS)
Intermittent pneumatic compression devices (IPC)
Venous foot pump (VFP)

- Generally less efficacious than anticoagulant thromboprophylaxis
- Important in high bleeding risk patient groups (if high bleeding risk resolves, consideration should be made for anticoagulant thromboprophylaxis)
- Useful as adjunct to anticoagulant thromboprophylaxis
- Devices are nonstandardized and may lack demonstrative evidence of efficacy prior to marketing
- Patient compliance often poor (recommended to be worn 18 and 20 hours a day)
- Greater effect shown on calf DVT than proximal DVT, effect on PE and death unknown
- Should be initiated prior to induction of anesthesia and continued postoperatively

ANTICOAGULANT THROMBOPROPHYLAXIS

See table on following page.

Anticoagulant Thromboprophylaxis

Agent	LDUH–*low-dose unfractionated heparin*	LMWH–*low-molecular-weight heparin* (enoxaparin, dalteparin)
Mechanism of action	Binds antithrombin III, inactivates factor Xa and thrombin	Selectively inhibits factor Xa
Notes (including neuraxial block recommendations)	Risk of heparin-induced thrombocytopenia (HIT) • No contraindication to neuraxial blockade, best to delay dose until after block placement	Less risk of HIT than LDUH • Enoxaparin: dose adjustment in renal insufficiency as may bioaccumulate • Delay neuraxial blockade for 12 h after last dose of LMWH
Dose for VTE prophylaxis	5,000 U SQ q8–12 h, start 2 h preoperatively	Enoxaparin: • Hip replacement: 30 mg SQ q12 h, start 12–24 h after surgery or 40 mg SQ q day, start 9–15 h prior to surgery • Knee arthroplasty: 30 mg SQ q12 h, start 12–24 h after surgery • Abdominal surgery: 40 mg q day, start 2 h prior to surgery Dalteparin: • Hip replacement: 2,500 U SQ 4–8 h after surgery, and then 5,000 U q24 h or 2,500 U 2 h prior to surgery and 4–8 h after surgery, and then 5,000 U q24 h or 5,000 U 10–14 h prior to surgery, 4–8 h after surgery, and q24 h • Abdominal surgery: 2,500 U SQ q24 h, start 1–2 h prior to surgery • For high risk: 5,000 U SQ q24 h starting the evening prior to surgery or 2,500 U SQ 1–2 h prior to surgery, at 12 h, and 5,000 U q24 h thereafter
Antidote	Protamine	None

Other Anticoagulants

Agent	Fondaparinux (Arixtra®)	Oral vitamin K antagonists (warfarin)	Rivaroxaban (Xarelto®)	Dabigatran (Pradaxa®)
Mechanism of action	Indirect factor Xa-specific inhibitor	Inhibits synthesis of factors II, VII, IX, X	Direct factor Xa inhibitor	Direct thrombin inhibitor
Notes (including neuraxial block recommendations)	• Low HIT risk • Long half-life (17 h) • May accumulate in renal insufficiency • Contraindicated if creatinine clearance <30 mL/min • Neuraxial blockade contraindicated	• Therapeutic monitoring required • Anticoagulant effects not achieved until third or fourth day of treatment • Multiple food and drug interactions • Neuraxial block may be placed if INR <1.2	• Caution in patients with renal or hepatic impairment. Contraindicated in patients with ClCr <30 mL/min or Child–Pugh classes B and C • Avoid use in patients with indwelling neuraxial catheters. Remove epidural catheter 18 h after last dose. Next dose no earlier than 6 h after catheter removal	• Reduce dose to 75 mg twice daily if ClCr 15–30 mL/min. Do not use if ClCr <15 mL/min. No dosage adjustment if ClCr >30 mL/min • Do not use if severe hepatic impairment. Reduce dose in elderly • Not recommended in patients with indwelling neuraxial catheters. Remove catheters 4–6 h before first dose
Dose for VTE prophylaxis	Adults >50 kg: 2.5 mg SQ daily, start 6–8 h postoperatively after hemostasis established	2–5 mg PO, adjust according to INR	10 mg PO q day	220 mg PO q day (in Canada; not FDA-approved for VTE prophylaxis as of early 2012)
Antidote	None Possibly rFVIIa	Vitamin K FFP	None Dialysis with charcoal hemofiltration PCC Possibly rFVIIa	None Dialysis with charcoal hemofiltration PCC

Special Patient Population Considerations and ACCP Recommendations

Surgical patient group	Consideration
Moderate-risk patients	• Should receive thromboprophylaxis until hospital discharge
Prior VTE	• May benefit from up to 28 days of LMWH thromboprophylaxis
Major cancer surgery	• May benefit from up to 28 days of LMWH thromboprophylaxis
Total hip replacement, total knee replacement, and hip fracture surgery	• Thromboprophylaxis for 10–35 days
Laparoscopic surgery[1]	• Low risk
Inpatient bariatric surgery[1]	• Moderate risk • Anticoagulant dosing is uncertain: higher than standard doses of LMWH and LDUH are recommended
Vascular surgery[1]	• Low risk
Thoracic surgery[1]	• Moderate risk
CABG surgery[1]	• LMWH, LDUH, GCS, or IPC
Elective spine surgery[1]	• Low risk
Isolated lower extremity injuries distal to knee[1]	• Low risk
Major neurosurgery[1]	• IPC or • Postoperative LMWH or LDUH in combination with IPC
Trauma	• Thromboprophylaxis if possible and when safe to do so
Acute spinal cord injury	• Thromboprophylaxis with LMWH once primary hemostasis is achieved
Burn patients	• Thromboprophylaxis if possible and when safe to do so, when additional risk factors present

[1]Without additional VTE risk factors.

IVC FILTERS

• ACCP guidelines recommend against IVC filter placement in trauma and spinal cord injury patients as thromboprophylaxis
• IVC filters are indicated for acute proximal DVT or PE if anticoagulation therapy is not possible because of bleeding risk. (If bleeding risk resolves, anticoagulation therapy should be initiated.)

REFERENCES

For references, please visit **www.TheAnesthesiaGuide.com**.

CHAPTER 68
Heparin-Induced Thrombocytopenia

Rita Parikh, MD

- **Type 1:** Isolated HIT develops early in heparin therapy and is benign. No resultant bleeding or thrombotic complications. Not mediated by the immune system: passive heparin binding to platelets resulting in a modest shortening of the platelet life span. The platelet count rarely falls below $100 \times 10^9/L$
- **Type 2:** Heparin-induced thrombocytopenia and thrombosis syndrome (HITTS) is associated with severe thrombocytopenia and paradoxically thrombotic episodes instead of hemorrhagic complications. Occurs in patients receiving heparin for more than 5 days; may occur within 1 day if prior heparin therapy exposure <100 days

Frequency varies widely depending on type of heparin used and the patient group:
- Unfractionated heparin is associated with a higher frequency of HIT than fractionated heparin
- Surgical patients have a higher frequency of HIT than either medical or obstetric patients with the same heparin exposure
- Postoperative orthopedic patients receiving unfractionated heparin have the highest HIT frequency (<5%), and require more intense platelet count monitoring
- Pregnant women receiving LMWH have an almost negligible risk

PATHOPHYSIOLOGY (FIGURE 68-1)

- Heparin exposure can induce the formation of pathogenic IgG antibodies that can cause platelet activation by recognizing complexes of platelet factor 4 (PF4) and heparin on platelet surfaces

FIGURE 68-1. Pathophysiology of HIT

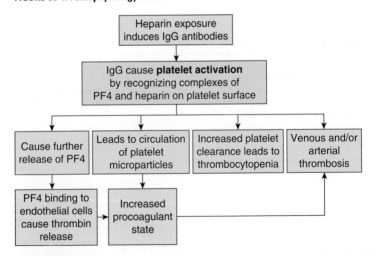

PF4: platelet factor 4.

- Platelet activation results in further release of PF4 and the appearance of platelet microparticles in circulation, both of which magnify the procoagulant state of HIT. PF4 complex binding to endothelial cells stimulates thrombin release. There is an increased clearance of platelets with resultant thrombocytopenia and venous and/or arterial thrombus formation with the potential for severe organ damage (loss of limbs, stroke, MI) and unusual sites of thrombosis (adrenal, portal vein, skin)
- Potential for severe organ damage (loss of limbs, stroke, MI) and unusual sites of thrombosis (adrenal, portal vein, skin)
- In rare cases, targets other than PF4 are involved (NAP-2, IL8)
- The risk of heparin-induced thrombosis is far lower than the incidence of antibody formation. Fewer than 10% of those who develop an antibody to the heparin–PF4 complex will exhibit a thrombotic event
- PF4 antibodies usually decline to undetectable levels within a few weeks or months of an episode of HIT, and there is no anamnestic response

LABORATORY DIAGNOSIS

- Testing should be performed when HIT is clinically suspected. HIT antibodies are detected using either PF4-dependent antigen immunoassays (PF4–heparin antibody ELISA) or functional assays (serotonin release assay) of platelet activation and aggregation. Both tests are very sensitive but specificity is poor
- Clinically insignificant HIT antibodies are common in patients who have received heparin 5–100 days earlier. In the ICU setting, HIT is uncommon (0.3–0.5%), whereas thrombocytopenia from other causes is very common (30–50%)

CLINICAL DIAGNOSIS

- The diagnosis of HIT should be based on clinical abnormalities (thrombocytopenia with or without thrombosis) and a positive test for HIT antibodies
- HITTS has an incidence of <1% of patients receiving heparin. Platelet counts as low as 20×10^9/L can result in arterial and venous thrombosis, with an incidence of morbidity and mortality of 20% of the patients who develop HITTS
- About 25% of HIT patients receiving a heparin bolus develop signs or symptoms—fever, chills, respiratory distress, or hypertension. Transient global amnesia and cardiorespiratory arrest have also been reported. About 5–15% of HIT patients develop decompensated DIC
- Thrombocytopenia does not usually develop until days 5–10 of heparin treatment and reaches a median nadir of 55×10^9/L. The platelet counts falls below 150×10^9/L in 90% of HIT cases
- Hemorrhage and platelet counts below 10×10^9/L suggest an alternative cause such as posttransfusion purpura
- Patients who have received heparin within the last 100 days may have a fall in platelet counts within 1 day of heparin reexposure

TREATMENT OF HIT

- **Stop heparin immediately, and do not readminister** in patients who develop thrombocytopenia to 100×10^9/L or if the original platelet counts falls by 50%
- Platelet counts should return to normal within 4–6 days
- As HIT is associated with thrombosis, an **alternative anticoagulant** should be initiated, initially with a parenteral agent, and then with warfarin:
  - ▸ Direct thrombin inhibitors—lepirudin and argatroban—and the heparinoid danaparoid (not approved in the United States) may be used. HIT patients can cross-react to danaparoid sodium (10% in vitro, less common in vivo). DTI administration should be continued until the platelet count has recovered to 100×10^9/L (at which point treatment with warfarin may be initiated) and until INR of 2–3 achieved with warfarin

- ‣ Bivalirudin and fondaparinux are investigational agents for the treatment of HIT:
  - ▪ Fondaparinux is a pentasaccharide that potentiates antithrombin and has anti-Xa activity. Despite being a synthetic heparin derivative, it does not generate HIT antibodies and has been used safely in those with suspected or confirmed HIT
- ‣ No antidote: bleeding that may occur with these treatments may not be easily corrected. Direct thrombin inhibitors have short plasma half-lives, so their effects resolve relatively quickly
- ‣ There is a 5–20% frequency of new thrombosis despite treatment of HIT patients with an alternative anticoagulant
- Prophylactic platelet transfusions are relatively contraindicated
- Oral anticoagulants should only be used while direct thrombin inhibitors are administered as well:
  - ‣ Patients with HIT, particularly those with associated thrombosis, often have evidence of increased thrombin generation that can lead to consumption of protein C. If these patients are given warfarin without a concomitant parenteral anticoagulant to inhibit thrombin or thrombin generation, the further decrease in protein C levels induced by the vitamin K antagonist can worsen thrombosis and trigger skin necrosis
  - ‣ Warfarin should be continued for at least 30 days, due to a persistent risk of thrombosis even after the platelet count has recovered. In patients in whom thrombosis has been documented, anticoagulation with warfarin should continue for at least 3 months

FIGURE 68-2. Treatment algorithm for HITTS

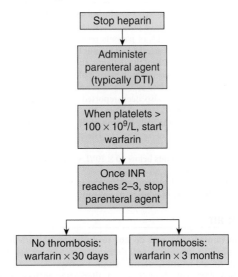

Agents Approved for the Treatment of HIT

Anticoagulant	Dosing (therapeutic range)	Pharmacokinetics ($t_{1/2}$)	Comment
Danaparoid sodium (Orgaran)	Bolus (adjust for body weight): <60 kg: 1,500 U 60–75 kg: 2,250 U 75–90 kg: 3,000 U >90 kg: 3,750 U	Renal metabolism 25 h anti–factor Xa activity 2–4 h anti–factor IIa activity	Approved for use in countries outside of the United States Withdrawn from the US market because of potential for in vivo cross-reactivity (rare, not predictable by in vitro testing)
	Infusion: 400 U/h × 4 h, then 300 U/h × 4 h, and then 200 U/h, with monitoring by anti–factor Xa levels (0.5–0.8 anti-Xa U/mL)		Anticoagulant monitoring not always necessary; preferred for very small or large patients, renal failure patients, and those with life- or limb-threatening thrombosis
Lepirudin (Refludan)	Bolus: 0.4 mg/kg Infusion: 0.15 mg/kg/h (target aPTT range 1.5–2.5 times baseline) In the absence of life-threatening thrombosis or when treating isolated HIT, may be prudent to omit the initial bolus and to aim for aPTT of 1.5–2 times baseline	Renal excretion: 80 min	Approved by FDA for the treatment of HIT-related thrombosis $t_{1/2}$ rises considerably in renal failure patients High rate of antihirudin antibodies (40–60%) that are not usually significant Anaphylaxis reported after lepirudin especially with a repeat treatment course
Argatroban (Novastan)	2 μg/kg/min without an initial bolus (target aPTT range 1.5–3 times baseline)	Hepatobiliary excretion 40–50 min	FDA approved for prevention and treatment of HIT-related thrombosis (identical therapeutic dose regimens used for both indications) Argatroban increases the INR, so a higher therapeutic range is reported during overlapping of argatroban and warfarin

Investigational Agents for the Treatment of HIT			
Bivalirudin (Angiomax)	0.15–0.2 mg/kg/h without an initial bolus (target aPTT range 1.5–2.5 times baseline)	Enzymatic > renal 25 min if normal renal function 57 min if severe renal insufficiency	Approved in the United States for anticoagulation during PCI (non-HIT) Short $t_{1/2}$ and enzymatic metabolism are theoretical advantages over lepirudin for cardiac surgery in patients with HIT (current investigation)
Fondaparinux (Arixtra)	Uncertain	Renal 17–20 h	Approved for DVT prophylaxis after orthopedic surgery Theoretically, lack of in vitro cross-reactivity with HIT antibodies suggests that it may be efficacious in patients with HIT (not yet studied for this indication)

REFERENCES

For references, please visit **www.TheAnesthesiaGuide.com**.

CHAPTER 69
Common PACU Problems; PACU Discharge Criteria

Jan Boublik, MD, PhD

Immediate Issues	
Airway	Pneumothorax, airway obstruction, hematoma
Breathing	Hypoventilation, PE, hypoxemia
Circulation	Hypotension/hypertension, MI, arrhythmias, CHF, cardiac tamponade
Endocrine/metabolic	SIRS/sepsis, adrenal insufficiency, thyroid issues, anaphylaxis, residual anesthetic effects
Miscellaneous	PONV, injuries, altered mental status/postoperative cognitive dysfunction

PONV 9.8%, upper airway obstruction 6.8%, and hypotension 2.8% are the most common.

Airway and Respiratory Issues		
Upper airway obstruction	**Hypoventilation**	**Hypoxemia**
Loss of pharyngeal muscle tone	Residual anesthetics or muscle relaxants	Atelectasis, diaphragmatic injury/paralysis
Residual muscle relaxation	Postoperative opioids, splinting due to pain	Aspiration
Airway edema/trauma	Obesity, OSA	Asthma/COPD exacerbation
Secretions	Premature infants/neonates	ALI/ARDS
Laryngospasm	Tight abdominal binder/abdominal compartment syndrome	PTX, pleural effusion
VC paralysis, arytenoid dislocation		Pneumonia
Foreign body		CHF, fluid overload
Anxiety		

A. Diagnosis and management (general)

- Assess airway, breathing, and circulation
- Deliver increased FiO_2; increase flow rate; consider NRB or shovel mask to goal of SaO_2 93–97% (PaO_2 80–100 mm Hg)
- Consider jaw thrust, chin lift, oral/nasal airway placement, or positive-pressure ventilation
- Review history, OR and postoperative course, fluids and medications administered
- Consider noninvasive ventilation (CPAP or BiPAP) or intubation
- Consider ABG, chest x-ray

B. Management of specific conditions

Common Respiratory Issues in PACU			
		Treatment	
Condition	**Diagnosis**	**Suspected cause**	**Treatment**
Hypoventilation	• Inadequate ventilation for sufficient gas exchange ($PaCO_2$ high and respiratory acidosis)	Residual muscle relaxant	Administer ACh inhibitor
		Opioid overdose	Consider 20–40 µg naloxone IV
		Residual inhaled/IV anesthetic	Arouse patient
		Tight abdominal binder	Release binder
		OSA/obesity	Reposition patient CPAP/BiPAP
		Splinting (due to pain)	Pain control
		Premature infants/ neonates	Avoid opioids, alternative techniques
Upper airway obstruction/ stridor	• Edema/trauma, VC paralysis, arytenoid dislocation • Secretions (blood/ fluid) • (Suspected) foreign body	• Humidified air, steroids, racemic epinephrine aerosol • Suction secretions/glycopyrrolate (drying agent) • Reintubation for severe edema/trauma • ENT consult for VC paralysis/arytenoid dislocation/foreign body removal	

(continued)

Common Respiratory Issues in PACU (*continued*)			
		Treatment	
Condition	Diagnosis	Suspected cause	Treatment
Asthma/COPD exacerbation	• Wheezing on auscultation	• Albuterol/Atrovent nebulizers, steroids, cromolyn sodium, aminophylline, epinephrine as last resort • CPAP/BiPAP, reintubation for severe bronchospasm	
Laryngospasm	• Involuntary tightening laryngeal constrictor muscles and vocal cords • Risk factors: young age, URI, GERD, OSA/obesity, ENT surgery	• Positive-pressure ventilation • If severe propofol (10–20 mg) or succinylcholine (0.1 mg/kg) • Watch for negative pressure pulmonary edema (4% patients)	
Atelectasis	• Decreased breath sounds, opacification on CXR	• Incentive spirometry • Reposition patient • Inhaled N-acetylcysteine, chest PT • CPAP/BiPAP	
Pulmonary embolism	• ECG (S1Q3T3) • Lower extremity Doppler • TTE/TEE • CT angiogram of chest • VQ scan (if high probability)	• Cautious fluids, invasive monitoring, consider inotropes/pressors • Consider anticoagulation, IVC filter • Consider embolectomy/lysis	
ALI/ARDS Transfusion-related ALI (TRALI)	• Acute respiratory failure without cardiac failure • Bilateral fluffy infiltrates on CXR • ALI Pao_2/FiO_2 ratio <200 versus ARDS <300	• Lung-protective ventilation (tidal volume 5–7 mL/kg) • Treat underlying cause	
Pneumothorax/ hemothorax, pleural effusion	• CXR diagnostic	• Needle decompression, chest tube • Surgical exploration if large hemothorax	
Anxiety stridor (Munchausen stridor)	• Episodic inspiratory stridor with normal flow loops • Risk factors: female, anxiety, GERD, type A personality	• Patient education, speech therapy, benzodiazepine (lorazepam)	

CARDIOVASCULAR COMPLICATIONS

A. Hypotension

Hypovolemic (low preload), distributive (low afterload), or cardiogenic (pump failure).

Cardiovascular Issues	
Intravascular volume depletion	Surgical bleeding Persistent fluid losses Third spacing of fluid Bowel preparation GI losses
Increased capillary permeability	Sepsis Burns TRALI
Decreased vascular tone	Sepsis Allergic reactions (anaphylactic, anaphylactoid) Adrenal insufficiency Spinal shock (cord injury, iatrogenic, high spinal) Medications (ACE-I)
Decreased cardiac output	Myocardial ischemia Cardiac dysrhythmias Valvular diseases Cardiac tamponade Pericardial diseases Pulmonary embolus Tension pneumothorax Drug induced (beta-blockers, calcium channel blockers)

Management of specific conditions

Common Cardiovascular Issues in PACU		
Condition	Diagnosis	Treatment
Hypovolemia	• Tachycardia, low BP • Low CVP/PWCP • Respiratory variation in arterial waveform • Low urine output	• Fluid resuscitation/transfusion • Assess for causes (bleeding, high NG output, diuresis)
Bleeding	• Tachycardia, hypovolemia • Anemia • Sanguineous drain output	• Fluid resuscitation/blood product transfusion • Consider return to OR
Sepsis	• Tachycardia, hypovolemia • Fever, leukocytosis • Lactic acidosis	• Fluid resuscitation • Cultures, broad-spectrum antibiotics • Pressors (norepinephrine 5–20 μg/min, vasopressin 0.01–0.1 U/min) if needed
Myocardial ischemia	• 12-lead ECG • Cardiac enzymes • TTE/TEE • Risk stratification ; low (<45 years old, no cardiac disease, no or one risk factor) versus high risk–in high risk evaluate despite absence of symptoms	• ASA, beta-blockers, and nitroglycerin if tolerated • Cardiology consult postoperatively • Cautious fluids • Consider heparinization after consultation with surgeon • Left heart catheterization as per cardiology • Consider inotropic/vasopressor/IABP support

(continued)

Common Cardiovascular Issues in PACU (*continued*)		
Condition	Diagnosis	Treatment

Arrhythmias	• 12-lead ECG cardiac enzymes
	• Check electrolytes, ABG
	• Atrial tachycardia—up to 10% major noncardiothoracic surgeries, not benign, associated with increased mortality and length of stay
	• Ventricular arrhythmias—most common PVCs due to increased sympathetic stimulation
	• Atrial fibrillation
	• Often iatrogenic (drugs—beta-blockers, anticholinesterase reversal, opioids, dexmedetomidine) or procedure/patient related (bowel distension, increased ICP/IOP, spinal anesthesia blocking T1–4 accelerator fibers)
		• Treat cause, ACLS protocol
		• Consider cardiology consult
		  ▸ Tachycardia: Electrical/chemical cardioversion Correct electrolytes
		  ▸ Atrial fibrillation: control ventricular response, beta-blockade or calcium channel blockers versus cardioversion in hemodynamic instability
		  ▸ Bradycardias: atropine/dopamine/epinephrine, transcutaneous/transvenous pacing

Pulmonary embolus	• ECG (S1Q3T3) • Lower extremity ultrasound • CT angiography • TTE/TEE	• Cautious fluids, invasive monitoring • Anticoagulation • Consider inotropes/pressors, • Consider embolectomy/lysis, IVC filter
Anaphylaxis	• Tachycardia, vasodilatory shock • Check serum tryptase and eosinophils	• Remove causative agent • Fluids • Diphenhydramine, epinephrine, steroids
Drugs		• Stop drug, give antagonist (e.g., naloxone for morphine)
Pneumothorax	• No breath sounds and lung markings on affected side	• Needle decompression (salvage procedure if tension pneumothorax), chest tube, surgical decompression if needed
Pericardial tamponade	• Back's triad (hypotension, JVD, muffled heart sound) • Pulsus paradoxus • Nonspecific ECG changes • Enlarged heart (CXR) • Echo	• High preload, high afterload, and tachycardia • Pericardiocentesis • Consider surgical drainage
Congestive heart failure	• Exam (bibasilar crackles, frothy sputum) • CXR (vessel cephalization, pulmonary edema) • Decreased CO and increased filling pressures	• Oxygen • Diuresis • Digoxin/inotropes
Error in measurement	• Wrong cuff size/transducer level • Poor waveform (underdampened/overdampened) • Malfunction transducer	• Appropriate cuff size • Manual measurement • Zero transducer at right level • Check A-line waveform

B. Hypertension

Most common following carotid endarterectomy and intracranial operations.

Causes of Postoperative Hypertension	
Preoperative hypertension	Increased sympathetic activity (pain, agitation, anxiety, urinary retention, bowel distension, hypercapnia)
Arterial hypoxemia	Drug rebound
Shivering	Increased intracranial pressure
Emergence excitement	Hypervolemia
Endocrine issues (thyroid storm, pheochromocytoma)	Error in measurement (e.g., incorrect cuff size)

Diagnosis and management (general)

- Treat underlying cause
- Resume home medication(s) as soon as possible
- For initial management consider labetalol 5–30 mg IV q10 minutes, hydralazine 2.5–20 mg IV q10–20 minutes, metoprolol 2.5–10 mg IV bolus q5 minutes
- For severe hypertension consider vasodilator infusion (sodium nitroprusside 0.25–10 μg/kg/min, nicardipine 5–15 mg/h); consider esmolol (loading dose 0.5–1 mg/kg followed by 50–300 μg/kg/min infusion) or diltiazem (loading dose 0.25 mg/kg over 2 minutes followed by 5–15 mg/h infusion)

POSTOPERATIVE RENAL DYSFUNCTION/ISSUES

Frequently multifactorial with preexisting renal dysfunction aggravated by intraoperative insult.

Etiologies of Renal Dysfunction		
Prerenal	**Intrarenal**	**Postrenal**
Hypovolemia	Ischemic acute tubular necrosis	Mechanical urinary catheter obstruction or malfunction
Low cardiac output	Radiographic contrast dye	Ureter obstruction (clots or lithiasis)
Intra-abdominal hypertension	Rhabdomyolysis	Surgical injury to ureter
Renal vascular obstruction/ disruption	Hemolysis	
Hepatorenal syndrome	Tumor lysis (uric acid crystals)	

A. Diagnosis and Treatment

Focus on readily reversible causes of oliguria (<0.5 mL/kg/h) such as urinary catheter obstruction, potential anatomical obstructions/disruptions/injuries (confer with surgical team).

- Fluid challenge for suspected intravascular volume depletion, rule out surgical bleeding and consider CBC
- Consider furosemide challenge to evaluate if tubular resorption affected by oliguria
- Consider bladder ultrasound to evaluate for obstruction

- Aggressive hydration for suspected contrast nephropathy (3 mL/kg/h of NaHCO₃ for 1 hour followed by 1 mL/kg/h for 6 hours) if not performed intraoperatively. Consider *N*-acetylcysteine (PO: 1,200 mg once before, or 600 mg q12 hours before and after contrast administration; IV: 150 mg/kg in 500 mL NS over 30 minutes immediately before contrast, followed by 50 mg/kg in 500 mL NS over 4 hours)
- Consider measurement of bladder pressure if abdominal compartment syndrome suspected
- Evaluate for possible rhabdomyolysis risk factors; consider aggressive hydration, alkalinization, loop diuretics, and mannitol

Neurologic Issues		
Delirium	• 10% of patients >50 years will experience delirium in first 5 postoperative days (35% of hip and 41% of bilateral knee replacements) • Risk factors: age >70, preoperative cognitive impairment, decreased functional status, alcohol abuse, previous postoperative delirium	• Diagnosis and treatment: ▸ Evaluate for underlying conditions and metabolic (hepatic and renal) derangements ▸ Rule out iatrogenic factors (pain, medications, inadequate hydration, hypoxemia/hypercapnia, electrolyte imbalances)
Emergence agitation	• Transient confusion state associated with emergence from general anesthesia (usually within 10 min of recovery), peak in children 2–4 years old • Possible etiologic factors: rapid emergence, type of surgery, postoperative pain, age, preoperative anxiety, underlying temperament, and adjunct medications	• Prevention is the best treatment. Decrease preoperative anxiety, treat postoperative pain, and provide stress-free environment for patients

Delayed awakening	**Metabolic causes**	**Neurologic causes**	**Pharmacologic causes**
	Hypothermia	Increased intracranial pressure	Residual neuromuscular block
	Hypoglycemia	Stroke	Residual sedation from opioids and benzodiazepines
	Electrolyte derangements	Seizure	Central cholinergic sedation

PONV

- Average incidence of about 20–30% in the absence of prophylaxis
- Can adversely affect patient satisfaction
- Increased cost because of prolonged PACU stay and unplanned admission
- Serious complications such as aspiration, wound dehiscence, esophageal rupture, and retinal detachment are also possible

A. Pathophysiology

- Multifactorial
- The emetogenic center of the brain is located in the lateral reticular formation of the medulla and receives input from the chemoreceptor trigger zone, the vestibular apparatus, the cerebellum, the solitary tract nucleus, and the cerebral cortex
- Receptors involved include dopamine, acetylcholine, histamine, and serotonin receptors

B. Recommended strategy for minimizing the incidence of PONV

Simplified Risk Factor Scale
• Female gender
• History of PONV or motion sickness
• Nonsmoker
• Postoperative opioid use anticipated

Recommended Intervention to Prevent PONV		
Number of risk factors	Risk of PONV without prophylaxis (%)	Recommended intervention
0	10	None
1	20	Dexamethasone
2	40	Dexamethasone + 5-HT3 antagonist
3	60	TIVA + dexamethasone + 5-HT3 antagonist
4	80	TIVA + dexamethasone + 5-HT3 antagonist + droperidol

- Dexamethasone: administer 10 mg IV after induction; avoid administration in an awake patient as it can cause a sensation of perineal pain and burning
- 5-HT3 antagonist: for example, ondansetron 4 mg IV about 30 minutes before the predicted end of the procedure
- TIVA: total intravenous anesthesia, using a propofol IV infusion with avoidance of volatile anesthetics and nitrous oxide
- Droperidol: 0.625 mg IV administered at the end of the procedure. *NB*: Droperidol carries an FDA black box warning regarding its association with a prolongation of the QT interval. However, the low doses used for PONV prevention (relative to doses used for antipsychotic purposes) have not been associated with significant QT prolongation

PACU DISCHARGE/TRANSITION OF CARE ISSUES

Discharge criteria should be tailored to the patient's disease/comorbidities, recovery course, and postoperative level of care. Certain general principles universally apply:
- Patients should be alert and oriented or at baseline mental status
- Airway reflexes and motor function returned to maintain patency and prevent aspiration, acceptable oxygenation, and ventilation with sufficient reserve
- Vital signs should be stable and within acceptable limits (usually within 20% of preoperative values)
- Discharge should only be performed when specific criteria have been met
- Outpatients should only be discharged in company of a responsible adult and after having received instructions for postoperative care as well as an emergency contact number
- Scoring systems can facilitate documentation of discharge readiness
- A physician needs to accept responsibility for the discharge from the unit
- Passing urine and the ability to drink and retain fluids is not a discharge requirement. There is no mandatory minimum length of stay

A. Scoring systems

Use clinical judgment due to large variability among patients.

| PACU Discharge Scoring Systems | |
Modified Aldrete Score	Postanesthesia Discharge Scoring System
Respiration 2: able to take deep breath and cough 1: dyspnea/shallow breathing 0: apnea	Vital signs 2: BP + pulse within 20% of baseline 1: BP + pulse within 20–40% of baseline 0: BP + pulse more than 40% off baseline
Oxygen saturation 2: maintains SpO_2 >92% on room air 1: needs O_2 inhalation to maintain O_2 saturation >90% 0: O_2 saturation <90% even with supplemental oxygen	Activity 2: steady gait, no dizziness or meets preoperative level 1: requires assistance 0: unable to ambulate
Consciousness 2: fully awake 1: arousable on calling 0: not responding	Nausea and vomiting 2: minimal/treated with PO medication 1: moderate/treated with parenteral medication 0: severe/continues despite treatment
Circulation 2: BP ± 20 mm Hg preoperatively 1: BP ± 20–50 mm Hg preoperatively 0: BP ± 50 mm Hg preoperatively	Pain Controlled with oral medications and acceptable to patient 2: yes 1: no
Activity 2: able to move four extremities 1: able to move two extremities 0: unable to move extremities	Surgical bleeding 2: minimal/no dressing changes 1: moderate/up to two dressing changes 0: severe/more than three dressing changes
Score of 9 or higher for discharge	Score of 9 or higher for discharge

REFERENCES

For references, please visit **www.TheAnesthesiaGuide.com**.

PART V

SPECIFIC PROCEDURES

CHAPTER 70

Orthopedic Procedures; Bone Cement Implantation Syndrome; Pneumatic Tourniquet

Arthur Atchabahian, MD

ORTHOPEDIC PROCEDURES

A. Ambulatory surgery

- Most peripheral procedures can be performed on an ambulatory basis
- Regional anesthesia, peripheral, or neuraxial:
  - Peripheral nerve blocks, single-injection or continuous, allow:
    - Performing surgery with block + MAC and bypassing PACU stage I
    - Postoperative pain control
  - Spinal: low-dose bupivacaine, chloroprocaine; no need for voiding prior to discharge
- PONV prevention: main cause of unplanned admission with pain

B. Positioning issues

- Supine:
  - Lumbar pain by hyperextension
  - Risk of ulnar nerve compression at the elbow
  - Shoulders not abducted more than 90°
- Fracture table (hip fracture, anterior hip replacement, hip arthroscopy):
  - Perineal pressure
  - Upper extremity of operative side positioned over the chest:
    - Padding
    - Ensure IV patency
- Lateral decubitus (hip replacement, shoulder surgery, elbow surgery):
  - Keep neck neutral
  - Ensure that dependent eye is free (highest risk of injury)
  - "Axillary roll" to release pressure on shoulder: placed low enough that a hand fits between axilla and roll
  - Nondependent arm on board: pad well to prevent nerve compression
- Prone (spine):
  - Head positioner (various devices) with eyes free of pressure and neck neutral; avoid lateral rotation
  - Risk of visual loss if prolonged surgery (see chapter 62)
  - Spread body weight on maximal surface

- Keep abdomen and chest free to avoid impeding respiration and venous return; supports by iliac crests and upper thorax
- Ensure that genitalia and breasts are not compressed
- Shoulders not abducted more than 90°
- Sitting (shoulder surgery):
  - Ensure that head and neck are stable
  - Improves respiratory function
  - Beware of the pressure differential between arm (or sometimes calf) BP cuff and brain at the level of the circle of Willis (level of external auditory meatus); risk of cerebral ischemia

C. Analgesia

- Bone and joint surgery especially painful
- Importance of multimodal analgesia:
  - Regional techniques
  - Opioids
  - NSAIDs, COX-2 inhibitors (avoid if spinal fusion)
  - Acetaminophen
  - Gabapentin/pregabalin
  - Low-dose ketamine
- Amputation:
  - Prevention of phantom limb pain
  - Use perineural catheters placed by anesthesiologist or surgeon
  - Multimodal analgesia

D. Blood loss

- Blood loss can be massive, especially in spine surgery, hip/shoulder surgery, and tumor surgery
- Discuss surgical plan with surgeon
- Ensure that blood is cross-matched and available prior to starting procedure with risk of major blood loss
- *Preoperative donation (±EPO), Cell Saver*; normovolemic hemodilution rarely used
- *Tranexamic acid* (antifibrinolytic for knee/hip replacement and spine surgery):
  - Multiple protocols, for example, 10 mg/kg IV bolus prior to incision, and then:
    - For spine, 10 mg/kg/h until end of procedure
    - For hip, 1 mg/kg/h until end of procedure
    - For knee, 1 mg/kg/h until 6 hours after end of surgery

E. Fat embolism

- Ten to 20% mortality
- Classically presents within 72 hours following long bone or pelvic fracture
- Triad of dyspnea, confusion, and petechiae
- Free fatty acid levels have a toxic effect on the capillary–alveolar membrane leading to the release of vasoactive amines and prostaglandins and the development of ARDS
- Neurological manifestations (agitation, confusion, stupor, or coma) due to capillary damage to the cerebral circulation and cerebral edema
- Diagnosis:
  - Petechiae on the chest, upper extremities, axillae, and conjunctiva
  - Fat globules in the retina, urine, or sputum
  - Thrombocytopenia and/or prolonged clotting times
  - Serum lipase activity may be elevated; no relationship to severity
  - Mild hypoxemia with normal CXR to severe hypoxemia and diffuse patchy pulmonary infiltrates
  - During GA, $\downarrow$ in $EtCO_2$ and SpO_2, $\uparrow$ PA pressures
  - EKG: ST changes and right-sided heart strain
- Treatment:
  - Prophylactic: early stabilization of fracture

‣ Supportive: O_2 with CPAP, intubation–ventilation with PEEP
‣ High-dose steroids, especially if cerebral edema

F. Iliac crest bone harvest

• Typically GA and drain for 24–72 hours
• Adverse effects relevant to the anesthesiologist:
  ‣ Pain (often worse than primary surgery for which bone is harvested)
  ‣ Nerve lesions (cluneal, lateral femoral cutaneous, subcostal, iliohypogastric), with possible evolution to chronic pain
• Analgesia options:
  ‣ Local infiltration
  ‣ Instillation of local anesthetic (catheter inserted next to bone, under periosteum, by surgeon during closure)
  ‣ TAP block ± catheter

BONE CEMENT

Methyl methacrylate (MMA) "cement" is used to secure implants into bone (knee and hip replacements), and occasionally to replace lost bone (pathological fractures, kyphoplasty). It is different from the phosphocalcic cements used as allografts.

A. Advantages

• Very biocompatible
• Polymerizes quickly to stiffness between cancellous and cortical bone
• Provides for even distribution of forces between prosthesis and bone
• Heat generated destroys nerve endings and provides local analgesia

B. Disadvantages

• Heat generated by chemical reaction kills adherent bone osteoblasts
• Severe potentially life-threatening adverse reactions may occur during implantation

C. Bone cement implantation syndrome

• Occurs most often during the impaction of MMA into the femoral canal during hip replacement surgery, but may occur at other times, e.g., cementing of acetabular component, or on deflation of tourniquet for knee arthroplasty
• Placement of cement into canal and subsequent forcing of femoral prosthesis into cement causes MMA to be forced into trabecular areas of femoral canal
• Direct intramedullary pressure within the femoral canal/reamed open bone may result in *embolization of MMA monomers, air, bone debris, bone marrow elements, fat, and thromboplastic elements (fibrin + platelets)*
• Histamine release and complement activation also play a role

D. Intraoperative signs (temporally related to cement placement)

• Hypotension
• Hypoxemia
• Vasodilation
• Bronchoconstriction
• Cardiovascular collapse/cardiac arrest
• Postoperative confusion associated with hypoxemia might have a similar pathophysiology

E. Risk factors

• Patient (increased severity)
  ‣ Pulmonary HTN
  ‣ Significant cardiac disease (NYHA 3 or 4)
  ‣ Osteoporosis
  ‣ Pathological fracture
  ‣ Intertrochanteric fracture

- Surgery (increased likelihood):
  ‣ Primary surgery
  ‣ Long stem arthroplasty
  ‣ Insertion of cement while still very fluid
  ‣ Absence of use of a plug in the femoral canal

F. Treatment

- 100% O_2, intubation/respiratory support if necessary
- Vasopressors (ephedrine, phenylephrine) as needed
- Aggressive fluid resuscitation (if hypovolemia is suspected)
- Bronchodilators (albuterol, ipratropium inhalers, terbutaline SC)

G. Prevention/mitigation:

- Anesthetic:
  ‣ Maintain high degree of vigilance during key periods; consider invasive monitoring in patients at risk
  ‣ Maintain euvolemia during case
  ‣ Increase FiO_2 to 100% prior to acetabular or femoral cementing; avoid N_2O
- Surgical:
  ‣ Medullary lavage
  ‣ Good hemostasis before cement insertion
  ‣ Minimizing the length of the prosthesis
  ‣ Using noncemented prosthesis (especially if using a long stem implant)
  ‣ Venting the medulla (but this might increase the risk of femoral fracture)
  ‣ Insertion with a cement gun and retrograde insertion
  ‣ Mixing cement in a partial vacuum

PNEUMATIC TOURNIQUET

- Used in orthopedic surgery to obtain a blood-free operating field:
  ‣ Typically exsanguination using an Esmarch band
  ‣ Then inflation of tourniquet to about 100 mm Hg above SBP, usually *250 mm Hg for upper extremity, 300 mm Hg for lower extremity*
  ‣ Limit duration to *90 minutes on upper extremity* and *120 minutes on lower extremity*
  ‣ *No evidence that deflation with subsequent reinflation decreases risk*
- *No evidence of positive impact on operative time* (except maybe for microsurgery), *or on blood loss: poor surgical hemostasis* and *fibrinolysis* (induced by hypothermia, hypoxia, and acidosis) *increases postoperative bleeding*
- *Tourniquet pain* with complex mechanism:
  ‣ Incompletely blocked by GA: ↑ HR and BP after 20–30 minutes
  ‣ Even under RA, the level of tourniquet pain rises and after 60–80 minutes, pain will typically be perceived despite an adequate level of anesthesia for the surgical procedure
  ‣ Possible postoperative hyperalgesia
- *Increased thromboembolic risk*:
  ‣ If DVT present preoperatively (immobilization, cast, etc.), embolization can happen on initial exsanguination, with possible massive PE and cardiac arrest
  ‣ Embolization on release, including of debris/fat from the surgical procedure, with *possible massive PE and cardiac arrest*
  ‣ Studies using TEE show that *embolization will happen even while tourniquet inflated* (through bone vessels), especially during femoral stem insertion during knee arthroplasty
  ‣ Pulmonary embolization will raise right-sided pressure, possibly reopening a PFO and leading to emboli crossing to the systemic circulation, with possible CVA and/or organ infarcts
- On tourniquet release, acidotic, cold blood is released, with *increase in PaCO₂*, which will take 4–5 minutes to normalize:
  ‣ Rarely, dysrhythmias can result

- Administered drugs will not reach limb after tourniquet inflation:
  - ‣ Give, for example, *antibiotics at least 5 minutes before inflation*
  - ‣ Also, *possible release on deflation of anesthesia drugs stored after induction*
- *Muscle ischemia*, with possible ischemia–reperfusion injury and compartment syndrome
- *Possible arterial occlusion*:
  - ‣ Atherosclerosis with plaque rupture
  - ‣ Sickle cell anemia
  - ‣ *Check pulses after deflation*
- Possible *neuropathy*:
  - ‣ Incidence related to duration of inflation and preexisting neuropathy ("double crush" injury)
- Because of local ischemia and hypothermia, *increased incidence of surgical infection*
- *Contraindications*:
  - ‣ PVD, especially if stent(s)/bypass vascular graft on the extremity
  - ‣ Sickle cell anemia
  - ‣ Preexisting neuropathy (DM, etc.)

REFERENCES

For references, please visit **www.TheAnesthesiaGuide.com**.

CHAPTER 71
ENT Procedures

Nasrin N. Aldawoodi, MD and Claude McFarlane, MD, MA

TONSILLECTOMY/ADENOIDECTOMY

A. Preoperative considerations

- Seek history of obstructive sleep apnea (OSA), bleeding disorders, loose teeth, sickle cell
- OSA and tonsillar hypertrophy = airway obstruction
- Inspect oropharynx: percentage of area occupied by hypertrophied tonsils correlates with ease of mask ventilation
- Check hematocrit, use of ASA or other anticoagulants
- High incidence of PONV
- Consider vigorous IV hydration to counteract dehydration due to poor oral intake

B. Anesthetic plan

- Aim: rapid emergence to alertness prior to leaving OR. Ability to clear secretions and protect airway is key
- Avoid sedative premedication in patients with OSA or large tonsils
- IV induction for adults. Mask induction with N_2O, O_2, and volatile agent for children
- Consider oral RAE
- PONV prophylaxis with ondansetron, dexamethasone
- Decompress stomach with orogastric tube prior to emergence (swallowed blood is a potent emetic)

C. Perioperative pearls

- Up to 8% experience postoperative hemorrhage. Usually occurs within 24 hours of surgery, may occur 5–10 days postoperatively
- Chronic hypoxemia, hypercarbia = increased airway resistance leads to cor pulmonale
- Note EKG for findings of RVH, dysrhythmias; CXR with cardiomegaly
- CXR or TTE may be indicated in patients with suspicion of cor pulmonale

BLEEDING TONSIL

A. Preoperative considerations

- Hemorrhage rate higher in adults, male gender, and presence of peritonsillar abscess
- Check Hgb, Hct (might not drop if acute bleeding; estimate bleeding clinically based on hemodynamic response), and coagulation
- Type and cross-match ready
- Hypotension a late symptom

B. Anesthetic plan

- Oxygenate and resuscitate first
- Dependable large-bore IV access
- Anticipate difficult laryngoscopy: clots, bleeding, swelling, and edema
- Use smaller ETT
- Rapid sequence induction (RSI): preferred but patient may inhale blood, CV depression on top of hypovolemia
- 2 wall suctions available
- Head-down position for intubation
- Decompress stomach with orogastric tube to clear blood after securing airway
- Extubate when fully conscious and able to protect airway

C. Perioperative pearls

- Rebleeds usually occur within 6 hours of surgery
- Bleeding may be occult
- Problems usually due to aspiration, hypovolemia, difficult laryngoscopy

MYRINGOTOMY/EAR TUBE INSERTION

- Pediatric patients with recurrent otitis media frequently have URIs as well
- Okay to do surgery on most patients with URI; just give postoperative O_2
- Short, same-day surgeries
- Avoid premedication due to short duration of surgery
- Consider mask ventilation with volatile anesthetic, N_2O, and oxygen for surgery
- The only case that can be performed without inserting an IV

TYMPANOPLASTY/MASTOIDECTOMY

A. Preoperative considerations

- High incidence of PONV
- Mastoid surgery: facial nerve usually monitored

B. Anesthetic plan

- Mask for IV induction for children; IV induction for adults
- Neck turned laterally. Be careful of positioning
- Facial nerve monitoring = no NMB during case
- Avoid N_2O: middle ear is air-filled, nondistensible spaces
- No NMB and no N_2O means high-dose volatile agent or propofol infusion
- Consider relative hypotension MAP 20% below baseline to avoid excessive bleeding; however, use pressor (phenylephrine infusion) if excessive hypotension from high-dose volatile agent/propofol

- Consider deep extubation, avoid straining, coughing on emergence
- PONV prophylaxis with ondansetron, dexamethasone

C. Perioperative pearls

- MAP <20% of baseline may diminish CPP. A potential issue in patients with previous CVA or TIA

LARYNGOSCOPY/BRONCHOSCOPY

A. Preoperative considerations

- Detailed preoperative airway evaluation, and discussion with surgeon
- Stridor at rest = critical airway obstruction
  - ▸ Stridor differential diagnosis: laryngotracheomalacia, vocal cord paralysis, masses, foreign body aspiration, tracheal stenosis
- Unable to lie flat: suggests critical airway obstruction
- Review clinic preoperative fiber-optic/mirror laryngoscopy
- Review relevant radiographs
- Intraoperative periods of intense stimulation followed by minimal stimulation. Consider propofol/remifentanil IV infusion
- Consider block of superior laryngeal nerve to minimize hemodynamic alterations

B. Anesthetic plan

- Avoid premedication: short surgical duration and risk of decreasing airway reflexes
- Goal: deep anesthesia and muscle relaxation during procedure to blunt airway reflexes
- Consider preoperative antacid: unprotected airway manipulation under anesthesia
- Consider antisialagogue
- Consider awake FOI or tracheostomy in cases of suspected difficult airway
- GETA: consider microlaryngeal tracheal tube (MLT)
- Mask or IV induction for children, IV induction for adults
- Induce patients with stridor in ideal breathing position (e.g., sitting position)
- Aim for rapid return of consciousness and airway reflexes at end of case
- Ventilate during bronchoscopy, via:
  - ▸ Side port on rigid bronchoscope
  - ▸ MLT
  - ▸ Technique with periods of mask or ETT ventilation followed by 2- to 3-minute apnea
  - ▸ High-frequency jet ventilation using a cannula in the pharynx
- Use high fresh gas flows, large tidal volumes, and high volatile anesthetic concentrations during procedure
- Consider inserting ETT at end of procedure to protect airway until emergence

C. Perioperative pearls

- Standby equipment for surgical tracheostomy
- Potential OR pollution

LARYNGOSCOPY/BRONCHOSCOPY VIA SPONTANEOUS VENTILATION

A. Preoperative considerations

- As per laryngoscopy/bronchoscopy surgical procedure

B. Anesthetic plan

- Avoid premedication: short surgical duration and risk of decreasing airway reflexes during spontaneous ventilation
- Consider preoperative antacid: unprotected airway manipulation under anesthesia
- Consider antisialagogue
- Consider mask induction with sevoflurane in oxygen to maintain spontaneous ventilation

- Induce patients with stridor in ideal breathing position (e.g., sitting position)
- Ventilation during bronchoscopy via: (1) insufflation techniques; (2) nasopharyngeal airway; (3) bronchoscope. Limitations: potential airway soiling, lack of controlled ventilation

C. Perioperative pearls
- OR pollution
- Consider total intravenous anesthesia (TIVA) after airway established

NASAL/SINUS SURGERY
A. Preoperative considerations
- Nasal polyps can potentially make mask ventilation difficult
- Nasal polyps are associated with asthma and CHF (Samter's syndrome)
- Nasal mucosa: high vascularity
- Inquire about anticoagulant use or blood clotting problems
- Assess for OSA, CAD, and potential effects of nasal vasoconstrictors

B. Anesthetic plan
- Consider local anesthesia, anterior ethmoidal and sphenopalatine nerve block with IV sedation for minor procedures
- GETA: consider oral RAE
- Consider inserting oral airway to mask-ventilate before intubation, as many of these patients have nasal obstruction
- Protect eyes of patient with pads and tape
- Epinephrine or cocaine-soaked pledgets in nose limit mucosal bleeding
- Extubation goal: minimal coughing or straining to minimize bleeding
- Ask surgeon to place nasal airway prior to emergence

C. Perioperative pearls
- If cocaine used as a nasal vasoconstrictor, be aware of toxic reactions. *Do not* use beta-blockers to treat hypertension (see chapter 52)

LASER AIRWAY SURGERY
See chapter 72.

HEAD AND NECK CANCER SURGERY
A. Preoperative considerations
- Detailed preoperative airway evaluation, and discussion with surgeons
- Read clinic notes about laryngoscopy and location of airway masses relative to vocal cords, arytenoids. Review CT scan if available
- Most of these patients have comorbid conditions that need to be optimized (COPD, CAD, HTN, malnutrition)
- Preoperative radiation, airway masses complicate mask ventilation and intubation
- Substantial blood loss can occur. Have at least type and screen
- Consider intra-arterial BP monitoring and placement of CVC

B. Anesthetic plan
- Avoid excessive premedication in patients with difficult airway
- Consider awake fiberoptic intubation or inhalational induction maintaining spontaneous ventilation
- Equipment, surgeons available for emergency tracheostomy
- Avoid NMB during neck dissection if CN VII monitored

- Microvascular free flap anastomosis: maintain normotension; avoid using phenylephrine and direct vasoconstrictors. Avoid direct vasodilators (SNP) that can decrease perfusion pressure to flap. Avoid diuresis and maintain Hct 27–30% for flap perfusion
- If carotid or jugular tumor, with head-up tilt, watch for venous air embolism. Maintain normotension to prevent decrease in CPP
- Plan for tracheostomy

C. Perioperative pearls
- Potential emergent tracheostomy
- Denervation of bilateral carotid sinuses and bodies can lead to postoperative hypertension and hypoxia
- Manipulation of stellate ganglion and carotid sinus can cause blood pressure fluctuations, arrhythmias, asystole, and other signs of CV instability
- Infiltration of carotid sheath with LA can attenuate CV instability

MAXILLOFACIAL/ORTHOGNATHIC SURGERY
A. Preoperative considerations
- Detailed preoperative airway evaluation and discussion with surgeons
- Check mouth opening, neck mobility, mandible size and protrusion, tongue size
- Substantial blood loss can occur
- Have at least a type and screen

B. Anesthetic plan
- Consider awake fiberoptic intubation or tracheostomy if evidence of difficult mask ventilation or intubation
- Consider nasal RAE
- Basilar skull fracture is a contraindication to nasal intubation
- Slight head-up position to minimize blood loss. If osteotomies, consider controlled hypotension (nicardipine or nitroprusside infusion, arterial BP monitoring) if safe given patient's other comorbidities
- Protect eyes (pads and tape)
- Watch for ETT kinking, disconnection, or cuff tear
- Remove throat pack and suction stomach at end of case to remove blood
- Assess for airway swelling; consider dexamethasone. Consider leaving patient intubated postoperatively
- Maxillomandibular fixation patients should have wire cutters nearby for emergency

EPIGLOTTITIS
A. Preoperative considerations
- Usually occurs in children aged 2–8, male gender, but possible in adults
- Etiology: *H. influenzae*
- Signs/symptoms: fever, drooling, insistence on sitting up, dysphagia
- Do not attempt to directly visualize epiglottis without anesthesia
- Pediatric patient: avoid IV insertion if possible prior to securing the airway to avoid airway obstruction from agitation

B. Anesthetic plan
- GETA
- Have personnel available for emergent tracheostomy
- Keep patient in sitting position prior to induction
- Mask induction with sevoflurane
- Choose ETT half size smaller than usually appropriate
- Avoid NMB if possible

C. Perioperative pearls

- Avoid airway manipulation without anesthesia
- Patient taken to ICU intubated postoperatively
- Patient returns to OR >48 hours for extubation after direct visualization to evaluate inflammation
- Check for cuff leak prior to extubation

CHAPTER 72
Anesthesia for Laser Surgery

Albert Ju, MD

BASICS

- Laser = light amplification by stimulated emission of radiation
- Focalized high energy → instant coagulation → reduced bleeding, sparing of healthy tissues

Type of Lasers			
Type of laser	Wavelength (nm)	Features	Type of surgery
CO_2	10,600	High vaporization superficially, little damage to deep tissues	Oropharyngeal surgery, vocal cord surgery
Nd:YAG	1,064	Further spread, greater coagulation versus vaporization	Tumor debulking, tracheal procedures
Ruby	694	Absorbed primarily by dark pigments	Retinal surgery
Argon	515	Transmitted by water, absorbed by hemoglobin	Vascular lesions

Vocal cord surgery:
- Complete NMB of vocal cords
- Inhibition of pharyngeal reflexes
- Decrease secretions (glycopyrrolate 0.2–0.4 mg IV)
- If intubation, prefer special laser ETT (metal-coated, double cuff, small diameter); inflate cuff(s) with colored saline
- If no intubation, typically transglottic jet ventilation

ANESTHETIC CONCERNS

Tissue injury:
- Iatrogenic injury to patient can be caused by laser:
  ‣ Pneumothorax, blood vessel puncture, hollow viscus (trachea) rupture
  ‣ Dental injury

- Eye injury is of special concern, to both patient and health care provider:
  ▸ Window to OR door should be covered
  ▸ Everyone in OR (including patient) should wear appropriate wraparound goggles (Table below on Appropriate Eye Protection)
  ▸ Place wet eye pads on taped patient's eyes and under goggles

Appropriate Eye Protection		
Type of laser	Structures damaged	Precautions
CO_2	Cornea	Clear lenses
Nd:YAG	Retina	Green goggles
Ruby	Retina	Red goggles
Argon	Retina	Amber goggles

Venous gas embolus:
- Gas is often used to cool laser probe tip
- Gas embolus can occur (especially during laparoscopic uterine surgery):
  ▸ Saline insufflation can be used, but fluid overload is possible
- Watch end-tidal CO_2 closely. If embolus suspected, cease use of laser, support hemodynamics until embolus resolves

Laser plume:
- Vaporized tissue can be inhaled by operating room personnel
- In theory, possible vector of infection (viruses) or malignant cells
- Consider use of high-efficiency filtration masks

Airway fire (ETT ignition):
- Prevention of airway fire:
  ▸ Limit FiO_2 to lowest amount compatible with adequate patient oxygenation (21–40%)
  ▸ Avoid N_2O (supports combustion)
  ▸ Use specially designed tube (if unavailable, wrap tube in metal foil)
  ▸ Encourage placement of moistened pledgets around cuff by surgeons
  ▸ Fill cuff with methylene blue–colored saline to provide surgeons with visible warning of cuff puncture
- Treatment of airway fire:
  ▸ Cease use of laser immediately
  ▸ Immediately disconnect tube from circuit. This should extinguish fire quickly:
    ▪ Extubate as soon as the fire is extinguished. If fire still persists after circuit disconnection, pour saline in mouth
  ▸ Place tube in water after extubation
  ▸ Reintubate patient:
    ▪ Airway damage may increase difficulty of intubation. Consider use of difficult airway equipment. Have surgeons prepare for tracheostomy if necessary
  ▸ Assess lung damage with bronchoscopy. Keep patient intubated postoperatively. Monitor arterial blood gases, chest radiograph; assess airway for swelling (consider steroid course)

REFERENCES

For references, please visit **www.TheAnesthesiaGuide.com**.

CHAPTER 73
Ophthalmology

Manuel Corripio, MD

BASICS

- Regulation of intraocular pressure (IOP). Normal intraocular pressure: 12–20 mm Hg

Factors Affecting IOP	
Variable	Effect on IOP
Central venous pressure	
Increase	↑↑↑
Decrease	↓↓↓
Arterial blood pressure	
Increase	↑
Decrease	↓
$PaCO_2$	
Increase (hypoventilation)	↑↑
Decrease (hyperventilation)	↓↓
PaO_2	
Increase	O
Decrease	↑

- Clinical pearl: Pressure from a tightly fitted mask, improper prone position or retrobulbar hemorrhage can lead to ↑ IOP

Effects of Anesthetics on IOP	
Drug	Effect on IOP
Inhaled anesthetics	
Volatile agents	↓↓
Nitrous oxide	↓
Intravenous anesthetics	
Barbiturates	↓↓
Benzodiazepines	↓↓
Ketamine	?
Opioids	↓
Muscle relaxants	
Depolarizing (succinylcholine)	↑↑
Nondepolarizers	O/↓

O, no effect; ↑, increase (mild, moderate); ↓, decrease (mild, moderate); ?, conflicting reports.

- Mechanisms for the decrease of IOP: a drop in BP reduces choroidal volume, relaxation of the extraocular muscles (EOM) lowers wall tension, and papillary constriction facilitates aqueous outflow

- ▸ Clinical pearl: Succinylcholine ↑ IOP by 5–10 mm Hg for 5–10 minutes, through prolonged contracture of the EOM. This may cause:
  - ▪ Extrusion of ocular contents through an open surgical or traumatic wound
  - ▪ Abnormal forced duction test for 20 minutes (test used in strabismus surgery)
- The oculocardiac reflex:
  - ▸ Pathway: Afferent trigeminal nerve (V1)/Efferent vagus nerve (X)
  - ▸ Most common scenarios: pediatric patients, strabismus surgery
  - ▸ Symptoms/Signs: Cardiac dysrhythmias ranging from bradycardia to ventricular ectopy to sinus arrest. In awake patients, somnolence and nausea
  - ▸ Prevention:
    - ▪ Anticholinergic medication. IV is more effective than IM
    - ▪ Retrobulbar block and/or deep inhalation anesthesia may also help
    - ▪ Local infiltration by surgeon
  - ▸ Management:
    - ▪ Immediately notification of surgeon and temporary cessation of surgical stimulus until hemodynamic stability
    - ▪ Confirm adequate ventilation, oxygenation, and depth of anesthesia
    - ▪ IV atropine (10 mcg/kg) if hemodynamic instability
    - ▪ If more than one episode, infiltration of the rectus muscle with local anesthetic
- Intraocular gas expansion:
  - ▸ The surgeon may inject air or gas into the posterior chamber to flatten a detached retina and allow better healing
  - ▸ The air bubble is usually absorbed in 5 days by diffusion
  - ▸ If the patient is breathing nitrous oxide (N_2O) the bubble will increase in size → ↑IOP
  - ▸ N_2O is 35 times more soluble than nitrogen (major component in air) in blood
  - ▸ Sulfur hexafluoride (SF_6) is an inert gas that is less soluble in blood than nitrogen, and less soluble than N_2O. It has a duration of action of 10 days
  - ▸ Bubble size doubles within 24 hours after injection because nitrogen from air enters the bubble more rapidly than the SF_6 diffuses into the bloodstream
  - ▸ Unless high volumes of SF_6 are injected, the slow bubble expansion will not increase IOP
  - ▸ However, if a patient is breathing N_2O, the bubble will rapidly increase in size and ↑ IOP
  - ▸ N_2O should be stopped at least 15 minutes before the injection of air and should be avoided until at least 5 days after the injection of air and 10 days after the injection of SF_6
- *Systemic side effects of ophthalmic drugs:*

Drug	Mechanism of action	Effect
Acetylcholine	Cholinergic agonist (miosis)	Bronchospasm, bradycardia, hypotension
Acetazolamide	Carbonic anhydrase inhibitor (decreases IOP)	Diuresis, hypokalemic metabolic acidosis
Atropine	Anticholinergic (mydriasis)	Central anticholinergic syndrome
Cyclopentolate	Anticholinergic (mydriasis)	Disorientation, psychosis, convulsions
Echothiophate	Cholinesterase inhibitor (miosis, decreases IOP)	Prolongation of succinylcholine and mivacurium paralysis, bronchospasm
Epinephrine	Sympathetic agonist (mydriasis, decreases IOP)	Hypertension, bradycardia, tachycardia, headache
Phenylephrine	α-Adrenergic agonist (mydriasis, vasoconstriction)	Hypertension, tachycardia, dysrhythmias
Scopolamine	Anticholinergic (mydriasis, vasoconstriction)	Central anticholinergic syndrome
Timolol	β-Adrenergic blocking agent (decreases IOP)	Bradycardia, asthma, congestive heart failure

PREOPERATIVE

- The selection of premedication may vary depending on the patient population
  - ▶ Pediatric patients: usually have congenital abnormalities (Down, Goldenhar, rubella)
  - ▶ Adults: usually elderly, with multiple systemic illnesses (hypertension, diabetes, coronary artery disease)

MONITORING

- Patient's head away from anesthesiologist, making pulse oximetry and capnography very important
- ETT kinking, circuit disconnection, and unintentional extubation are more likely
- Kinking and obstruction can be minimized by using a preformed oral RAE ETT
- Increased likelihood of arrhythmias (oculocardiac reflex): pulse tone audible and constantly monitoring of the EKG
- On infants the body temperature usually rises because of head to toe draping and insignificant body exposure

INDUCTION

- The choice of induction technique usually depends more on the patient comorbidities than on the type of surgery planned
- Patients with a ruptured globe or having open eye surgery will benefit with controlled IOP and a smooth induction
  - ▶ Coughing should be avoided by having a deep level of anesthesia and adequate paralysis
  - ▶ The IOP response to laryngoscopy can be blunted with prior administration of lidocaine (1.5 mg/kg) or an opioid
  - ▶ Rocuronium is used rather than succinylcholine because of the latter's effect on IOP
  - ▶ Most patients with an open eye injury have a full stomach, so a rapid sequence intubation may be required

MAINTENANCE

- The pain and stress of these types of surgeries are usually less than with other types of surgeries
- The lack of cardiovascular stimulation and the need for an adequate level of anesthesia can result in hypotension in elderly individuals. This can be minimized with adequate intravenous hydration, small doses of ephedrine (2–5 mg), and the use of non-depolarizing muscle relaxants with awareness monitor, for a lighter level of anesthesia
- Intraoperative administration of intravenous metoclopramide (10 mg in adults) or a 5-HT3 antagonist (e.g., ondansetron 4 mg in adults 30 minutes before end of surgery) decreases the incidence of PONV
- Dexamethasone (4 mg in adults after induction) should also be given to patients with strong history of PONV

POSTOPERATIVE

- A smooth emergence is desirable to decrease the risk of wound dehiscence
- Coughing on emergence can be avoided by extubating the patient "deep", in stage 3:
  - ▶ As the end of the surgical procedure approaches, muscle relaxation is reversed and spontaneous respiration allowed to return
  - ▶ N_2O is discontinued and lidocaine (1.5 mg/kg) can be given to blunt the cough reflex temporarily
  - ▶ Extubation proceeds 1–2 minutes after lidocaine and during spontaneous respiration with 100% oxygen
  - ▶ Alternatively, the ETT can be exchanged for an LMA (Bailey maneuver)
  - ▶ Proper airway control is crucial until the patient's cough and swallowing reflexes return
  - ▶ This technique is not suitable for patients at increased risk of aspiration
- Small doses of intravenous narcotics are usually sufficient for pain control. Severe pain may signal intraocular hypertension, corneal abrasion, or other surgical complications

REGIONAL ANESTHESIA

- Retrobulbar blockade (see Figure 73-1):
  - ‣ Local anesthetic is injected behind the eye into the cone formed by the extra-ocular muscles
  - ‣ A blunt-tip 25-gauge needle penetrates the lower lid at the junction of the middle and lateral one third of the orbit
  - ‣ The patient is instructed to stare upward and medially as the needle is advanced 3.5 cm towards the apex of the muscle cone
  - ‣ After aspiration to exclude intravascular injection, 2–5 mL of local anesthetic is injected and the needle is removed. Firm pressure is then applied on the eye for 90–120 seconds to reduce the risk of hemorrhage
  - ‣ Local anesthetics could be: lidocaine 2% and bupivacaine or ropivacaine 0.75%. Addition of epinephrine (1:200,000 or 1:400,000) may reduce bleeding and prolong the anesthesia
  - ‣ Hyaluronidase, a hydrolyzer of connective tissue polysaccharides, is frequently added (3–7 IU/mL), to enhance the spread of the anesthetic
  - ‣ A successful block is accompanied by anesthesia, akinesia, and abolishment of the oculocephalic reflex
  - ‣ A facial nerve block is occasionally required to prevent blinking (Figure 73-2)
  - ‣ Complications: retrobulbar hemorrhage, globe perforation, optic nerve atrophy, flank convulsions, oculocardiac reflex, acute neurogenic pulmonary edema, trigeminal nerve block, and respiratory arrest
  - ‣ The postretrobulbar apnea syndrome is probably due to the injection of anesthetic into the optic nerve sheath, with spread into the CSF. The CNS is exposed to high concentrations of anesthetic and causes apprehension and unconsciousness. Apnea occur within 20 minutes and resolves within an hour. Treatment is supportive, with positive pressure ventilation to prevent hypoxia, bradycardia and cardiac arrest
  - ‣ Contraindications: bleeding disorders, extreme myopia (the longer globe increases the risk of perforation), or open eye injury (the pressure from injecting fluid behind the eye may cause extrusion of extraocular contents through the wound)

FIGURE 73-1. Retrobulbar block

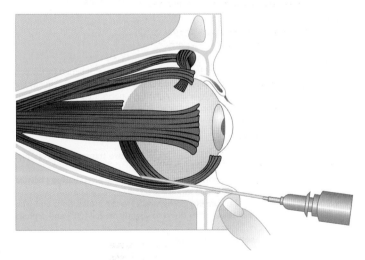

FIGURE 73-2. Techniques of facial nerve block

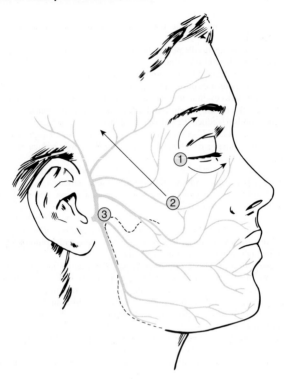

(1) van Lint, (2) Atkinson, and (3) O'Brien. Reproduced from Morgan GE, Mikhail MS, Murray MJ: *Clinical Anesthesiology*. 4th ed. Figure 38-2. Available at: www.accessmedicine.com. Copyright © The McGraw-Hill Companies, Inc. All rights reserved.

- Peribulbar blockade (see Figure 73-3):
  ‣ In contrast with the retrobulbar blockade, the needle does not penetrate the cone formed by the extraocular muscles. Both techniques achieve akinesia equally well
  ‣ Advantage of this block may include less risk of eye perforation, optic nerve and artery laceration, and less pain on injection
  ‣ Disadvantages include slower onset and an increase likelihood of ecchymosis
    ▪ The block is performed with the patient in the supine position and looking directly ahead
    ▪ After topical anesthesia of the conjunctiva, one or two transconjunctival injections are given
    ▪ As the eyelid is retracted, an infratemporal injection is given halfway between the lateral canthus and the lateral limbus
    ▪ The needle is advanced under the globe parallel to the orbital floor and when it passes the equator of the eye it is directed slightly medial (20°) and cephalad (10°)
    ▪ Five milliliters of anesthetic is injected

FIGURE 73-3. Peribulbar block

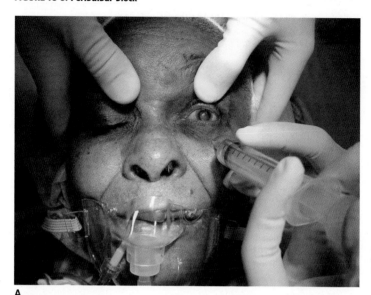

A

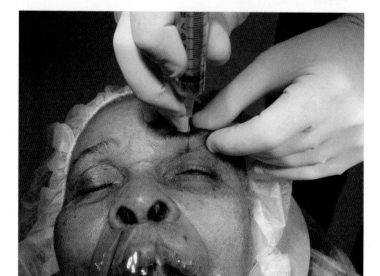

B

The classic technique of peribulbar anesthesia involves two injections. A: The first injection is inferior and temporal, the needle being introduced at the same site as for an RBA injection, but with a smaller "up-and-in" angle. B: The second injection is superior and nasal between the medial third and the lateral two thirds of the orbital roof edge. Reproduced from Hadzic A: *The New York School of Regional Anesthesia Textbook of Regional Anesthesia and Acute Pain Management*. Figure 21-4. Available at: www.accessanesthesiology.com. Copyright © The McGraw-Hill Companies, Inc. All rights reserved.

REFERENCES

For references, please visit **www.TheAnesthesiaGuide.com**.

CHAPTER 74
Endocrine Surgery

Brooke Albright, MD

THYROID

- **Hyperthyroidism**
  - Causes
    - Excess release of thyroid hormone as seen in Graves' disease, multinodular goiter, toxic adenoma, thyroiditis, pituitary thyrotropin (rare), iodine induced (amiodarone or angiographic contrast media), pregnancy induced
  - Signs and symptoms
    - Goiter
    - Sweating
    - Tachycardia, nervousness
    - Bowel or menstrual problems
    - Eye symptoms (ophthalmopathy)
    - Dermopathy
    - Skeletal muscle weakness
    - Vasodilation
    - Heat intolerance
  - Preoperative
    - Treat with anti-thyroid drugs, surgery, or radiation to reduce thyroid tissue
      - Propylthiouracil (PTU), methimazole, and carbimazole can be used to inhibit organification of iodide and synthesis of hormone
    - At least 6–8 weeks are required to regulate thyroid levels in most hyperthyroid patients
    - Optimal duration of anti-thyroid drug therapy for Graves' disease is 12–18 months with low dose therapy to prevent relapse
    - Beta-blockers should be used in all hyperthyroid patients to attenuate excessive sympathetic activity unless contraindicated. Goal is HR <90 bpm
      - Propranolol also impairs the peripheral conversion of T4 to T3 over 1–2 weeks
    - Potassium iodide can be used prior to surgery to reduce circulating thyroid hormone and cardiovascular symptoms
    - Glucocorticoids (dexamethasone 8–12 mg/day) can be used in severe thyrotoxicosis to reduce hormone secretion and peripheral conversion of T4 to T3
    - Thorough airway exam is necessary in anticipation of a difficult airway in those patients with goiters, especially substernal goiters. It may be necessary to perform an awake fiberoptic intubation or an inhalation induction
  - Intraoperative
    - All anti-thyroid medications should be continued through morning of surgery
    - General anesthesia with tracheal intubation and muscle relaxation is the most popular anaesthetic technique for thyroidectomy. A small reinforced tracheal tube may be needed if there is some degree of tracheal compression present
    - The incidence of temporary unilateral vocal cord paralysis resulting from damage to the recurrent laryngeal nerve (RLN) is 3–4%. Intraoperative

electro-physiological monitoring of the RLN can be done with the use of a tracheal tube with integrated EMG electrodes positioned at the level of the vocal cords. When the RLN has been identified, the nerve is stimulated until an EMG response is obtained
- Anesthetic goal is to keep patient deep enough to avoid exaggerated sympathetic response to surgical stimuli
  - Hyperthyroidism does NOT increase MAC requirements
- Avoid medications that may stimulate the nervous system, such as pancuronium and ketamine
  - Avoid histamine releasing drugs as well, such as atracurium and vancomycin
- Treat hypotension with direct-acting vasopressors, rather than those that indirectly release catecholamines
- May need to use reduced dose of muscle relaxant initially, and use a nerve stimulator to guide subsequent muscle relaxant doses
- Some surgeons perform thyroid surgery under MAC and cervical plexus block. Typically, a superficial cervical plexus block will be performed on the side with the smaller goiter or nodule, and both a deep and superficial cervical plexus block on the larger side. Avoid bilateral deep blocks, as this would block the phrenic nerve bilaterally
- Postoperative
  - Complications of thyroidectomy include recurrent laryngeal nerve damage, tracheal compression due to hematoma or tracheomalacia, and hypoparathyroidism
  - Iatrogenic hypoparathyroidism may result in hypocalcemia manifesting as laryngeal stridor progressing to laryngospasm within the first 24–96 hours post op
  - To assess recurrent laryngeal nerve damage, ask the patient to phonate before and after surgery by saying "ee". Bilateral recurrent laryngeal nerve damage causes aphonia and requires immediate reintubation. Unilateral damage causes hoarseness and is usually transient
- ALERT
  - **Thyroid storm:** Possible life-threatening exacerbation of hyperthyroidism. Manifestations include hyperthermia, tachycardia, dysrhythmias, MI, CHF, agitation, delirium, jaundice, abdominal pain, severe diarrhea, and coma. Treatment is largely supportive and includes large doses of PTU. It must be differentiated from malignant hyperthermia, pheochromocytoma, and light anesthesia
  - **Hyperthyroidism in pregnancy:** Increased risk of miscarriage, stillbirth, preterm birth, IUGR, severe pre-eclampsia, or placental abruption. Surgery usually not recommended. Avoid radioactive iodine treatment during pregnancy because it may destroy fetal thyroid resulting in permanent hypothyroidism in newborn. PTU was the drug of choice in pregnancy, as it is associated with fewer teratogenic effects than methimazole; however, with an increase in reports of liver damage in people taking PTU, some women may be treated with PTU in 1st trimester and then changed to methimazole

- **Hypothyroidism**
  - Causes
    - Primary: decreased production of thyroid hormone (i.e., Hashimoto's thyroiditis, autoimmune, radioablative, surgical, or idiopathic)
    - Secondary: hypothalamic or pituitary disease
  - Signs and symptoms: (See Table 74-1)
  - Preoperative
    - Treatment with L-Thyroxine (Levothyroxine, Synthroid)—onset is 6–12 hours, peak effect 10–12 days, half-life 7.5 days
    - Avoid premedication in patients with lethargy
    - Check lab work for electrolyte abnormalities
  - Intraoperative
    - Increased sensitivity to myocardial depressant effects of inhaled anesthetics, may require A-line placement

- Patients may have depressed ventilatory responsiveness to hypoxia and hypercapnia
- In patients with symptoms of skeletal muscle weakness, prolonged neuromuscular blockade is possible. Most NMB are acceptable at reduced doses. Guide dosing with a nerve stimulator
- Propensity for hypothermia: maintain active warming of patient intraop
- Possibility of decreased hepatic metabolism and renal elimination of drugs
- ▸ Postoperative
  - In patients with severe hypothyroidism, anticipate prolonged post op ventilation secondary to delayed emergence or depressed ventilation due to respiratory muscle weakness (hypothyroid myopathy), and impaired response to hypercarbia
- ▸ ALERT
  - **Myxedema Coma:** Rare severe form of hypothyroidism with 50% mortality rate characterized by delirium, unconsciousness, hypoventilation, hypothermia (cardinal feature, 80% of patients), bradycardia, hypotension, severe dilutional hyponatremia. Treatment is IV thyroxine

PARATHYROID

- **Hyperparathyroidism**
  - ▸ Causes
    - Primary: multiple endocrine neoplasia (MEN) type 1 or 2A, adenoma, carcinoma
    - Secondary: renal failure or pituitary adenoma
  - ▸ Signs and Symptoms
    - Reflect increased calcium such as skeletal muscle weakness, fatigue, anorexia, mental impairment, depression, GI upset, dehydration, nephrolithiasis, bone disease, cardiovascular disease
  - ▸ Preoperative
    - Preoperative imaging with high-quality sestamibi scans and/or ultrasound of the parathyroid gland is extremely important in guiding the surgeon's decision to perform a minimally invasive parathyroidectomy (MIP) or a complete bilateral neck exploration (BNE). For MIP, only the single dysfunctional gland is removed and the rest is left behind. Alternatively, some surgeons prefer BNE surgery, where all four parathyroid glands are explored, and macroscopically enlarged glands are excised
      - ◆ Exclusion criteria for minimally invasive parathyroidectomy includes large tumors, associated thyroid disease, suspicion of carcinoma, lithium treatment, chronic renal failure, and previous neck surgery
    - Obtain baseline EKG, compare with previous EKG for any changes
    - Correct electrolyte disturbances
    - Obtain baseline parathyroid hormone level, preferably on the day of surgery prior to administration of anesthetic
    - Document presence or absence of hoarseness preoperatively to eliminate confusion postoperatively when the integrity of the recurrent laryngeal nerve is evaluated
    - Patients presenting for surgery for secondary causes of hyperparathyroidism may present with significant cardiovascular and renal comorbidities requiring medical optimization and clearance
      - ◆ Active vitamin D therapy (calcitriol, paricalcitol) and phosphate binders may be used to suppress PTH levels preoperatively
  - ▸ Intraoperative
    - Regional anesthesia with a superficial cervical plexus block plus MAC sedation is the mainstay of anesthesia for MIP. Confirm with the surgeon that the patient is a candidate for a minimally invasive surgical approach before discussing the anesthetic plan with the patient

- One study reports patients under regional anesthesia were more likely to experience better energy levels and return to work earlier than those patients who received general anesthesia
  - Another advantage to regional with MAC is assessment of voice quality to confirm integrity of the recurrent laryngeal nerves
- For those in whom MIP is not possible or in those patients who cannot tolerate MAC with regional, general anesthesia with an LMA is a reliable alternative. It is best to avoid muscle paralysis in those patients since dosing can be unpredictable, the surgeries are usually short, and recurrent laryngeal nerve damage can be difficult to differentiate from residual muscle paralysis postoperatively
- For parathyroid cases, the surgical field is very close to the face and it is possible for high concentrations of oxygen to accumulate under the drapes. Because of oxygen's greater density compared to room air, it typically concentrates in the most dependent areas, usually along the patient's neck, closest to where the surgeon is using electrocautery. To avoid serious airway fires, low oxygen flows are preferred, and high flows of air circulating along the patients face may prevent build up of oxygen to dangerous levels
- Rapid intraoperative PTH assay after excision of the parathyroid adenoma should demonstrate exponentially decreased levels of parathyroid hormones in patients with adequate resection and cure of primary hyperparathyroidism. These blood samples should be obtained at time 0 (excision of gland), 5 minutes, 10 minutes, 15 minutes, and occasionally at 20 minutes according to the surgeon's discretion. If the levels of PTH remain elevated and fail to decrease exponentially, then re-exploration of the remaining parathyroid glands or alternative diagnoses should be considered
  - Because most patients are positioned for this surgery with their arms padded and tucked at their sides, obtaining frequent blood samples can be a challenge. The most reliable method for obtaining the samples is via an IV line placed in the antecubital vein. All samples can be drawn from this IV and save the patient from additional needle sticks, as well as the need for position changes intraop. Care should be taken to avoid diluting the sample with IV fluid and medications by discarding the first 10 mL of blood, as well as to avoid hemolysis by drawing on the IV line gently
  - Propofol was originally believed to interfere with PTH assay and in the past was avoided. However, recent randomized prospective trials suggest propofol sedation may be used
- Postoperative
  - Most studies show a decrease in hospital stay in patients undergoing MIP versus BNE. The majority of MIP patients are discharged home the same day or within 23 hours
  - Postoperative nausea and vomiting should be prevented with adequate prophylaxis if high dose alfentanil or other short acting opioids are used for MAC sedation. Some anesthesiologists advocate using at least 2–3 lines of prophylaxis (i.e., metoclopramide, ondansetron, and dimenhydrinate)
  - Assess integrity of recurrent laryngeal nerve by asking the patient to say "ee"
  - Most surgeons advocate the prophylactic administration of calcium carbonate in the immediate post op period to prevent hypocalcemia. If hypocalcemia is severe, vitamin D is added
- **Hypoparathyroidism**
  - Causes
    - Iatrogenic (inadvertent removal during thyroidectomy, neck surgery, or complication from radiation), idiopathic, or congenital (DiGeorge syndrome, autoimmune polyglandular failure syndrome, Ca^+-sensing receptor defect)
  - Signs and Symptoms
    - Reflect decreased calcium reabsorption by the kidneys and abnormalities in mineral metabolism including hypocalcemia, hyperphosphatemia, and hypomagnesemia. Clinical manifestations include neuromuscular irritability,

numbness, tetany (carpopedal spasm), laryngospasm, bone pain, fatigue, arthralgias, muscle cramping, osteoporosis, seizures, bradycardia, hypotension, and prolonged QT interval. Chronic hypercalciuria can lead to impairment of renal function, nephrocalcinosis, and renal insufficiency

▸ Preoperative
  ▪ Management of the disease includes replacement of mineral deficiencies, and recently, replacement of parathyroid hormone. Patients must be monitored for overtreatment as well, since hypercalciuria can lead to nephrocalcinosis and permanent renal damage
    • The only FDA approved treatment at this time is vitamin D analogs. Synthetic human PTH has recently been FDA approved for treatment of severe osteoporosis and is currently being used off-label for treatment of refractory hypoparathyroidism
  ▪ Laboratory studies should include calcium, phosphate, and magnesium – any disturbances should be corrected. Creatinine levels should be drawn to assess baseline kidney function as well
▸ Intraoperative
  ▪ Surgery for treatment of hypoparathyroidism is rare. However recently, allotransplantation of parathyroid fragments has become more popular again with the advent of transplant tissue devoid of immunogenic antigens, eliminating the need for immunosuppression
    • Allotransplantation is performed under local anesthesia with a tiny incision in the skin and subcutaneous tissue of the nondominant forearm. The arm is chosen for ease of monitoring transplant function and for the available well-developed vascular network
  ▪ Prolonged response to NMB, so conservative dosing is recommended
▸ Postoperative
  ▪ Patients s/p total thyroidectomy surgeries are at high risk of transient or prolonged hypocalcemia due to the inadvertent removal of the parathyroid glands intraop. Studies have shown that low levels of parathyroid hormone levels (PTH) can predict impending hypocalcemia. Some ENT surgeons believe Ca^+/Vitamin D supplementation should be given routinely postoperatively, while others believe a PTH level < 15 mg/dL should be treated with calcium, and the rest watch trends of calcium levels

PITUITARY

• Causes
  ▸ Pituitary adenoma, craniopharyngioma, result of bilateral adrenalectomy with inadequate negative feedback (Nelson's syndrome)
• Signs and Symptoms
  ▸ Clinical presentation is dependent upon whether the tumor is hormone secreting or not
    ▪ Non-secreting tumors present with problems of mass effect including visual changes (i.e., bitemporal hemianopsia) and headaches. They may also present with features of hypopituitarism (i.e., skin changes, loss of body hair, impotence, infertility, amenorrhea, hypothyroidism, and hypoadrenalism)
    ▪ Secreting tumors include:
      • **Growth Hormone (GH) secreting (acromegaly)**—hypertrophy of facial bones, soft palate, epiglottis, and turbinates. Soft tissue thickening of nose, tongue, and lips. Hoarseness should raise suspicion of possible laryngeal stenosis, vocal cord fixation, or recurrent laryngeal nerve palsy. Chronic acromegaly may result in severe CHF, overt DM, and renal insufficiency
      • **Adrenocorticotrophic Hormone (ACTH) secreting (Cushing's)**—HTN, ischemic heart disease, LVH, asymmetric septal hypertrophy, sodium and water retention, DM, thin skin, easy bruising, weakness and pain of pelvic girdle muscles, hypokalemia, severe osteoporosis
      • **Thyroid-stimulating Hormone (TSH) secreting**—symptoms of hyperthyroidism (see hyperthyroidism 'Signs and Symptoms' above)

- Preoperative
  - Preoperative blood work should include glucose, renal function tests, electrolytes including potassium, calcium, and sodium levels
  - Endocrine consult regarding function of the anterior pituitary, hormone activity of the lesion, and in cases of hypopituitarism, optimization of replacement therapy
    - In GH secreting tumors, it is advised to treat preoperatively with the somatostatin analogue octreotide (see chapter 75)—this may reverse some of the laryngeal changes, improve sleep apnea, and avoid the need for preop tracheostomy and post op respiratory depression. Furthermore, treatment with octreotide preoperatively may improve cardiac function in those with severe acromegaly-induced CHF
    - In ACTH and TSH secreting tumors, preoperative cortisol replacement may be needed for the stress response to surgery, as well as to suppress the release of hormone and help control signs and symptoms
    - In TSH secreting tumors, preoperative beta-blockers (propranolol) and anti-thyroid drugs may be needed
  - Ophthalmology consults in all patients with tumors extending into the suprasellar region for perimetric examination and testing of visual acuity
  - Prolactin level should be checked to rule out prolactinoma, which if diagnosed, should be medically managed with dopamine agonists instead of surgery
    - Prolactin, follicle-stimulating hormone (FSH), and luteinizing hormone (LH) secreting hormones do not seem to be associated with medical syndromes necessitating anesthetic consideration
  - Some institutions recommend preop medication with glycopyrrolate to help decrease secretions of the nasopharynx
  - Patients should be made aware of the post op placement of nasal packing and need to breathe through the mouth to avoid possible distress in the recovery period
- Intraoperative
  - 90% of pituitary tumors are resected via the transsphenoidal approach. The remaining 10% of tumors requiring transcranial resection are usually larger, have a less favorable prognosis, and higher complication rate
  - In GH secreting tumors, anticipate a difficult airway. In selected cases, an awake preoperative tracheostomy should be performed
  - In TSH secreting tumors, have a high suspicion for thyroid storm
  - After intubation of the trachea, it is customary to pack the oropharynx in order to absorb blood from the nasopharynx and prevent it from entering the trachea and esophagus
  - A-line placement for beat-to-beat blood pressure monitoring as well as blood draws is essential
  - Nitrous oxide should be avoided, especially if patients are placed in the semi-sitting position, because of the risk of venous air embolism
  - Anesthetic requirements for endoscopic endonasal transsphenoidal hypophysectomy include:
    - Hemodynamic stability
      - Be prepared to treat hypertension upon nasal infiltration of vasoconstrictors, and emergence
      - Aggressive control of painful stimuli is necessary to avoid sudden increases in blood pressure, particularly when the surgeon approaches the sellar floor through sphenoid sinus—short acting opioids (i.e., remifentanil) are recommended to prevent delayed emergence
    - Facilitation of surgical exposure
      - Excellent control of arterial pressure to limit bleeding is required due to the small and narrow operative field—even the smallest amounts of bleeding can complicate excision of the pituitary adenoma
      - To minimize potential bleeding from nasal mucosa, cocaine or lidocaine with epinephrine is usually infiltrated prior to insertion of surgical instruments through the nasal passage

- For tumors with significant suprasellar extension, a lumbar CSF drain can be placed to allow injection of 20–30 mL 0.9% saline, so as to raise the diaphragma sellae down toward the sphenoid sinus and facilitate more complete resection
  - Smooth and prompt emergence for neurologic assessment
    - The procedure is usually short so careful titration of neuromuscular blockade and opioids is essential
    - Patients should be fully awake upon extubation to prevent airway compromise due to nasal packing
  - Raised intracranial pressure is usually not a concern in transsphenoidal hypophysectomies, but can be a concern in transcranial resections if the tumor size is large and causing mass effect
  - Immediately prior to extubation, packing from the oropharynx should be removed and the oro-nasopharynx meticulously suctioned to avoid aspiration of blood
- Postoperative
  - Risk of potential airway difficulty due to nasal packing
    - Avoid excess opioids and assure adequate neuromuscular blockade reversal to prevent post op respiratory depression
  - Positive pressure ventilation in these patients post op should be avoided, as there is a risk of tension pneumocephalus, venous air embolism, and introduction of bacteria in the subarachnoid space
  - Postoperative check of visual acuity and visual fields, which may or may not normalize or improve after tumor resection
  - Possibility of new post op hormonal dysfunction or persistence of pituitary deficiency
    - Diabetes insipidus (DI) as a result of manipulation of pituitary stalk or hypothalamus is more common in transcranial surgery than following transsphenoidal
    - Inappropriate secretion of ADH leading to hyponatremia most commonly occurs a few days after the procedure
  - Injury to hypothalamus due to disruption of blood supply or direct surgical injury may manifest postoperative as DI, body temperature dysregulation, progressive obesity, loss of memory functions, and disruption of circadian sleep rhythms
  - CSF leak (seen as rhinorrhea) can be treated by placement of lumbar CSF drain to promote resolution of the leak
  - After resection, the patient will most likely be maintained on glucocorticoid and thyroxine replacements, both of which would need to be given in the perioperative period if the patient returned for subsequent surgeries. Since the posterior pituitary is usually spared, replacement of vasopressin or oxytocin in the future is not required
  - ALERT:
    - Pituitary apoplexy is an acute onset of hypopituitarism because of bleeding into the tumor or infarction. It is considered a surgical emergency, as it can lead to blindness, cranial nerve palsies, and increased intracranial pressure

PEARLS

- Three commonly used drugs to decrease peripheral conversion of T4-T3 in hyperthyroidism are PTU, propranolol, and glucocorticoids
- Hyperthyroidism does NOT increase MAC requirements
- Thyroid storm is a life-threatening exacerbation of hyperthyroidism. Treatment is supportive and includes large doses of PTU
- Myxedema coma is a rare severe form of hypothyroidism with 50% mortality rate. Treatment is IV thyroxine
- Anticipate a difficult airway in certain patients presenting for endocrine surgery (i.e., goiters, acromegaly)

- With advancements in imaging technology and the ability to localize parathyroid adenomas or dysfunctional parathyroid tissue, more selective and less invasive surgeries are being performed
- Before deciding on MAC with regional anesthesia as the final anesthetic plan for parathyroidectomies, it is important to confirm with the surgeon that the patient is a candidate for a minimally invasive surgical approach
- Prevent airway fires in parathyroidectomy surgeries by utilizing low oxygen gas flow, circulation of room air around the patients head and neck to avoid build up of oxygen under the drapes, and avoidance of nitrous oxide use
- Pituitary apoplexy is considered a surgical emergency, as it can lead to blindness, cranial nerve palsies, and increased intracranial pressure
- Replacement of glucocorticoids and thyroxine may be necessary in the perioperative periods in those patients s/p resection of the anterior pituitary

TABLE 74-1 Signs and Symptoms of Hypothyroidism

Mild	Moderate	Severe
• Fatigue	• Lethargy, apathy, listlessness	• Hypothyroid cardiomyopathy with decreased SV and contractility
• Weight gain	• Slowed speech, dulled intellect	
• Dry thickened skin	• Cold intolerance	
• Brittle hair	• Constipation	• Increased ventricular dysrhythmias
• Deep hoarse voice	• Menorrhagia	
• Large tongue	• Slowed motor function	• Increased SVR, decreased blood volume, pericardial and pleural effusions, decreased breathing and DLCO capacity
• Coarse facial features	• Periorbital and nonpitting edema	
	• Flattened T waves and low amplitude P waves/QRS complexes on ECG (from accumulation of cholesterol rich pericardial fluid around the heart)	
	• Bradycardia	

REFERENCES

For references, please visit **www.TheAnesthesiaGuide.com**.

CHAPTER 75
Carcinoid Tumor, Somatostatin and Octreotide

Ruchir Gupta, MD and Arthur Atchabahian, MD

PHYSIOPATHOLOGY

Abnormal secretion of vasoactive substances (i.e., histamine, kallikrein, serotonin) by carcinoid tumor.

Most common localization of tumor: small bowel, stomach, and ovaries.

Effects of Secreted Hormones			
	Serotonin	Kallikrein	Histamine
Clinical manifestation	Coronary artery spasm, HTN, diarrhea	Hypotension, flusing, bronchoconstriction	Vasodilation, bronchoconstriction, cardiac arrhythmias

PREOP

- Measurement of 5-hydroxyindoleacetic acid (5HIAA) is most commonly used to diagnose carcinoid
- Echocardiogram may help delineate the level of cardiac involvement (pulmonic stenosis and TR most common)
- If diarrhea, possible hypokalemia
- Octreotide 100 mcg SQ tid in the preceding 2 weeks; increase dose if needed until symptoms disappear, up to 500 mcg tid
- Monitor LFTs and blood glucose
- Patients on octreotide should continue their dose on the morning of surgery
- Anxiolysis with benzodiazepines should be given to prevent stress-induced release of serotonin
- H1 and H2 blockers should also be given (e.g., diphenhydramine 25 mg IV and ranitidine 50 mg IV)

ANESTHESIA

Monitors: A-line is useful because manipulation of the tumor can cause wide hemodynamic fluctuations.

CVL and PAC may also be helpful; consider TEE if altered cardiac function.

Induction: Etomidate or propofol can be used as long as hemodynamic stability is maintained. Succinylcholine should be avoided because of possible histamine release.

Intraoperative: All inhalation agents acceptable but desflurane may be preferable because of low hepatic metabolism in cases of liver metastasis of tumor.

Measure electrolytes frequently.

Volume expansion may be helpful with crystalloid or colloid.

Avoid drugs known to provoke release of mediators.
Octreotide 25–100 mcg should be used prior to tumor manipulation to attenuate hemodynamic effects.

Anesthetic Agents and Carcinoid	
Drugs provoking mediator release (Avoid)	Drugs not known to release mediators (Use)
Succinylcholine, mivacurium, atracurium, epinephrine, norepinephrine, dopamine, isoproterenol, thiopental, morphine	Propofol, etomidate, vecuronium, cisatracurium, rocuronium, sufentanil, alfentanil, fentanyl, remifentanil, volatile agents

Hypotension should be treated with volume expansion and octreotide and not with catecholamines/sympathomimetics.

Hypertension: deepen anesthesia, then IV esmolol.

POSTOP

ICU with invasive hemodynamic monitoring for 48–72 hours.

Taper octreotide over 3–4 days.

Pain control necessary to prevent stress-induced release of mediators; avoid morphine.

PEARLS AND TIPS

Carcinoid crisis can be precipitated by stress, tumor necrosis, or surgical stimulation, as well as from anesthetic drugs such as succinylcholine.

Octreotide infusion at 50–100 mcg/h can be given with boluses of 25–100 mcg for treatment of crisis.

SOMATOSTATIN AND OCTREOTIDE

Octreotide is a synthetic, long-acting analog of somatostatin, a naturally occurring hormone produced by δ cells of the pancreatic islet, cells of the GI tract, and in the CNS (pituitary). They inhibit a wide variety of endocrine and exocrine secretions, including TSH and GH from the pituitary, gastrin, motilin, VIP, glicentin, and insulin, glucagon, and pancreatic polypeptide from the pancreatic islet.

Octreotide is administered SQ tid. An extended release form of octretide, Sandostatin-LAR Depot®, is administered SQ only every 4 weeks.

Indications:
- Control of symptoms (diarrhea and flushing) in patients with metastatic carcinoid tumors
- Treatment of watery diarrhea associated with vasoactive intestinal peptide-secreting tumors (VIPomas)
- Treatment of acromegaly
- Variceal bleeding: reduction of portal BF and variceal pressures; mechanism poorly understood (off-label)
- Reduction of output from small bowel fistulas (off-label)
- Treatment of severe hypoglycemia related to sulfonylurea ingestion
- Prophylaxis and treatment of acute pancreatitis (off-label)
- "Dumping syndrome" seen in some patients after gastric surgery and pyloroplasty

Complications with long-term use:
- Gallbladder abnormalities (stones and biliary sludge)
- GI symptoms (diarrhea, nausea, and abdominal pain)
- Hypoglycemia or hyperglycemia
- Hypothyroidism and goiter

Somatostatin Versus Octeotride	
Somatostatin	Octreotide (Sandostatin®, 0.05 mg/mL)
Half life: 3–6 min	Serum half life: 1–2 h Duration of action: 12 h
Typical dose: 100–250 mcg/h IV infusion	50–100 mcg SQ tid, up to 500 mcg tid
Variceal bleeding: 250 mcg/h IV × 3–5 days	IV infusion 50 mcg/h × 3–5 days

REFERENCES

For references, please visit **www.TheAnesthesiaGuide.com**.

CHAPTER 76
Pheochromocytoma

Neelima Myneni, MD

BASICS

- Tumors of the adrenal medulla that produce, secrete, and store catecholamines
- Norepinephrine is predominantly secreted along with small amounts of epinephrine, and occasionally dopamine
- Perioperative mortality has been reported to be as high as 45% from cardiovascular causes, and directly correlates with tumor size and degree of catecholamine secretion. With appropriate management, mortality is very low
- Surgical exploration is curative in 95% of cases, with reduction in mortality to 3%
- Rule of 10s: 10% are malignant, 10% are extra-adrenal, 10% are bilateral
- Occasionally associated with syndromes: MEN IIA, MEN IIB, von Hippel-Lindau disease, or in rare cases, Von Recklinghausen's disease, tuberous sclerosis, and Sturge-Weber syndrome
- Typical presentation is a young adult in 30s to 50s with sustained hypertension (or occasionally paroxysmal), tachycardia, palpitations, tremor, sweating, flushing, hyperglycemia (secondary to α-stimulated inhibition of insulin secretion)
- Cerebral vascular accidents and myocardial infarction are possible
- In patients with chest pain and dyspnea, catecholamine-induced cardiomyopathy should be ruled out. The cardiomyopathy may be reversible if the catecholamine stimulation is removed early before fibrosis has occurred
- Diagnosis: elevated plasma levels of free catecholamines and elevated urinary vanillylmandelic acid (VMA) levels along with CT findings
- MIBG (methyl-iodo-benzyl-guanidine) scan may be needed to locate tumor(s)

PREOPERATIVE CONSIDERATIONS

- Evaluate for signs of end-organ damage and optimize medical treatment to minimize risk
- Continue α-adrenergic blockade for at least 10 to 14 days before surgery
  ‣ Both noncompetitive blockers (phenoxybenzamine) and selective α1 blockers (prazosin) have been shown to be equally effective in controlling blood pressure
- Continue beta blocker therapy (usually used in patients with persistent tachycardia or dysrhythmias), but only with concurrent alpha blockade to avoid unopposed α-mediated vasoconstriction

- Optimization of medical management indicated by the following:
  - No in-hospital blood pressure higher than 165/90 for 48 hours before surgery
  - Presence of orthostatic hypotension but blood pressure on standing no lower than 80/45 (and typically stuffy nose because of vasodilation)
  - ECG free of ST-T changes
  - No more than one premature ventricular contraction present every 5 minutes
- Preoperative workup should include
  - TTE to evaluate LV function and relaxation
  - Labs: Na, K, and glucose
- Normalization of intravascular volume and return of hematocrit toward normal is also recommended

Brief List of Drugs to Prepare Besides Usual GA Setup		
Medication	Dilution	Infusion range
Nitroprusside	50 mg in 250 mL = 200 mcg/mL	0.5–10 mcg/kg/min
Nitroglycerin	50 mg in 250 mL = 200 mcg/mL	0.5–10 mcg/kg/min
Nicardipine	25 mg in 250 mL = 100mcg/mL	Start at 5mg/h Increase as needed by 2.5 mg/h increments up to 15 mg/h
Esmolol	2.5 g in 250 mL = 10 mcg/mL	5–200 mcg/kg/min
Phenylephrine	20 mg in 250 mL = 80 mcg/mL	0.2–1 mcg/kg/min
Norepinephrine	4 mg in 250 mL = 16 mcg/mL	0.2–20 mcg/min

- Have in room
  - Phentolamine (Bolus: 2–5 mg, Infusion: 1–30 mcg/kg/min)
  - Lidocaine (Bolus: 100 mg, usual concentration 20 mg/mL)
  - Amiodarone (Give 150 mg slowly over 10 minutes, usual concentration 50 mg/mL)

MONITORING

- Pre-induction arterial line
- Central venous line TLC (preferably above the diaphragm), in addition to at least 2 large-bore peripheral IVs
- Pulmonary artery catheter or TEE depending on patient's comorbidities
- BIS will help decide whether sudden HTN is due to the tumor or to light anesthesia
- Foley catheter

INDUCTION OF ANESTHESIA

- Consider placing a mid thoracic (T7-9) epidural for postoperative pain control if open approach. Do not load epidural with local anesthetics until after tumor removal because of risk of profound hypotension
- Use a potent sedative-hypnotic in combination with an opioid analgesic and an NMB without cardiovascular effect (e.g., etomidate + fentanyl + rocuronium)
- Ensure an adequate depth of anesthesia before laryngoscopy
- Aim to minimize hemodynamic swings during induction and laryngoscopy; a low-dose nitroprusside infusion can be initiated or alternatively one can have short-acting drugs such as nitroglycerin or esmolol, and phenylephrine available to bolus based on A-line readings
- Avoid histamine-releasing agents (e.g., morphine); Also avoid drugs that stimulate the sympathetic system (desflurane) or anticholinergics (e.g., succinylcholine, pancuronium)
- Use sevoflurane for maintenance

ANESTHETIC MANAGEMENT

- Balanced anesthesia with combination of opioid analgesic and an inhalation agent
  - ‣ Critical periods: induction, intubation, incision, insufflation, tumor manipulation
  - ‣ Tumor manipulation
    - Can cause acute hypertensive crises (ask surgeon to stop) that can be treated with infusions of nitroprusside or phentolamine. Nitroglycerin is less effective. Watch for tachycardia when administering vasodilators
    - Can cause dysrhythmias; control with lidocaine or amiodarone or alternatively an infusion of short-acting beta antagonist esmolol as long-acting agents can cause persistence of bradycardia and hypotension after tumor removal
  - ‣ Tumor removal
    - Ligation of venous supply results in abrupt reduction in blood pressure can be corrected with preemptive fluid administration. If PA catheter in place, aim for wedge pressure of 16–18 mm Hg prior to this stage
    - Treat as needed with phenylephrine or norepinephrine
    - If no drop in BP, consider incomplete excision or other tumor
    - Monitor for hypoglycemia; change IV fluids to dextrose-containing fluids to prevent hypoglycemia
- If procedure performed laparoscopically
  - ‣ Typically 30° reverse Trendelenburg, with possible blood pooling in lower extremities
  - ‣ Initiate pneumoperitoneum with low pressure (8–10 cm H_2O)

POSTOPERATIVE MANAGEMENT

- ICU for at least 24 hours
- CXR to r/o pneumothorax
- Most patients become normotensive after surgery
- Watch for
  - ‣ Hypertension (50% patients remain hypertensive for several days after surgery, 25% remain hypertensive indefinitely)
  - ‣ Hypotension (secondary to decreased plasma catechols, third-space fluid losses, prolonged effects of phenoxybenzamine); most frequent cause of death
  - ‣ Hypoglycemia

REFERENCES

For references, please visit **www.TheAnesthesiaGuide.com**.

CHAPTER 77
Laparoscopic Surgery

Jennifer Wu, MD, MBA

BASICS

- Advantages
  - Small incisions
  - Minimal disruption of abdominal musculature
  - Faster postoperative recovery
  - Faster return of ventilatory function
  - Less postoperative pain
- Common procedures
  - Appendectomy
  - Cholecystecomy
  - Nephrectomy
  - Prostatectomy
  - Many gynecologic and gastrointestinal procedures
- Can be safely performed on children and pregnant women. Care should be taken to avoid hypercarbia and acidosis

PREOPERATIVE

- Keep in mind possible conversion to open procedure
- Neuraxial analgesia usually not necessary
- Adequate preoperative hydration: hypovolemia during insufflation of carbon dioxide may result in hypotension
- Patients at risk for cardiac events (CHF, CAD) or poor respiratory tolerance (restrictive or obstructive syndrome) should be optimized, as laparoscopy causes hemodynamic changes, including reduced cardiac output and increased SBP
- Thromboprophylaxis similar to open procedure
- Contra-indications to laparoscopy
  - Emphysema with large bullae
  - Recurring pneumothorax
  - Patient with ASD or VSD
  - VP shunt, peritoneo-jugular shunt
  - Increased ICP, acute glaucoma
  - Diaphragmatic hernia

MONITORING

- General anesthesia with careful monitoring of ventilation and $EtCO_2$
  - As CO_2 from insufflation is systemically absorbed, $EtCO_2$ will rise and minute ventilation needs to increase accordingly (usually by increasing RR)
  - $EtCO_2$ should plateau after about 30 minutes. Significant increases after this time suggest subcutaneous emphysema
  - Increased intra-abdominal pressures and Trendelenburg position may cause a reduction in Vt delivered, particularly if pressure-controlled ventilation is used. Frequent adjustments in ventilator settings may be necessary to maintain adequate ventilation
  - Especially if pulmonary disease or CHF, the gradient between $PaCO_2$ and $PEtCO_2$ will increase
- Invasive blood pressure monitoring, and even PAC/TEE, may be required for patients at risk for cardiac events or those who may not tolerate the reduced cardiac output and increased systolic blood pressure caused by laparoscopy

INDUCTION

- Endotracheal intubation and muscle relaxation necessary
- Careful attention to positioning
  ▸ Steep Trendelenburg position may result in pressure on shoulders and neck
  ▸ Arms tucked at sides or adequately secured to padded arm boards
- Insert OGT to decompress stomach prior to trocar insertion
- High risk of PONV. Unless contraindicated, give 10 mg dexamethasone IV after induction, then an HT5-inhibitor (e.g., ondansetron 4 mg IV) 30 minutes before extubation

MAINTENANCE

- Careful attention to HR early in case, as insufflation can elicit a vagal response
  ▸ Ask the surgeon to release abdominal pressure
  ▸ If bradycardia does not resolve, administer 0.5–0.7 mg atropine IV
  ▸ Typically, reinflation will not cause bradycardia, or the response will be attenuated
- Maintain adequate level of general anesthesia and muscle relaxation
- Over the length of the case, heart rate and blood pressure rise secondary to neuro-humoral factors. These will decrease upon cessation of laparoscopy. Overaggressive treatment of hypertension and tachycardia may lead to hypotension following the removal of the trocars
- BIS/Entropy monitors help in ensuring adequate levels of anesthesia
- Changes in Vt, PAP, and EtCO$_2$ should be closely monitored. Ventilation may need to be altered based on the intra-abdominal pressure, Trendelenburg position, and systemic absorption of end tidal carbon dioxide. Aim for PEtCO$_2$ ≤ 38 mm Hg (unless chronic hypercarbia) and PAP ≤ 25 cmH$_2$O. Use PEEP 5 cmH$_2$O to prevent atelectasis
- Aggressive hypothermia prevention
- Complications:
  ▸ Endobronchial intubation as the diaphragm rises
    ▪ Reassess BS after insufflation and Trendelenburg, pull back ETT if needed
  ▸ Subcutaneous emphysema and/or pneumothorax
    ▪ Increased PAP, hypotension
    ▪ Tension pneumothorax possible: STAT needle exsufflation, then chest tube insertion
  ▸ Carbon dioxide air embolism
    ▪ Can happen at any time; most common during insufflation
    ▪ Subacute: rise of PEtCO$_2$, unresponsive to increased ventilation
    ▪ Acute: tachycardia, hypotension, up to cardiac arrest, decreased EtCO$_2$
    ▪ Treatment: exsufflation, supportive
  ▸ Cardiovascular collapse
    ▪ Large blood vessel laceration (especially iliac vessels)
    ▪ Conjunction of decreased venous return, increased SVR and preexisting cardiac disease
  ▸ Dysrhythmias
    ▪ Usually due to hypercapnia

POSTOPERATIVE

- Prior to extubation, the chest and neck should be examined for subcutaneous emphysema
- Long time periods in the Trendelenburg position or large fluid shifts may result in edema of the airway, precluding extubation
- Shoulder pain may be a result of diaphragmatic irritation by peritoneal gas. If not contraindicated, NSAIDs are effective
- Prophylactic antiemetics and adequate fluid hydration can reduce risk of PONV
- Respiratory function is better following laparoscopy compared to open procedures. However, postoperative atelectasis is present, particularly in obese patients. PEEP and alveolar recruitment maneuvers are useful to increase oxygenation postoperatively

- Need for adequate NMB until near completion of procedure. Ensure adequate reversal prior to extubation; if needed, transport to PACU intubated for delayed extubation

PEARLS AND TIPS

- Complications from CO_2 insufflation of the peritoneum include endobronchial intubation, subcutaneous emphysema, CO_2 embolism, and pneumothorax
- Insertion of trocars and operating equipment may cause injury to large blood vessels or retroperitoneal hematoma

REFERENCES

For references, please visit **www.TheAnesthesiaGuide.com**.

CHAPTER 78
Robotically Assisted Laparoscopic Prostatectomy

Nitin K. Sekhri, MD and Ervant Nishanian, PhD, MD

BASICS

- Robots allow surgeons unprecedented control and precision of surgical instruments in minimally invasive procedures
- Benefits
  - ‣ Less pain
  - ‣ Less trauma
  - ‣ Less blood loss (mean 150 mL vs. 1200 mL for open) and transfusion
  - ‣ Shorter hospital stays (1 vs. 3 days)
  - ‣ Quicker recovery
  - ‣ Improved cosmetic and functional (sexual function, incontinence) results (not conclusively demonstrated)

PREOPERATIVE

- Relative contraindications
  - ‣ Because of intraoperative cardiovascular changes (see below), a thorough cardiac evaluation must be done
  - ‣ CHF (must be optimized)
  - ‣ Valvular disease (may require repair or replacement prior to surgery)
  - ‣ Hemorrhage could be difficult to control intraoperatively, therefore, anticoagulation and antiplatelet therapy must be held
  - ‣ Prior abdominal surgery may increase duration of surgery due to adhesions
- Prolonged Trendelenburg position may be relative contraindication in patients with history of stroke or cerebral aneurysm
- Patients with elevated PA pressure may not tolerate the position well

INTRAOPERATIVE

- GA with ETT because of pneumoperitoneum and positioning
- Monitoring
  - ‣ Arterial line for blood sampling and beat-to-beat BP monitoring

- Maintenance
  - ▸ Patient is placed in steep Trendelenburg position
    - Reduction of FRC, increased atelectasis
    - Increased pulmonary blood content causes further decrease in FRC and pulmonary compliance
    - Increases CVP, ICP, IOP, myocardial work, and pulmonary venous pressure
    - Upward displacement of the trachea: ETT may migrate into a main-stem bronchus
  - ▸ Thighs spread far apart to allow docking of the robotic system
  - ▸ The patient's arms will be tucked at the side and the drapes will keep the patient far away from the reach of the anesthesiologist; position and pad with care (risk of nerve injury)
  - ▸ Peripheral nerve injury is relatively common (most frequent: median nerve palsy)
  - ▸ IVs, monitoring lines, and ETT have to be secured in such a way that they will not kink or pull out
  - ▸ When robot is docked over the patient, no way to move the patient or to initiate resuscitative measures without removing the robot (which can take several minutes)
  - ▸ In the hands of an experienced surgeon, a straightforward prostatectomy can be done in two and a half hours of operative time
  - ▸ Large bore intravenous line as potential for large blood loss
  - ▸ Insufflation of carbon dioxide for production of a pneumoperitoneum
    - Increases CVP, PAOP, and PA pressures, and decreases cardiac output
    - Coexisting cardiovascular disease can cause even more pronounced impairment of cardiac function, which may thrust a compensated heart failure into decompensation or a marginally perfused myocardium into an ischemic episode
    - Insufflation reduces blood flow to organs within the abdominal cavity by direct mechanical compression
    - Bradycardia possible, usually responds to atropine; exsufflate if persists
  - ▸ Hypercarbia
    - CO_2 highly diffusible into the bloodstream from the peritoneal cavity
    - Only rarely is the hypercarbia severe enough to cause arrhythmias or unmanageable hypertension that requires conversion to an open procedure
  - ▸ No difference between VCV and PCV, as long as CO_2 and Vt monitored
  - ▸ Venous gas embolism (can occur with open procedure as well)
    - Suspected when sudden cardiovascular collapse
    - Treatment
      - ◆ Discontinue insufflation
      - ◆ Cardiopulmonary resuscitation if necessary
      - ◆ Only return the patient to horizontal position once robot is unlocked for resuscitation
  - ▸ Blood loss
    - Typical blood loss is 150–250 mL
    - However, as with all robotic procedures, blood loss may be difficult to control

POSTOPERATIVE

- Typically, ambulation the same day or the next
- Patient discharged home with very little discomfort the day after surgery
- Small percentage of patients will stay hospitalized because of complications such as ileus that is short lived and self-limited
- Clinical swelling of the face, eyelids, conjunctivae, and tongue along with a plethoric color of venous stasis in the head and neck is a common observation
- If significant upper airway edema is suspected, it will be prudent to delay extubation until such time as the edema has subsided to a safe degree
- Subcutaneous emphysema is commonly seen
  - ▸ Extension into the thorax, causing pneumothorax and pneumomediastinum, could occur if high insufflation pressures are used, but is rarely a clinical concern

PEARLS AND TIPS

- Once prepped and draped, the anesthesiologist will have limited access to the patient
  ‣ ETT and lines must be secured
- ETT may migrate distally when moving the patient into steep Trendelenburg position
- During the procedure, following prostate removal, the bladder and urethra are unattached
  ‣ At this time, any urine output will empty into field, making urine output estimation difficult
  ‣ Causing increased urine output, either in the form of diuretics or overhydration, before the anastomosis of the urethra to the bladder, will impede surgeon visualization

REFERENCES

For references, please visit **www.TheAnesthesiaGuide.com**.

CHAPTER 79
Bariatric Surgery

Jamey J. Snell, MD

BASICS

- *Indications*: BMI 30–35 kg/m² if co-morbidities, or BMI >35 kg/m² if no co-morbidities, after having failed non-surgical therapy
- *Procedures*: Roux-en-Y gastric bypass, gastric banding, sleeve gastrectomy, partial gastrectomy, gastroplasty—vast majority performed laparoscopically unless patient too large
- Weight loss achieved by mechanical (restricted volume) and/or metabolic (malabsorption) mechanisms
- Know pathophysiologic and pharmacologic implications of obesity (see chapter 14)
- Be aware of the anesthesiologist's role in assisting bariatric surgery and be vigilant regarding monitors and instruments

PREOPERATIVE

- Pre-surgical testing
  ‣ Assess co-morbid conditions of obesity; further work-up as indicated
  ‣ Some institutions allow patient to bring and use own NIPPV device on day of surgery
- Pre-operative holding
  ‣ History
    ▪ Many patients w/ OSA are undiagnosed (see chapter 13)
    ▪ If patient uses CPAP at night, obtain settings and have available in PACU. Also have available if highly suspected but not diagnosed
    ▪ Ask about ability to breathe lying flat for induction considerations
    ▪ Ask about GERD symptoms
    ▪ Prior bariatric surgery warrants evaluation for nutritional deficiencies & electrolytes. Determine whether patient is on liquid diet and/or had bowel prep to anticipate hypovolemia

- ‣ Physical examination
  - ▪ Assess for potential difficulties w/ vascular access
  - ▪ Mallampati ≥ 3, increased neck circumference (>40–60 cm), BMI > 30 highest predictors of difficult intubation
  - ▪ Chest auscultation important to determine baseline lung sounds and to assess for pulmonary congestion
- ‣ Labs/Studies
  - ▪ Elevated hematocrit and elevated bicarbonate suggestive of chronic hypoxemia and respiratory acidosis from sleep disordered breathing
  - ▪ Review EKG and CXR for evidence of cardiomegaly, right heart overload from pulmonary hypertension, or LV dysfunction; Echo if needed. Daytime, awake ABG on room air with evidence of hypoxia and hypercarbia is suggestive of obesity-hypoventilation syndrome (OHS) in addition to OSA, with even greater risk for post-operative respiratory complications
  - ▪ Review data pertinent to co-morbidities
- ‣ Discuss plan with patient and surgery team as additional time frequently needed for induction
- Pre-medication
  - ‣ If awake or sedated intubation planned, begin airway topicalization 30 minutes prior and administer glycopyrrolate 0.4 mg IV, as an antisialagogue, 10 minutes prior to surgery
  - ‣ Clonidine (2 mcg/kg PO the night before, and 2 hours before induction) has been shown to reduce intraoperative anesthetic and analgesic requirements

MONITORING

- BP cuff can be placed at wrist on forearm if arm circumference too large to prevent overestimation of blood pressure (inflatable bladder portion should be 80% of limb circumference)
- Invasive monitors only if co-morbid conditions suggest intolerance of large fluid shifts, decreased pre-load, or hypercarbia
- Place CVL if unable to obtain adequate peripheral access; usually poor landmarks, use US guidance
- Neuromuscular monitoring indicated
  - ‣ Muscle relaxation required for pneumoperitoneum, via CO_2 insufflation, of a sufficient volume (~3 L) for operative visualization with intra-abdominal pressure limited to <15–18 mm Hg due to impedance of flow through the IVC
  - ‣ Frequent discrepancy between surgical assessments of relaxation versus NMB monitor
  - ‣ Apply electrodes to facial nerve rather than ulnar/PT (subcutaneous adipose tissue increases electrical resistance)
- Avoid esophageal stethoscope/temperature probes to prevent accidental incorporation into the stomach by sutures or stapler
- Orogastric tubes (OGT) may be removed after initial suctioning or left in if required to assist during initial part of surgery, however, these may be accidentally incorporated as well and should be partially withdrawn or removed if not in use
- Processed EEG monitors can reduce anesthetic doses and speed recovery

INDUCTION

- Positioning
  - ‣ HELP (head-elevated laryngoscopy position): DL optimal when ear same height as sternum and chin higher than chest
  - ‣ Place OR table in 25–30° reverse Trendelenburg
  - ‣ Ensure all pressure points are padded, including strap
  - ‣ Ensure sequential compression devices on lower extremities—high risk for DVTs. OR table should have foot supports to prevent patient from sliding in reverse Trendelenburg position

- Pre-oxygenation/De-nitrogenation
  - Use head strap to facilitate adequate seal during spontaneous and bag-mask ventilation
  - Close APL valve to 5–10 cm H_2O to keep upper airway patent
  - Low FRC:closing volume ratio → rapid hypoxia w/ apnea
- Induction for patients not suspected to be difficult to ventilate
  - Standard IV induction; administer induction agent and NMB simultaneously
    - Hypoxemia is rapid, ventilation is often more difficult than intubation
  - RSI (not indicated for all patients—consider if GERD, not anticipated to be difficult to intubate)
  - Have oral and nasal airways, and LMAs on hand
- Induction for patients suspected to be difficult to ventilation (large chest, OSA, intolerance of supine position, etc.); awake/sedated fiberoptic bronchoscope assisted intubation
  - Topicalize thoroughly
  - Slow titration of short-acting opioids preferable to benzodiazepines or propofol as the former agents suppress laryngeal reflexes along with mild sedation while the latter only induce sedation and can cause disinhibition; use as little sedation as is practical
  - Use caution if combining narcotics and benzodiazepines or propofol due to nonlinear dose-dependent apnea thresholds and CO_2 response suppression
  - Remifentanil and dexmedetomidine infusions, as well as small boluses of droperidol or haloperidol, have been successfully used while maintaining spontaneous ventilation
    - Apply nasal prongs or a nasal airway to deliver O_2 while securing airway
- Intubation for patients not suspected to be difficult to intubate
  - Standard laryngoscopy (have straight blade on hand as back-up as excessive soft-tissue can create a floppy epiglottis)
  - Have a secondary method readily available
- Intubation for patients suspected to be difficult to intubate
  - Video or mirrored laryngoscope
  - Flexible fiberoptic bronchoscope w/ oral airway or laryngeal mask airway (oral or nasal approach)
  - Laryngoscope-assisted fiberoptic devices (rigid support facilitates anterior displacement of redundant soft tissue)
  - Intubating laryngeal mask airway

MAINTENANCE

- Anesthetics/Medications
  - GETA for laparoscopic procedures (majority), combined w/ neuraxial for postoperative pain and reduced anesthetic/analgesic requirements for laparotomy (rare)
  - No proven difference between volatile anesthetic agents; typically desflurane or sevoflurane
  - Avoid prolonged N_2O to prevent diffusion into abdominal or other air spaces
  - Utilize adjuncts intraoperative (ketorolac 30–60 mg IM/IV, acetaminophen 1 g IV, dexmedetomidine 0.2 mcg/kg/h) to minimize opioid requirements, if no contraindications
  - Re-dose NMB only if surgically indicated and TOF >2; minimal improvement in muscle relaxation w/with TOF <2, with risk of extubation issues
  - Know which drug dosages are based on TBW versus IBW (see chapter 14)
  - Cefazolin 2 g IV and heparin 5000 units SQ prior to incision if no contraindications
- Cardiovascular
  - *Hypotension:* Intra-abdominal insufflation and steep reverse Trendelenburg positioning both reduce pre-load and can cause hypotension. Treat with a limited volume of intravenous fluid then with short-acting vasopressors; avoid volume overload

- Respiratory
  ▸ *Ventilation modes*
    - Increased intra-abdominal pressure + heavy chest wall = restrictive physiology → reduced lung compliance → high airway pressures during mechanical ventilation
    - Volume-control (TV 8–12 mL/kg IBW) more convenient than pressure-control since consistent minute ventilation is achieved despite changes in compliance throughout case, preventing hypoventilation or volutrauma
  ▸ *Elevated airway pressures*
    - Tolerate up to 30 cm H_2O + intra-abdominal pressure
    - Barotrauma is a risk only with elevated trans-pulmonary pressures, not elevated plateau pressures alone ($P_{trans\text{-}pulmonary} = P_{alveolar} - P_{pleural}$; $P_{pleural} \approx Pi_{intra\text{-}abdominal}$)
  ▸ *Hypercarbia*
    - Increased RR required to maintain normal $EtCO_2$ due to CO_2 insufflation
    - High RR shorten exhalation times ⇒ breath-stacking → hypotension, hypoxemia, and paradoxical increase in CO_2
    - If suspected, prolong expiratory time (I:E 1:3 or 4) and/or reduce RR
  ▸ *Hypoxemia*
    - Treat hypoxemia by increasing FiO_2, utilizing PEEP (5-15 cm H_2O), and periodic recruitment maneuvers (maintain 40 cm H_2O for 8 seconds), keeping in mind that the latter options can increase intrathoracic pressure and decrease preload
    - Consider FOB to rule out mainstem intubation secondary to cephalad displacement of the diaphragm if refractory hypoxemia occurs after insufflation
- Renal
  ▸ *Oliguria/ATN*
    - Increased intra-abdominal pressure can impede flow through renal vessels and impair glomerular/tubular function → monitor urine output closely
- Surgical assistance (if requested for partial gastrectomy/bypass surgery)
  ▸ *Early*: advancement of the OGT to facilitate grasping of the stomach
  ▸ *Mid-case*: advancement of trans-oral metal anvil to facilitate creation of the gastric pouch. Use caution to avoid damage to teeth, pharynx, and esophagus
  ▸ *End*: Add 5 mL of 1% methylene blue to a 500 mL bottle of sterile water or normal saline and pour into a basin. Use 60 mL bulb syringe to flush in 100 mL of fluid through orogastric tube. Apply suction, then remove tube when no leaks are seen by surgeons at anastomosis

POSTOPERATIVE

- Extubation
  ▸ Reverse all non-depolarizing NMB. Even TOF of 4/4 may have up to 70–75% of receptors blocked by NMB. Administer only if TOF ≥2. Base dose (e.g., neostigmine 40–70 mcg/kg) on number of twitches/fade to prevent paradoxical weakness from overdosing
  ▸ Position in reverse Trendelenburg or back-up
  ▸ Use strict extubation criteria (fully awake, follows commands, 5-seconds head lift, TVs regular and equal to baseline or >6 mL/kg, vital capacity >10 mL/kg)
  ▸ Discriminate between vital capacity breaths (sporadic) and tidal volumes (regular) as mistaking the former for the latter will overestimate respiratory function/strength
  ▸ Use recruitment maneuvers and positive pressure prior to and during removal of tube
- PACU
  ▸ Call ahead for ventilator on stand-by if patient given NMB toward end of case or no twitches
  ▸ NIPPV
    - Call ahead for CPAP setup if prior diagnosis or if clinical suspicion of OSA. Initial settings of 10 cm H_2O, 50% FiO_2 if unknown. Adjust according to ABG
    - Bi-level PAP equally as effective. Initial settings of 10-12/4-5 cm H_2O, 50% FiO_2
    - Useful even for obese patients without OSA

- No evidence of negative outcomes on surgical anastomosis
  - Carefully dosed opioid IV PCA shown to be safe and effective
  - Admit patients with history of severe OSA for overnight observation
- ‣ Prolonged insufflation with CO_2 (>4 hours) carries a risk for subcutaneous, submucosal, and mediastinal emphysema
  - Implications include decreased upper airway diameter, delayed extubation, possible re-accumulation of CO_2 causing sedation, narcosis, and re-intubation in the PACU, and hemodynamic compromise
  - Assess periodically intraoperatively and postoperatively by pressing on skin in supraclavicular fossa for crackling, and perform an ETT leak test prior to extubation
- ‣ Position patient sitting up/reclined or lateral decubitus and encourage incentive spirometry to prevent atelectasis and pneumonia
- ‣ Be aware of other complications: anastomosis leak, gas embolism, thromboembolism, PONV (do not place NGT, call surgery), GI bleeding, pneumothorax, etc

PEARLS AND TIPS

- Communication with surgeon is key to preventing instrument-related complications. Document "removed with tip intact" for all orally inserted tubes for medicolegal protection
- Compromise between anesthesiologists and surgeons is required with regard to limitations on insufflation pressure or duration, degree of reverse Trendelenburg, or re-dosing of muscle relaxants
- If additional muscle relaxation requested toward end of the case, consider increasing volatile agent or administer 3–5mL of propofol (if BP allows) instead
- Airway-related complications occur more frequently in this patient population but are usually preventable. Avoid by having a well thought out plan, discuss with the patient and inform the surgical team, and have a LMA and secondary method for intubation readily available
- For any patient with potentially difficult intubation/ventilation, having another anesthesiologist in the room for intubation and extubation can be greatly beneficial
- Difficult intubation = difficult extubation. Have the same airway equipment used to secure the airway in the room for extubation. Inform the PACU team

REFERENCES

For references, please visit **www.TheAnesthesiaGuide.com**.

CHAPTER 80
Renal Transplant

Brooke Albright, MD

BASICS

- 5 stages of renal failure

Stage	Description	GFR (mL/min/1.73 m²)
1	Kidney damage with normal or increased GFR	≥90
2	Kidney damage with mild decrease in GFR	60–89
3	Moderate decrease in GFR	30–59
4	Severe decrease in GFR	15–29
5	Kidney failure	<15 (or HD)

- ▸ Most common causes of ESRD: DM, glomerulonephritis, polycystic kidney disease, and systemic HTN
- Renal blood flow: 3–5 mL/min/gm in normal tissue
  - ▸ If RBF <0.5 mL/min/gm, renal cells become ischemic and drug elimination is slowed
- Survival rate of patients after renal transplantation depends on the source of the donor kidney
  - ▸ Kidneys from a living donor seem to do better at 1 and 5 years post-transplantation compared to kidneys from a cadaver
- Common causes of morbidity and mortality in renal transplant recipients include hypertension (75%), coronary artery disease (15–30%), sepsis (27%), diabetes (16–19%), neoplasm (13%), and stroke (8%)
  - ▸ During the first year post-transplantation, most deaths are due to infectious causes

PREOPERATIVE

- Living related donor (LRD):
  - ▸ Need good bilateral renal function without h/o of diabetes, neoplasia, nor severe HTN
  - ▸ Similar HLA and ABO blood group antigens to kidney recipient
  - ▸ Start maintenance IV fluids (IVF) evening before surgery and double the rate 3–5 hours before surgery for adequate hydration
- Recipient:
  - ▸ Blood pressure control – most ESRD patients have HTN – if they present hypotensive, suspect profound extracellular volume depletion. Ideally, after HD, patients should be 2–4 kg above their dry weight
    - Antihypertensive meds: alpha blockers, such as clonidine and prazosin, can prove very useful, as well as nitroprusside and IV labetalol for acute HTN
  - ▸ Electrolyte disturbances: hyperkalemia, hypermagnesium, etc
  - ▸ GI disturbances: delayed gastric emptying, gastroparesis, N/V, GI bleeding, hiccups
  - ▸ Hematologic disturbances: anemia, platelet dysfunction, and thrombocytopenia
  - ▸ Cardiac disturbances: LVH, CHF, LV dysfunction, CAD, cardiac conduction abnormalities, and pericarditis associated with uremia

- Uremic pericarditis responds to dialysis and rarely leads to tamponade. Dialysis pericarditis is associated with pain, fever, and leukocytosis, and tamponade is more likely
- Assess airway
  - Difficult intubation more common in long term type 2 DM due to diabetic stiff joint syndrome, which is characterized by a short stature, joint rigidity, and tight waxy skin. This can be seen clinically by asking the patient to approximate their palms – if they cannot bend their fingers backwards ("prayer sign") then they may be at risk for difficult intubation
- Be aware of immunosuppressive treatment; some immunosuppressive drugs interact with anesthesia drugs (e.g., cyclosporine)
  - Calcium channel blockers and certain antibiotics (e.g., erythromycin, doxycline, ketoconazole) increase levels of cyclosporine and can lead to nephrotoxicity. Other drugs, including certain antibiotics (nafcillin, isoniazid) and anticonvulsants (e.g., phenytoin, phenobarbital), decrease levels of cyclosporine and predispose the patient to infection

MONITORING

- In addition to standard ASA monitors, invasive monitors are patient dependant
  - +/– CVP monitoring for guiding rate and volume of IVF intraoperative; prefer IJ, avoid side of AVF
  - A-line, if needed, best inserted in femoral position
- Arm with AVF protected; no IV, no BP cuff; SpO_2 best not measured on the AVF arm

INDUCTION

- Induce only after confirmation of graft adequacy, or once incision made for LRD
- General anesthesia
  - Sevoflurane is usually avoided due to its metabolism to inorganic fluoride, although no clinical renal toxicity has been demonstrated
  - Muscle relaxants – cisatracurium is usually selected since its clearance is not dependent on renal function
    - Avoid succinylcholine if possible: ventricular tachycardia and cardiac arrest has been reported in patients with uremic neuropathy after use of succinylcholine
  - RSI may be needed if significant gastroparesis is present
- Regional anesthesia
  - Evidence shows neuraxial anesthesia to be a comparable alternative to GA during renal transplantation with no significant difference in operative time or hemodynamic variables
  - Low thoracic epidural for living donor unless contraindicated. Insert catheter prior to inducing GA, do not use epidural until kidney out to avoid hypotension
- Pre-incision antibiotics prophylaxis is recommended along with prophylactic antibiotics coverage for 24 hours after donor nephrectomy to prevent wound infection

MAINTENANCE

- Living related donor:
  - Maintain normal blood pressure: use fluids, avoid vasopressors
    - A comparison between NS 0.9%, LR, and PlasmaLyte in early renal transplantation showed a superior benefit in metabolic profile (pH, lactate, kalemia) postoperative in patients receiving PlasmaLyte intraoperative
  - Maintain adequate UOP: if drops <1.5 mL/min, 12–25 gm of mannitol may be administered, although evidence of improved outcomes is lacking
  - Maintain eucarbia: hypo- and hypercarbia are potent inducers of renal artery spasm
  - Give mannitol 30 minutes prior to removal of kidney for renal protection, as well as before the ureter is cut, and during the resting period

- Heparin is injected before clamping of the renal vessels at the end of the rest period – protamine is administered slowly after removal of kidney
- Prior to extubation, obtain a chest X-ray to evaluate for pneumothorax (secondary to surgical retraction on diaphragm) and possible need for chest tube
- When reversing muscle relaxants, keep in mind the action of neostigmine may be prolonged in renal insufficiency
- Cadaveric donor:
  - Cadaveric donor kidney can be preserved by perfusion at low temperatures until transplantation for up to 48 hours
  - Anesthesia team supports the cadaveric donor until the aorta is cross-clamped
    - Important to maintain MAP > 60, UOP >0.5 mL/kg/h
      - "Rule of 100s": SBP >100 mm Hg, UOP > 100 mL/h, arterial PO_2 > 100 mm Hg
    - Support blood pressure by optimizing hydration first – may require large volumes of balanced salt solutions (up to 1000 mL/h), especially if diabetes insipidus is present. If absolutely necessary, dopamine up to 10 mcg/kg/min may be used
      - Caution is advised if vasopressors are required, as it increases the incidence of ATN and graft failure
- Recipient:
  - Be prepared for vascular clamp release after arterial anastomosis!
    - If hypotension results (release of chemicals from ischemic tissues), treat with IVF first
      - Cardiac arrest has been described upon clamp release due to sudden hyperkalemia caused by washout of potassium-containing preservative solutions of new kidney. Treat initially with bolus of 50 mEq of bicarbonate and CPR

POSTOPERATIVE

- Fluid resuscitation: replace U/O volume for volume to avoid hypovolemia
- If morphine IV PCA: no basal, increase lockout to 15 minutes (risk of buildup of morphine-3 and morphine-6 glucuronide)
- Avoid NSAIDs
- Regarding thromboprophylaxis and prevention of renal graft vein thrombosis in the postoperative period, no consensus currently exists. Treatment is highly dependent on the renal transplant center, as well as preoperative identified patient risk factors
  - An example of thromboprophylaxis in some institutions may consist of SQ heparin TID plus SCDs. LMWH is rarely used. Other agents are approached on a case by case basis
  - Aspirin 75 mg/day for 28 days postoperative has been shown in some studies to prevent renal transplant graft vein thrombosis
- Kidney rejection
  - Acute (anaphylaxis, shock, DIC) – Remove transplanted kidney
  - Delayed rejection (fever, local tenderness, decreased UOP) – High dose corticosteroids and antilymphocyte globulin Rx
  - Oliguria or anuria: renal artery Doppler, bladder US, r/o hypovolemia (TTE) and ATN (possibly biopsy); furosemide not shown to improve outcome. Consider HD if needed
- Wound infection – Antibiotics prophylaxis before incision to continue 24 hours postoperative
  - Opportunistic infections secondary to chronic immunosuppression after transplant can occur

PEARLS

- Regional or general anesthesia can be safely administered
- Remember drugs dependent on renal metabolism and elimination may be affected
- Control hypotension first with IVF and use mannitol to maintain kidney perfusion
- Be prepared to treat hyperkalemia and hypotension after vascular clamp release

REFERENCES

For references, please visit **www.TheAnesthesiaGuide.com**.

CHAPTER 81
Liver Transplant

Gebhard Wagener, MD

PREOPERATIVE

FIGURE 81-1. Indications for liver transplant

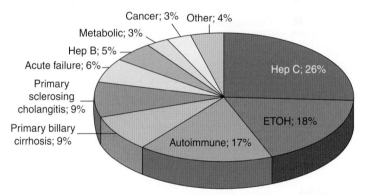

4000–600 liver transplants in the US/year over the last 10 years. Only 300–400 of these are living donor transplants.

CONTRAINDICATIONS

Absolute

Pulmonary hypertension: mean pulmonary artery pressure > 45 mm Hg
- Recidivism to alcohol and drug abuse
- Extrahepatic malignancies
- Systemic sepsis

Relative

- Pulmonary hypertension: mean pulmonary artery pressure > 35 mm Hg
- Significant cardiopulmonary disease
- Poor psychosocial support or compliance
- In the case of hepatocellular carcinoma ("Milan criteria")
  ‣ 1 tumor > 5 cm
  ‣ > 3 tumors < 3 cm
  ‣ Presence of extrahepatic tumors
  ‣ Presence of vascular invasion

TABLE 81-1	Liver Failure and Associated Morbidities
Neuro	• Encephalopathy • Increased intracranial pressure (with fulminant liver failure) • Coma
Respiratory	• Hepatopulmonary syndrome ‣ Transpulmonary shunts with paradoxical improvement of SaO_2 in supine position (orthodeoxia) • Atelectasis from ascites • Aspiration risk
Cardiac	• Hyperdynamic state of cirrhosis ‣ Low SVR, high cardiac output, splanchnic vasodilation • Portopulmonary hypertension • Mean PAP >35 mm Hg relative contraindication for liver transplantation
GI	• Delayed gastric emptying and increased intra-abdominal pressure (ascites) ‣ Rapid sequence induction • Esophageal varices

Renal	• Hepatorenal syndrome
	  ‣ Type I: doubling of serum creatinine within 2 weeks
	    ▪ Mean survival: 1 month
	  ‣ Type II: increase of serum creatinine > 1.5 mg/dL
	    ▪ Mean survival: 6 months
	• Relative hypovolemia
	• Hyponatremia

ID	• Immunosuppression • Spontaneous bacterial peritonitis

Hematology	• Myelosupression
	  ‣ Anemia
	  ‣ Leukopenia
	• Thrombocytopenia from hypersplenism
	• Coagulopathy of liver disease
	  ‣ Frequently hypo-/hypercoagulable disease

ANESTHESIA

Routine setup of liver room at Columbia University Medical Center (courtesy of Dr. Tricia Brentjens)

Drugs
Induction and maintenance

- Propofol
- Etomidate
- Midazolam (have 10 mg available)
- Fentanyl (have 3 mg available)
- Succinylcholine
- Cisatracurium (have 200 mg available)
- Isoflurane (have 2 full bottles available)

Vasoactive drugs

- Epinephrine 100 mcg/mL, 10 mL
- Epinephrine 10 mcg/mL, 10 mL
- Calcium chloride 1 g in 10 mL (have 10 vials available)
- Phenylephrine 40 mcg/mL, 10 mL syringe, and 250 mL bag

- Ephedrine 5 mg/mL, 10 mL
- Atropine 100 mcg/mL, 10 mL
- Sodium bicarbonate 50 mEq (have 10 vials available)

Others

- Magnesium sulfate 2 g (4 mL of the 0.5 g/mL solution): Not drawn up!
- Methylprednisolone sodium 500 mg
- Mannitol 12.5 g/20 mL: Not drawn up
- Acetylcysteine: discuss with your attending physician
  - Load: 150 mg/kg in 200 cc over 1 hour
  - Maintenance: 50 mg/kg in 500c c D5W over 4 hours
  - Then 100 mg/kg in 1 L D5W over 16 hours

Mandatory infusions

- Norepinephrine 4 mg/250 mL N saline
- Vasopressin 100 U/100 mL N saline
- Furosemide 100 mg/100 mL N saline

Have available

- Dopamine 200 mg/250 mL premix bag
- Dobutamine 250 mg/250 mL premix bag
- Nitroglycerin 50 mg/250 mL premix bottle
- Aminocaproic acid (Amicar) — antifibrinolytic: various protocols

Monitors
Routine monitors

- EKG 3 channels: I, II, V
- SpO_2
- NIBP cuff of medium, large, extra large sizes

Hemodynamic monitoring

- Do not heparinize pressure lines/bags!
- Three pressure transducers on the right: for right femoral artery, PA, CVP
- One pressure transducer on the left: for left radial artery
- Pediatric CVL kit [20 g] for femoral arterial line
- Assorted 20 G cannulas for radial arterial line placement
- Double lumen Cordis for IJ placement
- Oximetric PA catheter (needs to be calibrated prior to insertion)

IV setup

- All IVs are primed with PlasmaLyte except when otherwise indicated
- Rapid transfuser FMS2000 primed
- Two IV lines on warmers
- Venous infusion port (VIP) on microdrip with six ports for IV drips
- Call the blood bank and check on available products:
  - 10 PRBCs, 10 FFP, and 12 platelets

Others

- Point of care arterial blood gas (ABG) analyzer with at least 20 cartridges
- Multiple test tubes for complete blood count (CBC) and coagulation studies
- Two forced air warming machines with upper and lower body blankets
- For CVVHD: high-flow set for the blood warmer on the left side of the OR table to warm the returning limb of CVVH

MONITORING

- Arterial catheter (femoral and radial)
  ‣ Radial artery catheter often dampens during anhepatic phase
- PA catheter
  ‣ Maximize cardiac output
  ‣ Measure PA pressures
- Pulse pressure variation (PPV)
  ‣ Allows estimate of volume responsiveness
- Point of care arterial blood gas analyzer
  ‣ Measure pH, acidemia, hematocrit, potassium
- Point of care coagulation test: thrombelastography or rotational thromboelastometry (ROTEM®)
  ‣ Allows estimation of global *in vivo* hemostasis including coagulation factor defects, platelet function, abnormal fibrinogen polymerization, anticoagulant defects and hyperfibrinolysis

INDUCTION

- Rapid sequence induction for almost all patients (ascites)
- Patients are hyperdynamic with low SVR and maintain cardiac output with increased endogenous catecholamines: beware of hypotension after induction
- Most induction drugs will need a higher dose and have a delayed onset (larger volume of distribution) but have a prolonged half-life time (decreased hepatic metabolism)

MAINTENANCE

Surgical technique
Complete caval clamping

Vena cava is clamped completely above and below the liver and the donor cava is anastomosed end-end to the recipient.

Advantages:
- Fast
- Simpler (and possibly better) caval anastomosis

Disadvantages:
- Severe hypotension due to loss of preload during anhepatic phase
- Renal outflow obstruction and renal injury

Veno-venous bypass

Cannulation of portal vein and femoral vein with return of blood through a bypass pump either to a cannula in the axillary vein or the internal jugular vein. Anticoagulation is rarely required if heparin coated circuits are used.

Advantages:
- Hemodynamic stability during anhepatic phase
- Adequate renal venous drainage
- Less intestinal engorgement from portal occlusion

Disadvantages:
- Cumbersome
- Technical complications from access

Piggyback technique

Instead of replacing the vena cava with a typical bicaval approach, the recipient vena cava is preserved, and an anastomosis is created between the donor suprahepatic cava and a cuff of the recipient hepatic veins. Partial occlusion of the vena cava at the level of the hepatic veins. Partial caval blood flow is maintained throughout.

Advantages:
- Less hemodynamic instability
- Renal venous drainage is maintained

Disadvantages:
- Caval anastomosis is technically more difficult
- Portal occlusion may still cause intestinal engorgement (may be alleviated with temporal portocaval shunt)

FIGURE 81-2. Piggyback technique of liver transplantation

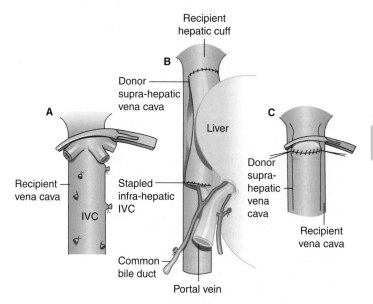

The recipient vena cava is preserved, and an anastomosis is created between the donor suprahepatic vena cava and a cuff of the recipient hepatic veins. Reproduced from Minter RM: *Current Procedures: Surgery*. Figure 32–7A–C. Available at: www.accesssurgery.com. Copyright © The McGraw-Hill Companies, Inc. All rights reserved.

TABLE 81-2	Four Phases of Liver Transplantation
Pre-anhepatic/ dissection phase	• Bleeding due to dissection in area of portal hypertension • Correct coagulopathy, anemia, and optimize volume status
Anhepatic	• Low preload and cardiac output despite low SVR • Acidosis: unable to metabolize lactate

Reperfusion	• Possibly sudden
	  ‣ Acidosis
	  ‣ Hyperkalemia
	  ‣ Pulmonary hypertension
	  ‣ Right ventricular distension and failure
	  ‣ Cardiac arrest

Neohepatic phase	• If the liver functions well: within hours improvement of
	  ‣ Acidosis
	  ‣ Coagulopathy
	  ‣ Vasodilatory state

PRE-ANHEPATIC/DISSECTION PHASE

Bleeding due to dissection in area of portal hypertension

- Treat only clinical bleeding, not laboratory numbers:
  - ‣ Increased INR can be associated with hypercoagulability (deficiency of liver derived protein C and S and other anticoagulant factors)
  - ‣ Thrombelastography/rotational thrombolastography (ROTEM) may detect specific coagulation defects
- Maintain isovolemia and optimize fluid status:
  - ‣ Occult blood loss from retroperitoneal dissection or bleeding from collateral veins
  - ‣ Acute fluid loss when ascites is drained
- Do not transfuse platelets unless platelet count low, clinical bleeding evident and after consultation with the surgery team
  - ‣ Platelets sequester in the spleen and platelet transfusion is associated with increased thrombotic complications
- Often furosemide is required to maintain urine output and create intravascular "room" for transfusion of coagulation factors (plasma)

ANHEPATIC

Low preload and cardiac output despite low SVR

- Requires adequate preload especially with caval cross-clamping
  - ‣ Goal CVP 12–15
- The anesthesiologist needs to be confident that he/she will be able to maintain adequate hemodynamics during the anhepatic phase before the liver is removed
- Often requires high doses of vasopressors
  - ‣ Norepinephrine 2–10 mcg/min
  - ‣ Vasopressin 1–4 units/h
  - ‣ Goal: MAP 60 mm Hg or within 20% of preoperative BP
  - ‣ No urine output during anhepatic phase may indicate worse renal outcome
- Acidosis: unable to clear lactate during anhepatic phase
  - ‣ Treat aggressively with sodium bicarbonate (50–100 mEq over 20 minutes) as acidosis will worsen with reperfusion
- Large fluid administration during the anhepatic phase will cause volume overload and possible right heart failure with reperfusion
  - ‣ Use preferentially vasopressors to maintain blood pressure
- We routinely give 2 g magnesium sulfate IV over 10 minutes during anhepatic phase to prevent arrhythmias during reperfusion
- Check arterial blood gas 20 minutes prior to reperfusion to detect treatable abnormalities: acidosis, hyperkalemia, hypocalcemia

REPERFUSION

Washout of graft often associated with sudden:
- Acidosis
- Hyperkalemia: closely watch T waves
- Pulmonary hypertension
- Right ventricular distension and failure
- Cardiac arrest
  - ‣ Reperfusion will be worse with prolonged cold or warm ischemic time, steatotic grafts or with organs after donation after cardiac death (DCD)
  - ‣ Consider requesting from surgeon to flush the graft with portal vein blood prior to finishing the caval anastomosis, or slow reopening of portal vein
  - ‣ Aggressively treat:
    - ▪ Hyperkalemia: Insulin/glucose, bicarbonate, $CaCl_2$
    - ▪ Hypocalcemia
    - ▪ Acidosis: bicarbonate and hyperventilation
    - ▪ Hypotension: vasopressors, epinephrine in 10–30 mcg intravenous boluses

NEO-HEPATIC

If the liver functions well: within hours, improvement of
- Acidosis
- Coagulopathy
- Vasodilatory state
  ‣ Excessive fibrinolysis possible due to graft reperfusion and release of tissue plasminogen activator (tPA): consider transfusion of cryoprecipitate
  ‣ Avoid platelet transfusions especially if hepatic artery or portal vein anastomosis is precarious. Discuss with surgical team

POSTOPERATIVE

Extubation in the operating room is possible but little benefit

TABLE 81-3	Early Complications after Liver Transplant

0–24 h	• Bleeding
	• Graft failure
	  ‣ Hepatic artery thrombosis
	  ‣ Portal vein thrombosis
	  ‣ Early graft failure/delayed graft function
	• Vasodilatory shock

1–5 days	• Acute kidney injury • Infection • Bile leak • Prolonged respiratory failure
>5 days	• Rejection • Malnutrition • Prolonged hepatic failure • "Failure to thrive"

Diagnostic features and therapy of early complications

Bleeding
Diagnosis:
- Increased drain output (consider checking drain fluid hematocrit)
- Increased abdominal girth (measure hourly)
- Increased intra-abdominal pressure (measure hourly)

Rx:

Correction of coagulopathy

If bleeding persists or substantial bleeding: re-exploration

Hepatic artery or portal vein thrombosis
Diagnosis
- Persistent
  ‣ Metabolic (lactate) acidosis
  ‣ Elevated total bilirubin
  ‣ Coagulopathy
  ‣ Ascites
  ‣ Vasodilatory state and high vasopressor requirements
  ‣ Low urine output and worsening acute kidney injury

- ▸ Late and severe cases:
  - ▪ Persistent hypoglycemia
  - ▪ Depressed mental status/encephalopathy
  - ▪ Hypothermia
- Diagnosis confirmed by Doppler ultrasound
- Elevated transaminases are due to (ischemic) injury to the liver and not necessarily a sign of dysfunction

Differential diagnosis
- Early allograft dysfunction due to
  - ▸ Primary non-function
  - ▸ Small for size syndrome

Rx:
- Re-exploration
- Rarely amenable to endovascular intervention

Bile leak

Diagnosis
- Persistent
  - ▸ Bilous fluid from drains
  - ▸ Increased total bilirubin, alkaline phosphatase (AP) and gamma-glutamyltrans-peptidase (γ-GT)
  - ▸ Fever, malaise
- Diagnosis confirmed by ultrasound (intra-abdominal fluid) and drain fluid total bilirubin concentration

Rx:
- Re-exploration (breakdown of biliary anastomosis often due to ischemic injury to the bile) and possibly Roux-en-Y revision
- Percutaneous drainage
- Endoscopic biliary stent placement

Acute rejection

Diagnosis
- Days after surgery
  - ▸ Worsening liver function
  - ▸ Increasing total bilirubin and transaminases
  - ▸ Malaise and fever
- Diagnosis confirmed by biopsy

Rx:
- Increased immunosuppression
- Pulse steroids
- OKT-3 (muromonab-CD3 antibody)

PEARLS AND TIPS

- Magnesium (2g IV over 20 minutes) during the anhepatic phase may stabilize membranes and ameliorate cardiac arrhythmias of reperfusion
- Avoid platelet transfusion postoperative if there is concern about the patency of the hepatic artery anastomosis

REFERENCES

For references, please visit **www.TheAnesthesiaGuide.com**.

CHAPTER 82
Electroconvulsive Therapy (ECT)

Tony P. Tsai, MD

BASICS

- Used to treat severe depression, mania, and schizophrenia
- Therapeutic effects thought to result from release of neurotransmitters or reestablishment of neurotransmitter levels
- Typically given three times a week for 2 to 4 weeks acutely, then as needed
- Typically started as inpatient, then possibly administered as outpatient if needed
- General anesthesia is preferred for ECT treatments

PREOPERATIVE

- Standard ASA NPO guidelines apply
- Have patient void before the procedure
- Contraindications:
  ‣ MI within past 3 months, severe angina
  ‣ CHF, aneurysm of any major vessel
  ‣ Pheochromocytoma
  ‣ Cerebral tumor, elevation of ICP
  ‣ Cerebral aneurysm
  ‣ Recent CVA
  ‣ Respiratory failure
- Precautions:
  ‣ Pregnancy
  ‣ Thyrotoxicosis
  ‣ Cardiac dysrhythmias
  ‣ Glaucoma and retinal detachment
  ‣ Pacemaker, ICD (to be deactivated before the procedure)
- Medications:
  ‣ Tricyclic antidepressants can increase the risk of HTN, rhythm and conduction problems, and confusion
  ‣ SSRIs and reversible MAOIs can increase the risk of prolonged seizure
  ‣ Lithium increases the risk of confusion, and can prolong the action of succinylcholine: maintain lithium level around 0.6 mEq/L
  ‣ Carbamazepine can prolong the action of succinylcholine
  ‣ Chronic benzodiazepine treatment can make it more difficult to induce seizures. Flumazenil 0.2–0.3 mg at induction is usually effective without causing withdrawal or prolonged seizures

INDUCTION

Medications needed are an induction agent and a muscle relaxant

Commonly Used Induction Medications for ECT		
Medication	Dose	Notes
Etomidate	0.15–0.3 mg/kg	Increased risk of PONV
Ketamine	0.5–2 mg/kg	Increased sympathetic discharge
Methohexital	0.75–1 mg/kg	Avoid in patients with porphyria
Propofol	0.75–1.0 mg/kg	Dose can be titrated up or down to achieve maximal seizure
Rocuronium	0.45–0.6 mg/kg	Use if succinylcholine is contraindicated
Succinylcholine	0.2–0.5 mg/kg	Avoid in bradyarrhythmias, watch for hyperkalemia

- Bite block placed to prevent injury to teeth and tongue during seizure (see Figure 82-1)
- Sequence of events: IV placement, pre-oxygenate, induction agent, muscle relaxant, place bite block, ECT, assist with ventilation if necessary; provide oxygen by mask or nasal cannula throughout
- ECT results in a generalized tonic-clonic seizure and brief parasympathetic discharge (PSD) followed by sympathetic discharge (SD). There is a brief cerebral vasoconstriction followed by vasodilatation, with increase in CBF, ICP, and oxygen consumption
- PSD results in bradycardia, possible asystole (rare), increased secretions, increased gastric and intraocular pressures
- SD results in tachycardia, hypertension, increased myocardial oxygen demand, and possible dysrhythmias
- Therefore, the following medications should be available immediately:
  ‣ Labetalol, esmolol, nicardipine, verapamil, atropine
- If the seizure is too short (<20 seconds):
  ‣ Decrease hypnotic dose or use different medication, hyperventilate before shock
- If the seizure is too long (>90 seconds):
  ‣ Administer more hypnotic (propofol), or midazolam
- Possible complications (besides those listed above):
  ‣ Laryngospasm, apnea
  ‣ Aspiration
  ‣ Tongue biting, mandible dislocation, long bone fracture, myalgias

FIGURE 82-1. Oral protector to prevent tongue biting or tooth fracture during seizure.

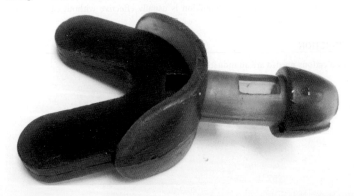

POSTOPERATIVE

- Surveillance in PACU. Same discharge criteria as surgical patients
- Side effects include:
  - ‣ Amnesia
  - ‣ Agitation
  - ‣ Confusion
  - ‣ Headache
  - ‣ Nausea and vomiting
- Rare complications include:
  - ‣ Myocardial ischemia and/or infarct
  - ‣ Transient neurologic deficits
  - ‣ Intracerebral hemorrhage
  - ‣ Blindness
  - ‣ Pulmonary edema
  - ‣ Splenic rupture

REFERENCES

For references, please visit **www.TheAnesthesiaGuide.com**.

CHAPTER 83
Off-site Anesthesia

Neelima Myneni, MD

CHALLENGES

- Remoteness of location and lack of trained personnel to assist in the event of an emergency
- Unfamiliarity with different equipment or specialized monitors
- At the end of the procedure, patients generally travel greater than usual distance to the PACU

REQUIREMENTS OF THESE LOCATIONS

- Immediate contacts with centrally located team when help is needed
- Adequate monitoring capability, ability to deliver supplemental oxygen, suction, equipment for mechanical ventilation, supply of drugs, scavenging capability
- Protection if radiation being used
- Backup equipment, personnel, and appropriate monitoring for transport

RADIATION SAFETY

- Intensity decreases with inverse square of the distance from emitting source
- Always wear a lead apron, thyroid shield, and remain 1–2 m from source
- Monthly radiation exposure not to exceed 50 mSv per FDA guidelines, as measured by radiation badges

ANESTHESIA

- Used for the sake of patient immobility and to minimize pain and anxiety
- Generally not necessary for adult patients, but for children and adults who cannot remain motionless (anxious, mentally retarded, demented, etc.)
- Either sedation or general anesthesia can be used
- Primary concern is airway management and maintenance of adequate oxygenation
- Comorbidities should be taken into consideration with special attention to airway as access is often limited
- Conscious sedation with continuous propofol infusions often used successfully
- Oversedation can lead to hypoventilation and airway obstruction, so ETT or LMA preferred by many
- Dexmedetomidine is often used, especially in patients likely to obstruct and become apneic, or those who require frequent assessment of mental status

MRI

Strength of the magnetic field of MRI unit ranges from 0.5 to 1.5 Tesla

Hazards of MRI

- Any ferrous-containing material may be drawn to magnet, often with lethal force (missile injury). It can injure patients or others in the room
- Pacemakers, ICDs, cochlear implants, orthopedic hardware, cerebrovascular clips also at risk of dislodgement, hemorrhage, or injury to adjacent vulnerable structures
- Magnetic metals (nickel, cobalt) most magnetic and dangerous while aluminum, titanium, copper, silver are not dangerous
- Alternative (MRI compatible) equipment and monitors
- Radiofrequency energy produced by scanner can be absorbed by tissue, producing heat that can cause tissue damage
- Loud sound (65–95 dB) generated, which can cause hearing loss; patients should wear ear plugs

MONITORING

- Extremely important as direct visualization is limited
- Should be placed at least 5–8 feet from the magnet bore to minimize magnetic pull
- EKG is often distorted by the radiofrequency energy and static magnetic field
- Monitoring sites, for example ECG pad sites, at risk for heating from the magnetic field, which can burn patients
- Electronic monitors can themselves generate radiofrequency waves that interfere with quality of MRI image
- MRI compatible fiber optic pulse oximeter should be used as standard oximeters can cause burns
- Radiofrequency pulsing can generate artificial spikes and generate erroneously high blood pressures on invasive blood pressure monitoring

RESUSCITATION

- Remove patient from MRI suite, call for backup, and initiate resuscitation at a different anesthesia station (that should be located right outside)
- If necessary, shut off magnetic field. It takes about 10 minutes to decrease magnetic field
- Restoring magnetic field takes 4 days and costs thousands of dollars; therefore, reserve for dire emergency

EXTRACORPOREAL SHOCK WAVE LITHOTRIPSY (ESWL)

- Utilization of high-intensity pressure waves of short duration to break renal or ureteral calculi into very small fragments that then wash out in urine
- Patients lie in a special table with water-filled cushions. This is a variation of the ancient method of immersion lithotripsy where patients were immersed in water bath
  - With immersion, peripheral venous compression can increase central intravascular volume, increasing central venous and aortic pressures
  - Work of breathing increased. Extrinsic pressure decreases FRC and VC that may not be tolerated in patients with preexisting pulmonary disease
  - Water temperature should be closely controlled. Warm water can cause vasodilatory hypotension
  - Immersion and emersion can cause cardiac dysrhythmias
  - In general, this method should not be used in patients at risk for CHF or MI
- Patient immobility is crucial for success of procedure; short-acting opioids are needed for pain at skin
- Minimal sedation with supplemental oxygen is sufficient
- Maintain adequate intravascular volume to allow passage of calculi fragments
- Risk of cardiac dysrhythmias (especially ventricular tachycardia). Minimized by initiating shock waves 20 milliseconds after the R wave (the absolute refractory period). Thus, the HR determines the rate of shocks and the duration of the procedure. On occasion, the anesthesiologist will be asked to increase HR (administer 0.2–0.4 mg of IV glycopyrrolate) to shorten the procedure
- Pacemakers are not contraindicated provided a back-up mode is available, but ICDs are (they should be turned off preoperative, with external defibrillator pads used during the case and kept on until ICD turned back on)

CARDIOVERSION

- Need a brief period of sedation and amnesia for the discomfort from electric shock
- Best achieved by reduced dose of propofol; if low EF, give repeated small boluses of propofol, waiting several minutes after each bolus to allow for long circulation time
- Ensure emergency drugs are available, provide preoxygenation, and, if necessary, provide assisted ventilation after shock
- Etomidate is not a good choice secondary to myoclonus. Avoid benzodiazepines because of slow onset and long duration of action

ENDOSCOPY/ERCP

- Upper endoscopy supine or lateral
- Lower endoscopy lateral
- Most endoscopies performed without anesthesiologist present. Typically needed for "difficult to sedate" patients, or medical issues
- ERCP most often prone + fluoroscopy; stimulating during bile duct dilatation
- Usually MAC (+ topicalization for upper endoscopy), but in some cases (full stomach, upper GI bleed, etc.), intubation may be needed

REFERENCES

For references, please visit **www.TheAnesthesiaGuide.com**.

CHAPTER 84
Cosmetic Surgery

Brooke Albright, MD

BASICS

- Outpatient cosmetic procedures have increased by 457% from 1997 to 2007
- Of these, 54% are performed in office-based settings, 29% in ambulatory-based settings, and 17% in hospital-based settings

PREOPERATIVE

- Because of the elective nature of cosmetic surgery, patients tend to be healthy ASA 1 and 2 patients, with no more than a single health problem
- Patients presenting for an office-based procedure must be medically optimized
- Preoperative history and physical examination must be within 30 days
- If the patient has significant comorbid conditions, anesthesiology consultation should be obtained prior to surgery scheduling
- It is recommended that ASA physical status patients greater than 3 have no more than local anesthesia (with no sedation) in an office-based setting

MONITORING

- Standard ASA monitors including EKG, non-invasive blood pressure, pulse oximetry, temperature, and capnography are required for cosmetic surgery procedures. Airways supplies, suction, emergency drugs, and a cardiac defibrillator should also be readily available

TOP FIVE COSMETIC SURGERIES

Liposuction

- Description
  - Percutaneous cannula aspiration of subdermal fat deposits through strategically placed small incisions
  - *Tumescent Liposuction*: Rapid pressure subcutaneous infiltration of several liters of wetting solution containing highly diluted lidocaine (0.05–0.10%) and epinephrine (1:1,000,000)
- Induction
  - A field block or use of tumescent local anesthesia is most commonly used
  - Some patients will request sedation and analgesia to relieve the brief discomfort of needle punctures for subdermal infiltration
  - Epidural and spinal anesthesia in the office setting is discouraged because of the possibility of vasodilation, hypotension, and fluid overload
- Maintenance
  - Fluid replacement and maintenance of normothermia
  - Improper fluid management in large-volume liposuction may lead to hypovolemic shock at one extreme, and hemodilution progressing to pulmonary edema at the other
  - About 60–70% of wetting solution is absorbed by hypodermoclysis; therefore, as much more wetting solution is infiltrated than fat aspirated, supplemental fluid may not be necessary
  - Avoid hypothermia due to infiltration of large volumes of room-temperature tumescent fluid solution by active warming of the patient intraoperatively

- Complications (overall rate 0.7%)
  - PE (23%), viscera perforation (14.6%), fat embolization (8.5%), local anesthetic toxicity leading to cardio-respiratory failure (5.4%), or vascular damage leading to hemorrhage (4.6%) by the suction wand
  - The liver drug clearance of lidocaine (estimated at 250 mg/h) is the limiting factor in drug disposition. If liver function is impaired, lidocaine will accumulate in circulation
  - The peak serum levels of lidocaine occur 12–14 hours after injection and decline over subsequent 6–14 hours

Breast Surgery

- Description
  - Augmentation, implant exchanges, breast reduction, and completion of transverse rectus abdominis muscle (TRAM) flaps
- Induction
  - MAC with paravertebral block using single-level (T4) injection and local anesthesia is being used more frequently in office-based settings
  - However, because of the pain associated with separating the pectoralis muscles from the chest wall during breast augmentation, general anesthesia with either an LMA or ETT is usually preferred
- Maintenance
  - Anti-emetics and postoperative analgesia
  - For postoperative pain control in first 48 hours, 3 methods have proven successful:
    - Intraoperative bupivacaine 0.25% using 10 mL placed in Jackson-Pratt drain prior to final subcuticular closure, allowed to dwell within the wound for 10 minutes
    - Paravertebral block
    - Preoperative steroids (dexamethasone 10 mg IV) and NSAIDS (e.g., Cox-2 inhibitors: rofecoxib 50 mg PO)
- Complications
  - Pneumothorax from surgical dissection
  - Uncontrolled postoperative pain

Blepharoplasty (eyelid surgery)

- Description
  - Surgical modification of the eyelid whereby excess skin and fat are removed or repositioned and surrounding muscles and tendons are reinforced
- Induction
  - Local anesthesia and oral sedation in office-based settings
  - Oral sedation may consist of diazepam 10 mg p.o. and propoxyphene with acetaminophen (100 mg/650 mg) given 30 minutes prior to the slow injection of each lid with 2 mL 1% lidocaine and 1:100,000 epinephrine
- Maintenance
  - MAC and/or local
- Complications
  - Complications within the immediate postoperative period include corneal abrasions and vision-threatening retrobulbar hemorrhage

Abdominoplasty ("tummy tuck")

- Description
  - Removal of excess abdominal skin and fat from the middle and lower abdomen to make the abdomen firmer. Occasionally, the rectus abdominis muscles require tightening by sutures as well. Sometimes combined with intra-abdominal procedures
- Induction
  - General anesthesia and conscious sedation with tumescent wetting solution have been used safely

- Maintenance
  - GA with inhalational or intravenous anesthesia, or conscious sedation
- Complications
  - Venous embolism and poor wound healing. Increased risk of venous embolism is related to length of surgery time, abdominal surgical site, and presence of cancer. Early ambulation can decrease the risk of postoperative complications
  - Smoking increases risk of poor wound healing
  - Overall risk of combining gynecologic and cosmetic abdominal surgical procedures is not substantially greater than risk of either performed alone

Facial Surgery

- Description
  - Laser resurfacing, rhytidectomy (face-lift), otoplasty (ears), mentoplasty (chin), rhinoplasty (nose), meloplasty (cheek), and others
- Induction
  - General anesthesia, conscious sedation combined with either topical EMLA cream and cooling techniques, or regional block with tumescent anesthetic infiltration have all been used
  - If GA is used for rhytidectomy, tape ETT in the midline in order not to distort the face, and in collaboration with the surgeon who will want the face maximally exposed; secure ETT well as the surgeon will move the head from side to side
- Maintenance
  - Usually anesthesia can be lightened up once block in place
  - When using GA, the lowest mixture of oxygen the patient will tolerate should be used. Avoid nitrous oxide during laser use
  - Avoid bucking/retching during awakening (risk of ecchymoses). Ensure that facial dressing does not constrict airway
  - Dexmedetomidine (1 mcg/kg IV over 10 minutes, then 0.2–0.6 mcg/kg/h maintenance) may reduce N/V postoperatively, maintain hemodynamic stability, and enable the patient to maintain spontaneous ventilation and oxygen saturation with room air, thus reducing concerns of fire hazard with use of supplemental oxygen
- Complications
  - Operating room fires due to the use of ignition sources (i.e., electrocautery) near the face where oxidizers (i.e., oxygen) are highest in concentration are one major concern in patients undergoing facial surgery

PEARLS

- FDA max adult dose of lidocaine + epinephrine for regional anesthesia is 7 mg/kg. Yet, when extremely dilute lidocaine (0.1%) with epinephrine (1 mg/L) is infiltrated subdermally for tumescent anesthesia, up to 35–55 mg/kg have been used safely
  - CNS symptoms (i.e., convulsions) may not be seen before cardiac symptoms (terminal asystole and other fatal arrhythmias) in lidocaine toxicity from tumescent liposuction
- Prevent operating room fires by limiting FiO_2 and turning off N_2O flows during laser use
- The face is the second most common surgical area injured by OR fire (tonsils the most common)

REFERENCES

For references, please visit **www.TheAnesthesiaGuide.com**.

PART VI

CARDIOVASCULAR AND THORACIC

CHAPTER 85
Basics of CPB

Jennie Ngai, MD

CARDIOPULMONARY BYPASS (CPB)

- Bypass blood circulation of the heart and lungs while still perfusing other organs
- Diversion of blood flow through a circuit located outside of the body, yet in continuity with it
- Primarily used for cardiac surgery, but also for major vascular surgery, neurosurgery, and transplant surgery

BASIC COMPONENTS (*SEE FIGURE 85-1*)

- Venous cannula to remove blood from the patient
- Venous reservoir
- Pump to return blood
- Oxygenator to add oxygen (and remove CO_2)
- Heat exchanger to warm or cool blood
- Filter to remove debris and air
- Arterial cannula to return blood to the patient

MONITORS USED DURING CARDIAC SURGERY

- Pulse oximetry—monitor for peripheral oxygen saturation
- EKG—monitor for dysrhythmias, ST segment changes
- Arterial line—necessary for cardiac surgery as noninvasive cuff measurement will not work during CPB (nonpulsatile flow)
- Central line—monitor for volume status, rhythm disturbances, superior vena cava (SVC) syndrome, and adequate venous drainage during CPB. Used for rapid volume resuscitation and medication administration
- Pulmonary artery (PA) catheter—should be placed in patients having off pump CABG, pulmonary hypertension, low EF. May not be routinely placed; depends on preference of surgical team for postoperative care
- Transesophageal echo (TEE)—if available, should be placed in every cardiac case. If limited availability, should be used preferentially for valve procedures. Monitor for contractility, volume status, valve competence, and presence of air prior to CPB separation. This is now becoming a standard of care
- Processed EEG monitor—level of anesthetic depth
- Cerebral oximetry—monitor for cerebral oxygenation and perfusion

FIGURE 85-1. Basic diagram of CPB machine

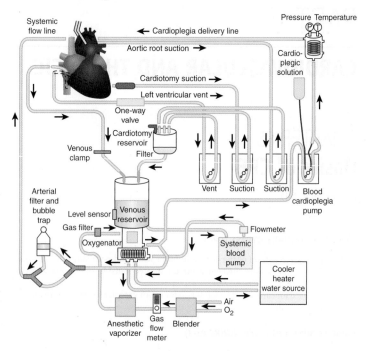

SPECIFIC PLACEMENT OF MONITORS

Arterial line placement

Arterial Line Location According to the Location of the Arterial Cannula	
Location of arterial cannula	Possible arterial line locations for monitoring
Ascending aorta	Right or left radial artery; right or left femoral artery
Axillary/innominate artery	Left radial artery; right or left femoral artery
Femoral artery	Right or left radial artery
Balloon endoclamp in ascending aorta	Two arterial lines, right and left radial artery

Arterial Line Location According to the Type of Surgery	
Type of surgery	Possible arterial line locations for monitoring
Coronary artery bypass surgery	Right or left radial artery, unless using radial artery graft; right or left femoral artery
Valve surgery	Right or left radial artery; right or left femoral artery
Ascending aorta surgery	Right or left radial artery; right or left femoral artery
Aortic arch surgery	Possibly need two arterial lines, discuss with surgeon about location

Central line placement

Central Line Locations	
Location of central venous pressure (CVP)	Rationale
Right internal jugular vein	Adequate monitoring of CVP; ease of PA catheter placement. If right internal jugular (RIJ) used for venous cannula, will need to find alternative site.
Left internal jugular vein	Adequate monitoring of CVP; more difficulty placing PA catheter
Subclavian vein	Able to monitor CVP; possible loss of line with sternal retractor; increased difficulty placing PA catheter
Femoral vein	Inaccurate monitor of adequate venous drainage from head during CPB; adequate for volume resuscitation

ANTIFIBRINOLYTIC

Aminocaproic acid (10 g load over 30 minutes, then 1 g/h for total dose of 15 g) is routinely used for cardiac cases, unless the risk outweighs benefits, that is, if the patient is prone to thrombosis. This is, however, institution- and surgeon-dependent. Antifibrinolytics should be started prior to sternotomy to increase benefit.

RE-OPERATION

- If the patient has had prior cardiac surgery, the risk of bleeding from injury to heart or major vessels on re-entry depends on surgical approach
- Sternotomy through prior sternotomy has higher risk than thoracotomy after previous sternotomy
- Plan for large venous access if re-operation, since risk of bleeding is greater. Have blood products readily available in the room

BEFORE GOING ON CPB

- Need to be able to monitor arterial BP and central venous pressure
- Need to have venous and arterial cannulae in place
- Need to be heparinized (initial dose 400 units/kg), for goal activated clotting time (ACT) >450
- If unable to reach goal ACT after 600 units/kg heparin, consider giving FFP or ATIII
- Give muscle relaxant and amnestic medications (as blood levels will be diluted by priming solution, possibly leading to awareness and movement)

Location of Arterial and Venous Cannulae According to Incision and Type of Surgery			
Surgical approach	Arterial cannulation	Venous cannulation	Comments
Sternotomy	Ascending aorta	Bicaval cannulation	Most common, standard approach
Thoracotomy	Ascending, axillary, femoral	Femoral (multiorifice cannula from femoral vein to SVC)	Arterial cannulation is surgeon preference. Femoral arterial cannulation increases risk of thromboemboli from retrograde perfusion
Re-operation	Ascending, axillary, femoral	Right atrial, bicaval, femoral	High risk of bleeding in re-operative, option to cannulate and go on CPB prior to opening chest. If massive bleeding prior to venous cannulation, use suction as venous return
Robotic cardiac surgery	Femoral	Femoral	
Ascending and arch aortic aneurysm/ dissection, calcified aorta	Axillary, femoral	Bicaval	If calcified aorta, try not to manipulate due to potential embolus

DURING CPB

- Give muscle relaxant and amnestic medications
- Stop ventilating when full flow on CPB, and after communicating with perfusionist to ensure there were no problems with CPB initiation
- Monitor MAP, usually between 50–70 mm Hg; if carotid stenosis or other pathology requiring higher perfusion pressures, maintain higher pressure, around 60–80 mm Hg
- Monitor BIS and cerebral oximeter
- Monitor ABG, Hct—should be lower to counter increased blood viscosity from hypothermia; glucose—should be in normal range, treat according to insulin protocol
- Flow during CPB depends on procedure and cannulation sites
  ‣ Some portions require low flow, that is, to clamp the aorta
  ‣ Flow index is typically 1.8–2.4 L/min/m^2
- Temperature dependent on procedure and previous cardiac surgery; usually cool to 32°C–34°C
  ‣ May need circulatory arrest if procedure involves head vessels (aortic aneurysm)
    ▪ If circulatory arrest is necessary, patient is cooled to 18°C–20°C
    ▪ Circulatory arrest time can be up to 45 min
  ‣ An alternative to circulatory arrest is selective cerebral perfusion to minimize cerebral ischemia
  ‣ May need lower temperature if previous CABG using internal mammary artery (IMA), as blood from the IMA (originating from subclavian artery, downstream from cross-clamp) will flush out cardioplegia solution

- Aorta will be cross-clamped when ready for cardiac arrest; procedures on right heart do not require arrest, and therefore no cross-clamp, and cardioplegia is not given
- Cardioplegia given after aortic cross-clamp. Solution is institution-dependent, most centers use a potassium-based cardioplegia. An alternative to depolarizing solution (potassium based) cardioplegia is nondepolarizing cardioplegia using adenosine, lidocaine, and magnesium. Cardioplegia can be given:
  ‣ Antegrade, into ascending aorta proximal to aortic cross-clamp, down the coronary arteries
  ‣ Individually to each coronary ostia
  ‣ Retrograde, through the coronary sinus; useful if moderate to severe AI or severe CAD

SEPARATION FROM CPB

Prior to separation from CPB, check for
- *Contractility*—if poor, add inotrope
  ‣ Epinephrine (0.01–0.1 µg/kg/min)
  ‣ Milrinone (0.3–0.7 µg/kg/min)
  ‣ Norepinephrine (0.01–0.1 µg/kg/min)
  ‣ Dobutamine (2–20 µg/kg/min)
- *Rate and Rhythm*—may need atrial and/or ventricular pacing wires if LVH and atrial contraction is beneficial. Should almost always have pacing wires, may need to temporarily pace postop if tissue edema, low risk to place pacing wires
- *Pressure*—if low, may need vasoconstrictor, but also check for SAM (see chapter 20); if high, add vasodilator ± β-blocker
  ‣ Vasopressin (0.04–0.08 units/min)
  ‣ Phenylephrine (25–200 mcg/min)
  ‣ Nitroglycerin (0.1–7 mcg/kg/min)
  ‣ Nitroprusside (0.1–2 mcg/kg/min)
- *Oxygenation and Ventilation*—make sure ventilator is on and working properly
- *Temperature*—OK to come off CPB when temperature is between 35–37°C, otherwise risk of arrhythmias and bleeding
- *Electrolytes*—should be in normal range, otherwise risk of arrhythmias
- *Hematocrit*—should be acceptable for patient before coming off, otherwise give blood

Reduce flow to about 2 L/min, and assess flow and function of heart; if good, wean off CPB

Administer protamine (SLOWLY) to reverse heparin based on heparin concentration assay, in a 1:1 mg-to-mg ratio.
- Anaphylaxis in 1% of diabetics who have received protamine-containing insulin (NPH or protamine zinc insulin), but possible in nondiabetics (especially if fish allergy)
- Less common reaction (thromboxane production due to heparin-protamine complexes): pulmonary vasoconstriction, right ventricle (RV) dysfunction, systemic hypotension, and transient neutropenia: stop infusion, give small doses of heparin to bind protamine, supportive care
- Protamine administration while on CPB can cause IMMEDIATE DEATH!

DIFFICULT SEPARATION FROM CPB

Issue	Action
Low oxygen saturation	Is anesthesia machine and ventilator on?
	Is oxygen flow adequate?
	Is endotracheal tube connected to circuit and machine?
	Is endotracheal tube obstructed? Suction and bronchoscopy
	Check echo for contractility, pulmonary embolus
	If patient is unstable, may need to return to CPB
Low tidal volume/high airway pressures	Perform bronchoscopy
	Adjust endotracheal tube as necessary
	If patient is unstable, may need to return to CPB
Abnormal end tidal CO_2	Is $EtCO_2$ monitor connected?
	Check for evidence of low cardiac output
	If BP low, see below
	Check endotracheal tube for obstruction
	Check echo for pulmonary artery obstruction
Poor contractility	Inotropic support
	If already high dose inotrope, consider intra-aortic balloon pump or ventricular assist device
Slow heart rate (HR <70)	Pace at higher rate
Fast HR >100, stable BP	Use β-blocker
Fast HR, unstable BP	Cardioversion (internal paddles 10–20 J, external paddles 200–300 J)
Low BP	Check echo for contractility and volume status
	Check echo for severe valvular abnormalities
	If poor contractility, add inotrope
	If empty ventricle (hypovolemic), give volume
	If dilated atrial and ventricular chambers, may need volume to optimize position on starling curve
	If normal/high cardiac output and low SVR, add vasopressor
	If already high dose vasopressor, consider methylene blue (2 mg/kg), an inhibitor of guanylate cyclase–mediated vasodilatation
	Check echo for systolic anterior motion (SAM)
SAM on TEE (Systolic anterior motion of anterior mitral leaflet, occluding LV outflow tract)	Decrease inotropes, consider β-blocker
	Increase volume
	Decrease heart rate
	Increase afterload with vasoconstrictors

TRANSPORT TO ICU

- Most patients will still be under GA and intubated at end of procedure
- When transported to ICU, should use monitors (EKG, SpO_2, A-line), oxygen, Ambu ventilation
- Watch that all lines and endotracheal tube (ETT) stay in place during transport
- Have venous access within reach to administer medications if necessary
- Continue all vasoactive medications during transport, and bring emergency medications and intubation equipment
- In the first 2 hours, determine if bleeding, hemodynamically stable, and ready for emergence and extubation (depending on patient and procedure)
- Fast track patients should be hemodynamically stable, no bleeding, on minimal vasoactive infusions, and ready to be extubated in the first 6 hours

REFERENCES

For references, please visit **www.TheAnesthesiaGuide.com**.

CHAPTER 86
Intraoperative TEE

Sanford M. Littwin, MD

Uses of Intraoperative Transesophageal Echocardiography (TEE)	
Noncardiac surgery	Cardiac surgery
• Assessment of regional wall motion abnormalities (RWMA) • Assessment of volume status	• Same as noncardiac • Basic TEE exam • Assessment of valve function, evaluation of repair/replacement • Assessment of tolerance of proximal aortic cross-clamping • Diagnosis and evaluation of therapy for difficulty weaning off cardiopulmonary bypass

BASIC TECHNIQUE

Relative contraindications: esophageal lesions (e.g., diverticulum, varices) or recent surgery, or unstable cervical spine lesion.

Lubricated probe inserted after stomach contents emptied with OG suction

Initially placed into mid-esophageal position approximately 25–30 cm.
- Probe manipulation (Figure 86-1)
  ‣ Rotation of probe
  ‣ Knobs
    ▪ Anteflexion/retroflexion
    ▪ Left/right flexion of probe tip
  ‣ Probe button(s)
    ▪ Scan angle: imaging array rotation from 0° to 180°
- Position of probe and views
  ‣ Position
    ▪ Upper esophageal
    ▪ Mid-esophageal
    ▪ Transgastric

FIGURE 86-1. Probe manipulation nomenclature

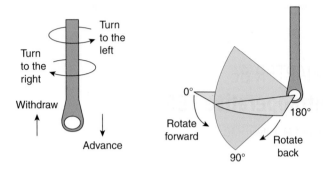

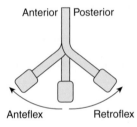 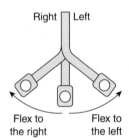

Reproduced with permission from Shanewise JS, et al. ASE/SCA guidelines for performing a comprehensive intraoperative multiplanetransesophageal echocardiography examination: Recommendations of the American Society of Echocardiography Council for Intraoperative Echocardiography and the Society of Cardiovascular Anesthesiologists Task Force for Certification in Perioperative Transesophageal Echocardiography. *Anesth Analg*. 1999;89:870.

- ‣ Views
  - ▪ Twenty standard views (see Figure 86-2)
- • Views performed systematically to gain information about cardiac pathology and performance
- • Subset of views most often used for noncardiac cases
  - ‣ Mid-esophageal 4 chamber view
    - ▪ Allows for assessment of overall chamber size (right and left atria, right and left ventricles)
    - ▪ Cardiac function (RWMA)
    - ▪ Valve pathology
      - ◆ Tricuspid regurgitation
      - ◆ Mitral regurgitation
  - ‣ Transgastric mid-papillary view
    - ▪ Assessment of RWMA
    - ▪ Volume status

FIGURE 86-2. Standard views

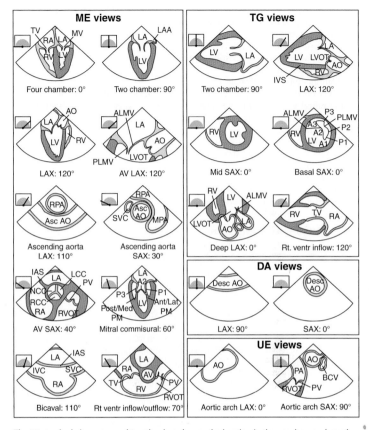

The 20 standard views grouped together based upon the location in the esophagus where they are obtained, upper esophageal (UE), middle esophageal (ME), transgastric (TG), and descending aortic (DA). Major cardiac structures are labeled including: right atrium (RA); left atrium (LA); mitral valve (MV); tricuspid valve (TV); right ventricle (RV); left ventricle (LV); left atrial appendage (LAA); aorta (AO); anterior leaflet of the mitral valve (ALMV); posterior leaflet of the mitral valve (PLMV); ascending aorta (Asc AO); right pulmonary artery (RPA); superior vena cava (SVC); main pulmonary artery (MPA); intra atrial septum (IAS); pulmonic valve (PV); right ventricular outflow tract (RVOT); noncoronary cusp of the aortic valve (NCC); right coronary cusp of the aortic valve (RCC); left coronary cusp of the aortic valve (LCC); posterior scallops of the mitral valve P1, P2, P3; anterior scallops of the mitral valve A1, A2, A3; posterior medial papillary muscle (Post/Med PM); anterior scallops of the mitral valve A1, A2, A3; posterior medial papillary muscle (Post/Med PM); anterolateral papillary muscle (Ant/Lat PM); inferior vena cava (IVC); descending aorta (Desc AO); left brachiocephalic vein (BCV). Reproduced from Wasnick JD, Hillel Z, Kramer D, Littwin S, Nicoara A. *Cardiac Anesthesia and Transesophageal Echocardiography*. Figure Intro–6. Available at: www.accessanesthesiology.com.

HEMODYNAMIC ASSESSMENT

Evaluation of patients undergoing noncardiac surgery by TEE allows for immediate assessment of cardiovascular pathologic processes.

- Cardiac ischemia
  - New onset during surgery: RWMA
  - Further advancement of existing cardiac compromise: decrease in EF
- Valve dysfunction
  - Regurgitation (color Doppler)
  - LVOT obstruction with systolic anterior motion (SAM) of the anterior leaflet of the mitral valve; clinical presentation similar to hypertrophic cardiomyopathy [HCM] (see chapter 20)
- Volume status (see below)
  - Assessment of ventricular size correlates with intravascular volume
  - Response to fluid administration can be evaluated
- Assessment of ejection fraction
  - Before, during, and after surgical procedure
  - Assurance that anesthetic management and surgical intervention do not negatively affect cardiac performance

Practical Assessment of Volume Status	
Surrogate	Evaluation for preload-dependence (i.e., hypovolemia)
LV size	• End-diastolic area (LVEDA) $<5 cm^2/m^2$ • Obliteration of LV cavity ("kissing papillary muscle sign") (also seen if decreased afterload and/or increased EF)
IVC size and collapsibility	Spontaneous ventilation: • Inspiratory collapse of IVC PPV: • Respiratory change in IVC diameter >12%[1] • IVC distensibility index >18%[2]
SVC collapsibility	SVC collapsibility >36%[3]
Aortic peak velocity	Respiratory variability of aortic peak velocity >12%[4]
Mitral flow	E/E' velocity ratio >8 (associated with left ventricular end-diastolic pressure [LVEDP] <15 mm Hg) E: transmitral wave inflow pattern E': tissue Doppler imaging of mitral annulus
Stroke volume (e.g., estimated through velocity-time integral (VTI) in LVOT[5])	Stroke volume variation with passive leg raise >12%

1. Respiratory change in IVC diameter $= \dfrac{IVC_{max} - IVC_{min}}{\dfrac{IVC_{max} + IVC_{min}}{2}}$

2. IVC distensibility index $= \dfrac{IVC_{max} - IVC_{min}}{IVC_{min}}$

   With IVC_{max} = maximal diameter of IVC during respiratory cycle, and IVC_{min} = minimal diameter of IVC during respiratory cycle.

3. SVC collapsibility index $= \dfrac{SVC_{max} - SVC_{min}}{SVC_{max}}$

   With SVC_{max} = maximal diameter of SVC during respiratory cycle, and SVC_{min} = minimal diameter of SVC during respiratory cycle.

4. Respiratory variability of aortic peak velocity $= \dfrac{V_{peak_{max}} - V_{peak_{min}}}{\dfrac{V_{peak_{max}} + V_{peak_{min}}}{2}}$

   With $V_{peak_{min}}$ and $V_{peak_{max}}$ the maximal and minimal, respectively, velocities in the aorta.

5. See Figure 86-3.

FIGURE 86-3. Measurement of CO based on volumetric flow across the LVOT

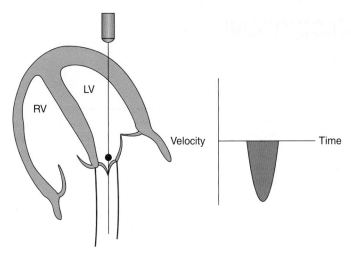

Note: This method should not be used in the setting of significant aortic valve disease. Using the deep transgastric view, the sample volume is placed in the left ventricular (LV) outflow tract just proximal to the aortic valve. This yields the spectral tracing shown to the right. The shaded area represents the velocity-time integral (VTI) The diameter of the LV outflow tract is measured by using a mid-esophageal long-axis view (ME AV LAX 120° in the standard views). Reproduced from Mathew JP, Swaminathan M, Ayoub CM. *Clinical Manual and Review of Transesophageal Echocardiography.* 2nd ed. Figure 6-2. Available at: www.accessanesthesiology. com.

Estimation of LV Filling Pressures	
Surrogate	Evaluation of LV filling pressures
LV size	• Calculation (Simpson rule) time-consuming • Unreliable if dilated cardiomyopathy
Mitral flow pattern	E/A velocity ratio >2 (associated with LVEDP >20 mm Hg): See Fig. 6-2.
Estimation of pressures based on continuity equation	• MPAP = 4 (peak PI velocity^2) + RAP • PADP = 4 (end-diastolic PI velocity^2) • LAP = Systolic BP–4 (peak MR velocity^2) • LVEDP = Diastolic BP–4 (end-diastolic AI velocity^2)

MPAP, mean pulmonary artery pressure; PI, pulmonary insufficiency; PADP, pulmonary artery diastolic pressure; LAP, left atrial pressure; MR, mitral regurgitation; LVEDP, left ventricular end-diastolic pressure; AI, aortic insufficiency.

REFERENCES

For references, please visit **www.TheAnesthesiaGuide.com**.

CHAPTER 87
CABG/OPCAB

Jennie Ngai, MD

BASICS

- Revascularization of coronary arteries to treat CAD
- Grafts used can be venous (saphenous, harvested from the legs) or arterial (radial, internal mammary, gastroepiploic artery)
- Can be done using CPB or off-pump (outcomes are equivocal, dependent on technique)
- Decision-making criteria for on-pump versus off-pump is evolving

PREOPERATIVE

- What is the exercise tolerance?
- What symptoms are present? Angina, dyspnea, fatigue
- What relieves the symptoms? Rest or medications?
- Results of cardiac catheterization, echo, stress test? What is the LVEF? Which vessels are occluded?
  - ‣ Knowledge of coronary anatomy (Figure 87-1)
    - ▪ Right coronary sinus anterior and left coronary sinus lateral and slightly posterior

FIGURE 87-1. Coronary anatomy

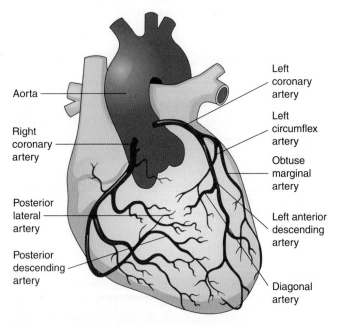

FIGURE 87-2. Typical perfusion beds of the epicardial coronary arteries

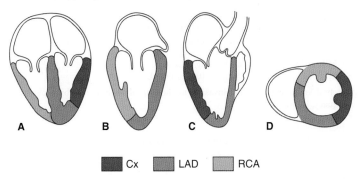

The above graphic demonstrates the midesophageal four-chamber view (A), the midesophageal two-chamber view (B), the midesophageal long-axis view (C), and the transgastric mid short-axis view. The different views provide the opportunity to observe the myocardium supplied by each of the three main coronary vessels, the left circumflex (Cx), the left anterior descending (LAD), and the right coronary artery (RCA). Areas of impaired myocardial perfusion are suggested by the inability of the myocardium to both thicken and move inwardly during systole. Image D is very useful for monitoring in the operating room because left ventricular myocardium supplied by each of the three vessels can be seen in one image. (Modified from: Shanewise JS, Cheung A, Aronson S, et al. ASE/SCA guidelines for performing a comprehensive intraoperative multiplane transesophageal echocardiography examination; recommendations of the American Society of Echocardiography Council for Intraoperative Echocardiography and the Society for Cardiovascular Anesthesiologists Task Force for Certification in Perioperative Transesophageal Echocardiography. *Anesth Analg.* 1999;89:870–884, with permission.)

- The left coronary artery (LCA) divides into the left anterior descending coronary artery (LAD) and left circumflex artery (LCx)
  - LAD gives rise to the diagonal branches and supplies the anterior wall of the right ventricle, the anterior two-thirds of the interventricular septum, the anterior wall of the LV, and the ventricular apex.
  - LCx gives rise to the obtuse marginal branches and supplies the left atrium, and the posterior and lateral walls of the LV.
  - "Left main" designates a significant lesion in the LCA (high risk for ischemia affecting a large portion of the LV, causing rapid hemodynamic collapse and cardiac arrest).
  - "Left main equivalent" designates high-grade obstructions in both the LAD and LCx: same risk as patients with left main disease.
- Other significant medical problems? DM, chronic obstructive pulmonary disease (COPD), renal insufficiency
- What medications are being taken? Should they be discontinued (e.g., metformin)

MONITORING/EQUIPMENT

- Pulse oximetry
- EKG
- Arterial line (usually placed pre-induction)
- Central venous line (usually placed post-induction)
- ± Transesophageal echo
- ± Pulmonary artery catheter (PAC)
- ± Bispectral index (BIS)
- ± Cerebral oximeter
- Urine output
- Temperature

- External pacemaker available
- Cell saver (for OPCAB)
- Typical medications to have available:
  ‣ Phenylephrine (100 mg/250 mL) (400 μg/mL)
  ‣ Epinephrine (2 mg/250 mL) (8 μg/mL)
  ‣ Norepinephrine (2 mg/mL) (8 μg/mL)
  ‣ Milrinone (20 mg/250 mL) (80 μg/mL)
  ‣ Vasopressin (40 units/250 mL) (0.16 units/mL)

Cerebral oximetry is a noninvasive method to determine cerebral perfusion adequacy. If low, consider:
- Increasing the hematocrit
- Increasing the FiO_2
- Decreasing the minute ventilation to allow the $PaCO_2$ to rise
- Increasing the systemic pressure

INDUCTION

- Goal is to maintain hemodynamic stability (blood pressure [BP] and HR)
- Choose induction agents that will have minimal effect on contractility, systemic vascular resistance (SVR), hemodynamics
  ‣ If preserved LVEF, propofol could be used
  ‣ If decreased LVEF, prefer to use etomidate to minimize decrease in contractility and SVR
  ‣ Key is to titrate medications
- Maintain coronary perfusion pressure through the stenotic portion by treating aggressively any hypotensive episode
  ‣ CPP = AoDBP-LVEDP (coronary perfusion pressure = aortic diastolic blood pressure-left ventricular end diastolic pressure)
- Insert transesophageal echo (TEE)
- Insert CVL ± PAC
- Insert Foley
- Obtain baseline ABG and activated clotting time (ACT)

MAINTENANCE

- Goal is to maintain perfusion through coronaries
- Inhalation agents can protect against myocardial reperfusion injury; no N_2O
- Use of antifibrinolytics can decrease bleeding and use of blood products
  ‣ Aminocaproic acid, tranexamic acid
- Use a balanced anesthetic technique to achieve fast-track status
  ‣ If no complications or significant comorbidities, decision can be made for fast track
  ‣ Patient should be able to be extubated within 6 hours of completion of surgery
- Use of high opiate doses reserved for critically ill cardiac patients
- Hold ventilation during sternotomy to reduce risk of lung injury
- Determination of inadequate coronary perfusion pressure:
  ‣ TEE—wall motion changes (most sensitive)
  ‣ EKG—ST changes
  ‣ PAC—increase in PA pressure, increase in pulmonary capillary wedge pressure (PCWP), large a waves, large v waves (least sensitive)
- Issues with on-pump CABG:
  ‣ Hemodilution from pump prime
  ‣ Release of inflammatory mediators from exposure to pump tubing
  ‣ Risk of awareness during CPB because of anesthetic dilution
  ‣ Movement during CPB
  ‣ Myocardial preservation
  ‣ "Pump head" (cognitive dysfunction following CPB, probably due to microdebris and microbubbles)

TABLE 87-1	Differences Between On and Off-pump CABG	
	On-pump CABG	Off-pump CABG
Monitors	A line, CVP, ±PAC, ±TEE, BIS, cerebral O_2, ECG, sPO_2, $ETCO_2$	A line, CVP, PAC, ±TEE, BIS, cerebral O_2, ECG, sPO_2, $ETCO_2$
Fluid administration	Restrict fluids; retrograde autologous prime; hemodilution when on-pump	Give fluids to prevent hemodynamic instability when lifting heart
Temperature	Let temperature drift down since cooling during CPB	Maintain temperature to keep patient normothermic
Ventilation	Turn off vent when full CPB, turn vent on before coming off CPB	Keep vent on during entire procedure
Blood pressure	Maintain CPP, mean arterial pressure (MAP) 50–70	Watch for drop in pressure when lifting heart; may need to change position of heart; if pt does not tolerate (Vfib), may need to go on CPB. Proximal anastomoses–SBP 80–90s. Distal anastomoses–SBP 110–120s
Heart rate	Not applicable	If HR is too high, can start esmolol (50–300 μg/kg/min) or diltiazem (3–5 mg/h) infusion to assist ease of anastomosis
Arrhythmias	Not applicable	May start lidocaine infusion to increase threshold for arrhythmias
Heparinization	Goal ACT >450; initial heparin dose 300 units/kg	Goal ACT 250–>450; surgeon preference; initial heparin dose 100–300 units/kg; check ACT q30 min
Heparin Reversal	Give protamine after completion of CPB to return to baseline ACT	Give protamine after completion of grafts to return to baseline ACT
Fast track	If no problems during case, should be fast tracked and extubated within first 6 h	If no problems during case, should be able to be extubated at end of case

NB: for further details on the management of CPB, refer to chapter 85.

- Even if the planned procedure is off-pump, you should still monitor, obtain vascular access, and anesthetize the patient as if you were going to go on-pump. If the patient does not tolerate the procedure off-pump, CPB will need to be initiated to complete the procedure safely
- Signs that patient is not tolerating OPCAB:
  ‣ Decreased systemic perfusion
  ‣ Increased PA pressure
  ‣ Wall motion changes
  ‣ EKG changes

May need to re-position the heart to allow better perfusion, administer fluid to decrease venous obstruction, or may need to institute CPB
- After revascularization:
  ‣ Check for ECG changes
  ‣ Check for wall motion abnormalities on TEE
  ‣ Check for elevated PA pressures
  ‣ Check flow through grafts with flow probe

POSTOPERATIVE

- Similar to other cardiac cases, transport to ICU with full monitoring
- Determine hemodynamic stability, bleeding, level of vasoactive medications needed
- Obtain labs and CXR
- Analgesia—opiates, IV acetaminophen, caution with NSAIDS due to risk of bleeding
- Ability to extubate
- If friable tissues, avoid higher BP to prevent excessive bleeding

REFERENCES

For references, please visit **www.TheAnesthesiaGuide.com**.

CHAPTER 88
Valve Surgery

Jennie Ngai, MD

VALVE LESIONS CAN BE CONGENITAL OR ACQUIRED

Congenital and Acquired Valvular Lesions	
Examples of congenital valvular disease	Examples of acquired valvular disease
• Bicuspid aortic valve—aortic stenosis (AS), aortic regurgitation • Congenital mitral stenosis • Marfan's—aortic regurgitation • Pulmonic stenosis • Mitral cleft (atrioventricular canal defect)—mitral regurgitation	• Rheumatic heart disease—mitral stenosis, mitral regurgitation, AS, aortic regurgitation • Mitral valve prolapse—mitral regurgitation • Myocardial infarct, papillary muscle rupture—mitral regurgitation • Mitral annular calcification—mitral stenosis, mitral regurgitation • Elderly—AS • Ascending aortic aneurysm—aortic regurgitation • Endocarditis—mitral regurgitation, aortic regurgitation

- Left-sided valve lesions are more poorly tolerated than right-sided lesions
- The valves can be either regurgitant or stenotic
  ‣ Regurgitation can be caused by a perforation, vegetation, chordal tear, prolapsed or redundant leaflet tissue, widened annulus, or coaptation failure due to restricted leaflets
  ‣ Stenosis is mainly due to calcified leaflets; if the valve is fused (e.g., bicuspid aortic valve), then it may become calcified

HEMODYNAMIC PARAMETERS

Hemodynamic Management of Patients with Valve Lesions				
Pathology	Afterload	Preload	Heart rate	Contractility
Aortic stenosis	Maintain	Maintain	Low normal (50–70 bpm)	Maintain
Aortic regurgitation	Decrease	Maintain	High normal (70–90 bpm)	Maintain
Mitral stenosis	Maintain	Maintain	Low normal (50–70 bpm)	Maintain
Mitral regurgitation	Decrease	Maintain	High normal (70–90 bpm)	Maintain

- Over 90% of pulmonic valve lesions are congenital
- Right-sided lesions will follow the same principles as left-sided lesions. However, if pulmonary hypertension is present, pulmonary vascular resistance (PVR) will be much more difficult to manipulate than systemic vascular resistance (SVR). Maintaining oxygenation and providing adequate ventilation is extremely important for these patients

Hemodynamic Management for Right-Sided Valve Lesions				
Pathology	Afterload	Preload	Heart rate	Contractility
Tricuspid stenosis	Maintain	Maintain	Low normal	Maintain
Tricuspid regurgitation	Decrease	Maintain	High normal	Maintain
Pulmonic stenosis	Maintain	Maintain	Low normal	Maintain
Pulmonic insufficiency	Decrease	Maintain	Normal (60–80 bpm)	Maintain

AORTIC STENOSIS (AS)

- Hypertrophy of left ventricle (LV) from increased workload
- Maintain afterload to perfuse the coronaries. Decreasing the afterload will decrease the coronary perfusion pressure. A higher perfusion pressure is also needed due to the LVH, with a thicker myocardium
- Keep the heart rate lower to allow more time in diastole to perfuse the coronaries, and to fill thick and stiff LV (LVH). The duration of systole does not change with HR
- It is also important to keep the patient in sinus rhythm. Patients with LVH are more dependent on atrial contraction (LV filling) for cardiac output. Normally, atrial contraction will contribute 20% to cardiac output, but in patients with LVH, it can contribute up to 40%
- In severe AS, a spinal anesthetic would be contraindicated because of the drop in afterload that usually occurs. Whether an epidural would be safe is controversial: the drop in afterload is somewhat less abrupt but still present
- Administering sedation would be appropriate, if carefully monitored. Increasing levels of sedation could result in dramatic decreases in afterload
- Appropriate monitoring should always be a consideration, no matter what the surgery. Minor surgery under GA in a patient with severe AS still requires invasive monitoring

AORTIC INSUFFICIENCY

- Dilated LV due to increased volume because of regurgitation
- Decreasing the afterload will decrease the amount of regurgitant flow back into the LV. However, sufficient afterload should still be maintained to allow adequate coronary perfusion pressure
- A higher heart rate is beneficial because it will shorten diastole, decreasing the regurgitation time
- The type of anesthetic and level of monitoring is not as critical as in AS

MITRAL STENOSIS

- Maintenance of afterload is extremely important, as it is for AS
- Patients may be in sinus rhythm, or atrial dysrhythmia due to an enlarged left atrium
- Usually the LV has a normal ejection fraction
- Very important to keep heart rate lower to allow more time for the ventricle to fill through a smaller mitral valve
- A spinal anesthetic would be contraindicated in a patient with severe mitral stenosis, because of the drop in afterload. Epidural anesthesia is controversial. A careful GA or local anesthesia with mild sedation would be more tolerable

MITRAL REGURGITATION

- Decreases in afterload are better tolerated, as in aortic insufficiency
- Higher heart rate is beneficial
- The type of anesthetic and level of monitoring will be determined by the surgical procedure

SURGICAL INDICATIONS

- Surgery to fix a valvular lesion should be performed when the lesion is severe, but prior to deterioration of the heart function
  ‣ For example, severe mitral regurgitation (MR) should be repaired prior to LV dysfunction
  ‣ Severe AS should be replaced if symptomatic, if having other cardiac surgery, or if LV systolic dysfunction is present
- Valves can be either repaired or replaced. This is determined by factors like age, comorbidities, compliance, and issues with anticoagulation
  ‣ Briefly, a repair of the valve leaves the native valve in place. The damaged portion of the valve is resected and repaired. The surgeon may place a band or ring in place at the level of the annulus. A repaired valve can last for many years. The patient is usually not anticoagulated. Usually, only valves that are regurgitant can be repaired
  ‣ Stenotic valves are always replaced, as the calcified leaflets are immobile and unrepairable. (If not calcified, surgical or balloon commissurotomy can be an option.) The native leaflets are removed, the annulus is debrided and the prosthetic valve is sutured in place
    • A bioprosthetic, or tissue valve, can last up to 10–15 years, and patients usually are not anticoagulated beyond a few weeks postoperatively
      ♦ Ross procedure: Aortic valve replaced by patient's own pulmonic valve; pulmonic valve replaced by bioprosthesis.
    • A mechanical valve can last up to 20 years (thus indicated in patients with longer life expectancy), but patients need to be anticoagulated indefinitely

For patients with valvular disease having noncardiac surgery:
- Determine severity of valvular disease
- If the valve lesion is severe, it is possible that the valve should be fixed prior to the nonemergent noncardiac surgery
- Level of monitoring should be determined by severity of valve lesion, not only by surgical procedure
- General anesthesia can be safely used for any valve lesion
- Local anesthesia with sedation can also be used if the surgical procedure is amenable
  ‣ Level of sedation should be carefully monitored
  ‣ Hypoventilation can increase PA pressures
  ‣ Increasing levels of sedation will decrease afterload
  ‣ Consider converting to general anesthesia if escalating level of sedation
- Regional anesthesia can be used safely if mild or moderate valve disease
- Neuraxial anesthesia should be avoided if severe aortic or mitral stenosis because of the resulting vasodilation

PREOPERATIVE

- Preoperative evaluation of patients should be similar regardless of what procedure the patient is about to have. It can indicate the severity and acuity of the lesions, and may require further workup
- What symptoms are present? Chest pain, dyspnea, fatigue
- What is the exercise tolerance?
- What relieves symptoms? Rest or medications
- Results of cardiac catheterization, echo, stress test
- Other significant medical problems

ECHO ASSESSMENT FOR SEVERE VALVE LESION

Echocardiographic Assessment of Severe Left-Sided Valve Lesions				
Valve lesion	Aortic stenosis	Aortic regurgitation	Mitral stenosis	Mitral regurgitation
Clinical Symptoms	Angina, dyspnea, syncope, heart failure, fatigue, ↓exercise tolerance	Dyspnea, fatigue, orthopnea	Fatigue, ↓exercise tolerance, dyspnea, cough, wheezing	Fatigue, chronic weakness, exhaustion
Valve area	<1 cm²		<1 cm²	
Mean gradient	>40 mm Hg		>10 mm Hg	
Vena contracta width		>0.6 cm		>0.7 cm
Regurgitant fraction		>50%		>50%

Right-sided lesions

Echocardiographic Assessment of Severe Right-Sided Valve Lesions			
Tricuspid stenosis	Tricuspid regurgitation	Pulmonic stenosis	Pulmonic regurgitation
Valve area <1 cm²	Vena contracta >0.7 cm	CW Doppler peak velocity >4 m/s	Color jet fills outflow tract
CW Doppler velocity >2.5 m/s CW mean gradient >5 mm Hg	Systolic flow reversal in hepatic veins	CW Doppler Peak gradient >60 mm Hg	Dense CW Doppler with steep deceleration slope

CW Doppler, continuous wave Doppler.

MONITORING

Monitoring is dependent on the type of anesthetic chosen and the planned procedure. The following list is for cardiac surgery.

- Pulse oximetry
- EKG (5 lead)
- Arterial line (pre-induction)
- Central venous line
- Transesophageal echo (standard of care for valve surgery)
- ± Pulmonary artery catheter
- ± Bispectral index (BIS)
- Cerebral oximeter (institution-dependent)
- Urine output
- Temperature

INDUCTION

- Goal is to maintain hemodynamic stability
- Choose induction agents that will manipulate the hemodynamics to favor the lesion
  - ▸ For example, if a patient has AS, etomidate may be a better induction agent because it preserves afterload and coronary perfusion pressure
  - ▸ If a patient has MR, propofol may be a good induction agent because it will decrease afterload, and thus decrease regurgitant flow
  - ▸ Careful titration of the induction agent is as important as the choice of agent

MAINTENANCE

- Choose an anesthetic technique that does not compromise cardiac function
- Maintenance can be achieved with a balanced technique using inhalation agent, opiate, and muscle relaxant
- Continue anesthetic technique that favors valvular lesion until cardiopulmonary bypass (CPB) initiated
- Monitor using ECG, transesophageal echo (TEE), PA pressures for signs of intolerance

POST BYPASS

- Use TEE to check
  - ▸ Valve function for residual regurgitation or stenosis
  - ▸ Left atrium and ventricle for presence of air
  - ▸ Ventricular function
- Check for bleeding, coagulopathy
- Correct activated clotting time (ACT) and ABG abnormalities
- Continue to warm patient to normothermia
- Stenotic lesions, once corrected, usually do not need inotropic support
- Regurgitant lesions, however, may need inotropic support

POSTOPERATIVE

- Transport to ICU intubated and monitored
- May need volume administration
- Continue to monitor for bleeding, pericardial tamponade

PEARLS AND TIPS

- A thorough echo examination should be performed before and after all valve repairs
- A low cardiac output may not always be from hypovolemia or decreased contractility. It could also result from systolic anterior motion of the mitral valve (SAM, see chapter 20). In this case, the anterior leaflet of the mitral valve gets swept into the left ventricular outflow tract during systole, preventing blood from flowing out of the heart. Increasing inotropic support will worsen the situation. An echo examination will show the anterior leaflet blocking the LVOT and turbulent flow instead of laminar flow in the LVOT. The treatment is volume, decrease in inotropy, beta-blockers if necessary
- The best way to determine if inotropic support is necessary is to look at ventricular function with the echo. If the function is poor, then an inotrope will be necessary to come off of CPB. Also, a cardiac output can be measured with the pulmonary artery (PA) catheter, either continuously or by thermodilution

REFERENCES

For references, please visit **www.TheAnesthesiaGuide.com**.

CHAPTER 89
Heart Transplantation

Meghann M. Fitzgerald, MD and Sumeet Goswami, MD, MPH

PREOPERATIVE REVIEW

- Routine work up including history of previous heart surgeries
- Presence and status of mechanical assist devices, pacemakers, and automatic internal cardiac defibrillators

INDUCTION AND MAINTENANCE

- Pre-induction: insert A-line using local anesthesia and minimal sedation if needed. Patients should receive immunosuppressive therapy, usually consisting of azathioprine and corticosteroids
- Consider "gentle" rapid sequence based on NPO status
- Induction should focus on minimizing negative inotropy; usually achieved with a combination of etomidate, opioids, and benzodiazepines
- Post-induction: Pulmonary artery catheter (prefer left IJ, as right IJ will be used for serial myocardial biopsies, and subclavian lines can kink with sternal retraction) and TEE
- Maintenance is achieved with a combination of volatile anesthetics on cardiopulmonary bypass (CPB) as tolerated, opioids, and benzodiazepines

BASIC SURGICAL TECHNIQUE

- Orthotopic transplantation: Standard biatrial or bicaval technique followed by end-to-end aortic and pulmonary anastomoses
- Pacemaker/ICD explanted as part of the surgery
- Heterotopic transplantation (rare) utilized in donor-recipient size disparity and irreversible pulmonary hypertension

SEPARATION FROM CPB

- Managing right ventricular failure and pulmonary hypertension is the key as the donor right ventricle is very sensitive to increased afterload
  - An inotrope (usually milrinone 0.375 µg/kg/min) is usually started prior to separation from CPB. Based on TEE findings, a second inotrope, such as dobutamine (3–5 µg/kg/min) or epinephrine (1–2 µg/kg/min) might be added
  - If, despite two inotropes, the patient continues to exhibit signs of RV failure (high CVP, low cardiac index, poor RV systolic function, high dose pressors), then pulmonary vasodilators such as inhaled nitric oxide and inhaled iloprost may be needed. The advantage of nitric oxide over iloprost is that it does not cause any systemic vasodilatation
  - Mechanical assist devices may be necessary to augment right heart function, if despite inotropes and pulmonary vasodilators, the patient continues to exhibit signs of RV failure
- Left ventricular failure can be similarly managed with inotropes and mechanical assist devices. Post-CPB management focuses on maintenance of adequate preload without right ventricular distention and management of coagulopathy

POSTOPERATIVE COURSE

- Extubation is achieved in the ICU, when hemodynamic stability is established and there is no bleeding requiring reexploration
- Inotropic support is gradually weaned over days and invasive monitoring withdrawn
- Antirejection and immunosuppressive regimens are instituted immediately

IMMUNOSUPPRESSIVE THERAPY

Triple therapy

- Calcineurin inhibitor that blocks interleukin-2 gene transcription (cyclosporine A, Tacrolimus [Prograf])
- Purine synthesis inhibitor (azathioprine [Imuran] or mycophenolatemofetil [Cellcept])
- T-cell dependent immunity suppression, inhibition of interleukin-2 production (methylprednisolone)

The adverse effects of these drugs consist of immunodeficiency resulting in infection and malignancy, and nonimmune toxicities such as diabetes, hypertension, and renal insufficiency. Monoclonal antibodies—interleukin-2 receptor blockers (basiliximab [Simulect], daclizumab [Zenapax]) have been used for induction therapy. They appear to decrease the risk of early postoperative rejection without increasing infection.

Grading and surveillance via serial endomyocardial biopsies.

Long-term course

- Median survival after heart transplant is 10 years
- Mortality risk is the highest in the first 6 months after transplant
- In the first year the common causes of death includes; non-CMV infection, graft failure, and acute rejection
- At 3–10 years the common causes of death include: graft failure, malignancy, and cardiac allograft vasculopathy

NONCARDIAC SURGERY IN HEART TRANSPLANT RECIPIENT

Physiology of transplanted heart

- The transplanted heart is a denervated organ but intrinsic cardiac mechanisms are preserved. With time some degree of functional reinnervation is reestablished
- The resting heart rate is high (90–110) as vagal tone is lost
- Tachycardia in response to stress is blunted
- The heart is also exquisitely sensitive to loading conditions
- Because of lack of afferent innervation, these patient's ischemia due to coronary allograft vasculopathy can be silent

Preoperative assessment

- ECG: Two P waves might be seen
- Echocardiography: To assess ventricular function
- Laboratory test: To assess: blood cell count to rule out bone marrow suppression, renal function, and main electrolytes
- Continue ongoing immunosuppression

Intraoperative management

- Both general and regional anesthesia can be performed as long as preload is maintained
- Medication must be based on degree of liver and renal dysfunction
- Drugs with direct pressor or chronotropic effects are required (e.g., avoid ephedrine and vagolytics)

Postoperative care
- Attention to preload, renal function, and infection
- Continue immunosuppression

REFERENCES

For references, please visit **www.TheAnesthesiaGuide.com**.

CHAPTER 90
Open AAA Surgery

Megan Graybill Anders, MD and Harendra Arora, MD

BASICS

- Large intra-abdominal surgery with rapid hemodynamic changes and potential for high blood loss
- Goal is to maintain intravascular volume and perfusion to brain, myocardium, kidneys, and central nervous system while controlling hemodynamics to prevent rupture
- Indications for repair include size >5.5 cm (>4.5 cm in women), expansion >0.5 cm in 6 months, or presence of symptoms
- Common comorbidities include CAD, PVD, chronic obstructive pulmonary disease (COPD), and HTN
- Mortality from elective repair <5% (outcomes better with vascular surgeons at high-volume centers), mortality from emergent repair of rupture >50%
- Endovascular repair has short-term mortality benefit for high-risk surgical candidates (e.g., severe CAD or COPD), although studies suggest equivalent long-term survival

PREOPERATIVE

- Evaluate and optimize coexisting disease to define and minimize risk
- Continue β-blocker therapy; if initiating therapy, titrate dose gently, to HR <70 while avoiding hypotension
- Continue or consider initiating statin therapy, which may reduce perioperative cardiovascular complications by reducing inflammation and stabilizing plaques
- Noninvasive evaluation of left ventricular (LV) function (e.g., echocardiogram) may be considered for patients with dyspnea of unknown origin or history of heart failure with worsening clinical status and no evaluation within 12 months
- Cardiac testing is recommended if it will change management; however, prophylactic coronary artery revascularization via percutaneous coronary intervention (PCI) or CABG before vascular surgery has not been shown to improve short- or long-term survival. (CARP trial, 2004)
- Brief list of equipment and drugs to prepare besides usual GA setup:
  - Possibly DL ETT if TAAA, with fiberoptic scope to check placement
  - Lumbar drain kit, if CSF drainage intended (discuss with surgeon)
  - A-line, CVL/Cordis, ± pulmonary artery catheter (PAC)
  - Transesophageal echo (TEE) if possible
  - Epidural kit

- ‣ Cell saver
- ‣ Rapid infuser device
- ‣ Upper-body warming device only (do not rewarm ischemic lower extremities)
- ‣ Nitroprusside (50 mg in 250 mL: 200 µg/mL; 0.5–10 µg/kg/min)
- ‣ Nitroglycerin (50 mg in 250 mL: 200 µg/mL; 0.5–10 µg/kg/min)
- ‣ Esmolol (2,500 mg in 250 mL: 10 mg/mL; 50–200 µg/kg/min)
- ‣ Norepinephrine (4 mg in 250 mL: 16 µg/mL; 1–10 µg/min)
- ‣ Phenylephrine (20 mg in 250 mL: 80 µg/mL; 0.2–1 µg/kg/min)

MONITORING

- Per ASA standards, plus preinduction arterial line (side with highest NIBP) and central venous line 8.5 Fr. at least
- Consider PAC for patients with systolic dysfunction (may help guide intra- and postoperative fluid therapy)
- Consider TEE for patients with at-risk myocardium on preop stress test (may help identify evolving wall motion abnormality) or severe LV dysfunction
- SSEP monitoring may help diagnose evolving spinal cord ischemia (especially with supraceliac cross-clamp, prolonged hypotension, known low origin of spinal accessory artery) and can help advise need for bypass or arterial reimplantation during procedure

INDUCTION OF ANESTHESIA

- Consider placing mid-thoracic (T8-9) epidural preop for postop pain control. Usually, epidural not used until after unclamping because of risk of extreme hypotension. Many vascular patients are on antiplatelet medications that will preclude neuraxial anesthesia
- Lumbar drain may be placed for patients at higher risk for paraplegia (Crawford type I or II aneurysm; see chapter 91)
- Select induction agent appropriate for patient's cardiac function
- Aim to minimize hemodynamic swings during induction and laryngoscopy (consider intratracheal lidocaine, have short-acting drugs such as nitroprusside, esmolol, and phenylephrine available for bolus)
- Double-lumen ETT may be required for lung isolation with higher (thoraco-abdominal) aneurysm repair

ANESTHETIC MAINTENANCE

- General or combined general-epidural anesthesia (intraoperative epidural dosing may be limited by hemodynamic instability)
- Anticipate blood loss; utilize cell salvage devices, and ensure availability of blood products
- Maintain normothermia due to association between hypothermia and perioperative myocardial infarction (MI), infection, and coagulopathy. Do not use forced-air warmers below the level of aortic cross-clamp due to increased injury to ischemic tissue. Upper-body warmers should be used
- Risk of acute renal failure 3–13%, even with infrarenal clamping. Renal function may be preserved by
  - ‣ Minimizing cross-clamp time (ideally less than 30 minutes)
  - ‣ Ensuring adequate intravascular volume
  - ‣ No evidence supports the administration of furosemide (Lasix), mannitol, or "low-dose" dopamine. Yet, it is common practice to give 12.5 g/70 kg of mannitol IV 10–15 minutes prior to cross-clamping and to initiate dopamine 3 µg/kg/min or fenoldopam 0.1 µg/kg/min

- Prevention of spinal cord ischemia (paraplegia 1% for low AAA to 7–40% for TAA and TAAA). The artery of Adamkiewicz originates most often between T9 and T12. Various strategies:
  - ‣ SSEP/MEP to identify spinal cord ischemia
  - ‣ Reimplantation of segmental vessels
  - ‣ Sequential aortic clamping
  - ‣ Shunt or bypass to maintain distal perfusion
  - ‣ CSF drainage via lumbar drain
  - ‣ Epidural cooling
  - ‣ Hypothermic circulatory arrest

FIGURE 90-1. Blood supply to the spinal cord

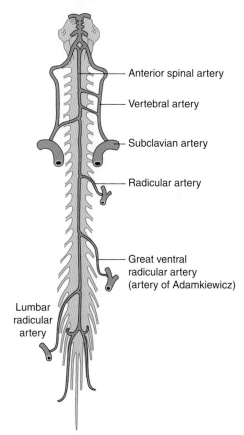

Reproduced from Waxman SG. *Clinical Neuroanatomy*. 26th ed. Figure 6-5. Available at: www. accessanesthesiology.com. Copyright © The McGraw-Hill Companies, Inc. All rights reserved.

FIGURE 90-2. Pathophysiology of aortic cross-clamping (AoX)

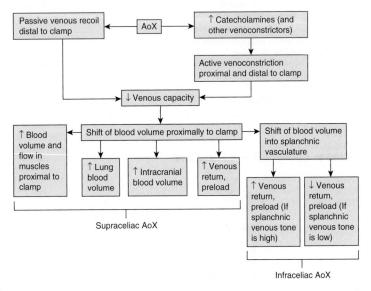

Reproduced with permission from Gelman S. The pathophysiology of aortic crossclamping and unclamping. *Anesthesiology.* 1995;82:1026.

- Aortic Clamping (Figure 90-2)
  ‣ Aortic cross-clamping causes an acute increase in afterload and LV strain, can cause LV failure or myocardial ischemia
  ‣ Nitroprusside (NTP 0.5–10 μg/kg/min) may be used to help to decrease afterload and blood pressure (BP)
  ‣ Nitroglycerin (NTG 0.5–10 μg/kg/min) decreases preload, leading to a decreased CO, and is a coronary vasodilator
  ‣ A combination of low-dose NTP and NTG infusion allows BP control and optimization of myocardial oxygen supply/demand balance; if good LV function, volatile agent alone can be enough
  ‣ Cross-clamp level affects intra- and postoperative course (renal microemboli and hypoperfusion, blood loss more severe with suprarenal clamp)
  ‣ Left heart bypass (aorto-femoral) may be used in high-risk patients (high clamp or low-cardiac reserve) to reduce afterload and improve distal perfusion
- Aortic unclamping (Figure 90-3)
  ‣ Release of cross-clamp results in reduced SVR, decreased venous return/ decreased CO, which often leads to hypotension, especially if hypovolemic; ensure adequate fluid administration, more or less vigorous depending on the level of the clamp
  ‣ Consider using norepinephrine (2–20 μg/min) or phenylephrine (0.2–1 μg/ kg/min) infusion. Caution as these will work better on vessels in the non-ischemic part of the body, causing blood redistribution
  ‣ Washout of products from anaerobic tissues below clamp can cause further vasodilation and hypotension
  ‣ With higher cross-clamp (and resultant liver/bowel ischemia), monitor pH closely and correct with sodium bicarbonate or tromethamine (THAM) if needed
  ‣ Gradual release of the clamp and reapplication have been recommended for fragile patients

FIGURE 90-3. Pathophysiology of aortic unclamping

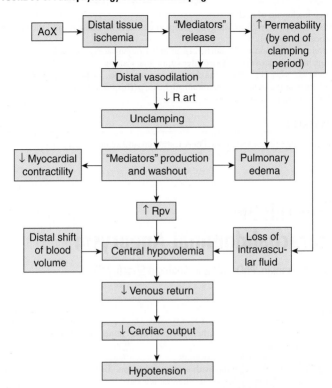

Cven, venous capacitance; Rart, arterial resistance; Rpv, pulmonary vascular resistance. Reproduced with permission from Gelman S. The pathophysiology of aortic crossclamping and unclamping. *Anesthesiology*. 1995;82:1026.

POSTOPERATIVE

- Consider early extubation if normal pH and temperature, no major ongoing fluid resuscitation, hemodynamically stable, and no severe underlying pulmonary disease
- Epidural analgesia if part of the plan. Epidural/intrathecal opioids have more downsides than advantages
- Follow renal function, support as needed
- Common and uncommon complications after AAA repair:
  ‣ Myocardial ischemia and infarction (most common)
  ‣ Renal insufficiency
  ‣ Respiratory failure
  ‣ Hemorrhage
  ‣ Gastrointestinal complications such as bowel ischemia
  ‣ Spinal cord ischemia
  ‣ Graft infection
  ‣ Sexual dysfunction
  ‣ Multiorgan failure
  ‣ Limb ischemia, commonly from distal embolization
  ‣ Stroke

PEARLS AND TIPS

- High likelihood of CAD
- Discuss the case with the surgeon preop, understand the anatomy and the planned procedure
- Level and duration of the aortic clamp affect organs at risk for ischemia/damage (e.g., higher risk of renal failure after suprarenal clamp)
- Avoid excessive HTN above the clamp to prevent stroke, LV failure, and myocardial ischemia; at the same time, maintain adequate perfusion to organs below the clamp (kidneys, bowel, spinal cord)

REFERENCES

For references, please visit **www.TheAnesthesiaGuide.com**.

CHAPTER 91
Thoracoabdominal Aneurysm

Ervant Nishanian, PhD, MD and Shahzad Shaefi, MD

BASICS

- Often associated with HTN, atherosclerosis, and connective tissue disorders such as Marfan syndrome
- Best surgical series has 10% mortality
- High risk of rupture along with aortic dissection. Untreated aortic dissection carries a 25–35% mortality within the first few days
- Comorbidities
  ‣ PVD
  ‣ CAD
  ‣ HTN
  ‣ Chronic obstructive pulmonary disease (COPD) (smokers)
  ‣ Renal impairment (independent predictor of postop renal failure and mortality)
- Anticipate potential for rapid large blood loss and hemodynamic shifts. Successful outcome requires maintenance of adequate cardiac output and flow to vital organs including the spinal cord while avoiding hypertension and aortic rupture
- Risk of paraplegia ≥3.5% blood as supply to the anterior spinal artery involved. Techniques to reduce incidence of paraplegia include:
  ‣ Epidural cooling of the spinal cord during surgery
  ‣ Cerebrospinal fluid drainage
  ‣ Reimplantation of intercostal arteries
  ‣ SSEP monitoring
  ‣ Provision of distal aortic perfusion during surgery with the use of atriofemoral (left atrium) bypass to the distal aorta
- Endovascular repairs are possible in patients that have appropriate anatomy. However, be prepared to convert to open procedure

FIGURE 91-1. Classification of aortic dissection and thoracoabdominal aneurysms

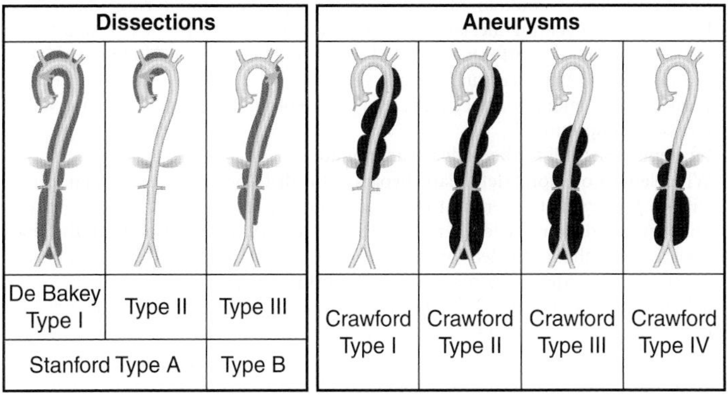

Dissections			Aneurysms			
De Bakey Type I	Type II	Type III	Crawford Type I	Crawford Type II	Crawford Type III	Crawford Type IV
Stanford Type A		Type B				

PREOPERATIVE

- Optimize comorbid conditions, anemia, renal function (consider HD if appropriate), pulmonary function (ideally stop smoking 4–6 weeks preop), and heart failure
- Coronary artery revascularization before elective vascular surgery does not change outcome and is not recommended. However, a cardiac echo is useful to evaluate other cardiac pathology; β-blockade and statins as appropriate
- The TAAA can distort the left mainstem bronchus; study CXR and CT-scan to predict difficulty with double-lumen ETT (DLETT) insertion
- Notify blood bank for extra RBCs, FFP, and platelets to be available
- Brief list of equipment and drugs to prepare besides usual GA setup:
  ‣ DLETT (or Univent, or bronchial blocker), with fiberoptic scope to check placement
  ‣ Lumbar drain kit, if CSF drainage intended (discuss with surgeon)
  ‣ A-line, CVL/cordis, ±pulmonary artery catheter
  ‣ TEE
  ‣ Epidural kit
  ‣ Cell saver
  ‣ Rapid infuser device
  ‣ Upper-body warming device only
  ‣ Nitroprusside (50 mg in 250 mL: 200 μg/mL; 0.5–10 μg/kg/min)
  ‣ Nitroglycerin (50 mg in 250 mL: 200 μg/mL; 0.5–10 μg/kg/min)
  ‣ Esmolol (2,500 mg in 250 mL: 10 mg/mL; 50–200 μg/kg/min)
  ‣ Norepinephrine (4 mg in 250 mL: 16 μg/mL; 1–10 μg/min)
  ‣ Phenylephrine (20 mg in 250 mL: 80 μg/mL; 0.2–1 μg/kg/min)

ACCESS AND MONITORING

- Right radial artery and femoral or dorsalis pedis pressure monitoring
- Internal jugular central line, large peripheral venous access with 7-Fr rapid infusion catheter (RIC), rapid infuser capable of 50 mL/min; consider a "double stick", that is, placing two introducers in the same vein
- Consider a pulmonary artery catheter if left ventricle (LV) systolic and diastolic function compromised
- Intraoperative TEE for hemodynamic monitoring
- When left atriofemoral (left heart) bypass to the distal aorta is used, a rapid infuser will keep up with the removal of blood from the left heart. The bypass circuit removes blood from the left heart and leaves it empty. The ejection from the heart is all the flow that is needed for the head and upper extremities. The rapid infuser provides for an adequate stroke volume to perfuse the brain
- Spinal drain placed at L4-5. Fluid is allowed to drain to keep CSF pressure <10–12 mm Hg. Be vigilant, as excess CSF removal can lead to subdural hematoma formation
- SSEP/MEP monitoring can warn that anterior spinal artery blood flow is compromised

INDUCTION OF ANESTHESIA

- Most people have cardiac pathology; a cardiac anesthesia induction with 10 µg/kg fentanyl and 0.1 mg/kg midazolam is prudent. The goal is to avoid large pressure swings across the aortic aneurysm wall
- Prevent unnecessary stimulation during laryngoscopy
- Insertion of double-lumen tube to facilitate surgical exposure through a left thoracotomy and collapsing the left lung is an absolute indication. Theoretical use of a right-sided DLT may be preferential due to surgical manipulation near the carina and/or aneurysmal encroachment. Fiberoptic confirmation of tube placement is mandatory. A Univent ETT or a bronchial blocker can be used, especially if the patient is to be kept intubated postop

MAINTENANCE OF ANESTHESIA

- Inhalational agents to maintain anesthesia if blood pressure allows
- Total intravenous anesthesia (TIVA) may be necessary if SSEP/MEP monitoring is being used (see spine surgery chapter)
- Consider acute normovolemic hemodilution if not anemic. Ensure adequate intravascular volume
- Monitor LV volume with TEE during LAFA (left atrial-femoral bypass, see below)
- Rapid infuser connected with large diameter tubing to peripheral RIC line and IJ line. Adjust vasopressors and vasodilators to fine-tune blood pressure (BP) at various points of surgery
- Have cell-saver device available in anticipation of large blood loss

AORTIC CROSS-CLAMPING

- Have rapid infuser circuit primed before cross-clamping aorta
- Cross-clamping will increase afterload; magnitude of effect depends on placement site
- Heart may fail, good to do test clamping to see if higher coronary perfusion pressure or an inotrope (like milrinone 0.375–0.75 µg/kg/min and or dobutamine 3–10 µg/kg/min) will be needed; common to see wall motion abnormalities and/or diastolic dysfunction on TEE
- BP and heart rate control. Sodium nitroprusside (0.3–10 µg/kg/min) and esmolol (50–200 µg/kg/min) are very short-acting and have a quick on/off effect. Nitroglycerin or nicardipine can also be used. Do not drop BP too much, as coronary and brain perfusion might suffer

- Pre-emptive venodilation with nitroglycerin (10–30 µg/min)
- Consider mannitol 0.5 g/kg prior to cross-clamp, may have renal protective effects (controversial). Fenoldopam (0.03–0.1 µg/kg/min) and bicarbonate have also been used for renal and mesenteric perceived effects
- Best outcomes with cross-clamp time less than 30 minutes
- Monitor spinal fluid pressure, as it may rise acutely with elevation of CVP during cross-clamping
- Once clamped, distal pressure monitored through pedal arterial line and nonpulsatile pressure controlled with the LAFA bypass circuit
- Pressure above the cross-clamp monitored with right radial arterial line and pressure adjusted with drugs, but this territory above the clamp does not have a great deal of smooth muscle to regulate pressure. Essentially, stroke volume and heart rate will determine CNS perfusion pressure

LEFT ATRIAL TO FEMORAL ARTERY BYPASS (LAFA)

- Initiate *before* aortic cross-clamping to off-load LV and minimize need for vaso-dilators
- LAFA provides distal flow at the expense of decreasing preload to left ventricle
- Coronary, brain, and upper extremity flow depends on intrinsic cardiac output during LAFA
- TEE assessment of LV filling helps guide fluid administration
- Rapid infusion of balanced RBC with FFP is essential to maintain preload during aggressive LAFA bypass
- Adequate distal aortic pressure along with spinal fluid drainage will prevent spinal cord ischemia
- Spinal cord cooling has also been successful in preventing spinal cord ischemia

AORTIC UNCLAMPING

- May produce hypotension and metabolic acidosis from the washout of ischemic lower body
- Maintain coronary perfusion pressure with volume (whole blood) and pressors (norepinephrine 1–10 µg/min)
- Follow ABG and lactate levels to ensure adequate systemic perfusion
- Correct any electrolyte issues and maintain adequate oxygen carrying capacity
- Keep SBP 105–120 mm Hg to avoid excessive stress on suture line

POSTOPERATIVE

- Particular note must be paid to cardiac, respiratory, renal, mesenteric, and neuro-logical systems
- Often multidrug antihypertensive management must be initiated in the short-term postoperative period
- Respiratory failure is common (50%) due to comorbidity, incision, and occasional hemidiaphragmatic paralysis
- Spinal drain kept in situ for 24–48 hours, or longer if neurology equivocal. CSF drainage has been shown to improve lower extremity paresis
- Frequent lower extremity exams (perfusion and neurologic function)
- Renal failure is a marker of poor prognosis

REFERENCES

For references, please visit **www.TheAnesthesiaGuide.com**.

CHAPTER 92
Anesthesia for Endovascular Procedures

Jamey J. Snell, MD and Brooke Albright, MD

NB: also see chapter on CEA in Neuro section for more details

BASICS

Endovascular Procedures			
	Carotid procedures	Aortic procedures	Peripheral/other vessel procedures
Types	Carotid artery stenting and angioplasty	Endovascular repair of abdominal (AAA), thoracic (TAA), or thoracoabdominal (TAAA) aortic aneurysms	Angiography, percutaneous transluminal angioplasty (PTA) ± stenting, intra-arterial thrombolytic therapy, embolectomy or stenting for subclavian, renal, iliac, femoropopliteal, or mesenteric arteries as well as venous procedures (TIPS,[1] inferior vena cava (IVC) stenting, etc.)
Indications	Revascularization for stroke prevention; endovascular is alternative to open CEA (e.g., if history of neck radiation)	Exclusion of aneurysms to prevent rupture or rupture repair	Revascularization from atherosclerotic or thromboembolic etiology to treat limb claudication, peripheral vascular disease, congestion, and organ hypoperfusion
Open vs. endovascular	Similar long-term risk of major stroke, slightly higher risk of minor stroke in endovascular; therefore, CEA still considered standard-of-care	Endovascular compared to open surgical approach may offer advantage of reduced postop pain, recovery time, and morbidity related to cross-clamping and large incisions; however, device failure and complications from device placement are unique complications; especially superior when significant comorbidities are present	
Morbidity and mortality	Typically secondary to cardiac, renal, and neurologic insults		

[1]Transjugular intrahepatic portosystemic shunt.

PREOPERATIVE

Preoperative Assessment for Endovascular Procedures			
	Carotid procedures	Aortic procedures	Peripheral/other vessel procedures
History and physical	Ask about exercise tolerance, comorbidities, preexisting neurologic deficits, iodine/contrast allergies; examine heart, lungs, and nervous system		
Cardiac risk assessment	• Review workup of clinical risk factors increasing perioperative morbidity and mortality (ischemic heart disease, cerebral vascular disease, Cr > 2, heart failure, etc.) and pulmonary function • Request additional workup if patient has limited functional capacity with >1 risk factor, information would change management, if data are missing or not updated since functional decline • Prophylactic coronary revascularization prior to surgery not superior to perioperative maintenance of medical therapy of CAD (β-blockers, statins, aspirin) in all patients; wait 6 weeks if pt underwent recent revascularization		
Labs	• Coagulation—pts may be on anticoagulants and will receive heparin intra-op • Creatinine—assess presence of acute or chronic renal insufficiency; also keep in mind the possibility of contrast-induced nephrotoxicity during the procedure • Hemoglobin/Hematocrit—to determine maximal allowable blood loss, especially if aneurysm rupture is suspected. Transfusion threshold of Hb 10 g/dL for patients with IHD (ischemic heart disease) or suspected CAD • Activated clotting time—need a baseline prior to heparinization • Type and cross—ensure active; may need 2 units available for larger procedures or if preop anemia		
Radiography	Cerebral angiography and duplex ultrasonography should be reviewed to assess for patency of Circle of Willis, contralateral carotid disease, and lesion characteristics	Review to appreciate size, location, involved branches, and plaque burden	Often does not change anesthetic management but assessment of disease extent and plaque burden may be of use if severe
Rx	Continue CAD therapy, except angiotensin-converting enzyme inhibitors (ACEI), hold oral hypoglycemic agents; insulin glargine dose should be halved the night before. If on antiplatelets, usually maintain perioperatively; however, consult w/surgeons and be mindful with regard to impact on neuraxial procedures (see chapter 119)		
Perioperative β-blockers	• Shown to reduce morbidity and mortality (most extensively studied in AAA patients). Mechanisms suggested: decrease myocardial oxygen demand, reduced pulsatile force on vessel walls, anti-inflammatory, plaque stabilization. • Greatest effect with longer duration of therapy before and after surgery; increased ischemic events when chronic therapy ceased prior to surgery • Class I recommendation to continue therapy for pts already on them • Class IIa recommendation to initiate therapy for pts deemed to be at high cardiac risk, titrated to HR (<85 bpm) and BP (based upon pt's baseline). Initiate low-dose titration >1 week prior to surgery. • Class III recommendation regarding routine initiation of high-dose β-blockers w/o titration • Most critical method to preserve efficacy is to avoid hypotension and relative bradycardia (<60–70 bpm) • Clonidine has been suggested as an alternative if β-blockers are contraindicated		
OR Safety	• Ensure adequate radiation protection equipment is available: lead apron, thyroid shield, transparent mobile lead shield, and radiation goggles • Survey the room beforehand to ensure that mobile fluoroscopic C-arms and OR tables do not interfere with or risk disconnecting anesthesia equipment		

ACCESS AND MONITORING

Access and Monitoring for Endovascular Procedures			
	Carotid procedures	Aortic procedures	Peripheral/other vessel procedures

Vascular access	• 2 Large bore (14–18G) peripheral IVs
	• Arterial line
	  ▸ Use right radial to allow left brachial access if needed for more proximal access
	  ▸ Indicated for continuous blood pressure monitoring and periodic blood sampling (ABG, activated clotting time (ACT), lactate, glucose for diabetics)
	  ▸ Consider placement prior to induction of anesthesia for pts w/ cardiac dysfunction
	• CVC or PAC
	  ▸ If indicated due to heart failure, valvular disease, pulmonary HTN, or other condition
	  ▸ May be used in TAAA or TAA repair since CVP≈CSFP (cerebrospinal fluid pressure) to calculate spinal cord perfusion pressure (SCPP) in lieu of lumbar drain		

Renal monitoring	Foley catheter to ensure urine output >0.5–1.0 mL/kg/h to prevent contrast-induced nephrotoxicity		
Neurologic monitoring	• Transcranial Doppler of the middle cerebral artery • Cerebral oximetry useful in patients undergoing carotid surgery under GA to dx ipsilateral ischemia from embolic phenomenon	• Lumbar drain to prevent anterior spinal cord syndrome for TAAA or TAA (see below) • Somatosensory and motor-evoked potentials may be employed to monitor for signs of spinal cord ischemia for TAAA or TAA • Requires avoidance of NMBDs (no re-dosing after intubating dose for MEPs); maintenance with total intravenous anesthesia (TIVA)—typically propofol (50–150 μg/kg/min) and remifentanil infusions (0.1–0.5 μg/kg/min)	
	Processed EEG (e.g., bispectral index [BIS]) monitoring useful in vascular procedures under GA with TIVA or to minimize volatile gas requirements due to hypotension or elderly pts sensitive to volatile anesthetics		
Anti-coagulation monitoring	ACT: point-of-care assay to determine anti-coagulation. Ensure you are familiar with the ACT device and it is functional and calibrated beforehand. "Normal" value based upon pt's baseline		
Cardiac monitoring	TEE: may be useful in TAA/TAAA to aid in identification of aneurysm anatomy, graft deployment, and graft leak		

Lumbar spinal drain
• Perfusion to spinal cord provided by 1 anterior spinal artery and 2 posterior spinal arteries—branches from the vertebral arteries
• Fed by contributions from segmental intercostal arteries from the thoracic aorta (artery of Adamkiewicz is the largest [T8-L1], which can be blocked or hypoperfused during TAAA or TAA repair)

- Consider prophylactic placement for high-risk TAAA or TAA repairs; risk of paraplegia as high as 8%
  - ▸ Extensive repair planned
  - ▸ History of prior aortic repair
  - ▸ Severe atherosclerosis of thoracic aorta
- Place at L3–5 with 17G Tuohy, secured 8–10cm beyond the tip of the needle, and connect to pressure transducer and sterile drainage bag. Zero at the level of the RA
- Traumatic placement: consider placement the day before to allow enough time for hemostasis in the event of a bloody tap; if occurs on day of surgery, delay 1–24 hours depending on urgency/circumstances
- Complications:
  - ▸ ICH (most morbid), hematoma, infection, catheter fracture, PDPH
  - ▸ Higher risk of ICH if excessive fluid drained, vascular anomalies, prior hx of cranial bleed, or atrophy
  - ▸ Safe to use in the setting of intraoperative anticoagulation when atraumatic
  - ▸ Use ASRA guidelines re: timing of placement after last dose of anticoagulation and removal
  - ▸ Do not leave in place >48–72 hours postop due to infection risk

INDUCTION

Induction of General Anesthesia for Endovascular Procedures

	Carotid procedures	Aortic procedures	Peripheral/other vessel procedures
General anesthesia	• Allows decreasing cerebral metabolic rate/oxygen consumption via anesthetic agents, hyperventilation, and redistribution of blood flow to ischemic regions • Avoid succinylcholine, coughing, or bucking due to increase in ICP • Avoid hypotension to prevent cerebral hypoperfusion	• Avoid tachycardia, hypertension, coughing, or bucking to reduce risk of aneurysm rupture • GA preferable in high-risk procedures, if massive transfusions anticipated, or risk for extensive groin or retroperitoneal dissection • Consider placement of DLT or Univent ETT for possible thoracotomy • Some retrospective studies suggest mortality benefit in high-risk pts, decreased LOS, and ICU admissions with local or regional. However, potential selection bias prevents clear demonstration of superiority	Typically chosen if pt unwilling or unable to tolerate regional or sedation (i.e., OSA) or for airway protection.

	• Increase risk of hypotension, increased IVF/pressor requirements, and postoperative pulmonary dysfunction in at-risk patients
	• Maintain hemodynamic stability
	  ▸ Goal is to avoid significant hypotension or hypertension (within 20% of baseline MAP)—although the former is more deleterious so err on the higher side
	  ▸ Slow administration of propofol (1–1.5 mg/kg) or etomidate (0.2 mg/kg) ± augmentation with volatile anesthetic during bag-mask ventilation
	  ▸ Fentanyl (2–4 μg/kg) to blunt cardiovascular response to laryngoscopy
	• Laryngeal mask airway (LMA) is acceptable in appropriate patients		

MAC and Regional Anesthesia for Endovascular Procedures

	Carotid procedures	Aortic procedures	Peripheral/other vessel procedures
MAC/local + sedation	Allows for communicating with patient to monitor cerebral function	MAC may be unpleasant for pt due to length of procedure, position intolerance, abdominal pain w/ adequate aortic dilatation or angioplasty	Typically done under local ± sedation if tolerated.
	• Vascular access via the femoral artery at the groin allows for infiltration of local anesthetic w/ MAC for most endovascular procedures • MAC offers advantage of being most hemodynamically stable • Be prepared to convert to general if pt becomes uncooperative/disinhibited during MAC • Pts may suffer discomfort from urethral catheterization, limb ischemia at clamping the access artery, or vessel angioplasty		
Regional/ neuraxial	Cervical plexus block + light sedation allow best neuromonitoring with patient awake	• Safe w/ intra-op anticoagulation if placement is not traumatic and other risk factors not existent • Usage of epidural may allow for usage for postop pain if converted to open w/ GETA; however, thoracic level typically needed • Neuraxial anesthesia via thoracic epidural may provide myocardial protection in patients with CAD by decreasing myocardial oxygen demand	• Studies for open procedures suggest regional anesthesia increases duration of graft patency (unclear whether this applies to endovascular procedures) • Most often, patients present on Plavix/ Ticlid and neuraxial block is contraindicated
	• Lumbar epidural can be placed to achieve a T10 dermatomal level for groin access • Titrate local anesthetic slowly for hemodynamic stability • Regional offers advantage of shorter hospital stay, less cardiopulmonary compromise, and more hemodynamic stability than general • Safe to perform despite anticoagulation if guidelines followed		

All anesthetic modalities available for most procedures–choice of modality ultimately based upon pt's surgical considerations, patient preference, and comorbidities.

MAINTENANCE

Maintenance of Anesthesia for Endovascular Procedures

	Carotid procedures	Aortic procedures	Peripheral/ other vessel procedures
Heparinization	Required prior to arterial access, (100 IU/kg in divided doses to check ACT or single bolus) to achieve ACT 250–300s to prevent thrombosis activation by intravascular devices		
Vascular access	Femoral or brachial artery	Femoral artery	
	All endovascular procedures present the risk of retroperitoneal bleeding and hemorrhage, requiring open conversion and potentially massive transfusion of blood products		

(continued)

Maintenance of Anesthesia for Endovascular Procedures (*continued*)

	Carotid procedures	Aortic procedures	Peripheral/ other vessel procedures
Surgical events	Retractable sieve or umbrella may be placed upstream of the angioplasty or stent prior to deployment to reduce traumatic release of microemboli	• Transient endoluminal obstruction of the aorta occurs at the time of stent-graft deployment (or aortic balloon inflation), which may create rapid increase in afterload • Hypotension may be requested during stent placement, down to MAPs of 50 mm Hg for the thoracic and 60–70 mm Hg (or SBP <100 mm Hg) for the abdominal aorta • Be aware of any branch vessels (i.e., renal, mesenteric, etc.), which may be compromised by graft to monitor for organ ischemia	
Cardiovascular	• *Bradycardia:* may occur at the time of carotid dilation, treat w/ glycopyrrolate or atropine • *Hypotension:* treat w/ α-agonist to maintain baseline MAP/SBP at or above preinduction baseline (~60–70/ 120–160 mm Hg)	• *Hypertension:* use nitroglycerin, nitroprusside, nicardipine, or esmolol to maintain MAPs 50–70 mm Hg • *Aneurysm rupture:* conversion to open with massive transfusion of blood products • *Endograft leak:* may require re-op or conversion to open	• *Hypertension:* avoid to reduce bleeding at access site • *Ischemic reperfusion syndrome:* hypotension, acidosis, hyperkalemia, myoglobinuria, and ATN
	If history of CAD/IHD, monitor ST changes on EKG, keep HR <100 with β-blockers		
Renal	• Contrast-induced nephropathy: most effective treatment is adequate hydration • Consider using *N*-acetylcysteine, sodium bicarbonate, acetazolamide, or mannitol in high risk patients		
Neurologic	• *Cerebral ischemia:* As a result of air, cholesterol emboli, or hypotension. Monitor via direct patient communication, cerebral oximetry, SSEPs, or TCD. Treat by decreasing cerebral metabolic rate/oxygen consumption and increasing cerebral perfusion. Treat seizures w/ benzodiazepines, barbiturates, or propofol.	• *Spinal cord ischemia:* ▸ maintain CSFP <10 mm Hg or SCPP >60 mm Hg ▸ 10–15 mL/h of CSF drained intermittently	

POSTOPERATIVE

Postoperative Management After Endovascular Procedures	
	Potential complications
General	• Significant incidence of complications in immediate postop period with potential for immediate re-op • Continue β-blockers and statins; antiplatelet therapy per surgical team • *Hematologic:* obtain initial postop coags and CBC for potential trending of occult bleeding; reversal of heparin with protamine may be indicated. Check groin site for swelling/hematoma/hemostasis or abdomen for distention/tenderness, suggesting retroperitoneal bleed • *Cardiac:* if prior history of cardiac dysfunction, check EKG, troponins; monitor closely for signs of CHF or myocardial ischemia; avoidance of hypothermia is important to reduce postop myocardial ischemia • *Renal:* continue to measure urine output as a marker for occult bleeding and reduce contrast-induced nephropathy • *Neuro:* establish baseline neurologic exam to allow for assessment of stroke or ischemic neuropathy
Carotid procedures	• *Postoperative hyperperfusion syndrome:* characterized by headache, seizure, focal deficits, edema, and potential intracranial bleed as a result of prolonged hypertension. Treat by lowering BP • Neurologic complications as mentioned above
Aortic procedures	• *Postimplantation syndrome:* noninfectious hyperinflammatory response, characterized by fever, leukocytosis, and coagulopathy • *Spinal cord ischemia:* may require emergent therapeutic placement of lumbar drain in addition to raising blood pressure to increase SCPP. Discuss anticoagulation with surgical team first • If spinal drain in use, continue to monitor for need for continued drainage. Remove within 48–72 h according to ASRA guidelines, or start prophylactic antibiotics • Endoleak, graft migration, occlusion of branch vessels, and aneurysmal rupture, all require emergent surgical intervention
Peripheral vascular procedures	• *Thrombosis:* temperature, color, pain, neurologic exam, and Doppler can all be used to assess for continued vascular patency.

PEARLS AND TIPS

• Always be prepared for the possibility of converting to an open procedure
• Be aware of your institution's massive transfusion protocol
• Optimal management requires involvement of the anesthesiologist extending beyond the typical perioperative period
• Surveillance of multiple physiologic monitors, lab values, and devices can be overwhelming if aortic procedures become complex—use of a time table may help to organize tasks and ensure parameters are not exceeded
• Have a high index of suspicion and low threshold for imaging and contacting surgical teams for postop complications

REFERENCES

For references, please visit **www.TheAnesthesiaGuide.com**.

CHAPTER 93
Tamponade

Tony P. Tsai, MD

PATHOPHYSIOLOGY

- Occurs when fluid or clots accumulate *rapidly* in the pericardial space, decreasing pericardial compliance; a large amount of pericardial fluid can accumulate over an extended period of time without causing tamponade
  - ‣ Ventricular compliance is decreased, leading to *decreased diastolic filling and decreased stroke volume*
  - ‣ *Systemic venous return is impaired* and as RA and RV collapse occurs, blood accumulates in the venous circulation, which further decreases cardiac output and venous return
  - ‣ In the extreme, *pressures equalize* in all heart cavities, with no blood flow
- Compensatory mechanisms:
  - ‣ Tachycardia to maintain cardiac output
  - ‣ Increased vascular resistance to maintain BP
  - ‣ Spontaneous ventilation, by decreasing intrathoracic pressure on inspiration, facilitates RV filling and ejection
- Three phases of hemodynamic changes
  - ‣ Phase I: Increased stiffness of ventricle due to pericardial fluid accumulation, requiring a higher filling pressure (LV and RV filling pressures >intrapericardial pressure)
  - ‣ Phase II: Pericardial pressure increases above ventricular filling pressure, resulting in decreased cardiac output
  - ‣ Phase III: Cardiac output decreases even more because of equilibration of pericardial and LV filling pressures
- Medical emergency, needs to be treated immediately to avoid death
- *Any acute hemodynamic deterioration in a patient post cardiac surgery should lead to an emergent re-exploration*, unless another obvious cause is present

DIAGNOSIS

Symptoms include
- Dyspnea, tachypnea; patient typically sitting
- Tachycardia
- Peripheral hypoperfusion with oliguria
- Pulsus paradoxus, with decreased pulse amplitude on inspiration
- Beck's triad: increased jugular venous pressure, hypotension, and diminished heart sounds

Echocardiogram: *best diagnostic tool.*
- There can be a circumferential fluid collection, or sometimes a single clot compressing the RA
- Right heart compression
- Interventricular septum flattening (RV impairing LV filling)

CXR: cardiomegaly, water-bottle-shaped heart, or pericardial calcifications; often normal 12-lead EKG findings suggestive of pericardial tamponade:
- Sinus tachycardia
- Low-voltage QRS complexes
- Electrical alternans (very specific but rare)
- PR depression in all leads

If the patient has a pulmonary artery catheter (PAC) (no indication to insert a PAC emergently)
- Low CO
- Equalization of CVP = RVEDP = PAP (diastolic)

TREATMENT

- Hemodynamic collapse
  - ▸ Emergent drainage at the bedside, ideally ultrasound-guided needle drainage (usually removing 100–200 mL of fluid is sufficient to relieve hemodynamic signs and symptoms)
  - ▸ Sternotomy re-exploration at bedside if post cardiac surgery
- If less critically ill, or after emergent drainage, a pericardial window or sclerosing of the pericardium can be performed surgically
- Supplemental oxygen
- Volume expansion to maintain preload
- Inotropic drugs can be useful to increase CO without increasing SVR (see Table 93-2)
- Avoid positive pressure ventilation because of the associated decrease in venous return; keep patient breathing spontaneously
- Repeat the echocardiogram and CXR within 24 hours

Anesthesia for pericardial window
- PreOp
  - ▸ Assess patient and stabilize hemodynamic status with goals of maintaining HR, preload, and afterload (i.e., fast, full, and tight) by giving crystalloids and using inotropes
  - ▸ Consider placing arterial line and PAC
  - ▸ Discuss type of procedure with surgeon and what depth of anesthesia is needed (local with minimal sedation or GA), consider draining fluid percutaneously prior to induction
- Intra-Op
  - ▸ If GA is planned, place standard ASA monitors, connect the arterial line and PAC (if placed), and make sure the surgical site is prepped and draped prior to induction
  - ▸ Consider inducing GA with ketamine at 0.5 mg/kg (max dose 2 mg/kg) and maintaining spontaneous ventilation over ETT (or LMA); also consider etomidate at 0.15 mg/kg (max dose 0.3 mg/kg) as an induction agent
  - ▸ Avoid inhalational anesthetics due to vasodilation, and avoid positive pressure mechanical ventilation until tamponade is relieved
- PostOp
  - ▸ If hemodynamically stable after drainage of pericardial effusion and meets criteria for extubation, remove the LMA or ETT
  - ▸ Maintain OR monitors in PACU or ICU (standard ASA, arterial line, PAC)
  - ▸ Patient may need continued inotropic support postoperatively

TABLE 93-1	Causes of Cardiac Tamponade
Cause	Percentage
Malignancy	30–60%
Uremia	10–15%
Idiopathic pericarditis	5–15%
Infectious diseases	5–10%
Connective tissue disorder	2–6%
Post-pericardiotomy syndrome	1–2%

TABLE 93-2	Vasopressors Used for Pericardial Window
Medication	Dose
Epinephrine	Start at 1 μg/min Max dose 20 μg/min
Norepinephrine	Start at 8–12 μg/min Max dose 30 μg/min
Vasopressin	Start at 2–4 U/h

CHAPTER 94
One-lung Ventilation

Jennie Ngai, MD

Indications for One-Lung Ventilation (OLV)	
Absolute	Relative

• Prevent contamination of healthy lung
  ▸ Purulence
  ▸ Bleeding
• Need for separate ventilation of lungs
  ▸ Bronchopleural fistula
  ▸ Unilateral bullae
  ▸ Tracheobronchial disruption
• Bronchoalveolar lavage (alveolar proteinosis)
• Video-assisted thoracic surgery
	• Lung resection
	• Thoracic aortic aneurysm surgery
	• Thoracic spine surgery
	• Esophageal surgery

DLETT Versus Bronchial Blockers	
DLETT	Bronchial blocker

• Allows separate ventilation/exclusion of lungs
• Complete and easy lung deflation
• Stable (but check position each time patient repositioned)
• If patient kept intubated, must be exchanged for SLETT at the end of surgery, or retracted into trachea
	• Allows exclusion of one lung, or ventilation of both lungs through the ETT lumen, but not separate ventilation
	• Small lumen; lengthy, incomplete deflation
	• Unstable
	• Becomes SLETT when bronchial blocker not in place
	• Specific relative indications:
	  ▸ Expected difficult intubation
	  ▸ Need for RSI
	  ▸ Severe hypoxemia
	  ▸ Postop ventilation

DLETT

Single-Lumen Tubes		
SLT size	ID (mm)	OD (mm)
7.0	7.0	9.6
7.5	7.5	10.2
8.0	8.0	10.9
8.5	8.5	11.5

For comparison, the inner (ID) and outer (OD) diameters (mm) of single-lumen and double-lumen tubes are listed.

Double-Lumen Tubes				
DLT size	Bronchial ID (mm)	Tracheal ID (mm)	OD (mm)	Patient height
35	4.3	5.0	11.7	<62 in.
37	4.5	5.5	12.3	63–68 in.
39	4.9	6.0	13	69–72 in.
41	5.4	6.5	13.7	>72 in.

There are left- and right-sided DLT—this refers to the bronchus the bronchial port should be in
• The right-sided DLT has a fenestrated bronchial cuff with a hole for the RUL

Left-sided DLT are most commonly used
• Easier to position
• Longer left mainstem bronchus between the carina and the left upper lobe (less likely to occlude LUL)
• Right bronchus shorter in length, risk of obstructing right upper lobe with bronchial balloon is much higher

Indications for right-sided DLT: Surgery involving left mainstem bronchus, or left pneumonectomy

FIGURE 94-1. Left-sided (on the left) and right-sided (on the right) double-lumen ETT

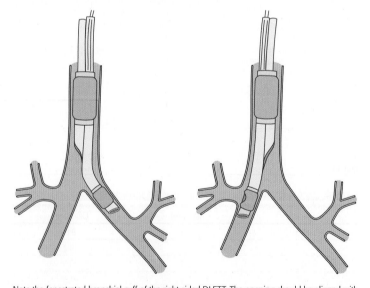

Note the fenestrated bronchial cuff of the right-sided DLETT. The opening should be aligned with the right upper lobe bronchus. Reproduced from Morgan GE, Mikhail MS, Murray MJ. *Clinical Anesthesiology*. 4th ed. Figure 24-6. Available at: www.accessmedicine.com. Copyright © The McGraw-Hill Companies, Inc. All rights reserved.

FIGURE 94-2. Technique of insertion of DLETT

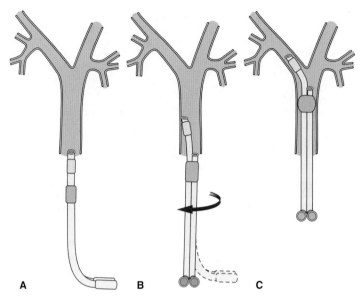

A　　　　　**B**　　　　　**C**

(A) The tube is inserted with the distal convexity facing down. (B) Once through the vocal cords, it is advanced AND rotated 90°C: the bronchial tip enters the left bronchus and resistance is felt when the DLT is in correct position. Reproduced from Morgan GE, Mikhail MS, Murray MJ. *Clinical Anesthesiology*, 4th ed. Figure 24-7. Available at: www.accessmedicine.com.

Placement of DLT can be more difficult than placement of SLT because of its larger size.

It can be placed using direct laryngoscopy, video laryngoscopy, or fiberoptic bronchoscope (FOB).

Be careful not to tear the tracheal balloon on the teeth while guiding the tip of the bronchial side into the trachea.

If using FOB, remove ETT connector prior to inserting FOB (to decrease ETT length)

Typically, the DLT will be at *29–31 cm on the lips in its final position*.

Correct position can be confirmed with *auscultation* of the lungs or with the *fiberoptic scope. Auscultation is not reliable*, and a FOB verification should always be performed (if FOB available).

Correct position should be *checked again each time the patient is repositioned* (e.g., from supine to lateral).

Auscultation technique to confirm placement of left-sided DLT (Figure 94-3)
- Inflate both balloons
  ‣ Check if DLT is in trachea; breath sounds should be heard on both sides
  ‣ DLT inserted too far
    ▪ If breath sounds are heard only on left side, both lumens are in the left bronchus
    ▪ If breath sounds are heard only on the right side, both lumens are in the right bronchus

FIGURE 94-3. Auscultation technique to confirm placement of left-sided DLT

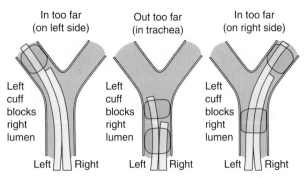

Procedure	Breath sounds heard		
Clamp right lumen (both cuffs inflated)	Left	Left and right	Right
Clamp left lumen (both cuffs inflated)	None or very ↓↓	None or very ↓↓	None or very ↓↓
Clamp left lumen (deflate left cuff)	Left	Left and right	Right

- Clamp the tracheal side
  ▸ Breath sounds should only be heard on the left side
  ▸ DLT not inserted far enough
    ▪ If breath sounds are heard only on the right side, the bronchial lumen is on the right
    ▪ If breath sounds are heard on both sides, the bronchial lumen is in the trachea
- Clamp the bronchial side
  ▸ Breath sounds should only be heard on the right side
  ▸ DLT not inserted far enough
    ▪ If breath sounds are heard only on the left, the bronchial lumen is on the right
    ▪ If breaths sounds are heard on both sides, the bronchial lumen is in the trachea

Fiberoptic technique to confirm placement of left-sided DLT (Figure 94-4)
- Place scope through tracheal lumen
- When exiting the DLT, the carina should be seen
- Bronchial lumen should be in left bronchus, and the bronchial balloon should be just visualized. Ideally, only inflate bronchial cuff under vision
- Direct the scope into the right bronchus to see the *RUL bronchus*
- It should be only 1–2 cm from the carina, have a very sharp angle as it comes off the right bronchus, and have *three divisions instead of two*
- Place the scope into bronchial lumen
- Ensure that the bronchial cuff does not herniate forward and occlude the bronchial lumen
- Ensure that the LUL bronchus is free

FIGURE 94-4. Fiberoptic technique to confirm placement of left-sided DLT. View from the tracheal lumen

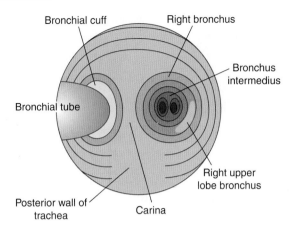

The bronchial lumen is seen in the left bronchus, and the bronchial balloon is just visualized, without herniation obstructing the right bronchus. Reproduced from Morgan GE, Mikhail MS, Murray MJ. *Clinical Anesthesiology*. 4th ed. Figure 24-9. Available at: www.accessmedicine.com. Copyright © The McGraw-Hill Companies, Inc. All rights reserved.

BRONCHIAL BLOCKERS

Bronchial blockers can be used with a regular ETT (Arndt and Cohen blockers) or be integrated into the ETT (Univent) (Figure 94-5)

They can *ONLY be placed with FOB guidance* (Figure 94-6)

FIGURE 94-5. Close-up of the tip of the Univent tube showing two lumens

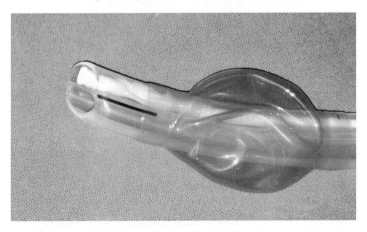

The small tube is retracted into the small lumen before intubation.

FIGURE 94-6. Sequential steps of the fiberoptic-aided method for inserting and positioning the Univent bronchial blocker in the left mainstem bronchus

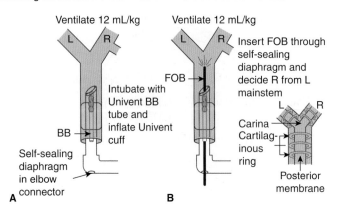

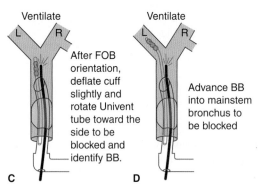

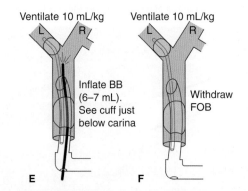

One- and two-lung ventilations are achieved by simply inflating and deflating, respectively, the bronchial blocker balloon. FOB, fiberoptic bronchoscope. Reproduced from Longnecker DE, Brown DL, Newman MF, Zapol WM. *Anesthesiology*. Figure 53-18. Available at: www.access anesthesiology.com. Copyright © The McGraw-Hill Companies, Inc. All rights reserved.

The Arndt blocker has a wire loop through which the FOB is passed in order to guide to blocker into the desired bronchus.

The Cohen blocker has a wheel proximally that allows deflecting the tip of the blocker.

EFFECTS OF LATERAL POSITION ON VENTILATION AND PERFUSION

- In lateral position, up to two-thirds of perfusion shifts to the dependent lung
- During spontaneous ventilation, a smaller increase in ventilation also occurs in the dependent lung→ limited ventilation-perfusion mismatch
- Under GA and mechanical ventilation, however, up to two-thirds of ventilation goes to the nondependent lung (path of least resistance)
- Opening the nondependent thorax further reduces ventilation to the dependent lung by facilitating expansion of the nondependent lung
- The net effect of these changes is
  ▸ Overperfusion relative to ventilation (or shunting) in the dependent lung
  ▸ Overventilation relative to perfusion (or dead-space ventilation) in the nondependent lung
- Left thoracotomy yields a higher PaO_2 during OLV than does right thoracotomy because the left lung normally receives 10% less blood flow than the right lung
- During OLV, all ventilation goes to the dependent lung, but all perfusion through the nondependent lung constitutes a shunt
- Hypoxic vasoconstriction (not opposed by anesthetic agents), lung collapse, and surgical occlusion of blood flow (pulmonary artery [PA] clamping, pneumonectomy) to the nondependent lung can reduce shunt and improve PaO_2 during OLV

MANAGEMENT OF OLV

Initial management of OLV anesthesia:
- Maintain two-lung ventilation as long as possible
- Use $FIO_2 = 1.0$
- Tidal volume, 8 mL/kg (8–12 mL/kg); keep peak pressures low, risk of barotrauma
- Adjust RR (increasing 20–30%) to keep $PaCO_2 = 40$ mm Hg
- No positive end-expiratory pressure (PEEP) (or very low PEEP, <5 cm H_2O)
- Continuous monitoring of oxygenation and ventilation (SpO_2, ABG, and ET CO_2)
- Hypoxic pulmonary vasoconstriction takes 20–30 minutes to shunt blood to ventilated lung

If severe hypoxemia occurs, the following steps should be taken
- Check DLT position with FOB
- Check hemodynamic status
- *CPAP (5–10 cm H_2O, 5 L/min) to nondependent lung, most effective (but can impair surgical exposure)*
- PEEP (5–10 cm H_2O) to dependent lung, least effective; can decrease BP, can worsen V/Q mismatch
- Intermittent two-lung ventilation
- Clamp pulmonary artery of operative lung ASAP
- NO or almitrine not effective

Other causes of hypoxemia during OLV
- Mechanical failure of O_2 supply or airway blockade
- Hypoventilation
- Resorption of residual O_2 from the clamped lung
- Factors that decrease SvO_2 (decreased CO, increased O_2 consumption)

POSTOPERATIVE VENTILATION

In some instances, the patient will need postoperative ventilation, yet not need separate lung ventilation via a double lumen tube.

Changing DLT to SLT:
- Perform direct laryngoscopy with standard laryngoscope or GlideScope to visualize airway for edema
- If vocal cords not visualized, keep DLT (see below)
- Suction oropharynx
- Place tube exchanger through tracheal lumen of DLT
- Deflate both the bronchial and tracheal cuffs
- Under direct visualization, pull DLT out and place SLT over tube exchanger

If there is too much edema, leave the DLT in:
- Suction oropharynx
- Deflate the bronchial and tracheal balloons
- Under direct visualization, pull the DLT back a few centimeters
- Both the tracheal and bronchial cuffs should be in trachea
- Reinflate tracheal cuff
- Elevate head of bed to decrease edema
- This is *uncomfortable* and *unstable*, and the patient should be kept well sedated
- At later time, the DLT can be exchanged for SLT, or the patient might be ready for extubation

Rarely, a patient may need *independent lung ventilation (ILV)* (Figure 94-7)
- ILV means that each lung is ventilated separately by a separate ventilator because of different compliance or airway resistance
- A DLT is indispensable
- Main indications: asymmetric lung disease or single-lung transplant

FIGURE 94-7. Each lumen of a double-lumen tube connected to separate ventilators

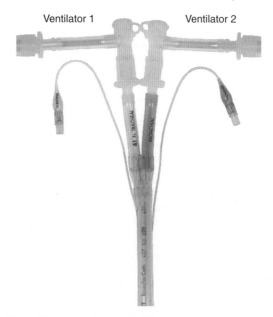

Ventilator 1   Ventilator 2

REFERENCES

For references, please visit **www.TheAnesthesiaGuide.com**.

CHAPTER 95
Thoracic Surgery

Meghann M. Fitzgerald, MD and Sumeet Goswami, MD, MPH

GENERAL CONSIDERATIONS

Preoperative

- Preoperative evaluation with cardiac risk stratification
  - Smoking history common
  - Impact of preoperative smoking cessation on outcome is unclear, but smoking cessation should be encouraged
  - Co-existing cardiovascular disease (CAD, HTN)
- If tumor
  - Review imaging studies (CT-scan) to assess extent of tumor spread, tracheal/bronchial deviation or compression, lung atelectasis
  - Assess for paraneoplastic syndrome

Intraoperative

- Monitoring
  - At least one large bore IV
  - A-line
  - CVL not routine; if significant blood loss anticipated, or for major lung resection, place CVL on side of thoracotomy (reduces impact of possible pneumothorax)
  - Pulmonary artery catheter (PAC) if indicated (significant pulmonary HTN, cor pulmonale, LV dysfunction); ensure that PAC tip is in the dependent lung, and especially not in the area to be resected; if pneumonectomy performed, inflate balloon carefully, as significant hemodynamic compromise can ensue (reduced vasculature cross-section)
- Analgesia: Thoracic epidural, paravertebral block, intercostal blocks
  - Very intense pain for 3–4 days following thoracotomy
  - Epidural gold standard for postop analgesia. Place at intended thoracotomy level, or 1–2 levels lower, prior to induction. Test-dose 3 mL 1.5% lido with 1:200K epi to rule out intravascular placement. Do not load preoperatively
  - Paravertebral block has the advantage of less/no sympathectomy and of not threatening the spinal cord; catheter placement possible
  - Intercostal blocks, level of thoracotomy and 2 level up and down (ropi 0.5% 5 mL/level), can be performed by surgeon under direct vision; limited duration
  - Cryoneurolysis takes 24–48 hours to be effective, but analgesia for over 1 month
- AFib prophylaxis:
  - Continue β-blockers if patient already on them; reduce dose if epidural (Class I)
  - Diltiazem reasonable if not on β-blocker preoperatively (Class IIa)
  - Amiodarone reasonable except for pneumonectomy (toxicity concerns) (Class IIa)
    - Lobectomy: 1,050 mg IV infusion over the first 24 hours after surgery (43.75 mg/h) then 400 mg PO BID × 6 days
    - Esophagectomy: 43.75 mg/h IV infusion (1,050 mg daily) × 4 days
  - Magnesium supplementation reasonable in combination with other medications (Class IIa)
  - Flecainide and digitalis not recommended (Class III)

- Induction: preoxygenation, IV induction adapted to patient's cardiovascular status
- Typically intubation first with SLETT to allow flexible bronchoscopy by surgeon; then exchange to DLETT
- One-lung ventilation: see chapter 94
  - ‣ Have multiple size DLETT available, FOB (for difficult airway as well as to verify ETT position), videolaryngoscope, etc. as needed
- Positioning: thoracic procedures (except for bilateral lung transplant) are performed in lateral decubitus. Dependent arm flexed, axillary roll, nondependent arm placed above head to pull scapula away from operative area; protect eyes and dependent ear, maintain neck neutral
- Maintenance: typically inhalational agent (minimal effect on hypoxic pulmonary vasoconstriction under 1 MAC) + opioid (sparingly if COPD) + NMB (to facilitate retraction); use high FiO_2 and no N_2O
- "Light" GA + epidural (load with 0.25% bupi/ropi in 5 mL aliquots)
- Deep anesthesia during rib spreading; possible vagal response at beginning of case, responsive to cessation of surgical stimulus, or IV atropine if fails
- Fluid management: restrict fluid as much as possible (only maintenance fluid + blood loss replacement), especially if lung resection; potential for dependent lung gravity-dependent transudation edema, and nondependent lung edema following surgical trauma and re-expansion
- End of case: re-expand manually all segments of collapsed lung; continue mechanical ventilation until chest tubes connected to suction

Postoperative

- Early extubation minimizes tension on suture lines and risk of pneumonia; if need to maintain intubated, consider replacing DLETT with SLETT
- Keep semi-upright, use incentive spirometry to minimize atelectasis
- Analgesia
  - ‣ Thoracic epidural: typically 0.125% bupi with 2–5 μg/mL of fentanyl, 3–4 mL/h with 3 mL bolus q15 minutes; monitor for hypotension (treat with pressors rather than fluids, unless prerenal ARF develops)
  - ‣ Epidural morphine (risk of respiratory depression, best avoided)
  - ‣ NSAIDs (risk of bleeding and renal injury)
  - ‣ Dexmedetomidine can be used as well (infusion 0.2–0.5 μg/kg/h IV)
- Thoracic drains kept in place until output less than 20 mL/d (surgeon-dependent) and no air leak
- Complications
  - ‣ Atrial fibrillation (10%)
  - ‣ Atelectasis, occasionally necessitating FOB suctioning
  - ‣ Air leak (7.2%); usually resolves after a few days, occasionally develops into bronchopleural fistula necessitating repair
  - ‣ Pneumonia (2.0%)
  - ‣ Respiratory failure (2.0%)
  - ‣ Empyema (1.3%)
  - ‣ DVT (0.7%)
  - ‣ Phrenic, vagus or left recurrent laryngeal nerve injury
  - ‣ Thoracic duct injury with chylothorax

LUNG RESECTION

Preoperative

- Lobectomy through the fifth or the sixth intercostal space is the procedure of choice for most lesions
  - ‣ Segmental or wedge resections are performed in patients with either small lesions or poor pulmonary reserve
  - ‣ Pneumonectomy is usually reserved for tumors extending into hilum or into the right or left main stem bronchus

- Poor prognosis criteria for high-risk patients undergoing pneumonectomy (also see Figure 4-5)
  - $PaCO_2$ >45 mm Hg, PaO_2 <50 mm Hg on room air
  - FEV_1 <2 L, Predicted postoperative FEV_1 <0.8 L
  - FEV_1/FVC <50% of predicted
  - Maximum breathing capacity <50% of predicted
  - Maximum oxygen consumption (VO_2) <10 mL/kg/min

Intraoperative considerations

- IV fluid restriction: lobectomy without significant blood loss typically receives no more than 1–2 L of crystalloid
- No chest tube after pneumonectomy; occasionally chest tube placed to withdraw fluid as needed to maintain mediastinum midline

Postoperative considerations

- Specific postoperative complications
  - Postoperative bleeding (rare)
  - Torsion of the lobe or segment (rare)

VIDEO-ASSISTED THORACOSCOPIC SURGERY (VATS)

- More and more procedures performed by VATS rather than open thoracotomy
- Indicated for lung biopsy, segmental or lobar resections, pleurodesis, and pericardial procedures such as pericardial window or pericardiectomy
- One-lung ventilation is mandatory for most procedures
- Usually no need for thoracic epidural

MEDIASTINOSCOPY

- Biopsy of mediastinal lymph nodes; establish either diagnosis or resectability of intrathoracic tumors
- Performed under general anesthesia with large bore intravenous access + A-line (left radial)
- Complications include:
  - Compression of the innominate artery (scope inserted between trachea and innominate artery) causing cerebral ischemia. Detected with pulse oximeter on the right hand
  - Recurrent laryngeal and phrenic nerve injury
  - Hemorrhage
  - Vagally mediated reflex bradycardia due to compression of the trachea
  - Pneumothorax
  - Air embolism

LUNG-VOLUME REDUCTION SURGERY (LVRS)

- Lack of demonstrated efficacy (NETT trial), but still being performed
- Explain risks to patient (lengthy, fluid shifts, possible transfusion)
- Thoracic epidural, A-line, and CVL ± PAC; TEE available, especially if poor cardiac function
- Avoid sedatives and limit systemic opioids
- Stress-dose steroid if indicated
- Ventilate with high VT, low RR, and long expiratory time (I:E ratio 1:3.5–4)
- Avoid hypothermia
- Extubate in OR, or as soon as possible
- Noninvasive ventilation with BiPAP if $PaCO_2$ >70 mm Hg postoperatively

ESOPHAGEAL SURGERY

- Common surgical procedures include endoscopy, esophageal dilatation, esophagectomies and ant reflux operations such as Nissen fundoplication
- High risk of aspiration due to obstruction, abnormal sphincter function or altered motility. Administer metoclopramide +H2-blocker or PPI preoperatively
- Rapid sequence induction for patients with moderate or severe GERD, or awake FOB intubation if difficult airway
- Esophagectomy
  - ▸ Depending on tumor location
    - Upper third: no thoracotomy; supine, abdominal, and cervical incision, gastric pull-through
    - Middle-third: combined laparotomy and right thoracotomy
    - Lower third: either esophagogastrectomy through left thoracotomy, or transhiatal esophagogastrectomy with gastric pull-through
    - If insufficient stomach length (upper third) or gastric disease, colon interposition in two stages
  - ▸ Typically malnourished patient, possibly dehydrated
  - ▸ Possible considerable blood loss and hemodynamic instability; A-line and 2–3 large bore IVs mandatory
  - ▸ Thoracic epidural if thoracotomy, consider even if abdominal and cervical incisions
  - ▸ Observe overnight in PACU or ICU, depending on co-morbidities
  - ▸ Usually need postop mechanical ventilation. If large amount of fluid administered, an easy airway can become difficult; ensure that vocal cords visualized by DL/videolaryngoscopy prior to exchanging DLETT for SLETT; otherwise, retract DLETT into trachea
  - ▸ Complications: injury to phrenic, vagus, and left recurrent laryngeal nerves

TRACHEAL RESECTION

- Airway obstruction: avoid sedatives, perform inhalation induction
- Left radial A-line preferable because of risk of innominate artery compression
- Either sterile ETT to ventilate lower portion of trachea after resection and before anastomosis (Figure 95-1), or HFJV
- Maintain neck flexed (often suture chin to chest) for 24–48 hours (Figure 95-2)
- Low tracheal lesions can necessitate CPB

FIGURE 95-1. Airway management of a high tracheal lesion

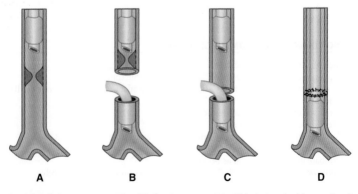

A B C D

FIGURE 95-2. Position of the patient before (A) and after (B) tracheal resection and reanastomosis with the patient's neck flexed for the first 24–48 hours

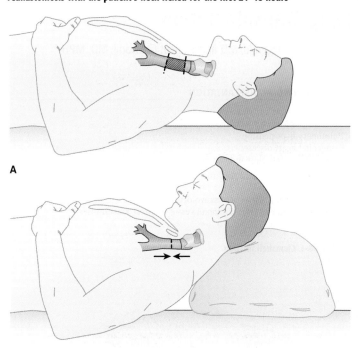

A

B

MEDIASTINAL MASSES

- Respiratory and cardiovascular compromise:
  - ‣ Airway obstruction, lung compression
  - ‣ Compression of PA, heart, SVC (SVC syndrome)
  - ‣ Involvement of recurrent laryngeal nerve and mediastinal sympathetic chain
  - ‣ Spinal cord compression
- Upright and supine flow-volume loops help evaluate the extent of airway obstruction
- If possible, obtain biopsy under local; if radiosensitive or chemosensitive, treat appropriately to decrease size preoperatively
- As a rule, *maintain spontaneous ventilation even under GA (ketamine induction/ maintenance)*
  - ‣ Loss of muscle tone might make ventilation impossible
- *Have rigid bronchoscope and CPB standby*
- *If possible, position patient semi-sitting*
- *Ensure ability to rapidly change position to lateral or prone in case of poor tolerance*

REFERENCES

For references, please visit **www.TheAnesthesiaGuide.com**.

CHAPTER 96
Lung Transplantation

Meghann M. Fitzgerald, MD and Sumeet Goswami, MD, MPH

BILATERAL LUNG TRANSPLANTATION

Often performed in candidates with:
- Chronic pulmonary infections
- Pulmonary hypertension
- Congenital heart disease
- Cystic fibrosis (absolute indication)

Usually performed via clamshell incision (Figure 96-1) and sequentially rather than en bloc as
- Cardiopulmonary bypass can be avoided
- Fewer complications with bronchial versus tracheal anastomoses

FIGURE 96-1. Clamshell incision

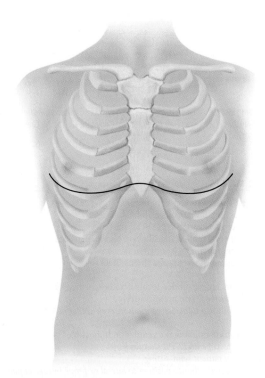

SINGLE-LUNG TRANSPLANTATION

Traditionally performed in candidates with
- COPD
- IPF

Poses challenges in postoperative ventilation and perfusion due to the discrepant compliance in the transplanted versus native lungs. Performed via thoracotomy in the fifth intercostal space.

PREOPERATIVE ASSESSMENT

Consider thoracic epidural for postoperative pain management in patients with lower likelihood of needing cardiopulmonary bypass during the procedure

Usually at least 6 hours notice prior to induction: patient NPO as for elective case

ANESTHETIC INDUCTION AND MAINTENANCE

Preinduction: A large bore IV and an arterial line.

Induction
- Consider 'gentle' rapid sequence induction based on NPO status
- Induction goals are to avoid increases in pulmonary vascular resistance and myocardial depression
- Induction is usually performed with a combination of midazolam, fentanyl, and etomidate
- PAC and TEE placed post-induction
- A single lumen endotracheal tube should be placed to enable an initial bronchoscopy to clear secretions, which will facilitate single-lung ventilation
- One-lung ventilation via a double lumen endotracheal tube

Maintenance
- Maintenance is achieved with cautious titration of volatile anesthetics, opioids, and benzodiazepines
- One-lung ventilation is needed to avoid cardiopulmonary bypass when performing sequential double-lung transplant or single-lung transplant
- One-lung ventilation may result in hypoxemia, hypercarbia, acidosis, and subsequent pulmonary hypertension and right ventricular compromise
- Clamping of the pulmonary artery, while improving oxygenation by decreasing shunt, may further increase pulmonary arterial pressures and compromise right ventricular function
- Norepinephrine and vasopressin may be required to maintain systemic hemodynamics
- In patients with pulmonary hypertension, milrinone (0.25–0.375 μg/kg/min) may be added to lower pulmonary vascular resistance and augment right ventricular function
- In case milrinone is insufficient, inhaled nitric oxide (20 ppm) may be added. Inhaled nitric oxide also helps improve V/Q mismatch and may reduce hypoxemia during one-lung ventilation
- Following pulmonary anastomosis, retrograde flow to wash out the pneumoplegia solution ensues, which may result in profound hypotension due to systemic vasodilation;
  ‣ Vasoactive support is usually necessary
  ‣ Avoid hypertension as it might result in pulmonary edema due to capillary leak
  ‣ Blood transfusion is helpful in maintaining blood pressure. Maintain hematocrit around 30
- Reinflation of the donor lung should be done manually on room air with low tidal volumes to minimize reperfusion injury and pulmonary edema
- During one-lung ventilation, SpO_2 >85% is tolerated to avoid cardiopulmonary bypass

- Later FiO_2 may be increased to maintain SpO_2 >94%
- Indications for initiating cardiopulmonary bypass
  - Severe hypoxemia
  - Hemodynamic instability
- If patient is hypoxemic after transplant, extracorporeal membrane oxygenation may be needed temporarily

POSTOPERATIVE COURSE

Immediate postoperative intensive care focuses on

- Maintaining intravascular volume and renal perfusion without causing pulmonary edema and compromising graft function
  - Aim for CVP of 6–8 and/or urine output of about 0.5 mL/kg/h
- Patients are usually kept intubated for about 12 hours or longer depending on the donor lung function
- May need bronchoscopy prior to tracheal extubation

IMMUNOSUPPRESSION

- Induction agents
  - IL-2 receptor blockers (basiliximab [Simulect], daclizumab [Zenapax])
  - Polyclonal antibodies (rabbit [Thymoglobulin] or horse [Atgam] anti-thymocyte globulin)
  - Monoclonal antibodies (muronomab CD3 [OKT3], alemtuzumab [Campath])
- Maintenance
  - Calcineurin inhibitors, blocks interleukin-2 gene transcription (cyclosporine A [Neoral, Sandimmune, Gengraf], Tacrolimus [Prograf])
  - Antimetabolites, purine synthesis inhibitors (azathioprine [Imuran], mycophenolatemofetil [Cellcept], mycophenolic acid [Myfortic])
  - Corticosteroids, T-cell dependent immunity suppression, inhibition of interleukin-2 production (methylprednisolone, prednisone)
  - m-TOR inhibitors (sirolimus [Rapamune])

Complications of Lung Transplantation	
Early	Late
Hyperacute rejection	Acute rejection
Acute rejection	Chronic rejection/bronchiolitis obliterans
Demyelinating disease (due to tacrolimus	(Bronchiolitis obliterans syndrome)
or cyclosporine)	Colonic perforation
Seizure disorder	Hyperlipidemia
Ectopic atrial tachycardia	Infection (EBV, CMV, HHV6, HHV9)
Infection (bacterial, viral, fungal, other)	Diabetes
	Hypertension
	Renal insufficiency/failure
	Post-transplant lymphoproliferative disease
	Kaposi sarcoma
	Osteoporosis
	Photosensitivity

SURVIVAL AND MORBIDITIES

Median survival after transplant is 5.3 years.

Leading causes of death in the first year are graft failure and non-CMV infections.

Leading causes of death following the first year are bronchiolitis obliterans syndrome and non-CMV infections.

REFERENCES

For references, please visit **www.TheAnesthesiaGuide.com**.

CHAPTER 97
Minimally Invasive Cardiac Surgery

Brad Hamik, MD and Ervant Nishanian, PhD, MD

BASICS

- Large range of surgical approaches, including:
  - Mini sternotomy, minimally invasive/thoracotomy, percutaneous valves (trans-femoral/transapical aortic valve insertion)
- Anesthetic management:
  - Need to accommodate surgical requirements
  - Be prepared to convert to open procedure

PROS AND CONS OF MINIMALLY INVASIVE TECHNIQUE

Pros and Cons of Minimally Invasive Technique	
Potential advantages	Potential problems
• Less trauma, smaller incisions	• Technically more difficult
• Reduced postoperative pain (except thoracotomy)	• If arterial or venous injury, need for expeditious full exposure
• Faster extubation, shorter ICU/hospital stay	• One-lung ventilation for some procedures and associated complications
• Faster return to normal activities	• Pain management issues if thoracotomy
• Cost savings	• Percutaneous valves: vascular injury, arrhythmias, device malfunction, device malpositioning, coronary occlusion, stroke
• Expanded patient inclusion	• Valvuloplasty: vascular injury, creation of regurgitant lesions, embolic events, short duration of symptom relief

Mini sternotomy: Open heart procedure with smaller incision

No significant difference from standard sternotomy procedure

MINIMALLY INVASIVE/THORACOTOMY

Thoracotomy approach mainly for aortic and mitral valve surgery

- Physiologic consideration—similar to mini sternotomy with some additional concerns
  - Neuro: potential cerebral blood flow changes with one-lung ventilation
  - Cardiovascular
    - Dysrhythmias
      - Hypercapnia may cause decrease in myocardial contractility and lower arrhythmia threshold
    - Right ventricular failure with one-lung ventilation and increased pulmonary vascular pressures

- Pulmonary
  - One-lung ventilation
  - Splinting and hypoventilation if thoracotomy pain not well controlled

Preoperative

- Double lumen ETT may improve surgical exposure
- Be prepared for standard sternotomy and need for cardiopulmonary bypass
- Arterial line and central venous access as with normal cardiac surgery

Induction

- Specific goals for blood pressure and heart rate will depend on specific patient and pathology
- Additional airway equipment available such as tube exchanger and fiberoptic scope

Maintenance

- Thorough transesophageal echo (TEE) evaluation pre-, intra-, and postoperatively
- Careful management of one-lung ventilation
- Vasoactive agents readily available
- Be prepared to convert to cardiopulmonary bypass (CPB) at any time

Postoperative

- TEE evaluation for adequacy of surgical repair
- Recovery in ICU
- More pain from thoracotomy
  - Multimodal analgesic regimen
  - Opioids, nonsteroidal anti-inflammatory drugs
  - Consider epidural and local anesthetics

PERCUTANEOUS VALVES

Transapical or transfemoral aortic valve
- Physiologic considerations
  - Neuro
    - Concern for embolic events during valve manipulation and deployment
    - Potential for one-lung ventilation and changes in cerebral blood flow with changes in $PaCO_2$
  - Cardiovascular
    - Dysrhythmias
      - Mechanical stimulation with guide wire during percutaneous procedures
      - Ventricular fibrillation initiated prior to valve deployment will cause changes in blood pressure which need to be anticipated
      - Hypercapnia may cause decrease in myocardial contractility and lower arrhythmia threshold.
    - Left ventricular failure with acute aortic insufficiency with valvuloplasty
    - Coronary ischemia if percutaneous valve deployment occludes coronary ostia
    - Right ventricular failure with one-lung ventilation and increased pulmonary vascular pressures
  - Pulmonary
    - One-lung ventilation and thoracotomy pain for transapical
  - Renal/Fluids/Electrolytes
    - Renal injury if dye used during percutaneous procedures

Preoperative

- Thorough history and physical
  - Evaluate pulmonary and cardiovascular status, acquire prior echo and catheterization reports
  - Evaluation of the size, tortuosity and calcification of peripheral arteries by angiography, CT, or MRI assists in choosing between transfemoral and transapical approaches
- Usually GETA. Double lumen ETT may improve surgical exposure for transapical aortic valve insertion AVR. Some centers perform transfemoral percutaneous procedures with sedation
- Peripheral vasculature needs to be evaluated to determine if patient is appropriate for transfemoral approach
- Prepare for standard sternotomy and need for cardiopulmonary bypass
- Obtain blood in room from blood bank (at least 2 U RBC)
- Clopidogrel 300 mg PO and ASA 325 mg PO prior to procedure

Monitoring

- Right radial A-line, TEE, and PAC
- External defibrillator pads applied
- TEE used to determine annulus size, degree of mitral regurgitation (MR), left ventricle (LV) function, and aortic root pathology
- Fluoroscopy and TEE is used to correctly position the introducer catheter in the aortic annulus
- Acute blood loss may occur during deployment device removal

Induction

- Short-acting opioid with midazolam (or etomidate) and rocuronium for smooth intubation, but possible extubation at end of case
- Avoid tachycardia and maintain coronary perfusion pressure. If moderate to severe aortic insufficiency (AI) present, avoid bradycardia as well
- Insertion of double lumen tube is NOT needed for transapical since apex of heart is close to 5th intercostal space

Maintenance

- Consider short acting agents (e.g., remifentanil) and inhalational agents (as tolerated) for percutaneous procedures
- Thorough TEE evaluation pre-, intra-, and postoperatively; mobile atherosclerotic plaques in the aorta may direct to a transapical instead of a transfemoral approach
- Careful management of one-lung ventilation
- Prepare for CPB at any time
- Keep patient warm

Intraoperative Course

- Femoral vein and artery access is obtained by the cardiologist/surgeon for anticipatory preparation for cardio pulmonary bypass (femoro-femoral CPB)
- Regardless of the approach, there are three rapid ventricular pacing (200 bpm) events; the first is testing of lead capture, followed by rapid pacing for balloon valvuloplasty and finally for prosthetic valve deployment. Vasopressor bolus (phenylephrine 40–80 µg) is commonly given prior to rapid pacing to offset hypotension
- Postimplantation TEE
  - Perivalvular and transvalvular regurgitation can be detected and quantified. These lesion if severe can be addressed with further balloon dilatation (perivalvular) or placing a second valve within the first (transvalvular)
  - Assess for aortic dissection, MR and LV function

Comparison of Retrograde Transfemoral Approach and Antegrade Transapical Approach for Aortic Valve Implantation		
	Retrograde transfemoral approach	Antegrade transapical approach
Method	• A ventricular pacing wire is passed into the right heart via groin access • 12F sheath inserted into femoral artery and a 20–23 mm balloon tipped valvuloplasty catheter is advanced over a wire that crosses the AV annulus. Blood pressure is artificially elevated with vasopressors prior to rapid pacing. Rapid ventricular pacing at 200 bpm will abolish forward cardiac output for 10 seconds and allow for proper valvuloplasty of the AV. 12F sheath exchanged for a 24 or 26F sheath and the device deployment catheter advanced retrograde across the AV annulus. Prosthesis position is finely tuned using fluoroscopy and TEE guidance prior to prosthetic final valve deployment during rapid ventricular pacing. Shortly after rapid pacing the heart function returns to baseline. • Valve function, location, and leaks are assessed immediately for any needed intervention	• Anterolateral mini-thoracotomy in 5th intercostal space over LV apex. Once the heart is exposed, epicardial pacing wires are placed A guide wire is placed into the LV apex and antegrade across the AV with fluoroscopy and TEE guidance. Wire should *not* enter mitral chordal apparatus! • 16F introducer sheath is placed over a wire and directed into the LVOT A valvuloplasty catheter is advanced through the LV apex and deployed during rapid ventricular pacing • A 33F sheath is exchanged and the device deployment catheter advanced and prosthetic valve deployed • Sheath removed and apical purse string sutures closed
Special precautions	• Fluoro root contrast injection and TEE monitoring for AI deterioration or aortic dissection!	• TEE monitoring for AI deterioration or aortic dissection!
Comments	Patch repair of femoral artery and or iliac vessels to close	• Intercostal nerve block with local anesthetic prior to closure of thoracotomy

Postoperative

- Patients can be extubated barring any intra-operative complication
- If uneventful, discharge after 1–2 days
- Patients receive clopidogrel 75 mg PO q day and ASA 81 mg PO q day for 6 months
- Significant mortality and morbidity in elderly patients with multiple comorbidities (typical candidates); comparison with surgical aortic valve replacement inappropriate
- Long-term outcomes not yet known

REFERENCES

For references, please visit **www.TheAnesthesiaGuide.com**.

PART VII

NEUROANESTHESIA / NEUROCRITICAL CARE

CHAPTER 98
ICP Monitoring, Acute ICP Increase

Alan W. Ho, MD and Mark Weller, MD

PATHOPHYSIOLOGY

- Intracranial pressure (ICP) = pressure exerted by the contents of the skull on the dura mater
- Normal ICP varies with age, body position, and clinical condition. Normal ICP is 5–15 mm Hg in a supine adult, 3–7 mm Hg in children, and 1.5–6 mm Hg in term infants
- Skull content includes brain tissue (compressible, ~83% by volume), blood (incompressible, ~6% by volume), and CSF (incompressible, ~11% by volume). In the event of increased ICP, compensation can occur by shifting either CSF or blood out of the intracranial compartment
- Intracranial hypertension over a critical threshold of 20 mm Hg is an independent predictor of poor neurological outcome after severe head injury

INDICATIONS FOR ICP MONITORING

- Pathological CT scan of the head with a Glasgow Coma Scale Score (GCS) of <9. Example of a pathological CT scan is one that shows hematomas, contusions, edema, herniation, or compressed basal cisterns (Figure 98-1)
- Normal CT scan and GCS <9 accompanied by two of the following: age >40, unilateral or bilateral motor posturing or systolic blood pressure <90 mm Hg

NB: A large body of clinical evidence supports the use of ICP monitoring to guide therapeutic interventions, detect intracranial mass lesions early, and assess prognosis in the setting of TBI.

FIGURE 98-1. Devices for ICP monitoring

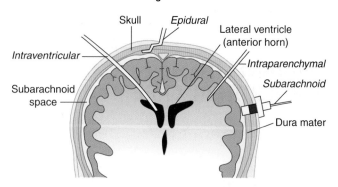

Various anatomic sites to monitor intracranial pressure: Extradural/epidural, subdural, intrapa-renchymal, intraventricular, lumbar subarachnoid. Reproduced from Hall JB, Schmidt GA, Wood LDH: *Principles of Critical Care*, 3rd Edition. Figure 65-8. Available at: www.accessmedicine.com. Copyright © The McGraw-Hill Companies, Inc. All rights reserved.

- *Intraventricular catheter/drainage (IVD)*
  - ‣ Gold standard for ICP monitoring. Thought to be the most accurate method
  - ‣ Requires placement of a catheter through a burr hole into the lateral ventricle; non-dominant hemisphere placement preferred (bleeding complications from insertion less likely to cause language disturbance)

Pros and Cons of Intraventricular Catheter	
Advantages:	Disadvantages:
• Direct pressure measurement	• Rate of infection ~5%
• Measures global pressure	• Risk of bleeding ~2%
• Accurate and reliable	• Placement can be difficult if the ventricles are shifted
• Allows therapeutic CSF drainage	out of place or compressed due to increased ICP
• In-vivo calibration possible	• Potential for leaks/blockages in the system →
• Allows adminstration of drugs	underestimates ICP
(i.e., antibiotics)	• Invasive method
• Relatively inexpensive	• Transducer adjustment needed with head
	movement

NB: Transduction of ICP while the CSF chamber is open to drainage is meaningless. The ICP should be transduced with the ventricular drain closed to drainage at least every 30–60 minutes for a 5- to 10-minute period with a recording of the ICP and CPP at the end of that time.
- *Subdural, subarachnoid screw/bolt*
  - ‣ Indicated if insertion of intraventricular drainage is difficult or impossible
  - ‣ Hollow screw inserted via a burr hole into the subarachnoid/subdural space

Pros and Cons of Subarachnoid Bolt	
Advantages:	Disadvantages:
• Placement is technically easier in circumstances of midline shift or compression of the intra-cerebral ventricles • Brain parenchyma is spared • Allows sampling of CSF • Lower infection risk than IVD	• Less reliable and accurate than IVD • Can be occluded → damped inaccurate trace and underestimate ICP • Transducer adjustment needed with head movement

- *Extradural transducer/Epidural catheter:*
  ‣ Indicated if insertion of intra-ventricular drainage is difficult or impossible
  ‣ Pressure sensor placed directly in contact with the dural surface

Pros and Cons of Extradural Transducer	
Advantages:	Disadvantages:
• Avoids penetration of the dura • Lower infection risk • No transducer adjustment needed with head movement	• Can be difficult to place—Irregularity of the dura prevents the transducer from lying flat against dural surface • Overestimates ICP if coplanarity with dura not achieved • Increasing baseline drift over time → questionable accuracy and reliability • Recalibration of system is not possible • Unable to drain CSF

NB: *In the past, measurement of lumbar CSF pressure was used to estimate ICP. However, it does not provide reliable ICP measurements and may be dangerous in the presence of increased ICP (risk of herniation).*
- *Parenchymal devices/microtransducer-tipped ICP monitors*
  ‣ Indicated if insertion of intra-ventricular drainage is difficult or impossible
  ‣ Can be placed in the brain parenchyma, subdural, subarachnoid, or intraven-tricular spaces via a burr hole, skull bolt, or during a neurosurgical procedure
  ‣ Includes the fiberoptic catheter tip transducer, strain gauge catheter tip transducer, and implantable devices

Pros and Cons of Parenchymal Devices	
Advantages:	Disadvantages:
• Can be placed in the brain parenchyma, subdural, subarachnoid, or intraventricular spaces • Minimal artifact and drift → accurate and reliable ICP measurements • No transducer adjustment needed with head movement • Easy to transport • No irrigation → less risk for infection	• Cannot be recalibrated after placement • Injury to brain tissue if placed in parenchyma or intraventricular space • Measures local pressure if placed in parenchyma • Cable/wire liable to breakage • Relatively expensive

NB: *Subdural or epidural placement of a pressure transducer do not have any major advantages over the parenchymal placement of a pressure monitoring device and do record ICP less reliably.*

Dangers of elevated ICP: brain ischemia and herniation (Figure 98-2)

FIGURE 98-2. Schematic drawing of brain herniation patterns

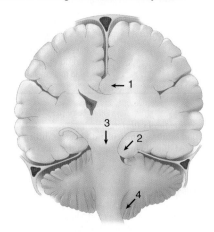

(1) Subfalcine herniation: The cingulate gyrus shifts across midline under the falx cerebri.
(2) Uncal herniation: The uncus (medial temporal lobe gyrus) shifts medially and compresses the midbrain and cerebral peduncle.
(3) Central transtentorial herniation: The diencephalon and midbrain shift caudally through the tentorial incisura.
(4) Tonsillar herniation: The cerebellar tonsil shifts caudally through the foramen magnum.
Reproduced with permission from Wilkins RH, Rengachary SS, eds. *Neurosurgery*. 2nd ed. New York: McGraw-Hill; 1996:349. Copyright © The McGraw-Hill Companies, Inc. All rights reserved.

CLINICAL SIGNS OF INCREASED ICP

- Headache
- Nausea and vomiting
- Progressive mental status decline
- Cushing's triad (late): hypertension, bradycardia, and irregular respiration
- Focal neurologic deficits such as hemiparesis if focal mass lesion
- Papilledema
- Unilateral papillary dilatation
- Oculomotor or abducens palsy

Head CT should be performed as soon as possible if elevated ICP is suspected

NB: lethargic or obtunded patients often have decreased respiratory drive, leading to a $PaCO_2$ increase, cerebral vasodilation, and worsening of ICH → "crashing patient" rapidly loses airway protection, becomes apneic, and herniates

Emergent intubation and ventilation to reduce $PaCO_2$ to roughly 35 mm Hg can reverse the process and save the patient's life.

MANAGEMENT OF INCREASED ICP

- Semi-upright position:
  ‣ Patient positioned 30° head up to optimize venous return
- Sufficient sedation:
  ‣ Sedation goals include analgesia, control of anxiety and agitation, reduction of stress response, and tolerance of positive pressure ventilation. Sedation reduces cerebral oxygen demand and thus can favorably influence the cerebral oxygen demand and supply balance

- Keep cerebral perfusion pressure (CPP) greater than 50 mm Hg:
  - Keep CPP between 50 and 60 mm Hg. Higher perfusion pressures might lead to an increase in vasogenic edema. Reduction of ICP is preferred over increase in arterial pressure to maintain CPP
- CSF drainage:
  - Fastest method to decrease ICP and thus optimize perfusion pressure. Vigorous drainage of CSF should be avoided, however, as it can increase filtration pressure and thus increase cerebral edema
- Hyperventilation:
  - Hyperventilation lowers arterial CO_2 and increases arterial pH and thus leads to cerebral vasoconstriction. The reduced intracranial blood volume lowers ICP. Cerebral vasoconstriction can also cause cerebral ischemia and therefore hyperventilation should be limited to decreasing arterial CO_2 to 35 mm Hg. When more aggressive hyperventilation is necessary, brain oxygenation should be monitored measuring jugular bulb oxygen saturation or direct brain tissue oxygenation
- Administration of mannitol/hypertonic saline:
  - Leads to an osmotic fluid shift from the brain parenchyma to the intravascular space. Diuresis is increased and thus ICP reduced
  - Typically 1 g/kg mannitol IV bolus (avoid if Na > 160 or serum osmolarity > 340)
  - Or 7.5% hypertonic saline (2 mL/kg IV over 20 minutes)
- Barbiturates:
  - Decrease brain metabolism and oxygen consumption. There also seems to be an effect to control free radical formation and lipid peroxidation. Some of this effect is due to a coupling effect on brain metabolism and perfusion
    NB: Thiopental is no longer marketed in the US
- Mild hypothermia:
  - The effects of hypothermia on the outcome after traumatic brain injury and increased ICP are unclear at present, with studies showing conflicting results
- Decompressive craniectomy:
  - Can lead to effective control of intracranial hypertension
  - Currently, however, it is unclear whether it leads to an improvement in outcome

REFERENCES

For references, please visit **www.TheAnesthesiaGuide.com**.

CHAPTER 99
Neuromonitoring (Transcranial Doppler (TCD), EEG, Carotid Stump Pressure (SP), Near Infrared Spectroscopy (NIRS), SjO₂)

John G Gaudet, MD

Three types of neuromonitoring devices:
- Monitors of cerebral hemodynamics (TCD, stump pressure)
- Monitors of cerebral oxygen metabolism (NIRS, SjO₂)
- Monitors of cerebral functional state (EEG, evoked potentials)

Awake (nonsedated) patient monitoring is the gold standard of neuromonitoring, but difficult to match during surgery.

FIGURE 99-1. Autoregulatory curve

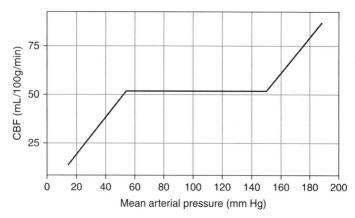

Flow is generally shown as being stable between mean arterial pressures (or more strictly, perfusion pressure) of 50 and 150 mm Hg. However, although this expresses the concept of autoregulation well, it does not depict reality. Reproduced from Longnecker DE, Brown DL, Newman MF, Zapol WM: *Anesthesiology.* Figure 50-10A. Available at: www.accessanesthesiology.com. Copyright © The McGraw-Hill Companies, Inc. All rights reserved.

Cerebral autoregulation (CAR): maintenance of constant CBF over a range of systemic BP (Figure 99-1)
- Lower limit of autoregulation (LLA): BP under which CBF decreases with BP (here about 50 mm Hg)
- Upper limit of autoregulation (ULA): BP above which CBF increases with BP (here about 150 mm Hg)
- CAR shift: modification of LLA and/or ULA set points, associated with altered relationship between systemic BP and CBF (LLA right shift in chronic HTN and anemia)

TRANSCRANIAL DOPPLER (TCD)

- Measures cerebral blood velocity (Vx), which correlates with cerebral blood flow (CBF)
- Relative changes over time are more accurate than absolute values
- Three main sites to obtain Doppler signal (Figures 99-2 and 99-3): temporal (most common, used essentially to measure Vx in MCA), suboccipital (posterior cerebral circulation), orbital (anterior cerebral circulation)

FIGURE 99-2. Sites to obtain TCD signal

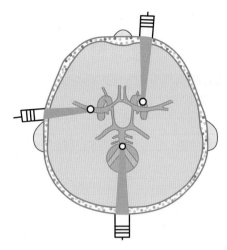

FIGURE 99-3. *Circle of Willis*

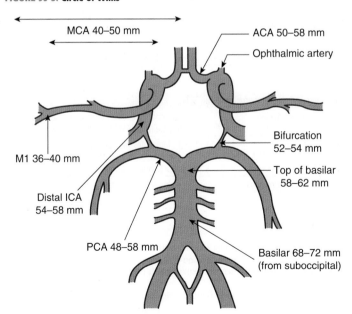

MCA 40–50 mm

ACA 50–58 mm

Ophthalmic artery

Bifurcation
52–54 mm

M1 36–40 mm

Top of basilar
58–62 mm

Distal ICA
54–58 mm

PCA 48–58 mm

Basilar 68–72 mm
(from suboccipital)

Problems encountered with TCD monitoring: no acoustic window (5%–15%), probe dislocation

Specific measurements
- Peak systolic velocity (PsVx) and End-diastolic Velocity (EdVx): measured directly
- Mean velocity (MVx): derived from PsVx and EdVx

Factors Affecting Velocity	
Factors associated with increased Vx signals	Factors associated with decreased Vx signals
Hypercapnia	Hypocapnia
Anesthetic inhalational agents	Anesthetic induction agents (except ketamine)
Vasopressors, hypertension with loss of CAR	Vasodilators, hypotension with loss of CAR
Increasing age, anemia, pre-eclampsia	Hypothermia, liver failure, pregnancy
Intracranial vascular abnormality	Raised ICP, brain death
Vasospasm, hyperemia	

- Pulsatility index (PI): maximal variation of Vx from systole to diastole, weighted by MVx
- Used to study changes in distal cerebral vascular resistance if HR and systemic BP pulsatility are maintained constant

Factors Affecting Pulsatility Index	
Factors associated with increased PI	Factors associated with decreased PI
Any cause of intracranial HTN	Vasospasm, hyperemia
Brain death	AVM
Portosystemic encephalopathy (hepatic failure)	Rewarming following hypothermia

Evaluation of Cerebral Perfusion Using TCD	
Cerebral hypoperfusion	50% reduction in MVx relative to baseline Absolute MVx in MCA <25 cm/s
Lindegaard ratio (LR) • Ratio of MVx in the MCA to MVx in the ICA	• Differentiates vasospasm from hyperemia in presence of elevated Vx (>120 cm/s) • LR >3: vasospasm, LR <3: hyperemia
Hemispheric PI asymmetry (>0.5)	• Asymmetry of cerebral hemodynamics

Clinical applications:
- General applications
  - Detection of cerebral hypoperfusion (relative or absolute decrease in Vx)
  - Detection of cerebral hyperperfusion (doubling of MVx in MCA)
  - Optimization of blood pressure management (identification of CAR range: LLA and ULA)
  - Detection of cerebral emboli (embolic signals: sudden interruptions of Doppler waveform)
  - Prediction of tolerance to carotid artery occlusion (quantification of CAR)
- Specific applications

CEA	• Intraoperative detection of cerebral ischemia during ICA clamping (40% of baseline signal cutoff associated with EEG changes) • Intraoperative quantification of hyperemic response after release of ICA clamp as a predictor of postoperative neurologic complications
SAH	• Early detection of postoperative vasospasm (very sensitive, not very specific, more likely and more severe in patients with higher Fisher grade) • Absolute Vx >120 cm/s with LR >3 indicative of vasospasm
AVM	• Improvement of TCD indices (autoregulation and cerebral perfusion) indicative of successful partial (embolization) or complete (resection) treatment of AVM
TBI	• Noninvasive diagnosis of intracranial HTN • Distinction between vasospasm and hyperemia in presence of elevated Vx (LR >3 indicative of vasospasm, LR <3 indicative of hyperemia)

CAROTID ARTERY STUMP PRESSURE

- One-time measurement of internal carotid artery (ICA) intraluminal pressure
- Mean CASP equivalent to CPP (normal range: 70–90 mm Hg)
- After cross-clamping of ICA, reflects back pressure from collateral cerebral flow

Artifacts: MAP, $PaCO_2$, type and dosage of anesthetic agents, incomplete ipsilateral ICA occlusion

Zero reference level should be placed at common carotid bifurcation

Applications: tolerance of carotid artery cross-clamping (indication to shunting)

Mean stump pressure <40 mm Hg after cross-clamp	Predictive of need to shunt during CEA
Mean stump pressure 25 mm Hg after cross-clamp	Equivalent to NIRS drop of 30%
Mean stump pressure 50 mm Hg after cross-clamp	Equivalent to NIRS drop of 10%

Presence of cross-filling from the anterior communicating artery on TCD is associated with good tolerance of cross-clamping

EEG

- **Monitoring of Depth of Anesthesia (Level of Consciousness): See chapter 44**

Level of consciousness	Observed EEG patterns	Frequency
Awake	fast frequencies ($\beta2/\gamma, \beta$) with small amplitude and minimal synchronicity	
Drowsy (superficial sedation)	anterior shift of medium frequencies (α)	
Light anesthesia (deep sedation)	medium slow frequencies (θ) with fast spindles	
Deep anesthesia	slow frequencies (δ), progression from slow spindles to burst suppression	

• **Detection of Cerebral Ischemia (Figure 99-4)**

Cerebral blood flow (CBF)	Functional impact on EEG signal
CBF < 50 mL/100 g/min	Normal CBF – normal EEG
CBF 22–50 mL/100 g/min	Mild hypoperfusion – normal EEG
CBF 15–22 mL/100 g/min	Moderate hypoperfusion – decrease in EEG amplitude and/or EEG slowing
CBF < 15 mL/100 g/min	Severe hypoperfusion – flattening of the EEG signal

Any significant decrease in CBF (cerebral ischemia) is associated with:
• A decrease in total power (decrease in relative α and β power, increase in relative θ and δ power)
• A decrease in relative α and β power
• An increase in relative θ and δ power
• Hemispheric asymmetry

FIGURE 99-4. Algorithm for evaluation and treatment of abnormal EEG

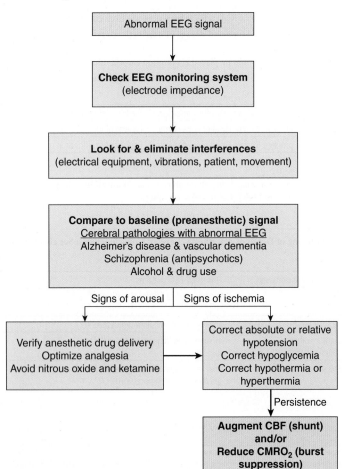

CEREBRAL OXIMETRY: NIRS AND SjO$_2$

Monitoring of regional (NIRS) or global (SjO$_2$) cerebral metabolic rate of oxygen (CMRO$_2$)

Factors Influencing CMRO$_2$	
Oxygen transport	Ventricular function, BP, anemia, oxygen desaturation Cerebral hypoperfusion, vasospasm
Cerebral oxygen metabolism	Cerebral ischemia (increased oxygen extraction) Brain death, hypothermia, burst suppression

- Near Infrared Spectroscopy (NIRS)
  - ‣ Noninvasive continuous monitor of regional cerebral tissue oxygen saturation (rSO$_2$)
  - ‣ Optimal placement of electrodes: one on each side, high on forehead to avoid frontal sinuses
  - ‣ 85% of rSO$_2$ is derived from cortical tissue (spatial resolution: subtraction of superficial saturation)

Artifacts: abnormal NIR absorption (hematomas, edema, jaundice), excessive ambient light

With such artifacts, absolute values may be incorrect but relative changes from baseline remain valid

Applications: NIRS is still considered experimental; it is mainly used to optimize cerebral perfusion

Optimization of Cerebral Perfusion	
Impact on postoperative stroke rate, cognitive function, incidence of major organ morbidity or mortality, hospital stay	
Detection of hypoperfusion (BP below LLA) during procedures affecting cerebral perfusion	10–20% relative decrease in rSO$_2$
Detection of hyperperfusion (BP above ULA) essentially after CEA	105–110% relative increase in rSO$_2$
Early detection of vasospasm after SAH	Unilateral NIRS signal reduction

- Jugular Venous Oxygen Saturation (SjO$_2$)
  - ‣ Obtained by retrograde cannulation of the internal jugular vein
  - ‣ Reflects the balance between the cerebral blood flow and the cerebral metabolic rate for oxygen
  - ‣ Normal SjO$_2$ range: 55–75%

Artifacts: incorrect catheter placement, resulting in contamination from external jugular vein

PEARLS

- The introduction of intraoperative cerebral monitoring has helped reduce the rate of intraoperative stroke, but not the rate of postoperative stroke after CEA
- TCD:
  - ‣ Identification of ACA, MCA, PCA via temporal window:
  - ‣ Identify ICA bifurcation into ACA and MCA (55–65 mm: bidirectional flow signals)
  - ‣ From ICA bifurcation: identify M1 (40–55 mm: unidirectional positive [towards probe] signal)

- ▶ From ICA bifurcation: identify A1 (60–75 mm anteriorly: unidirectional negative signal)
- ▶ From ICA bifurcation: identify P1 (60–75 mm slightly posteriorly: unidirectional positive signal)
- Changes in Vx during CPB do not reflect changes in CBF because of nonpulsatile flow
- The impact of inhalational agents on CAR is amplified by hypercapnia, reversed by hypocapnia
- EEG:
  - ▶ During the procedure, verify consistency of EEG with apparent state of the patient (clinical signs), administered anesthetic doses, and degree of surgical stimulation
  - ▶ Do NOT rely on EEG ALONE to manage the depth of anesthesia. EEG can adequately assess level of consciousness ONLY IF there is adequate analgesia and IF anesthetic agent concentrations are at steady state
- NIRS:
  - ▶ New generation NIRS monitors can also estimate cerebral blood volume (CBV)

REFERENCES

For references, please visit **www.TheAnesthesiaGuide.com.**

CHAPTER 100
Interventional Neuroradiology

Nicolai Goettel, MD, DESA

Intervention Types		
Intervention	Type of anesthesia	Approximate duration (h)
Diagnostic angiography		
Cerebral angiography	MAC	1
Medullar angiography	MAC	1½
Carotid angiography	MAC	1
Wada test[1]	MAC/no sedation	1½
Interventional angiography		
Cerebral aneurysm repair (endovascular "coiling")	GA	3–4
Cerebral artery angioplasty (dilatation)	MAC or GA	1½
Cerebral AVM embolization	GA	2½
Medullar artery embolization	MAC	1½
Cerebral intra-arterial thrombolysis	MAC or GA	1½
Cerebral artery angioplasty ("cerebral stenting")	GA	2
Carotid artery angioplasty ("carotid stenting")	MAC	1½

[1]selective injection of a barbiturate into each internal carotid artery to determine which hemisphere is responsible for vital functions such as speech and memory, prior to ablative surgery for epilepsy.

NB: see diagram of Circle of Willis in chapter 99 to identify the vessel where the procedure is being performed.

PREOPERATIVE CONSIDERATIONS

- Standard preoperative medical evaluation and anesthetic risk stratification (ASA score)
- Baseline neurologic status: GCS, pupils, focal neurologic deficits, seizures, grade Hunt/Hess, WFNS, Fisher (see pp. 454–455)
- Monitor specifically for changes in level of consciousness and/or focal neurologic deficits
- Monitor for signs of raised ICP
- Cardiac status: ECG, arrhythmia, HTN, cardiac enzymes as indicated
- Consider insertion of arterial line prior to induction if hemodynamic instability or risk of hypertensive peak during induction/laryngoscopy
- Avoid premedication with benzodiazepines and neuroleptics (impairment of baseline neurologic status)

INTRAOPERATIVE CONSIDERATIONS

Monitoring and Equipment			
Standard monitoring	Standard equipment	Invasive monitoring (if clinical indication)	Other (if clinical indication)
Pulse oximetry	Peripheral	Arterial line	Foley catheter
5-lead ECG	venous line		(if procedure
NIBP	Supplemental		>4 hours)
Capnography	oxygen		Central venous line
NMB monitoring (for GA)	(for MAC)		Transcranial Doppler

Induction

If MAC, consider low-dose sedation (propofol, midazolam, fentanyl)

If GA:

General considerations	Pre-oxygenation Full stomach: rapid sequence induction Avoid hypertensive peaks at induction, laryngoscopy
Induction drugs	Propofol 2–3 mg/kg IV, or etomidate 0.3 mg/kg IV, or thiopental 3–5 mg/kg IV Fentanyl 3–5 µg/kg IV, or sufentanil 0.3–0.5 µg/kg IV Succinylcholine 1–1.5 mg/kg IV, or rocuronium 0.6 mg/kg IV

Maintenance	
General considerations	• Sufficient anesthesia depth and neuromuscular blockade! • N_2O contraindicated!
Maintenance drugs/ volatiles	• Propofol 60–200 µg/kg/h IV, or sevoflurane (avoid high %: vasodilatory effect!) • Fentanyl 1–2 µg/kg/h IV, or sufentanil 0.1–0.2 µg/kg/h IV, or remifentanil 0.125 µg/kg/h IV infusion • Rocuronium 0.15 mg/kg IV bolus
Ventilation strategy	• Normoventilation • Hyperventilation causes cerebral vasoconstriction, potentiates cerebral ischemic lesions • Moderate and transient hyperventilation $PaCO_2$ 4.5 kPa (35 mm Hg) only if intracranial hypertension (ICH)
Hemodynamic strategy	• Control BP to maintain cerebral perfusion pressure >60 mm Hg (CPP = MAP – ICP) • BP at induction/until endovascular treatment of lesion: normal arterial blood pressure, CPP >60 mm Hg, MAP 70–90 mm Hg • BP after endovascular treatment of lesion: minimal HTN to favor brain tissue perfusion, CPP >60 mm Hg, MAP 90–120 mm Hg
Anticoagulation if warranted (discuss with neuroradiologist)	• Initial heparin 2,000–5,000 IU IV bolus • Consider heparin 1,000 IU/h IV bolus

POSTOPERATIVE CONSIDERATIONS

- Ambulatory or regular floor hospitalization usually appropriate for diagnostic cases
- Consider hospitalization in neurologic step-down unit or intensive care unit for interventions
- Extubate if possible for best neurologic monitoring
- Monitor specifically for changes in level of consciousness and/or focal neurologic deficits
- Supine and flat patient positioning for 4 hours (femoral artery puncture)
- Control arterial blood pressure: post-interventional MAP ≥ pre-interventional MAP
- Minimal postinterventional pain medication required
- Treatment of PONV

Basics, Special considerations	Complications
Cerebral aneurysm repair (endovascular "coiling") Positioning of a thin and flexible platinum coil to occlude the aneurysm. Indications: • Ruptured cerebral aneurysm with acute or sub-acute subarachnoid hemorrhage (SAH) • Nonruptured cerebral aneurysm (with risk of rupture) • Preventive treatment before triple-H-therapy (hypertension, hypervolemia, hemodilution); triple-H is controversial; arterial HTN is the main factor in maintaining CBF and tissue oxygenation (See further information below) Need NMB	(See below for details) Vasospasm Aneurismal rebleeding Arterial dissection/rupture or cerebral ischemia Hydrocephalus ICH Seizures Heart failure Electrolyte disturbances Hyperthermia Neurogenic pulmonary edema

(continued)

Basics, Special considerations	Complications
Cerebral artery angioplasty (dilatation) Indication: • Vasospasm after SAH	
Cerebral AVM embolization AVMs may enlarge over time; significant risk for rupture and intra-cranial hemorrhage Indications: • Prior to radio-surgery treatment or surgery, patients with multiple AVMs or lesions larger than 3 cm usually require embolization. The goal is to diminish the amount of blood flowing into the AVM by filling it with specially designed particles, microcoils, or glue	AVM rupture or cerebral ischemia Cerebral hyperperfusion syndrome Normal-perfusion-pressure-breakthrough edema
Cerebral intra-arterial thrombolysis Indications: • Acute ischemic stroke • If symptoms <3 h, presence of clinical criteria and absence of contra-indication: systemic IV thrombolysis with alteplase (Actilyse) 0.9 mg/kg in 1 h • If symptoms <6 h, or no clinical amelioration after IV thrombolysis: cerebral intra-arterial thrombolysis with alteplase (Actilyse) • Recent advances in neurointerventional techniques now allow effective intra-arterial treatment of stroke past the 6-hour limit	Subarachnoid hemorrhage
Cerebral artery angioplasty ("cerebral stenting") Indication: Acute stroke: cerebral artery stenosis or other pathology of the cerebral vasculature Platelet anti-aggregation (usually started before intervention) • Clopidrogel (Plavix) • Aspirin • Consider GP IIb/IIIa inhibitors tirofiban (Aggrastat), abciximab (Reopro) if acute ischemic stroke	Subarachnoid hemorrhage Arterial rupture/dissection Cerebral ischemia (stroke)
Carotid artery angioplasty ("carotid stenting") Indication: Symptomatic carotid artery stenosis (alternative to surgical carotid endarterectomy) Unlike cerebral angioplasty, carotid angioplasty is best performed under MAC (best neurologic monitor available!) Platelet anti-aggregation (usually started before intervention) • Clopidrogel (Plavix) • Aspirin • Consider GP IIb/IIIa inhibitors tirofiban (Aggrastat), abciximab (Reopro) if acute ischemic stroke	Arterial rupture/dissection Cerebral ischemia (stroke) Cerebral hyperperfusion syndrome Bradycardia, hypotension

Cerebral aneurysm repair (endovascular "coiling") additional information

Aneurismal SAH—Hunt and Hess

Grade	Signs and symptoms
I	Asymptomatic, mild headache, slight nuchal rigidity
II	Moderate-to-severe headache, nuchal rigidity, no neurologic deficit other than cranial nerve palsy
III	Drowsiness/confusion, mild focal neurologic deficit
IV	Stupor, moderate–severe hemiparesis
V	Coma, decerebrate posturing

Aneurismal SAH—WFNS: World Federation of Neurological Surgeons Grading Scale for aneurismal SAH

Grade	GCS score	Focal neurological deficit
I	15	None
II	13–14	None
III	13–14	Present
IV	7–12	Present or none
V	3–9	Present or none

Aneurismal SAH—Fisher

Grade	Appearance of hemorrhage on CT scan
1	None evident
2	Less than 1 mm thick
3	More than 1 mm thick
4	Any thickness with intraventricular hemorrhage or parenchymal extension

Site of cerebral aneurysms (see diagram of Circle of Willis in chapter 99)

Location	Percentage
Anterior communicating artery	30–35%
Bifurcation of the internal carotid and posterior communicating artery	30–35%
Middle cerebral artery bifurcation	20%
Basilar artery bifurcation	5%
Remaining posterior circulation arteries	5%

Coexisting Disease/Risk Factors	
Risk factor	Comments
Arterial hypertension	In 80% of cases with SAH
Smoking	
Alcohol abuse	
Drug abuse	e.g., cocaine
Genetic factors	Incidence of cerebral aneurysm in patients with family history of aneurysm: 4% (General incidence of cerebral aneurysm: 2%)
Polycystic kidney disease (PKD)	Incidence of cerebral aneurysm in patients with PKD: 16%
Aortic coarctation	
Fibromuscular dysplasia	

Complications of SAH and/or Endovascular Aneurysm Repair		
Complication	Comments	
Vasospasm	Major risk in between the 5th and 14th day after SAH Secondary ischemic cerebral lesions "Angiographic" vasospasm: 60–70% "Symptomatic" vasospasm: 20–30%	
	Therapeutic options	Intra-arterial nimodipine (Nimotop) Intra-arterial papaverine Triple-H (hypertension, hemodilution, hypervolemia); controversial Cerebral artery angioplasty (dilatation)
Aneurismal rebleeding		
Arterial dissection/ rupture or cerebral ischemia		
Hydrocephalus	May require insertion of an external ventricular drainage (EVD) device	
ICH		
Seizures	Prophylactic and/or therapeutic phenytoin	
Heart failure	Myocardial stunning/ischemia due to excessive sympathetic activity ECG changes Cardiac enzymes	
Electrolyte disturbances	SIADH	
Hyperthermia	Of central origin	
Neurogenic pulmonary edema		

REFERENCES

For references, please visit **www.TheAnesthesiaGuide.com**.

CHAPTER 101
Craniotomy

Nicolai Goettel, MD, DESA

BASICS

Cranial contents
- Skull represents a closed, non-expandable unit containing three compartments (CBV, CSF, brain tissue) determining ICP
- Any increase in volume of one of the cranial compartments must be compensated by a decrease in volume of another to maintain the pressure equilibrium (Monro-Kellie doctrine)
- Small increases in intracranial volume will lead to large increases in ICP once this buffer mechanism is exhausted (Figure 101-1), compromising CBV

Blood and cerebral vasculature (cerebral blood volume, CBV)
- Two carotid arteries (70% blood flow to the brain)
- Two vertebral arteries (30% blood flow to the brain)
- Arterial anastomosis through Willis circle and anastomosis with external carotid arteries through branches of facial and ophthalmic arteries
- Venous return through cortical veins (superficial drainage), and basilar and ventricular veins (profound drainage) essentially into the IJ veins

Cerebro-spinal fluid (CSF)
- Produced by choroid plexus, reabsorbed by granules of Pacchioni
- Total volume of CSF in the adult: 140–270 mL
- Production of 0.2–0.7 mL/min or 600–700 mL/day

FIGURE 101-1. ICP as a function of IC volume

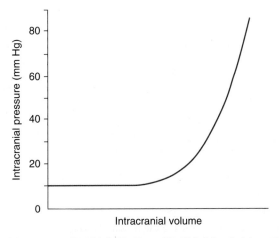

Physiologic Background: Cerebral Perfusion and Autoregulation

Cerebral blood flow (CBF), cerebral metabolic requirement of oxygen (CMRO₂), and cerebral perfusion pressure (CPP)

- CBF (normal: 50 mL/min/100 g of brain) is coupled with $CMRO_2$ and determined by cerebral autoregulation and cerebrovascular reactivity to CO_2
- Cerebral perfusion pressure (CPP) is the difference between mean arterial pressure (MAP) and ICP
- Cerebral autoregulation is the capacity of the cerebral arterioles to maintain a relatively constant CBF by alteration of their vascular resistance (vasoconstriction over a wide range of blood pressures (between MAP of approximately 50–150 mm Hg). At the extreme limits of MAP or CPP (high or low), CBF is directly proportional to CPP (Figure 101-2)
- CO_2 is a potent vasodilator, showing a relationship between $PaCO_2$ (30–80 mm Hg) and CBF that is nearly linear
- Autoregulation and cerebrovascular reactivity to CO_2 may be altered in various pathological states (TBI, severe focal ischemia, brain tumor), as well as by administration of anesthetics

FIGURE 101-2. Influence of PaO₂, PaCO₂, and MAP (green line) on cerebral blood flow

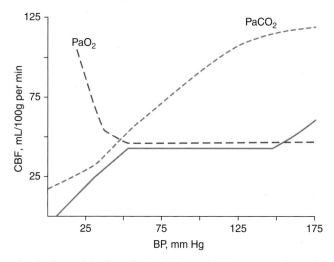

Reproduced with permission from Shapiro HM. Intracranial hypertension: Therapeutic and anesthetic considerations. *Anesthesiology*. 1975;43:445.

Influence of Anesthetic Agents on CBF, ICP, and CMRO$_2$

Medication	CBF and ICP	CMRO$_2$
Propofol	↓	↓
Thiopental	↓	↓
Etomidate	↓	↓
Ketamine	↑	↑
Nitrous oxide	↑	↑
Volatile anesthetics[1]	↑	↓
Opioids[2]	=	Slight ↓

[1]Do not exceed 0.8 MAC to maintain CO$_2$ reactivity and cerebral autoregulation.
[2]Opioids can increase CBF and ICP if allowed to cause hypercarbia.

Indications for craniotomy

Vascular surgery
- Repair of intracerebral aneurysm ("clipping"): carotid or vertebro-basilar circulation
- Cerebral arterio-venous malformation (AVM)
- Extracranial-intracranial micro-vascular anastomosis
- Carotid-cavernous fistula

Oncologic surgery
- Malignant tumors (astrocytoma, glioblastoma, or metastatic)
- Benign tumors (meningioma, acoustic neurinoma)
- Transsphenoidal hypophysectomy

Epilepsy surgery
- Ablative surgery of epileptic foci (lobectomy)
- Intracranial implantation of electrodes for electrocorticography

Functional stereotaxy of the brain
- Deep brain stimulator insertion (DBS)
- Intracranial implantation of chronic surface electrodes

Cranio-cerebral injuries
- Intracerebral hematoma (subarachnoid hemorrhage): ruptured aneurysm, spontaneous intracerebral hemorrhage
- Epidural hematoma
- Subdural hematoma (acute or chronic)
- Reduction of skull fracture
- Decompressive craniectomy
- Removal of foreign body from brain

Other
- Intracranial abscess
- Intracranial cyst
- Brain tissue biopsy (e.g., to diagnose prion disease)
- Microvascular decompression for trigeminal neuralgia
- CSF Shunting/drainage procedures
- Repair of skull defect

Primary goals in neuroanesthesia for craniotomy
• Maintain sufficient anesthesia depth (balanced anesthesia) • Maintain relaxed and compliant brain tissue • Maintain optimal brain oxygenation and perfusion • Maintain cerebral homeostasis (cerebral protection)
Understand the patient's neurological condition and planned procedure • Thorough and targeted preoperative assessment • Communication with the surgical team
Prevent secondary insult though brain ischemia AVOID: • Hypoxemia • Hypercapnia • Hyperthermia • Anemia • Hemodynamic instability
Respect cerebral homeostasis • Normovolemia • Normoglycemia • Treat and/or prevent any increases in ICP • Maintain cerebral autoregulation • Maintain adequate cerebral perfusion
Provide cerebral relaxation • Create optimal operating conditions for the neurosurgeon • Reduce the likelihood of perioperative cerebral ischemia
Plan for fast and predictable recovery from anesthesia • Enable neurological assessment in the immediate postoperative period

PREOPERATIVE CONSIDERATIONS

- Baseline neurologic status: GCS, pupils, focal neurologic deficits, seizures, grade Hunt/Hess, WFNS, Fisher (see pp. 454–455)
- Monitor specifically for changes in level of consciousness and/or focal neurologic deficits
- Monitor for signs of raised ICP
- Consider insertion of arterial line prior to induction if hemodynamic instability or risk of hypertensive peak during induction/laryngoscopy
- Avoid premedication with benzodiazepines and neuroleptics (impairment of baseline neurologic status, risk of hypoventilation, and raised ICP)

Pre-operative Assessment Before Craniotomy

Cerebral imaging	Chart	Patient

• **All masses**
Location and size of lesions
Surrounding structures at risk
Hydrocephalus
• **Raised ICP**
Midline shift
Herniation
Effacement of sulci and gyri,
loss of differentiation
• **Tumors**
Vascularization
Vascular lesions
Isolated versus multiple
Evidence of vasospasm
Evidence of hemorrhage
• **TBI**
Evidence of cervical instability?
	• Hb, Ht, Platelets
	• PT, PTT, ABO
	• Na, K, Osm, Glycemia
	• SpO$_2$ (room air)
	• **Epileptic patients**
	▸ Drug levels
	▸ LFTs, BUN, Cr, Ca
	• **Medication list**
	▸ Anti-epileptic drugs
	▸ Anti-Parkinsonian drugs
	▸ Psychotropes
	▸ Anti-platelet agents
	▸ Anti-coagulants
	▸ Anti-hypertensive
	  agents
	▸ Corticosteroids
		• GCS and Cognitive
		  function
		• Baseline neurologic status
		• Hemodynamic status
		• Difficult airway predictors
		• **Traumatic brain
		  injury (TBI)**
		▸ Expect difficult airway
		  in presence of facial
		  trauma
		▸ Cervical spine unstable
		  until proven otherwise
		  (maintain cervical collar)
		• **Awake craniotomy**
		Patient selection

INTRA-OPERATIVE CONSIDERATIONS

Monitoring

Standard equipment	Other equipment if indicated

• Pulse oximetry
• 5-lead ECG
• NIBP
• Capnography
• NMB monitoring
• Arterial line
	• Foley catheter
	• Central venous line
	• Precordial Doppler ultrasound
	• Neurophysiologic monitoring: evoked potentials, EEG, EMG, BIS
	• Lumbar CSF drainage catheter (if indicated by neurosurgeon)
	• Other (neuroICU): transcranial Doppler sonography (TCD),
	  jugular bulb venous oximetry, cerebral microdialysis,
	  near-infrared spectroscopy (NIRS)

Induction

General
considerations
	• Preoxygenation
	• Full stomach: rapid sequence induction
	• Avoid hypertensive peaks at induction, laryngoscopy; have
	  vasoactive medications ready (phenylephrine, esmolol) to maintain
	  hemodynamic stability
	• For non-intubated patients with increased ICP: encourage
	  spontaneous hyperventilation

Induction drugs	• Propofol 2–3 mg/kg IV, or etomidate 0.3 mg/kg IV, or thiopental
	  3–5 mg/kg IV
	• Fentanyl 3–5 mcg/kg IV, or sufentanil 0.3–0.5 mcg/kg IV, or
	  remifentanil 0.5–1 mcg/kg IV
	• Succinylcholine 1–1.5 mg/kg IV, or rocuronium 0.6 mg/kg IV, or
	  atracurium 0.5 mg/kg IV

Maintenance	
General considerations	• Sufficient anesthesia depth and neuromuscular blockade! • Avoid N_2O
Maintenance drugs/volatiles	• Propofol 60–200 µg/kg/h IV as TIVA, or sevoflurane (avoid high MAC%: vasodilatory effect!) • Fentanyl 1–2 mcg/kg/h IV, or sufentanil 0.1–0.2 mcg/kg/h IV, or remifentanil 0.125 mcg/kg/h IV infusion • Rocuronium 0.15 mg/kg IV bolus, or atracurium 0.1 mg/kg IV bolus
Ventilation strategy	• Normoventilation (check ABG if doubt on arterial-end-tidal gradient) • Hyperventilation causes cerebral vasoconstriction, potentiates cerebral ischemic lesions • Moderate and transient hyperventilation $PaCO_2$ 4.5 kPa (35 mm Hg) only if intracranial hypertension
Hemodynamic strategy	• Control BP to maintain cerebral perfusion pressure >60 mm Hg (CPP = MAP − ICP) • BP at induction: normal arterial blood pressure, CPP >60 mm Hg, MAP 70–90 mm Hg • As a general rule maintain normal BP; treat hypotension or HTN according to clinical context

Intraoperative reduction of a brain bulk = Treatment of acute intracranial hypertension
• Place patient's head up (30°, neutral neck position) • Mild to moderate hyperventilation (goal: $PaCO_2$ 32–35 mm Hg) • Optimize oxygenation and ensure low airway pressures, no PEEP • Osmotic diuresis: mannitol 0.5–1 g/kg IV • Consider loop diuretics: furosemide 0.25–1.0 mg/kg IV • Maintain normovolemia, normoglycemia • Decrease or stop volatile agents and switch to TIVA • Surgical drainage of CSF and/or surgical decompression

Emergence

- Avoid HTN (esmolol, labetalol, nitroglycerine)
- Avoid coughing-associated raise in ICP (intratracheal or IV lidocaine)
- Head elevated at 30° in neutral position
- Delayed emergence: extubation criteria not met within 30 minutes after end of surgery: Consider emergent CT-scan

Additional criteria for extubation (be ready to reintubate after removal of ETT)
• Stable hemodynamics, normothermia, normoglycemia, and normovolemia
• Reversal of muscle relaxants
• No gross swelling of face or neck
• Pupils equal in size
• Patient is awake and obeying simple commands (eye opening, moves limbs)
• Neurological examination shows no new deficits and presence of gag reflex
• Normal lab results (ABG, Hb/Hct, Na/K/Ca/Osm, glycemia)

POSTOPERATIVE CONSIDERATIONS

- Usually transfer to neuro ICU
- Extubate if possible for best neurologic monitoring
- Monitor specifically for changes in level of consciousness and/or focal neurologic deficits
- Control arterial blood pressure
- Treatment of postoperative pain (goal: EVA <3) but avoid sedation that interferes with adequate examination of the patient's neurological status
- Prophylaxis/treatment of PONV
- Early diagnosis of pneumocephalus/tension pneumocepalus, and adequate treatment
- Early diagnosis of seizures, and treatment

Special Considerations for Craniotomy in the Sitting Position			
Indications	Patient positioning	Contraindications	Complications
• Brainstem surgery • Surgery of the cerebellum • Surgery of 4th ventricle • Infratentorial craniotomy	• Sitting position • Prone position ("Concorde") • Half-sitting position, head turned	• Advanced age • Acute or chronic heart failure • Para- or tetraplegia • Uncorrected hypovolemia • Intraatrial or intraventricular communication (e.g., PFO)	• Venous air embolism

Ensure patient positioning on table that makes it possible to rapidly lower head below heart level in case of venous air embolism.

PEARLS AND TIPS: COMPLICATIONS

Acute intracranial hypertension (see above, and chapter 98, for treatment)

Venous air embolism (VAE)

Pathophysiology
- Consider whenever head >5 cm above heart (classically in the sitting position)
- Transected veins in cut edge of bone or dura may not collapse
- Air→RV→pulmonary circulation
- Paradoxical (air) embolism into coronary or cerebral circulations via patent foramen ovale (PFO; 20–30% of adults have probe-patent PFO)

Respiratory effects	**Diagnosis**	**Treatment**
$ETCO_2\downarrow$ • Acute ventilation-perfusion mismatch (dead space ventilation) • Hypoxemia • Hypercarbia • Bronchoconstriction • Acidosis **Cardiovascular effects** • Acute right heart failure and obstructive shock • Pulmonary arterial and peripheral vascular resistance ↑ • Cardiac output ↓ • Carotid output ↓ • Cerebral perfusion pressure ↓ • Cardiac arrhythmia and cardiac arrest • Arterial hypotension	• Look out for clinical signs and symptoms • Precordial Doppler ultrasound near right upper sternal border is most sensitive non-invasive monitor (detects 0.25 mL) • Transesophageal echocardiography is more sensitive, but more invasive and cumbersome • Sudden decrease in $ETCO_2$ • Gasping, hypotension, dysrhythmias, cyanosis, "mill-wheel" murmur	• Potentially life-threatening: ABC approach • 100% oxygen ventilation • Trendelenburg positioning and/or left side down • Normal saline irrigation of the operating field by the surgeon • Apply occlusive material (bone wax) to bone edges • Uni- or bilateral jugular vein compression • Aspiration of embolized air through central venous line • Inotropes may be needed • Stop surgery until patient stabilized • **BEWARE:** PEEP, by reversing RA-LA pressure gradient, may lead to paradoxical air emboli via PFO

REFERENCES

For references, please visit **www.TheAnesthesiaGuide.com**.

CHAPTER 102
Awake Craniotomy

Nicolai Goettel, MD, DESA

BASICS

Indications for awake craniotomy
See table on following page.

Indications for awake craniotomy
Brain tumor (located either in or close to areas of eloquent brain function, such as speech, motor, and sensory pathways) • Surgical advantages: optimal tumor resection, minimization of the risk of neurologic injury • Brain mapping (electrocorticography) for accurate localization of eloquent brain function before tumor resection
Epilepsy surgery • Resection of epileptogenic foci (intractable lesional epilepsy) • Brain mapping (electrocorticography) for accurate localization of eloquent brain function before resection of epileptogenic foci
Functional stereotaxy of the brain • Implantation of deep brain stimulation (DBS) electrodes: classically Parkinson's disease, but other simple or complex central movement disorders, Alzheimer's disease, psychiatric disease, pharmacoresistant depression, and eating disorders are increasingly considered for DBS insertion
Minor craniotomy • Drainage of acute/chronic subdural hematoma • Intracranial catheter placement

Poor candidates for awake craniotomy
Poor understanding or cooperation • Children • Mental retardation • Psychiatric conditions • Extreme anxiety • Claustrophobia • History of poorly tolerated sedation • Severe dystonia • Language barrier
Difficult airway • Anticipated or documented difficult airway • Morbid obesity • Obstructive sleep apnea (OSA) • Intractable epilepsy: watch for rare syndromes associated with airway abnormalities
Hemorrhagic risk • Coagulopathy or anticoagulation agents • Thrombocytopenia, thrombopathy, or antiplatelet agents

CONDUCT OF ANESTHESIA FOR A STANDARD AWAKE CRANIOTOMY

Preoperative considerations

- Routine assessment and preparation as for any patient undergoing a craniotomy (cf. chapter 101)
- Patient preparation: give detailed explanation of procedure, inquire about expectations and fears
- Premedication: minimal/no preoperative sedation, nausea prophylaxis
- Continuation of all preoperative medications including anti-epileptics and steroids (Exception: For DBS insertion anti-Parkinsonian drugs may need to be stopped for better intraoperative evaluation of electrode placement)
- Establishment of good collaborative rapport with the patient

Intraoperative considerations

- The goal is to provide a comfortable environment to the patient, who is able to stay immobile on an operating room table for the duration of the procedure, and yet be alert and cooperative with cortical mapping

Installation and monitoring

- Limited access to airway: GA setup ready, fiberoptic available, treatment of complications available
- Patients position themselves in such a way as to have some freedom of movement of the extremities to allow for intraoperative mapping
- Provide comfortable environment (padding, quiet, and warm OR)
- Neuronavigation is usually used, necessitating rigid fixation of the head (pins are inserted under local anesthesia with sedation)
- Maintain continuous communication and visual contact with patient and surgical team
- Standard monitoring, capnography, supplemental O_2, large-bore IV
- Fluids should be kept to a minimum, a urinary catheter is not routinely needed, but to be considered if procedure exceeding 4 hours
- Invasive monitoring (arterial line) not routinely used

Anesthetic technique

- The decision for the choice of the technique of anesthesia will depend on the preferences of the institutional team including surgeon and anesthesiologist

Scalp anesthesia for craniotomy

- Long-acting agents such as bupivacaine with epinephrine are used
- Infiltration of the craniotomy site with a "ring block" or scalp nerve blocks of the auriculotemporal, occipital, zygomaticotemporal, supraorbital, and supratrochlear nerves may be used
- Lidocaine should be used for addition painful areas during surgery
- Respect non toxic doses of each local anesthetic agent used

Anesthetic technique for awake craniotomy	
Conscious sedation/fully awake technique	AAA: Asleep-awake-asleep (General anesthesia is induced at the beginning for the craniotomy, the patient is then fully awoken for cortical mapping, and GA is resumed for tumor resection and closure.)

• Infiltration, scalp blocks (neurosurgeon), placement of head frame
 • Craniotomy:
   ▸ Sedation with propofol, midazolam, or dexmedetomidine
   ▸ Analgesia with fentanyl or remifentanil
   ▸ Close monitoring of capnography, continuous communication with patient
 • Cortical mapping: stop propofol and remifentanil, maintain/decrease dexmedetomidine infusion rate
 • Closure of craniotomy:
   ▸ Sedation with propofol or dexmedetomidine
   ▸ Analgesia with fentanyl or remifentanil
	• Infiltration, scalp blocks (neurosurgeon), placement of head frame
	 • Craniotomy:
	   ▸ GA and airway management: preferably LMA, but ETT, nasal/oral airway can be used
	   ▸ Either inhalation or intravenous anesthetic agents may be used with or without controlled ventilation
	 • Cortical mapping: fully awake patient, removal of airway
	 • Closure of craniotomy: GA with propofol and remifentanil
	 • Emergence: prompt extubation for immediate neurologic examination

Tip: Nonpharmacologic measures including frequent reassurance, warning the patient in advance about loud noise (drilling bone) and painful areas are also useful.	**BEWARE:** Avoid hypoxemia, hypercarbia and hypertension that may increase ICP and/or cause bleeding.

Postoperative considerations
- Please refer to the chapter 101

Complications

Complications During Awake Craniotomy	
Complication	Treatment
Respiratory function	• Airway obstruction and hypoxia may result from oversedation, seizures, mechanical obstruction, or loss of consciousness from an intracranial event	• Immediate! • Can include stopping or decreasing sedation, use of jaw thrust or insertion of an oral or nasal airway, LMA, or endotracheal tube
Pain or discomfort	• May occur during pin fixation, dissection of the temporalis muscle, traction on the dura, and manipulation of the intracerebral blood vessels	• Additional analgesia or sedation or infiltration of local anesthesia
Seizures	• May occur in patients who have or have not had preoperative seizures • Most commonly occur during cortical stimulation	• Small dose of propofol (20–30 mg), or midazolam (1 mg) • Surgeons can also treat seizure by irrigating cold solution on the cortex • Anti-epileptics (phenytoin)
Conversion to GA	• This may be required for the management of ongoing complications and catastrophic intracranial events including loss of consciousness and bleeding	• Airway management may include LMA, standard endotracheal intubation, or via video laryngoscopy or fiberoptic bronchoscopy
Other complications	• Uncooperative or disinhibited patient • Brain bulge • Nausea and vomiting	• According to intraoperative situation

PEARLS AND TIPS

- Ensure that the head frame does not create a drape pocket around the patient's face, with dangerous accumulation of CO_2
- Careful airway management is paramount, in particular in patients with sleep apnea or difficult airways. Intubation is virtually impossible once the head frame is in place. Conversion to from MAC to GA is very difficult intraoperatively. Do not oversedate!
- Carefully document patient's neurological status preoperatively, as postoperative neurological and/or cognitive deficits can develop
- Although most patients generally tolerate the procedure well, some individuals may experience the awake craniotomy in a negative way. Adequate sedation (without inducing apnea) is advisable. In this context, the importance of a good patient-caregiver relationship cannot be overly stressed!

REFERENCES

For references, please visit **www.TheAnesthesiaGuide.com.**

CHAPTER 103
Neurovascular Surgery

Zirka H. Anastasian, MD

BACKGROUND

Major types of neurovascular disease:
- Cerebral vessel stenosis (i.e., carotid stenosis): See chapter 104
- Cerebral aneurysm
- Cerebral arteriovenous malformation (AVM)

Pathophysiology		
	Cerebral aneurysm	Cerebral AVM
Epidemiology	About 1–6% of asymptomatic adults	About 0.1% of population, usually present between ages 10 and 40 years
Location (most common)	About 85% are in anterior circulation (especially circle of Willis)	About 90% are supratentorial
Mechanism	*Saccular*: thin-walled protrusions from the intracranial arteries with thin or absent tunica media (most responsible for SAH) Fusiform: dilation of entire circumference of vessel *Mycotic*: from infected emboli *Causes*: multifactorial, hemodynamic stress, and turbulent flow cause damage *Risks*: HTN, smoking, connective tissue disease	Pathogenesis unclear: considered sporadic congenital developmental vascular lesions, higher rate with hereditary hemorrhagic telangiectasia. About 20% of patients with AVMs also have cerebral aneurysms due to flow rate disruptions
Treated when:	Depends on size of aneurysm (5-year rupture rate 7–12 mm: 2.6%, >25 mm: 40%), risk of rupture (also location dependent: posterior have highest risk of rupture, cavernous carotid artery aneurysm are the lowest risk, anterior circulation: intermediate risk) and patient's age Preferred treatment modality (endovascular versus open surgical clipping) depends on size, location, neck: dome ratio, and medical status of patient	Acute or chronic hypertension does not seem to increase risk of hemorrhage Risk factors for hemorrhage: hemorrhage as initial clinical presentation, deep venous drainage, deep brain location, increased patient age. Tx. Depends on patient's age, lesion size and location, and prior history of intracerebral hemorrhage (annual risk of hemorrhage with 0 factors: 0.9%, risk with 3 factors: 34.4%)

Preoperative Evaluation/Considerations		
	Cerebral aneurysm	Cerebral AVM
Past medical history	Hx of headaches? Hx of smoking? Determine *normal* baseline BP Cardiac history?	Determine *normal* baseline BP Did the patient have embolization (successful or attempted) of vessels preoperatively?
Physical examination	Baseline neurological examination (compare deficits)	Baseline neurological examination (compare deficits) Evaluate for symptoms of large shunts: congestive heart failure
Medication history	Antihypertensive medication history, Weight loss supplements? CHF meds? (mannitol often requested by surgeon)	CHF meds?
Studies to review	CT, MRI, Angiography	CT, MRI, Angiography
Specific questions	How many aneurysms? What is their size (assess rupture potential)? For how long have they been managed? What was the date of the last MRI/angiography? Has coiling/clipping been done in the past?	What is the size of the AVM? What was the medical plan?

Anesthesia and Intraoperative Issues		
	Cerebral aneurysm	Cerebral AVM
Monitors	Standard monitors/lines: EKG, BP cuff, pulse oximeter, esophageal/bladder temperature probe (especially, important if cooling), peripheral IVs (2 or more) Additional monitors/lines: arterial line (preferably pre-induction to monitor BP changes during laryngoscopy), possible spinal drain (if ruptured), Foley catheter, neuromuscular blockade monitor, consider central line	Standard monitors/lines: EKG, BP cuff, pulse oximeter, esophageal/bladder temperature probe, peripheral IVs (2 or more) Additional monitors/lines: arterial line (preferably pre-induction to monitor BP changes during laryngoscopy), Foley catheter, neuromuscular blockade monitor, consider central line
Induction	Avoid hypertension by giving induction agent accordingly, doing test laryngoscopy, and have fast-acting antihypertensive (i.e., esmolol) ready.	Avoid hypertension by giving induction agent accordingly, doing test laryngoscopy, and have fast-acting antihypertensive (i.e., esmolol) ready.
Airway management	Avoid prolonged intubation attempt: avoid prolonged laryngoscopy	Consider possibility of co-present aneurysm: avoid prolonged laryngoscopy
Blood pressure goals	Avoid hypertension and avoid sudden fluctuations in blood pressure (which put stress on the walls of the aneurysm)	Meticulous BP control: avoid hypertension due to risk of aneurysm

(continued)

Anesthesia and Intraoperative Issues (*continued*)

	Cerebral aneurysm	Cerebral AVM
Intraoperative surgical issues	Prevent retraction injury by brain "relaxation" measures: hyperventilation, mannitol, steroid Key points in the open surgical clipping are temporary clip placement or aneurysm rupture Temporary clip placement: Surgeon will try to minimize time of temporary clamp (will decrease perfusion to tissue distal to clamp). May be necessary to aid in peri-aneurysm surgical dissection. Cerebral protection may be provided by increasing blood pressure or by infusing barbiturate Aneurysm rupture: induce burst suppression with barbiturate and consider hypothermia (though has to be commenced prior to acute rupture) for cerebral protection. During open surgical procedure, will need acute hypotension (to be able to place temporary clip proximal to rupture to stop the bleeding) and then hypertension (for collateral flow). Acute blood loss can be marked: increase fluid rate Key point in endovascular treatment is aneurysm rupture: Aneurysm rupture: reverse heparin with protamine, burst suppression, consider hypoventilation, consider emergent surgical management, depending on location	Prevent retraction brain injury by hyperventilation and steroid (consider mannitol: but causes acute hypervolemia) Key point in the surgery is bleeding during AVM resection or aneurysm rupture AVM resection bleeding: can be significant. Patient may be a candidate for vessel embolization prior to the surgical resection to minimize intra-operative bleeding. Monitor blood loss carefully and don't forget to look at the surgical field (loss may be collected into a bag at the head of the bed) Aneurysm rupture: induce burst suppression with barbiturate. Consider immediate surgical management of aneurysm, depending on location
Emergence	Avoid hypertension, sudden changes in BP Avoid large doses of long-acting agents that may compromise ability to perform neurological testing	Avoid hypertension, sudden changes in BP Avoid large doses of long-acting agents that may compromise ability to do neurological testing
Possible agents to consider having on-hand	Short-acting beta blockers, calcium channel blockers, opioids for smooth emergence, protamine (if using heparin: endovascular tx)	Short-acting beta blockers, calcium channel blockers, opioids for smooth emergence

Postoperative (Complications)		
	Aneurysm	AVM
Complication	Aneurysm rupture: (often there are multiple aneurysms) Obstruction of arterial flow due to clip placement (neurological changes postoperatively)	Aneurysm rupture AVM bleed Residual AVM Normal perfusion pressure breakthrough syndrome: immediately following surgical excision of a cerebral AVM, even normal brain tissue surrounding the lesion may hemorrhage Occlusive hyperemia: venous outflow obstruction by surgical ligation with incomplete occlusion of arterial feeders
Acute management	Rupture: If time of rupture known, induce burst suppression with barbiturate, consider hypothermia, consider immediate surgical intervention Obstruction: Blood pressure management (consider increasing blood pressure to provide collateral blood flow), Angiography, consider returning to OR to replace/re-position clip. Some surgeons do routine intra-operative angiography to prevent this complication	Avoid hypertension during emergency Immediate angiography/other imaging to determine etiology of mental status change, consider emergent surgery, decompressive craniotomy Some surgeons do routine intraoperative angiography to prevent occlusive hyperemia

PEARLS AND TIPS

Surgical management may vary substantially based on hospital resources, individual preferences, and individual patient history for neurovascular surgery. Have a discussion with the surgical team about their planned management (including preoperative and intraoperative interventions, where applicable).

REFERENCES

For references, please visit **www.TheAnesthesiaGuide.com**.

CHAPTER 104
Carotid Artery Endarterectomy (CEA)

John G. Gaudet, MD and Yann Villiger, MD, PhD

FIGURE 104-1. Algorithm showing evaluation and treatment of patient with suspected carotid stenosis (also see chapter 108)

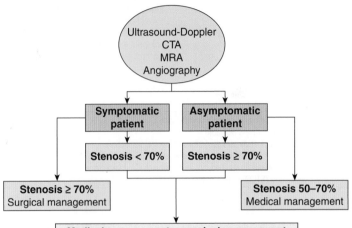

Medical management	Surgical management
ASA + ACEI/ARB + Statin ± β-blocker	Carotid artery endarterectomy (CEA)
≥2 events: add Clopidogrel or Dipyridamole	Carotid artery stenting (CAS)

Preoperative Assessment		
Imaging	Chart	Patient
Indication	BP normal range (both arms)	Baseline neurologic status
Degree of stenosis on operative side	Glycemic profile	Baseline cognitive function
	Hb/Hct/ABO typing	Level of cooperation
Collaterals	Platelets/PT/PTT	Effect of head positioning
Degree of stenosis in contralateral carotid and vertebral vessels	No ACEI/ARB the day of surgery	Tolerance to supine position
	Maintain antiplatelet agents	Orthostatic hypotension
	Maintain β-blockers and statins	Difficult airway predictors
	• Follow ACC/AHA guidelines for cardiac evaluation (see chapter 7)	

Before the procedure starts:
• Make sure drugs, shunt, and monitoring are ready or available

Intraoperative Equipment	
Drugs and shunt	Monitoring
• **Vasopressors and vasodilators** *Available for immediate use:* Phenylephrine Ephedrine Nitroglycerin Atropine *Available in room:* Clonidine 15 mcg/mL (0.5–1 mcg/kg) Nicardipine 1 mg/mL (5–15 mg/h) • *Heparin available for immediate use* • *Protamine available in room* • *Shunt available in room* • *Lidocaine available to surgeon for carotid sinus infiltration*	• *SpO_2, 5-lead ECG, NIBP* • *2 IV lines (at least one large-bore)* • *Arterial line* • A glucometer should be available • Central venous catheter not required. If necessary (unstable patient): ▸ Avoid carotid injury, favor subclavian ▸ US guidance, placed by senior staff • Foley not required Confirm patient has voided
If procedure performed under general anesthesia: • Confirm neuromonitoring is available • Measure baseline CO_2 (RA) as a guide for mechanical ventilation *If procedure performed under regional anesthesia:* • Have all equipment and drugs ready for conversion to GA if necessary • Monitor ventilation ($ETCO_2$ in face mask)	

Neuromonitoring		
Neuromonitor *Signs of cerebral hypoperfusion*	Pros	Cons
Awake evaluation *New neurologic deficit* *Loss of consciousness*	Gold standard	**Requires good cooperation** Affected by presence of preexisting neurologic deficits
EEG *Hemispheric asymmetry* *Decrease in total power*	Sensitive for cortical ischemia Complete map of cortical activity Continuous	Not very specific Requires trained technician
SSEP *≥50% relative decrease* *(amplitude or latency)*	Sensitive for subcortical ischemia Few leads necessary	Affected by medullary dysfunction Requires trained technician
TCD *≥50% relative decrease* *MCA velocity <25 cm/s*	Measures MCA flow continuously Detects microemboli Quantifies cerebral autoregulation	TCD impossible in 5–15% of cases Probe dislocation Insonating jelly drying
NIRS *≥20% decrease in rSO_2*	Non-invasive, easy Postoperative monitoring possible	Contribution of scalp perfusion 70% cortical perfusion is venous
Stump pressure *Mean pressure <40 mm Hg*	Assesses quality of collateral flow	Invasive, discontinuous assessment

Intraoperative Management		
	General anesthesia	Regional anesthesia
Pros	• Airway and ventilation control • Optimal surgical conditions	• Hemodynamic stability • Awake neuromonitoring
Cons	• Hemodynamic instability • Indirect neuromonitoring	• Difficult conversion to GA • Patient may move
Outcome	No significant differences in morbidity and mortality	

Technique	Short-acting premedication if
	    necessary
	
	Induction: avoid hypotension
	Etomidate or titrated propofol
	Vasopressor as needed
	Short-acting opioids best
	Avoid histamine-releasing
	    NMBAs
	Airway: smooth intubation
	Spray cords with lidocaine
	ETT secured on opposite side
	Maintenance: IV or inhalational
	*Ventilation: maintain CO_2
	    near baseline (as measured
	    at RA)*
	
	Normothermia
	Normoglycemia
	
	Smooth extubation
	Avoid hemodynamic instability
	Avoid excessive coughing
	Immediate neurological exam
		No premedication
		
		Confirm patient:
		• is not sedated,
		• is cooperative
		• understands procedure
		• has empty bladder
		Supplemental oxygen
		CO_2 monitoring
		Maintain access to airway
		
		US-guided cervical plexus block
		Superficial block with or without
		    deep block
		
		*Combine cervical plexus block
		    with infiltration below horizontal
		    branch of mandible*
		
		If patient not comfortable:
		Supplemental local infiltration
		Consider remifentanil
		(0.05–0.1 mcg/kg/min)
		Convert to general anesthesia

BP control	Maintain BP within baseline range While carotid cross-clamp is in place: • Upper baseline range • Max 20% above baseline After unclamping or while carotid shunt is in place: • Lower baseline range • Min 20% below baseline	

FIGURE 104-2. Flowchart showing anesthetic concerns during CEA

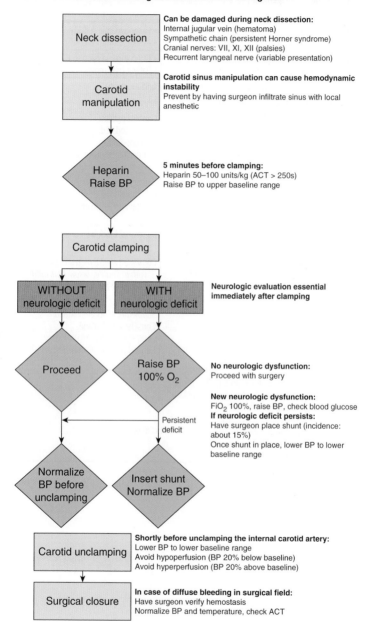

Neck dissection

Can be damaged during neck dissection:
Internal jugular vein (hematoma)
Sympathetic chain (persistent Horner syndrome)
Cranial nerves: VII, XI, XII (palsies)
Recurrent laryngeal nerve (variable presentation)

Carotid manipulation

Carotid sinus manipulation can cause hemodynamic instability
Prevent by having surgeon infiltrate sinus with local anesthetic

Heparin Raise BP

5 minutes before clamping:
Heparin 50–100 units/kg (ACT > 250s)
Raise BP to upper baseline range

Carotid clamping

WITHOUT neurologic deficit

WITH neurologic deficit

Neurologic evaluation essential immediately after clamping

Proceed

Raise BP 100% O₂

No neurologic dysfunction:
Proceed with surgery

New neurologic dysfunction:
FiO_2 100%, raise BP, check blood glucose
If neurologic deficit persists:
Have surgeon place shunt (incidence: about 15%)
Once shunt in place, lower BP to lower baseline range

Persistent deficit

Normalize BP before unclamping

Insert shunt Normalize BP

Carotid unclamping

Shortly before unclamping the internal carotid artery:
Lower BP to lower baseline range
Avoid hypoperfusion (BP 20% below baseline)
Avoid hyperperfusion (BP 20% above baseline)

Surgical closure

In case of diffuse bleeding in surgical field:
Have surgeon verify hemostasis
Normalize BP and temperature, check ACT

POSTOPERATIVE MANAGEMENT

All patients: 4–6 hours surveillance in PACU

Any complication: prolonged stay in PACU or transfer to ICU

Regular (every hour or more) surveillance of:
- Neurological and cognitive status
- Vitals and blood glucose
- Neck wound

Neurologic complications following CEA	
Stroke New neurologic deficit	**Hemorrhagic stroke** • Reduce systemic BP • Normalize ACT
Organize native head CT if symptoms persist after • Correction of hypotension • Exclusion of occlusion (carotid Doppler)	**Ischemic stroke** Hypotension: • Exclude myocardial infarction • Vasopressors and fluids Carotid occlusion: • Emergent revascularization Distal embolization: • Consider intra-arterial thrombolysis
Cognitive dysfunction New/progressive deficit in: • Orientation • Attention • Memory • Language • Organization	**Look for contributing factors** Hypo/Hypertension Hypoxemia Hypo/Hyperthermia Hypoglycemia Hypo/Hypernatremia

Cardiac complications following CEA	
Hypertension BP higher than baseline range	**First, exclude MI or stroke** Consider urinary retention and pain
Hyperperfusion syndrome: • Headache • Visual trouble • Seizure	**Treat hypertension** β-blockers (labetalol, metoprolol) if indicated Vasodilators (nicardipine, NTG, NTP)
Hypotension BP lower than baseline range with or without organ ischemia	**First exclude MI or stroke** **Treat hypotension** First-line therapy: vasopressors Second-line therapy: fluids
Myocardial ischemia Frequently asymptomatic Watch for atypical symptoms: • Hemodynamic instability • Abnormal neurologic status	O_2, aspirin EKG, enzymes Normalize BP, HR, Hct Cardiology consultation ASAP

Surgical Complications Following CEA	
Neck hematoma Non-expanding	Contact surgeon Mark hematoma borders
Expanding *without* airway compression	• Contact surgeon ASAP • Be ready for difficult airway

Expanding
 with airway compression
	• Emergent intubation:
	   ▸ Be ready for difficult airway
	   ▸ Consider *opening cervical incision at bedside*
	     to release pressure
	 • Contact surgeon ASAP, back to OR

Recurrent laryngeal nerve dysfunction Unilateral injury • Dysphonia • Dysphagia	ENT consult Prepare for emergent intubation Be ready for difficult airway
Bilateral injury • Stridor • Dyspnea	Consider tracheostomy

PEARLS

- Carotid occlusion is *not* an indication to surgery. Optimize medical therapy
- Patients with insufficient collateral circulation and/or abnormal cerebral autoregulation are less likely to tolerate carotid artery cross-clamping. Carefully discuss strategy, consider non-selective placement of carotid shunt
- Use beta-blockers (labetalol, esmolol) with caution during manipulation of carotid sinus due to significant risk of profound bradycardia
- In patients with previous stroke, use non-paretic limb to monitor neuromuscular function
- Irrespective of anesthetic technique, TCD or NIRS can be used to optimize BP postoperatively
- The introduction of intraoperative cerebral monitoring has helped reducing the rate of intraoperative stroke, not the rate of postoperative stroke

REFERENCES

For references, please visit **www.TheAnesthesiaGuide.com.**

CHAPTER 105
Spinal Surgery and Neurophysiologic Monitoring

John G. Gaudet, MD and Christopher Lysakowski, MD

- Evaluation of risk depends on several factors:
  - ▸ Elective versus emergent versus staged surgery
  - ▸ One versus several vertebral levels
  - ▸ Primary versus repeat procedure
- ALL cases of spine surgery associated with:
  - ▸ Risk of medullary injury
  - ▸ Risk of significant blood loss
  - ▸ Rare occurrence of significant venous emboli (beware if PFO)
  - ▸ Higher prevalence of chronic pain and drug dependence
- Prone positioning associated with:
  - ▸ Cardiovascular instability
  - ▸ Positioning injuries: pressure points and nerve damage, rarely rhabdomyolysis
  - ▸ Visual loss
  - ▸ Difficult access to airway
- Patients with previous high (above T5) spinal cord injury (See chapter 32)
  - ▸ Abnormal autonomic responses (hypertensive crisis or hypotension and bradycardia)
  - ▸ Vasoplegia (relative hypovolemia)
  - ▸ Atelectasis from inefficient cough and/or hypoventilation
  - ▸ Bladder spasticity
  - ▸ Creatinine does not correlate with renal function
  - ▸ Intramuscular injections may have delayed absorption

PREOPERATIVE CONSIDERATIONS

- Severe scoliosis: assess for MH susceptibility and latex allergy
- Baseline neurologic status: *document* any preexisting neurologic deficit, look for symptoms appearing during/exacerbated by neck motion (especially in presence of rheumatoid arthritis or spinal stenosis with cervical myelopathy)
- Discuss type of neuromonitoring with surgeon and specialized personnel
- Baseline visual status: *document* any preexisting visual defect
- Cardiopulmonary comorbidities and physiological reserve
  - ▸ Noninvasive cardiac testing in patients with major AHA/ACC risk factors, or intermediate AHA/ACC risk factors and limited exercise tolerance
  - ▸ Risk of blood loss: blood work (Hb/Hct, platelets, PT/PTT, ABO typing), assess vascular access, order blood products if necessary
  - ▸ Severe scoliosis with pulmonary HTN: obtain baseline ABG and PFTs, look for cor pulmonale, possible need for postoperative ventilation
  - ▸ Anti-hypertensive drugs: no ACEIs and/ARBs the day of surgery; no diuretics the day of surgery if history of orthostatic hypotension
- Diffuse articular disease
  - ▸ Assess ROM in neck and TMJ (high incidence of difficult airway)
  - ▸ Assess ROM in limbs (risk of difficult positioning)
- Chronic pain and drug dependence: consider placement of epidural catheter by surgeon during procedure and specialized pain consultation
- Anticipate need for ICU after surgery

- *All patients* should receive following information:
  - ‣ Risk of neurologic injury, importance of neurologic evaluation immediately after surgery (ETT sometimes still in place), rare necessity to perform wake-up test during procedure (patient maintained in prone position)
  - ‣ Risk of blood loss, possible necessity to transfuse blood products
  - ‣ If prone position: risk of visual loss (see postop complications chapter 62)
  - ‣ If long procedure (>6 hours), especially if prone and/or cervical, possible necessity to maintain sedated after surgery with ETT in place until safe to extubate
  - ‣ If awake fiberoptic intubation: give usual information
  - ‣ If major surgery in elderly patient: risk of postoperative cognitive dysfunction

INTRAOPERATIVE CONSIDERATIONS

Before induction:
- Prone positioning: make sure specialized table is available with adequate padding
- Usual GA setup plus two large-bore IV lines, A-line, CVL if patient with limited reserve or if high risk of venous air embolism, Foley
- Hemodynamic monitoring to guide fluid administration or if high risk of blood loss
- Have vasopressors, fluid warmers, and blood transfusion sets available. Consider intraoperative blood salvage techniques

Induction:
- Awake fiberoptic intubation if limited cervical and/or temporo-mandibular ROM
- Low-pressure ETT cuffs for long procedures (risk of airway edema)
- Congenital scoliosis, residual paralysis or autonomic hyperreflexia: avoid succinylcholine
- Patients with prior high (above T5) spinal cord injury: fluid preloading (vasoplegia)

Positioning:
- Surgeon *must* be present during positioning
- Venous access and hemodynamic monitoring must be in place *before* prone positioning
- Confirm position of endotracheal tube after positioning
- Make sure and *document* eyes are not compressed and eyelids fully closed (verify periodically during surgery)
- Objectives:
  - ‣ Avoid thoracic and abdominal compression (venous engorgement) by having the patient rest on well-padded bony prominences (iliac crests, clavicles)
  - ‣ Maintain head in neutral position
  - ‣ Genitalia and breasts free of compression
  - ‣ Provide liberal padding
  - ‣ Avoid extreme positioning of the limbs (e.g., keep shoulder abduction <90°)
- Always have stretcher immediately available outside OR to turn patient supine emergently
- Motor evoked potentials: place bite block, ensure tongue midline

Before the procedure starts, consider:
- Preemptive analgesia (ketamine 0.25 mg/kg IV, clonidine 0.2 mcg/kg up to 150 mcg IV)
- Antifibrinolytics (tranexamic acid 10–15 mg/kg IV) to reduce intraoperative blood loss

Maintenance: do not interfere with neurophysiologic monitoring
- Maintain steady state: carefully select limited number of drugs, avoid boluses, favor infusions
- TIVA often preferred: propofol (titrate to BIS/entropy) and sufentanil or remifentanil
- No inhalation agent, or very low levels (<1% desflurane); discuss with neuromonitoring team
- Discuss muscle relaxant use with neuromonitoring team: often 2 twitches on TOF adequate for SSEP, but occasionally request for no NMB
- Maintain hemodynamics, temperature, and glycemia within normal range
- Beware of occult blood loss and acidosis: frequent blood gas analyses

Emergence:
- Facial/airway edema: assess feasibility of extubation (cuff leak test)
- Immediate neurologic and visual status: document any new deficit
- Anterior cervical procedures: look for dysphagia, hoarseness, stridor, hematoma

NEUROPHYSIOLOGIC MONITORING: EVOKED POTENTIALS AND EMG

- Amplified recording of electrical potentials produced after stimulation of specific neural structures. Expressed as voltage versus time plots, with biphasic polarity (peaks and valleys)
- Set up and analyzed by certified neurophysiologists
- Interpretation may be less reliable in patients with preexisting neurologic deficits
- Analysis: modifications of *amplitude* (peak/valley voltage) and/or *latency* (time from initial stimulation to peak/valley) not due to external factors (drugs, hemodynamics and temperature, electrical noise, defective connections)

Neurophysiologic Monitoring Modalities			
Structure at risk	Dorsal column-medial lemniscus (posterior spinal cord)	Corticospinal tract (anterior spinal cord)	Spinal nerve roots
Monitored with	Somatosensory evoked potentials (SSEPs)	Motor evoked potentials (MEPs)	Electromyography (EMG)
Principle	Stimulation at periphery Recording upstream	Stimulation of motor cortex Recording downstream	Recording of muscle activity with (triggered) or without (spontaneous) electrical stimulation
Hypoxemia Anemia	AVOID	AVOID	
Hypothermia	AVOID	AVOID	
Hypotension	AVOID	AVOID	
Hypoglycemia	AVOID	AVOID	
Electrolyte disorders	AVOID	AVOID	
Inhalational agents	SAFE up to 0.5 MAC	AVOID	
Nitrous oxide	AVOID	SAFE up to 50%	
Opioids	SAFE in infusion avoid large boluses	SAFE in infusion avoid large boluses	
Neuromuscular blockers	SAFE	AVOID except at induction	
Propofol	SAFE in infusion avoid large boluses	SAFE in infusion avoid large boluses	
Etomidate	Paradoxical changes[1]	AVOID	
Thiopental Midazolam	SAFE avoid large boluses	AVOID[2]	
Ketamine	Paradoxical changes[3]	Paradoxical changes[3]	
Dexmedetomidine Clonidine	SAFE	SAFE	

[1]*amplitude amplification often coincident with myoclonus.*
[2]*MEP depression can be long-lasting despite presence of only mild EEG changes.*
[3]*amplitude amplification with ketamine can compensate for mild depressant effect of propofol.*

- Baseline SSEPs are abnormal in presence of MS, vitamin B12 deficiency, tabes dorsalis
- Baseline MEPs are abnormal in presence of MS, vitamin B12 deficiency, ALS, poliomyelitis
- Baseline EMG is abnormal in presence of myasthenia gravis, Lambert–Eaton syndrome, muscular dystrophies, botulinum toxin
- Contraindications to MEPs: deep brain stimulators, cochlear implants, ICD, epilepsy, increased ICP

FIGURE 105-1. Stepwise approach to abnormal neuromonitoring signal

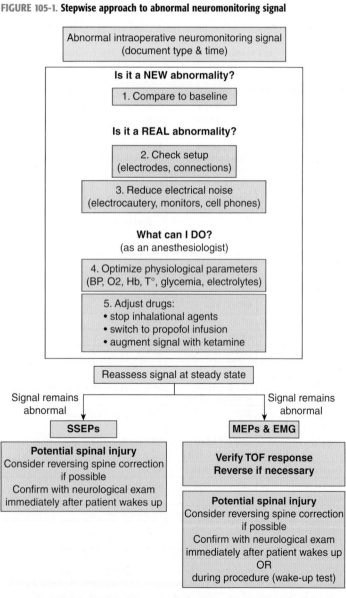

- Patients with severe scoliosis: look for pulmonary restrictive syndrome, pulmonary HTN with cor pulmonale, underlying neuromuscular disease with higher risk of malignant hyperthermia and latex allergy
- Patients with previous high (above T5) spinal cord injury: risk of abnormal autonomic responses (hypertensive crisis or hypotension and bradycardia), atelectasis from inefficient cough and/or hypoventilation, aspiration from gastroparesis, hypothermia from abnormal vasoconstriction. Regional anesthesia preferred, maintain adequate depth if GA
- Patients with rheumatoid arthritis: beware of dynamic spinal compression from cervical axial instability (positional neurologic abnormalities)
- Patients with ankylosing spondylarthropathy: look for pulmonary restrictive syndrome
- Spine surgery for tumors or vascular lesions: preoperative embolization can help reduce intraoperative blood loss
- Staged surgery: follow-up procedures often performed after one week; watch for coagulation abnormalities!

REFERENCES

For references, please visit **www.TheAnesthesiaGuide.com.**

CHAPTER 106
Anticonvulsants: Seizure Prophylaxis and Chronic Treatment

Harsha Nalabolu, MD

PREOPERATIVE

- Prophylactic anticonvulsant therapy prior to neurosurgery is controversial
- Patients should continue their preoperative anticonvulsants as long as they have therapeutic drug levels
- Phenytoin 100 mg Q8 hours or levetiracetam 500 mg are the most common regimens
- Levetiracetam is now being used more often due to broad-spectrum seizure coverage and lower side effects, and serum therapeutic levels do not need to be checked

Common Preoperative Anticonvulsant Regimens and Side Effects		
Drug	Dose	Side effects
Carbamazepine (Tegretol®)	400 mg po tid	Blurred vision, ataxia, sedation, hyponatremia, rash
Ethosuximide (Zarontin®)	500 mg po q day	Nausea, vomiting, ataxia, GI distress, drowsiness
Gabapentin (Neurontin®)	300–1200 mg po tid	Drowsiness, weight gain, peripheral edema
Lamotrigine (Lamictal®)	200 mg po bid	Rash, Stevens–Johnson's, red cell aplasia, DIC, hepatic or renal failure
Levetiracetam (Keppra®)	1000 mg po bid	Irritability, somnolence
Oxcarbazepine (Trileptal®)	600 mg po bid	Hyponatremia, rash, interactions with oral contraceptives
Phenobarbital (Solfoton®)	100 mg po q day	Drowsiness, confusion, slurred speech, ataxia, hypotension, respiratory depression, nystagmus
Phenytoin (Dilantin®)	300–400 mg po q day	Vertigo, somnolence, ataxia, gingival hyperplasia, hirsutism
Topiramate (Topamax®)	150–200 mg po bid	CNS side effects, nephrolithiasis, open-angle glaucoma, weight loss
Valproate (Depakene®)	250–500 mg po tid	GI disturbance, sedation, weight gain, somnolence, hair loss, thrombocytopenia

INTRAOPERATIVE

Anesthetic choice

- Inhalational anesthetics are primarily antiepileptic
- Nitrous oxide tends to inhibit seizure spikes
- Benzodiazepines and propofol are antiepileptic
- Ketamine, etomidate, and methohexital can be proconvulsant with low dosages and should be avoided
- High doses of fentanyl and alfentanil can trigger epileptiform spike activity on EEG
- Large doses of meperidine, atracurium, or cisatracurium should be avoided due to epileptogenic metabolites normeperidine and laudanosine
- Regional anesthesia is encouraged as long as optimal surgical environment is maintained

If seizure occurs
- Treat with small dose of thiopental 2 mg/kg, midazolam 2–5 mg, or propofol 1–2 mg/kg
- Consider phenytoin 500–1000 mg IV slow loading dose (or the equivalent as fosphenytoin: less likely to cause hypotension) for prevention of recurrent seizures
- If seizures refractory to above, administer general anesthetic doses of inhalational or IV anesthetics

POSTOPERATIVE

- Drug levels of older antiepileptics such as phenytoin need to be monitored
- If patient cannot take po postoperatively, convert to IV and adjust dose

REFERENCES

For references, please visit **www.TheAnesthesiaGuide.com**.

CHAPTER 107
Status Epilepticus
Victor Zach, MD and Roopa Kohli-Seth, MD

BACKGROUND

- Seizures persisting for more than 5 minutes, or seizure occurring during the postictal state from a prior seizure
- Can be convulsive, non-convulsive, and/or refractory (continuing despite two intravenous agents)
- Etiologies:
  - ▸ Known seizure disorder: poor compliance, drug interaction, lack of sleep
  - ▸ First seizure:
    - ▪ CVA, brain abscess or tumor, meningitis, head trauma
    - ▪ Metabolic (hypoglycemia, hyponatremia, hypocalcemia, porphyria)
    - ▪ Withdrawal (alcohol or drug), toxic (antidepressants, salicylates, ethylene glycol)

INITIAL MANAGEMENT

ABCs as needed, supplemental oxygen

Do not use bicarb to correct metabolic acidosis unless extreme (pH ≤ 6.9).

HISTORY AND PHYSICAL

- Is there a history of epilepsy? Is the patient on anti-epileptics? (Dose, obtain plasma levels)
- Time of onset (when was the patient last seen normal?)
- Drugs (agents that lower the seizure threshold; illicit drug abuse?)
- Mental status (if not awake without twitches for more than 30 minutes, get EEG to rule out non-convulsive status; get CT-scan to rule out evolving brain lesion such as a stroke or hemorrhage)
- Check for focal neurologic findings (if present, suggest underlying focal lesion)

CALL

- Epilepsy or neurology consult
- EEG – arrange for continuous monitoring if available
- Call CT scanner and request a STAT head CT w/o (and possibly with, depending on clinical picture and suspicion of other lesion) contrast

LABS

CBC, electrolytes, liver function panel, urinary toxicology screen, anti-epileptic drug levels, PT/INR, PTT

LP if immunosuppressed, fever, or no etiology found

TREATMENT

PRIMARY:
- Thiamine 100 mg IV
- 50 mL of D50 IV, unless finger stick >60
- Lorazepam (Ativan) 0.1 mg/kg IV over 2 minutes (can repeat three times q5 minutes) OR 20 mg PR (if no IV access; can also use nasal midazolam 0.1–0.5 mg/kg) *and* Fosphenytoin (Cerebyx) 20 mg/kg IV (maximum of 150 mg/min) OR phenytoin (Dilantin) 20 mg/kg IV (maximum of 50 mg/min)
- If Dilantin allergy, give valproic acid (Depacon) 20 mg/kg IV

SECONDARY: (if seizures persist, give one of the following)
- Fosphenytoin (Cerebyx) 10 mg/kg IV (additional)
- Valproic acid (Depacon) 40 mg/kg IV over 15 minutes
- Levetiracetam (Keppra) 1000 mg IV (can repeat up to a maximum of 4000 mg)
- Phenobarbital 20 mg/kg IV (maximum of 100 mg/min)

TERTIARY: (if seizures persist, intubate the patient, if not already done, and treat with one of the following)
- Midazolam (Versed): load 0.2 mg/kg IV (maximum 2 mg/kg), then continuous drip 0.5–2.0 mg/kg/h
- Propofol (Diprivan): load 1 mg/kg IV (maximum 15 mg/kg, avoid >5 mg/kg for >24 hours), then continuous drip 1–15 mg/kg/h
- Titrate agents towards maximum until seizure cessation or EEG burst-suppression pattern

QUATERNARY: (if seizures persist clinically or on EEG)
- Pentobarbital (Nembutal): load 5 mg/kg IV (maximum 10 mg/kg/h), then continuous drip 0.5–10 mg/kg/h

REFERENCES

For references, please visit **www.TheAnesthesiaGuide.com.**

CHAPTER 108
Asymptomatic Cerebrovascular Disease (For Non-neurosurgery)

Zirka H. Anastasian, MD

BACKGROUND

Major types of neurovascular disease:
- Cerebral vessel stenosis (i.e., carotid stenosis)
- Cerebral aneurysm
- Cerebral vessel arteriovenous malformation

PATHOPHYSIOLOGY

See Neurovascular surgery (chapter 103)

Preop Evaluation/Considerations

	Carotid stenosis	Cerebral aneurysm	Cerebral AVM
Past medical history	Hx of TIA? Determine NORMAL baseline blood pressure Cardiac hx? (high likelihood of CAD) Hx of MI? Angina? Exercise tolerance?	Hx of headaches? Hx of smoking? Determine NORMAL baseline blood pressure Cardiac history?	Determine NORMAL baseline blood pressure
Physical exam	Baseline neurological exam (compare deficits)	Baseline neurological exam (compare deficits)	Baseline neurological exam (compare deficits) Evaluate for symptoms of large shunts: congestive heart failure, etc.
Medication history	Antihypertensive medication history (class, last dose timing), anticoagulation history (aspirin, etc.)	Antihypertensive medication history, weight loss supplements?	CHF meds?
Studies to review	Doppler US, angiography, EKG, stress test	CT, MRI, angiography	CT, MRI, angiography
Specific questions	How significant is the stenosis? Is the patient symptomatic? Is it unilateral or bilateral?	How many aneurysms? What is their size? For how long have they been managed? What was the date of the last MRI/Angio?	What is the size of the AVM? What was the medical plan?

Anesthesia

	Carotid stenosis	Cerebral aneurysm	Cerebral AVM
Monitors	Standard monitors/ lines: EKG, BP cuff, pulse oximeter, temperature probe, peripheral IV Additional monitors/ lines: arterial line (preferably preinduction to monitor BP changes during induction and laryngoscopy)	Standard monitors/ lines: EKG, BP cuff, pulse oximeter, esophageal/bladder temperature probe (especially important if cooling), peripheral IVs (2 or more) Additional monitors/ lines: arterial line (preferably preinduction to monitor BP changes during induction and laryngoscopy), Foley	Standard monitors/ lines: EKG, BP cuff, pulse oximeter, esophageal/bladder temperature probe (especially important if cooling), peripheral IVs (2 or more) Additional monitors/ lines: arterial line (preferably preinduction to monitor BP changes during induction and laryngoscopy), Foley

(continued)

Anesthesia (*continued*)

	Carotid stenosis	Cerebral aneurysm	Cerebral AVM
Induction	Avoid HYPOtension by either using agents such as etomidate, or following induction agent with a vasopressor	Avoid HYPERtension by doing induction agent accordingly, doing test laryngoscopy, and have fast-acting antihypertensive (i.e., esmolol) ready	Avoid HYPERtension by doing induction agent accordingly, doing test laryngoscopy, and have fast-acting antihypertensive (i.e., esmolol) ready
Airway management	Avoid pressure on the carotid, avoid excessive neck manipulation (to avoid dislodging possible emboli)	Avoid prolonged intubation attempt: avoid prolonged laryngoscopy	Consider possibility of co-present aneurysm: avoid prolonged larygoscopy
Blood pressure goals	Maintain adequate cerebral perfusion pressure: keep patient's pressure on the high side of what THEIR normal pressure is	Avoid hypertension and avoid sudden fluctuations in blood pressure (which put stress on the walls of the aneurysm)	Meticulous BP control: avoid hypertension due to risk of aneurysm
Emergence	Avoid hypercarbia (which can decrease cerebral blood flow)	Avoid hypertension, sudden changes in pressure	Avoid hypertension, sudden changes in pressure
Possible agents to consider having on-hand	Phenylephrine infusion Ephedrine Etomidate (to avoid hypotension during induction)	Short-acting β-blockers, calcium channel blockers, opioids for smooth emergence	Short-acting β-blockers, calcium channel blockers, opioids for smooth emergence

Postoperative (Complications)

	CEA	Aneurysm	AVM
Complication	TIA Ischemic stroke Hyperperfusion	Aneurysm rupture	Aneurysm rupture/ AVM bleed
Acute management	Immediate angiography Consider intra-arterial thrombolysis and clot extraction vs open surgical clot extraction Anticoagulation For hyperperfusion, follow transcranial Doppler and carefully decrease blood pressure	If time of rupture known, induce burst suppression with barbiturate, consider hypothermia, consider immediate surgical intervention	Immediate angiography/ other imaging to determine etiology of mental status change, consider emergent surgery, decompressive craniotomy

PEARLS AND TIPS

Carotid stenosis in patients undergoing CABG:
- Asymptomatic carotid stenosis prior to CABG: no change in incidence of perioperative stroke
- Stroke rate is the same for combined CABG-CEA versus CABG alone in pts with asymptomatic bruit (but if the degree of stenosis is HIGH, this significantly increases stroke probability)
- Stroke rate is lower for combined CEA-CABG versus CABG alone in pts with history of stroke or TIA

REFERENCES

For references, please visit **www.TheAnesthesiaGuide.com.**

CHAPTER 109
Management of Patient with Intracerebral Hemorrhage (ICH)

Aditya Uppalapati, MD and Roopa Kohli-Seth, MD

INCIDENCE

- 12–31 per 100,000 people
- 10–30% of all strokes
- Six-month mortality rate of 30–50%
- Only 20% regain functional independence at end of 6 months

MAJOR RISK FACTORS

- Men
- African-Americans, Japanese
- Low LDL cholesterol, Hypertension
- Excessive alcohol consumption
- Anticoagulation

SECONDARY CAUSES

- Ischemic stroke with hemorrhagic conversion
- Amyloid angiopathy (age >60 years)
- Chronic hypertension
- Coagulopathy
- AV malformation, cavernous angioma, neoplasm, dural sinus thrombosis with hemorrhage
- Vasculopathy
- Trauma

PATHOPHYSIOLOGY

- Hemorrhages continue to grow and expand over several hours after onset of symptoms (hematoma growth)
- Most of the brain injury and swelling that happens after ICH is the result of inflammation caused by thrombin and other coagulation end-products

CLINICAL EVALUATION

- *Determine if any predisposing illness* – cancer, hypertension, smoking, trauma, dementia (amyloid), vascular malformations (aneurysm, AVM), anticoagulation (warfarin, heparin, LMWH), anti platelet medications, renal disease (uremic platelets), liver disease (abnormal coagulation parameters – prothrombin time), hematologic disease, recreational drug abuse (cocaine), seizure disorder, CVA, hemophilia, von Willebrand's disease
- *History* – sudden onset of focal neurological deficit, which progresses over minutes to hours, headache, vomiting
- *Physical examination*
  ‣ Vitals: elevated systolic blood pressure > 160 mm Hg, temperature > 37.5°C associated with growth of hematoma
  ‣ HEENT: look for signs of injury (laceration, fracture, scars) on the head
  ‣ Cardiovascular: rule out atrial fibrillation and other arrhythmias
  ‣ CNS: detailed neurological exam-assess mental status, cranial nerves, sensory, motor, and cerebellar exam

LABS (SEE CLINICAL EVALUATION)

- PT for patients on warfarin
- PTT to rule out von Willebrand's disease
- Platelet count for thrombocytosis or thrombocytopenia
- Liver function test, fibrinogen, D dimer,
- Chemistry
- Urine toxicology screen
- Type and cross match sample

DIAGNOSTIC EVALUATION

- *Imaging*
  ‣ Non-contrast computed tomography (CT) scan or magnetic resonance imaging (MRI) (whichever is faster to obtain) to assess:
    ▪ Location of blood (deep, superficial, cerebellar, intraventricular)
    ▪ Volume of blood ($[A \times B \times C]/2$)
    ▪ Presence of hydrocephalus, midline shift
  ‣ CT scan is better at evaluating ventricular extension
  ‣ CT angiography for aneurysm, arteriovenous malformation
  ‣ MRI is better at detecting underlying structural lesions and delineating perihematomal edema and herniation
- *ICP monitoring (see chapter 98)*
  ‣ Especially helpful in patients with decreased level of consciousness

TREATMENT

- *Emergency management*
  ‣ Airway evaluation for rapid neurological decline and necessity for endotracheal intubation
    ▪ Failure to recognize leads to aspiration, hypoxemia, hypercapnia (with increased ICP and downward spiral)
    ▪ For rapid sequence intubation, choose sedatives (propofol) and neuromuscular blockers (rocuronium; cisatracurium if indicated) that do not raise ICP. Consider topical lidocaine to suppress cough reflex
    ▪ Avoid excessive hyperventilation to PCO_2 below 28 mm Hg as it leads to increased vasoconstriction and brain ischemia
- *Blood pressure*
  ‣ Maintain SBP between 160 and 180 mm Hg or MAP < 130 mm Hg
    ▪ Cardene   infusion, 5–15 mg/h *or*
    ▪ Labetalol   5–20 mg bolus and infusion at 2 mg/h *or*
    ▪ Esmolol   250 mcg/kg IV loading, maintenance at 25–300 mcg/kg/min
    ▪ Avoid nitroprusside (can raise ICP)

- ‣ Hypotension
  - ▪ Isotonic fluid bolus
  - ▪ Vasopressors (norepinephrine or phenylephrine) if needed to maintain a CPP of >60–80 mm Hg
- *Lowering ICP (See chapter 98)*
  - ‣ Head of bead >30°
  - ‣ Head midline
  - ‣ Sedation
  - ‣ Osmotic dieresis with hypertonic saline or mannitol
  - ‣ Optimize CPP
  - ‣ Ventriculostomy for obstruction from intraventricular hemorrhage
- *Stopping or slowing the bleeding*

• Vitamin K	10 mg IV over 10 min for patients on warfarin
• If INR/PT prolonged	In addition to vitamin K, treat with 15–20 mL/kg of FFP. Consider prothrombin concentrate complex (PCC) 50 IU/kg in patients with no recent thrombotic event or DIC.
• Heparin, enoxaparin	Use protamine 1 mg for 100 U of heparin or 1 mg of enoxaparin
• TPA	Check fibrinogen – if <100, give 0.15 U/kg of cryoprecipitate, may consider platelet transfusion
• Direct thrombin inhibitors	Argatroban, lepirudin: no reversal agents
• Renal failure patients	With increased creatinine: DDAVP – 0.3 mcg/kg IV
• Platelet inhibitor	Aspirin, plavix use: DDAVP – 0.3 mcg/kg IV, may consider platelet transfusion
• Thrombocytopenia	Transfuse to keep platelets >50,000
• Hemophilia	Factor VIII, IX

- *Seizure*
  - ‣ Acute seizure: lorazepam – 0.05–0.1 mg/kg (repeat as needed) followed by anti -epileptics (fosphenytoin 20 mg/kg IV, valproic acid 15–45 mg/kg, or pheno-barbital 15–20 mg/kg)
  - ‣ Patients with large supratentorial bleed and decreased level of consciousness might benefit from prophylactic antiseizure medications
- *General measures*
  - ‣ Position – head of bed >30° (to decrease ICP and risk of pneumonia in intubated patients)
  - ‣ Fluids: isotonic. Avoid fluids containing dextrose or hypotonic (increases cerebral edema and ICP)
  - ‣ Temperature: treat any source and lower the temperature to normothermia with antipyretics, cooling devices. Mild hypothermia (35°) if elevated ICP
  - ‣ Nutrition and blood glucose – Early enteral nutrition within 48 hours. Maintain euglycemia
  - ‣ DVT prophylaxis – Sequential compression devices. Can consider heparin or LMWH on day 2 of ICH
- *Surgery:* Indications vary with site of bleed
  - ‣ Cerebellar hemorrhage >3 cm in diameter with neurological deterioration or her-niation or hydrocephalus cerebellar decompression with removal of hematoma
  - ‣ Can consider open craniotomy in supratentorial ICH with lobar clots >30 mL within 1 cm of the surface
  - ‣ Intraventricular hemorrhage – if hydrocephalus from obstruction ventriculos-tomy and external ventricular drainage

REFERENCES

For references, please visit **www.TheAnesthesiaGuide.com.**

CHAPTER 110
Management of Subdural and Extradural Hematomas

Lisa E. Vianna, DO and Roopa Kohli-Seth, MD

NB: For the management of craniotomy or burr hole for SDH or EDH, see chapter on Craniotomy (chapter 101).

FIGURE 110-1. Anatomy of subdural and epidural hematomas

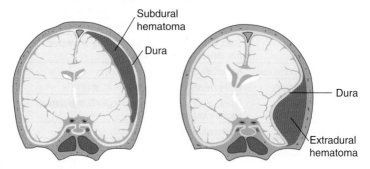

Subdural Versus Extradural Hematoma		
	Subdural	Extradural
Anatomic location	**Under dura mater** Bridging veins between the brain and dura tear	**Outside of dura mater** Can occur in the spine (epidural hematoma)
		Tears in small arteries (predominantly the middle meningeal artery)
		Higher pressure in arteries leads to more rapid bleeding; often in temporal or temporal–parietal region
Bleeding	Venous	Arterial
Time course	**Acute/subacute** (minutes to hours) or **chronic** (days to weeks)	**Acute**
Causes	• Head injury/trauma • Malignancy • Spontaneous	Head trauma

(continued)

Subdural Versus Extradural Hematoma (*continued*)		
	Subdural	Extradural
Risk factors	• Extremes of age (very old or very young) • Use of anticoagulants (clopidogrel [Plavix], Aspirin, warfarin [Coumadin]; dabigatran [Pradaxa]) • Chronic alcohol use/abuse • Frequent and recurrent falls	
Symptoms	Adults • Headache • Balance disturbances • Weakness or paresthesias • Seizures • Slurred or confused speech • Nausea/vomiting • Change in level of consciousness (mild delirium to obtundation) Infants • Bulging fontanelles/change in head circumference • Seizures • Irritability or lethargy • Vomiting or difficulty feeding	• Headache–often intense/severe • Change in mental status–unconsciousness; can have a *"lucid interval"* with rapid decline thereafter ("talk-and-deteriorate") • Cranial nerve III (oculomotor)–*fixed and dilated pupil on the same side* as the injury/bleed; eye will appear inferior and laterally deviated (unopposed CN VI) • Abnormal cerebral posturing • Weakness of the extremities *on the same side* as the lesion • *Loss of vision on the contralateral side* • Respiratory arrest possible (due to transtentorial or uncal herniation–compression on the medulla)

Imaging appearance (noncontrast CT brain or MRI)	• Classically appears *crescent shaped* with concave surface away from the skull
	  ▸ Extra-axial collections with increased attenuation
	  ▸ When large enough, may cause effacement of the sulci and midline shift
	  ▸ Can cross suture lines
	• May have a convex appearance particularly in the early stages of bleeding but distinguished from epidural bleeds by *ability to cross suture lines*
		Often appears as a *biconvex lens*

Treatment	Indications for surgery: • SDH with thickness greater than 10 mm or midline shift greater than 5 mm • Comatose patient (GCS <9) with lesion less than 10mm or midline shift less than 5 mm, if GCS decreased by 2 or more points between time of injury and hospital presentation • Patient presents with an asymmetric/fixed or dilated pupil • ICP exceeds 20 mm Hg (normal ICP ~5–15 mm Hg)	Surgical removal of blood. • Burr hole–less often utilized due to small access and limited visibility • Craniotomy–preferred • Procedure chosen determined by the surgeon, the size/location of the lesion and the anatomic access required of the underlying pathology

(*continued*)

Subdural Versus Extradural Hematoma (*continued*)

	Subdural	Extradural
Treatment	Surgical procedures: Procedure chosen determined by the surgeon based on the size/location of the lesion and the anatomic access required of the underlying pathology. • Burr hole–or keyhole craniotomy; small dime size; minimally invasive procedure • Craniotomy–removal of a larger portion of skull • Shunts (subdural to peritoneal)– particularly chronic subdural ‣ more often in infants and young children; rarely in adults	

	Medications:
	To reduce swelling and decrease intracranial pressure:
	• Corticosteroids: Dexamethasone 150 mg total over 9 days; 16 mg/day)
	• Mannitol : 0.25 to 2 g/kg IV once 60 to 90 min before surgery
	Antiepileptics/seizure prophylaxis to be considered: No prospective randomized control trials; often given for 1 month, then tapered off if no seizure activity
	
	• Phenytoin[Dilantin]: 4 to 6 mg/kg/day IV divided BID–TID
	• Levetiracetam (Keppra): 500 mg IV BID
	• Carbamazepine (Tegretol): Available orally, 800 to 1200 mg/day divided BID–QID
	Reversal of bleeding diathesis:
	• Fresh frozen plasma
	• Cryoprecipitate
	• Platelet transfusion
	• Vitamin K: 10 mg IV/IM/SC once
	• Protamine: 1 to 1.5 mg IV per 100 units heparin
	• DDAVP–for anti-platelet agents: dosing 0.3 µg/kg IV (approximately 20 µg for adults)
	• Recombinant activated Factor VIIa [NovoSeven]:
	  ‣ Intended to limit growth of hemorrhage
	  ‣ Not FDA approved; ongoing clinical investigation
	  ‣ No proven survival or functional outcome benefit to date
	  ‣ Utilized within 4 h of symptoms and 1 h post-CT imaging
	  ‣ Dose of 40, 80, and 160 µg/kg body weight IV have been used
		Correct coagulation status if needed

REFERENCES

For references, please visit **www.TheAnesthesiaGuide.com.**

CHAPTER 111
Management of Patient with Ischemic Stroke

Victor Zach, MD and Roopa Kohli-Seth, MD

HISTORY

- Determine the time of onset (time the patient was last seen normal). This is extremely important, as thrombolysis is possible only within 3–4.5 hours of the onset
- Was there any repetitive movement to suggest a seizure, as it is a contraindication to thrombolysis?

PHYSICAL

- Check vitals; BP must be <185/105 for treatment with intravenous tPA (Alteplase)
- Check FAST
  - F – face (droop?)
  - A – arm (drift or paresis?)
  - S – speech (aphasic or dysarthric?)
  - T – time last seen normal
- Assess for dysphagia – if present, insert nasogastric tube
- Calculate NIH Stroke Scale

NIH Stroke Scale (0–30)		
1a Level of consciousness	0	Alert
	1	Drowsy
	2	Stupor
	3	Coma
1b What month is it?	0	Both correct
How old are you?	1	One correct
	2	Both incorrect
1c Make a fist	0	Both correct
Close your eyes	1	One correct
	2	Both incorrect
2 Best gaze	0	Normal
	1	Partial gaze palsy
	2	Forced deviation
3 Visual fields	0	No visual loss
	1	Partial hemianopia
	2	Complete hemianopia
	3	Bilateral hemianopia

(continued)

NIH Stroke Scale (0–30) (*continued*)		
4 Facial paresis	0	Normal
	1	Minor paresis
	2	Partial paresis
	3	Complete palsy
5, 6, 7, 8 Motor (each arm and each leg)	0	Normal
	1	Drift
	2	Some effort against gravity
	3	No effort against gravity
	4	No movement
9 Ataxia	0	Absent
	1	Present in one limb
	2	Present in 2 or more limbs
10 Sensory	0	Normal
	1	Partial loss
	2	Dense loss
11 Best language	0	No aphasia
	1	Mild-moderate aphasia
	2	Severe aphasia
	3	Mute
12 Dysarthria	0	Normal
	1	Mild-moderate dysarthria
	2	Unintelligible
13 Neglect	0	No neglect
	1	Partial neglect
	2	Complete neglect

NIHSS <3 is a relative contraindication to thrombolysis, unless deficit highly disabling (e.g., an isolated severe aphasia).
NIHSS >24 has a high risk of hemorrhage; consider endovascular options.
NIHSS also has a prognostic value: a score ≥ 16 forecasts a high probability of death or severe disability, whereas a score of ≤ 6 forecasts a good recovery.

Call

• Emergent vascular neurology consult
• CT scanner – STAT non-contrast Head CT to rule out intracranial hemorrhage

Labs: CBC, electrolytes, liver function, glucose, PT/INR, PTT, urine toxicology, ABG

Management: Revascularization				
Modality	Time window	Dose	Pros	Cons
Intravenous-tPA (Alteplase)	0–4.5 h	0.1 mg/kg bolus, then 0.8 mg/kg drip over 1 h; maximum = 90 mg	Availability No specialty staff needed	Contraindications (see below)
Intraarterial-tPA (Alteplase)	0–6 h	2–20 mg intra-arterially	Longer window Lower dose	Highly trained team needed
Thrombectomy via MERCI, PENUMBRA, SOLITAIRE FR	0–8 h		Up to INR of 3.0 Longest time window	Highly trained team needed Highest procedural risk

CONTRAINDICATIONS TO INTRAVENOUS TPA

- Time of onset >4.5 hours
- Time of onset shortened to >3 hours when any of the following occur
  - Age > 80
  - History of both diabetes and stroke
  - Head CT with stroke >1/3 of vessel territory
  - Current anticoagulant use regardless of INR/PTT
- Serious head trauma, MI or stroke >3 months
- History of non-compressible site of hemorrhage <21 days ago (major surgery <14 days ago)
- Any prior or current intracranial hemorrhage
- BP >185/105 mm Hg after attempted treatment (>180/100 during IV rTPA infusion)
- Active bleeding or fracture
- PTT elevated or INR >1.7; heparin use within the last 48 hours; platelet count <100,000
- Blood glucose <50
- Seizure
- Rapidly improving symptoms

Management: BP Control		
	Blood pressure	Treatment
Candidates for thrombolysis Pretreatment	SBP > 185 or DBP >110 mm Hg	• Labetalol 10–20 mg IVP repeated every 10–20 min, or Nicardipine 5 mg/h, titrate by 2.5 mg/h every 5–15 min, maximum 15 mg/h; when desired blood pressure reached, lower to 3 mg/h or Enalapril 1.25 mg IVP
Candidates for thrombolysis Post-treatment	DBP > 140 mm Hg	• Sodium nitroprusside (0.5 mcg/kg/min)
	SBP >230 mm Hg or DBP 121–140 mm Hg	• Labetalol 10–20 mg IVP and consider labetalol infusion at 1–2 mg/min, or • Nicardipine 5 mg/h, titrate by 2.5 mg/h every 5–15 min, maximum 15 mg/h; when desired blood pressure reached, lower to 3 mg/h
	SBP 180–230 mm Hg or DBP 105–120 mm Hg	• Labetalol 10 mg IVP, may repeat and double every 10 min up to maximum dose of 300 mg
Non-candidates for thrombolysis	DBP > 140 mm Hg	• Sodium nitroprusside 0.5 mcg/kg/min; may reduce approximately 10–20%
	SBP >220, or DBP 121–140 mm Hg, or MAP > 130 mm Hg	• Labetalol 10–20 mg IVP over 1–2 min; may repeat and double every 10 min up to maximum dose of 150 mg or nicardipine 5 mg/h IV infusion and titrate, or • Nicardipine 5 mg/h, titrate by 2.5 mg/h every 5–15 min, maximum 15 mg/h; when desired blood pressure reached, lower to 3 mg/h
	SBP <220 mm Hg, or DBP 105–120 mm Hg, or MAP < 130 mm Hg	• Antihypertensive therapy indicated only if acute myocardial infarction, aortic dissection, severe CHF, or hypertensive encephalopathy present

SBP, systolic blood pressure; DBP, diastolic blood pressure; IVP, IV push; MAP, mean arterial pressure. Adapted from 2005 Advanced Cardiac Life Support (ACLS) guidelines and 2007 American Stroke Association Scientific Statement.

AFTER REVASCULARIZATION

- Maintain BP <180/105, check BP q15 minutes during infusion and 2 hours after infusion, then q30 minutes for 6 hours, then q1 hour for 16 hours
  - Labetalol (Trandate) 10–20 mg intravenous over 1–2 minutes (may repeat q10–20 minutes to maximum 300 mg)
  - Nicardipine (Cardene) infusion, 5 mg/h, titrate up by 0.25 mg/h at 5- to 15-minute intervals
- Avoid antiplatelets, anticoagulants, venipuncture, NG tube placement for 24 hours

PATIENTS THAT DO NOT QUALIFY FOR REVASCULARIZATION

- ABCs
- Start antiplatelet therapy
- Start high-intensity statin therapy
- Start enoxaparin 1 mg/kg q24 hours for DVT prophylaxis
- Avoid hypotonic fluids
- Keep head of the bed up 30°
- Order an MRI and an MRA of the brain
  - Repeat head CT and CT angio brain in 24–48 hours if MRI contraindicated
- Frequent neuro checks
- Labs: thyroid studies, HgbA1c, lipid profile, B12, homocysteine
- Echocardiography
- Carotid duplex
- Holter monitor
- Further work-up as per neurology
- If age <60 and Glasgow Coma Scale <8 or not following commands, contact neurosurgery for a decompressive hemicraniectomy (life-saving procedure with a number needed to treat of 2)

REFERENCES

For references, please visit **www.TheAnesthesiaGuide.com.**

CHAPTER 112
Glasgow and Liège Scales

Elisabeth Falzone, MD and Jean-Pierre Tourtier, MD

GLASGOW SCALE

Evaluation of a patient's consciousness and its evolution over time
- *Score from 3 to 15*
  - Under 8: coma
  - Between 12 and 8: critical, case-by-case evaluation
- *Limits*
  - Pediatric patients (adapted scale)
  - Deaf patients
  - Patients with paralysis

Glasgow Scale for adults

Glasgow Coma Scale

	1	2	3	4	5	6
Eyes	Does not open eyes	Opens eyes in response to painful stimuli	Open eyes in response to voice	Opens eyes spontaneously		
Verbal	Makes no sounds	Incomprehensible sounds	Utters inappropriate words	Confused, disoriented	Oriented converses normally	
Motor	Makes no movements	Extension to painful stimuli (decerebrate response)	Abnormal flexion to painful stimuli (decorticate response)	Flexion/ withdrawal to painful stimuli	Localizes painful stimuli	Obeys commands

Glasgow Scale for pediatric patients (under 5 years)

Pediatric Glasgow Coma Scale

	1	2	3	4	5	6
Eyes	No eye opening	Eye opening to pain	Eye opening to noise	Eyes open spontaneously		
Verbal						
0–23 month	No verbal response	Grunts or is agitated or restless	Persistent inappropriate crying when pain	Irritated, crying but consolable	Normal: smiles or coos appropriately	
2–5 years	No verbal response	Grunts	Persistent cries or screams	Inappropriate words	Appropriate words or phrases	
Motor	No motor response	Stereotyped extension to pain	Stereotyped flexion to pain	Withdrawal from pain	Withdrawal from touch	Spontaneously

NB: applied pain: noxious stimulus in an uninjured area.

Example: nail bed pressure with a hard object, or pressure behind vertical branch of mandible.

LIÈGE SCALE

Glasgow scale insufficient when deep coma because spontaneous eye opening is insufficiently indicative of brainstem arousal system activity

Better predictive value of cerebral trunk function than motor response

Glasgow–Liège Scale	
Reflex	Score
Fronto-orbicular	5
Vertical oculocephalic	4
Pupillary light	3
Horizontal oculocephalic (or oculovestibular)	2
Oculocardiac	1
No brainstem reflex	0

Score from 3 to 20 (Glasgow score + 0–5)

- Fronto-orbicular = percussion of the glabella (area of the forehead between the eyebrows) produces contraction of the orbicularis oculi muscle
- Oculocephalic reflex (doll's eyes) = present when deviation of at least one eye can be induced by repeated neck flexion and extension (vertical) or side-to-side movement (horizontal)
- If the reflexes are absent or cannot be tested (e.g., immobilized cervical spine), an attempt is made to elicit ocular motion by external auditory canal irrigation using iced water (i.e., oculovestibular reflex testing); contra-indicated if tympanic perforation
- Oculocardiac reflex = present when pressure on the eyeball causes the heart rate to slow down
- The best response determines the brainstem reflex score. The selected reflexes disappear in descending order during rostro–caudal deterioration

REFERENCE

For references, please visit **www.TheAnesthesiaGuide.com.**

CHAPTER 113
Management of Traumatic Brain Injury

Karim Tazarourte, MD, Eric Cesareo, MD, and David Sapir, MD

TRIAGE

- GCS <9 or a motor scale <5 = severe traumatic brain injury
- 9 <GCS ≤13: "moderate" but beware! Treat like a severe traumatic brain injury until proved otherwise
- GCS 14–15: minor head injury
- Beware of "talk-and-deteriorate" patients, whose GCS drops within 48 hours. Usually subdural or extra-dural hematoma

INITIAL MANAGEMENT OF SEVERE TRAUMATIC BRAIN INJURY

Airway

- C-collar until C-spine "cleared" (see trauma chapter)
- Tracheal intubation (in-line stabilization, or even fiberoptic)
  ‣ Unclear whether prehospital intubation improves outcome
- *Avoid*
  ‣ *Decreases in MAP during intubation*: use RSI with succinylcholine and ketamine or etomidate. Control MAP strictly. Use ephedrine or norepinephrine if necessary
  ‣ Also avoid large increases in MAP during intubation: topical lidocaine, "soft hands", IV esmolol if needed

Breathing

- Ventilation for SpO_2 >95% and $ETCO_2$ = 35 mm Hg

Circulation

- Insert A-line
- Bring MAP >80 mm Hg with isotonic crystalloids (fluid will not increase ICP in a hypotensive TBI patient)
- If needed, initiate norepinephrine infusion through a CVL
- Bring Hb >8 g/dL
- If severe hemorrhage due to other lesions, emergent surgical hemostasis might be necessary

Neuro

- Sedation-analgesia by midazolam (also prevents initial seizures) and opioids as infusion
- Emergent CT-scan without contrast; neurosurgery involvement depending on results
- Fixed dilated pupil (uni- or bilateral) = *emergency, incipient herniation*
  ‣ Neurosurgical consult STAT
  ‣ Acute hyperventilation to $PaCO_2$ of 25 mm Hg
  ‣ Mannitol 20% 2 mL/kg in 10 minutes IV or 7.5% hypertonic saline (HSS) 125 mL IV en route to CT-scan
  ‣ If the pupils are still fixed and dilated, repeat mannitol 20% 4 mL/kg
- Patient on warfarin
  ‣ Give prothrombin complex concentrate (PCC 1 mL/kg) or 25 IU/kg factor IX
  ‣ Give Vitamin K 10 mg IV
- If possible, perform transcranial Doppler (TCD) of MCA
  ‣ Normal values: PI <1.4 and Vd (diastolic velocity) >20 cm/s
  ‣ If abnormal, consider increasing MAP and Hb, administering mannitol or HSS

OPTIMAL TIMING FOR PERFORMING CT-SCAN

- Immediately if GCS <15 or GCS = 15 but associated injuries or patient on warfarin
- Delayed at 6 hours after the trauma if GCS 15 with initial loss of consciousness
- Repeat CT-scan if any neurological deterioration
- Repeat CT-scan after 6 hours if normal initially (in 20% of patients with initially normal CT scans, the repeat scan performed beyond the 6th hour is abnormal)

FURTHER MANAGEMENT GOALS

- Prevent secondary injury (ischemic, metabolic, excitatory neurotransmitters, reperfusion)
- Maintain a cerebral perfusion pressure above 60 mm Hg (CPP = MAP − ICP)
  ‣ Monitor ICP if possible; see chapter 98
- Maintain normocapnia
- Maintain normal osmolarity (290–300 mmol/l). Avoid dextrose or hypotonic fluids
- Seizure prophylaxis: fosphenytoin 13–18 phenytoin equivalents/kg
- Depending on underlying lesion:
  ‣ Neurosurgery if indicated (extra-dural/subdural hematoma, ventriculostomy, craniectomy if uncontrollable increase in ICP)
  ‣ Factor VIIa if persistent intra-cranial bleeding; controversial, very expensive

MANAGEMENT OF MINOR HEAD INJURY

- GCS 15 without warfarin, loss of consciousness or associated injury: no CT-scan, send home with monitoring instruction sheet
- GCS 15 with loss of consciousness without warfarin nor associated injury: CT-scan 8 hours after trauma; if normal, send home
- GCS 15 with warfarin: CT-scan immediately to rule out asymptomatic intracranial hemorrhage and CT-scan at 6 hours if the first one was normal. Emergent reversal if any intracranial hemorrhage
- GCS < 15: CT-scan immediately; repeat after 6 hours if first one was normal

REFERENCES

For references, please visit **www.TheAnesthesiaGuide.com.**

CHAPTER 114
Initial Management of Spinal Cord Injury (SCI)

Karim Tazarourte, MD, Eric Cesareo, MD, and David Sapir, MD

BASICS

Always suspect spine injury in significant trauma, even if no initial neurologic sign
DO NOT WORSEN LESIONS: immobilize, treat as unstable spine until cleared.

Beware of secondary SCI due to mechanical trauma (spine lesions) and/or ischemia

Spinal cord injury above C4 will block the diaphragm; high thoracic lesion will block abdominal and thoracic accessory muscles and weaken cough.

INITIAL DIAGNOSIS

Conscious patient: motor or sensory deficit often obvious.

Comatose patient: diagnosis more difficult. *Treat as unstable spine until cleared (CT-scan).* Additional suspicion if hypotension without tachycardia.

Be thorough.

Do not miss other lesions.

INITIAL MANAGEMENT: FOLLOW ATLS GUIDELINES

- Spine immobilization by *cervical collar and spinal board systematically*
- Only exception: alert, normal neurologic status, AND no pain: no imaging needed, remove collar

Airway
- Assess need for intubation: in-line stabilization with RSI. FOB or video laryngoscope if available
- Consider retrograde intubation if facial trauma
- No nasal intubation in trauma patient
- Avoid succinylcholine, especially if neurogenic shock (risk of extreme bradycardia); if necessary, administer atropine prior to succinylcholine

Breathing
- Ventilation for SpO_2 >95% and $ETCO_2$ = 35 mm Hg
- Gastric atony and distention: decompress stomach to facilitate ventilation

Circulation
- Insert A-line and CVL
- MAP >80 mm Hg with isotonic crystalloids (fluid will not increase ICP in a hypotensive TBI patient)
- If needed, initiate norepinephrine infusion through a CVL
- Transfuse as needed for Hb >8 g/dL
- If severe hemorrhage due to other lesions, emergent surgical hemostasis might be needed

Neuro
- Thorough clinical examination to document neurologic deficit, including assessment of anal sphincter tone and contraction
  ▸ Level of lesion? (Not always the same on both sides)
  ▸ Complete or incomplete lesion? (Any sensory/motor preservation below lesion, and/or anal sphincter tone maintained = incomplete lesion)
  ▸ ASIA score (see scoring sheet = Figure 114-1)
- 30% spinal cord injuries are at multiples levels
- Assess for traumatic brain injury (see chapter 113): GCS, neurological exam
- Whole body (vertex to pelvis) CT scan to diagnose associated lesions
- Transfer the patient to a specialized center as soon as possible
- Methylprednisolone probably not helpful, but still widely used as there is no effective therapy

Methylprednisolone Dosage	
Within 3 h of trauma	30 mg/kg, followed by 5.4 mg/kg/h for 24 h
3 to 8 h after trauma	30 mg/kg, followed by 5.4 mg/kg/h for 48 h
8 h or more after trauma	No benefit

FIGURE 114-1. ASIA Spinal Cord Injury Scoring Sheet

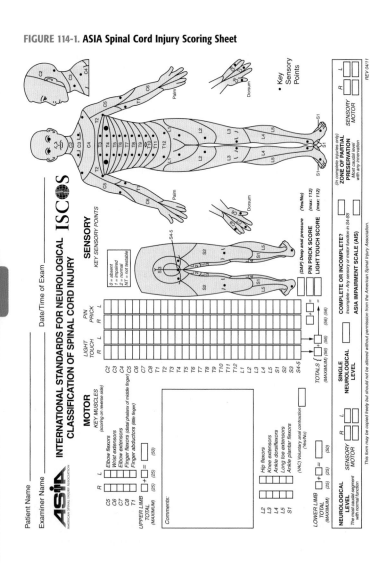

Muscle Function Grading

0 = total paralysis

1 = palpable or visible contraction

2 = active movement, full range of motion (ROM) with gravity eliminated

3 = active movement, full ROM against gravity

4 = active movement, full ROM against gravity and moderate resistance in a muscle specific position.

5 = (normal) active movement, full ROM against gravity and full resistance in a muscle specific position expected from an otherwise unimpaired peson.

5* = (normal) active movement, full ROM against gravity and sufficient resistance to be considered normal if identified inhibiting factors (i.e. pain, disuse) were not present.

NT = not testable (i.e. due to immobilization, severe pain such that the patient cannot be graded, amputation of limb, or contracture of >50% of the range of motion).

ASIA Impairment (AIS) Scale

☐ **A = Complete.** No sensory or motor function is preserved in the sacral segments S4-S5.

☐ **B = Sensory Incomplete.** Sensory but not motor function is preserved below the neurological level and includes the sacral segments S4-S5 (light touch, pin prick at S4-S5: or deep anal pressure (DAP)), AND no motor function is preserved more than three levels below the motor level on either side of the body.

☐ **C = Motor Incomplete.** Motor function is preserved below the neurological level**, and more than half of key muscle functions below the single neurological level of injury (NLI) have a muscle grade less than 3 (Grades 0-2).

☐ **D = Motor Incomplete.** Motor function is preserved below the neurological level**, and at least half (half or more) of key muscle functions below the NLI have a muscle grade ≥ 3.

☐ **E = Normal.** If sensation and motor function as tested with the ISNCSCI are graded as normal in all segments, and the patient had prior deficits, then the AIS grade is E. Someone without an initial SCI does not receive an AIS grade.

**For an individual to receive a grade of C or D, i.e. motor incomplete status, they must have either (1) voluntary anal sphincter contraction or (2) sacral sensory sparing with sparing of motor function more than three levels below the motor level for that side of the body. The Standards at this time allows even non-key muscle function more than 3 levels below the motor level to be used in determining motor incomplete status (AIS B versus C).

NOTE: When assessing the extent of motor sparing below the level for distinguishing between AIS B and C, the *motor level* on each side is used; whereas to differentiate between AIS C and D (based on proportion of key muscle functions with strength grade 3 or greater) the *single neurological level* is used.

Steps in Classification

The following order is recommended in determining the classification of individuals with SCI.

1. Determine sensory levels for right and left sides.

2. Determine motor levels for right and left sides.
   Note: in regions where there is no myotome to test, the motor level is presumed to be the same as the sensory level, if testable motor function above that level is also normal.

3. Determine the single neurological level.
   This is the lowest segment where motor and sensory function is normal on both sides, and is the most cephalad of the sensory and motor levels determined in steps 1 and 2.

4. Determine whether the injury is Complete or Incomplete.
   (i.e. absence or presence of sacral sparing)
   If voluntary anal contraction = **No** AND all S4-5 sensory scores = **0** AND deep anal pressure = **No**, then injury is COMPLETE. Otherwise, injury is incomplete.

5. Determine ASIA Impairment Scale (AIS) Grade:

Is injury Complete?

NO → If **YES**, AIS=A and can record ZPP (lowest dermatome or myotome on each side with some preservation)

↓

Is injury motor Incomplete?

If **NO**, AIS=B
(Yes=voluntary anal contraction OR motor function more than three levels below the motor level on a given side, if the patient has sensory incomplete classification)

YES ↓

Are at least half of the key muscles below the single neurological level graded 3 or better?

NO → AIS=C   YES → AIS=D

If sensation and motor function is normal in all segments, AIS=E
Note: AIS E is used in follow-up testing when an individual with a documented SCI has recovered normal function. If at initial testing no deficits are found, the individual is neurologically intact; the ASIA Impairment Scale does not apply.

Surgical indication
- Risk of spine instability and spinal cord compression depends on intensity and mechanism of trauma

Risk Stratification for Spine Instability and Spinal Cord Compression			
Very high risk	High risk	Moderate risk	Mild risk
Rotation	Compression (burst)	Extension (deceleration)	Flexion (retropulsion)
Facet dislocation	Bone extrusions	Ligament tears	Disk herniation
Fracture-dislocation (usually unstable)	Ligament tears (often unstable)	Severe SCI in presence of spinal spondylosis	Stable unless combined w/ dislocation

- Complete versus incomplete SCI: look for presence of *any residual neurologic function*
- Complete SCI: poor prognosis, attempt closed reduction if possible, irreversible after 48 hours
- Incomplete SCI: frequently requires early (<24 hours) surgery, especially if spine unstable
- Indications for early surgery (within 24 hours) following spinal trauma
  ‣ Unstable spine with incomplete spinal cord injury
  ‣ Stable spine with progressive incomplete spinal cord injury
  ‣ Unstable spine with uncooperative/agitated patient
  ‣ Unstable spine with rotational facet dislocation (high risk of neurologic deterioration)

Other
- Avoid dextrose containing IV fluids; hyperglycemia worsens neurologic injury
- Thromboprophylaxis as soon as possible
- See chapter 217 (trauma) for criteria for cervical spine "clearing"

Early complications

Respiratory
- Respiratory distress when lesion above C4; poor cough with thoracic lesion
- Anticipate difficulty weaning from mechanical ventilation
- Lesion above C6: absent or insufficient ventilation (tracheotomy)
- Lower cervical/high thoracic lesion: inefficient ventilation and coughing (postoperative positive pressure ventilation [PPV])
- Assess for neurogenic pulmonary edema

Neurologic worsening with secondary SCI
- Maintain MAP >80 for at least a week (IV fluids, norepinephrine if needed)
- Consider spinal cord cooling to limit edema and apoptosis (experimental)

Intraoperative hemorrhage
- Consider using tranexamic acid (1 g IV in 10 minutes)
- Optimize coagulation
- Transfuse RBC if Hct <24% (or 30 if h/o CAD [or high likelihood: elderly, long-standing DM, etc.])
- Transfuse FFP if RBC given. Start with 1 U FFP/3U RBC, but if >10 U RBC, give 1 U FFP/1 U RBC

REFERENCES

For references, please visit www.TheAnesthesiaGuide.com.

CHAPTER 115
Meningitis

Lisa E. Vianna, DO and Roopa Kohli-Seth, MD

Inflammation of the protective membranes (meninges) covering the brain and spinal cord.

CAUSES

- Bacterial: streptococci; *Neisseria*; gram negative bacilli, staphylococci; *Neisseria meningitides*; *Haemophilus influenzae*; *Listeria monocytogenes*
- Lyme (*Borrelia burgdorferi*)
- Syphilis – spirochete (*Treponema pallidum*)
- Viral: late summer and early fall: enterovirus; arboviruses, West Nile; also Herpes viruses, HIV, mumps, rabies
- Mycobacterial (MTB and MAI)
- Fungal: cryptococcal; *Coccidioides immitis* or *Coccidioides posadasii*, *Cryptococcus neoformans*, *Histoplasma capsulatum*, *Coccidioides immitis*, *Blastomyces dermatitides*
- Parasitic: *Toxoplasma gondii*, *Taenia solium* (cysticercosis)
- Eosinophilic meningitis: *Angiostrongylus cantonensis*, baylisascariasis, and gnathostomiasis
- Drugs: NSAIDs, antimicrobials (e.g., trimethoprim–sulfamethoxazole, amoxicillin, isoniazid), Muromonab-CD3 (Orthoclone OKT3), azathioprine, IVIG, intrathecal methotrexate, intrathecal cystine arabinoside, vaccines, allopurinol
- Neoplastic: infiltration of the subarachnoid space by cancer cells; can be metastatic or from a primary brain tumor like medulloblastoma
- Foreign bodies: CSF shunts, external ventriculostomy
- Systemic illness: sarcoidosis, leptomeningeal cancer, post transplantation lymphoproliferative disorder, systemic lupus erythematosus, Wegener granulomatosis, CNS vasculitis, Behçet disease, Vogt–Koyanagi–Harada syndrome

SIGNS AND SYMPTOMS

- Fever
- Headache
- Stiff neck
- Photophobia
- Nausea/vomiting
- Altered mental status
- Rash/purpura may be present, particularly in meningococcal meningitis
- Seizures possible

MANAGEMENT

Early recognition, rapid diagnosis, and urgent antimicrobial and adjunctive therapy are paramount; multidisciplinary treatment team should be involved: neurology, infectious diseases, etc.

- Head CT to evaluate for mass lesion and evaluate signs of elevated intracranial pressure, especially in immunocompromised patients, history of CNS disease, papilledema, change in level of consciousness, focal neurologic deficits
- SAH is part of the differential and should be excluded by CT
- Emergent culture sampling – blood and CSF analysis; LP contraindicated if CT signs of elevated ICP, as it may precipitate herniation

CSF Characteristics According to Meningitis Etiology				
Test	Bacterial	Viral	Fungal	Tubercular
Opening pressure	Increased	Normal	Variable	Variable
Glucose (CSF to plasma ratio)	Normal to decreased	Normal	Decreased	Decreased
Protein	Mild to moderate increase	Normal to increased	Increased	Increased
Cell differential predominance	PMNs	Lymphocytes	Lymphocytes	Lymphocytes
WBC count	>1000 per mm³	<100 per mm³	Variable	Variable

- Presumptive antibiotherapy; if imaging and CSF sampling delayed, presumptive antimicrobial therapy should be given immediately, recognizing this may diminish yield in culture sampling
  - Ceftriaxone 2 mg IV q12 hours *or* Cefotaxime 2 gm IV q6–8 hours
  - Vancomycin 1 gm IV q12 hours—in light of increasing resistance of streptococci to cephalosporin therapy
  - Ampicillin should be considered in young children, patients over 50, and immunocompromised patients to target *Listeria monocytogenes*
- Dexamethasone (0.15 mg/kg q6 hours for 2–4 days, to be initiated before antibiotic therapy) if proven or suspected pneumococcal meningitis
- Anti-epileptics if seizures are a presenting symptom
- Anti-fungals: Amphotericin B and Flucytosine in combination
  - Amphotericin B liposomal (Ambisome) 6 mg/kg/day IV for 11–21 days
  - Flucytosine 50–150 mg/kg/day po divided q6 hours
- Anti-virals: for herpes meningitis/encephalitis
  - Acyclovir 10 mg/kg IV q8 hours (using ideal body weight)
- Anti-tubercular drugs:
  - Isoniazid 5 mg/kg po/IM daily
  - Rifampin 10 mg/kg po/IV daily
  - Pyrazinamide 20–25 mg/kg po daily
  - Addition of a fourth drug dependent on local resistance patterns
  - Rifater (combination of Isoniazid/Rifampin/pyrazinamide)—weight-based dosing

REFERENCES

For references, please visit **www.TheAnesthesiaGuide.com**.

CHAPTER 116
Brain Abscess

Lisa E. Vianna, DO and Roopa Kohli-Seth, MD

PATHOGENESIS

- Direct extension from a local infection: ear infection, dental abscess, infection of paranasal sinuses or mastoid air cells, epidural abscess
- Direct inoculation: head trauma or surgical procedures
- Remote or hematogenous spread: bacteremia, endocarditis, and congenital heart disease

CAUSES

- Bacterial: often polymicrobial; gram-negative and gram-positive: Staphylococcus, Streptococci, Bacteroides, Prevotella, Fusobacterium, Enterobacteriaceae, Pseudomonas species, and anaerobes. Less common: *Haemophillus influenzae*, *Streptococcus pneumoniae*, and *Neisseria meningitides*; Nocardia in immunosuppressed hosts
- Mycobacterial (*M tuberculosis*, *Mycobacterium avium* intracellulare)
- Protozoan (*Toxoplasma gondii*, *Entamoeba histolytica*, *Trypanosoma cruzi*, Schistosoma, Paragonimus)
- Helminths (Taenia solium)
- Fungal: mainly immunocompromised patients (Aspergillus, Candida, Cryptococcus, Mucorales, Coccidioides, *Histoplasma capsulatum*, *Blastomyces dermatitidis*)
- Secondary to underlying tumors/malignancy

SYMPTOMS

- Alterations in mental status: anywhere along a continuum from confusion/inattention to coma
- Fever/chills
- Stiff neck
- Symptoms of increased intracranial pressure: headache, vomiting, visual disturbances
- Seizures
- Decreased motor skills or sensation perception
- Language difficulty

DIAGNOSTIC WORK-UP/TESTING/IMAGING

- Blood cultures
- CT and MRI of brain: Diffusion-weighted imaging (DWI) is helpful to distinguish abscess versus necrotic tumor (sensitivity and specificity over 90%)
- Antibody testing (*Toxoplasma gondii* and *Taenia solium* if epidemiology consistent with diagnosis)
- CXR: look for images suggesting septic emboli
- EEG
- Needle sampling (CT-guided, stereotactic) of collection for causative agent if feasible

TREATMENT

- Identification of causative organisms(s) is paramount to successful therapy. Initial therapy should be commenced with broad-spectrum antibiotics that cross blood–brain and blood–CSF barriers; choice of surgical procedure needs to be tailored to and specific for each patient
  - Empiric antibiotics:
    - Dental origin: amoxicillin + ornidazole (or metronidazole)
    - Ear, mastoid, unclear origin: cefotaxime + ornidazole (or metronidazole)
    - Immunocompromised: imipenem + trimethoprim/sulfamethoxazole
- Surgical options:
  - Twist drill craniotomy
  - Therapeutic burr-hole drainage
  - CT-guided stereotactic procedure: for most superficial and large abscesses; allows drainage and identification of causative pathogen
  - Craniotomy (rare)
- Combination approach:
  - Surgical aspiration or removal of all abscesses larger than 2.5 cm in diameter
  - 6 weeks or longer course of intravenous antibiotics
  - Weekly CT or MRI
  - Cure rate of more than 90% serial imaging until radiographic resolution
  - Any enlargement or failure to resolve should lead to further surgical aspiration or excision

- Medical approach favored in clinical situations of:
  - Multiple abscesses
  - Small abscess (less than 2 cm)
  - Toxoplasma: very amenable to medical therapy alone
  - Tuberculous abscesses often can be managed medically
  - Abscess anatomically very deep: difficult to access and may be harmful to attempt surgical approach
- Target treatment to culture data; removal of the primary focus paramount; treat for at least 6 weeks
- Antiepileptics—in high-risk patients—initiated immediately and continued for at least 1 year
- Outcome
  - Mortality is 50% to 90% and morbidity is even higher if severe neurologic impairment is evident at the time of presentation (or with extremely rapid onset of illness), even with immediate medical treatment
  - Pneumococcal abscess has the highest mortality among bacterial etiologies (20–30% in adults, 10% in children) and morbidity (15%)
  - Viral meningitis (without encephalitis) mortality rate is less than 1%
  - Prognosis worse for patients at extremes of age, with significant comorbidities and immunosuppression

REFERENCES

For references, please visit **www.TheAnesthesiaGuide.com.**

CHAPTER 117
Diabetes Insipidus

Ananda C. Dharshan, MBBS and Roopa Kohli-Seth, MD

Diabetes insipidus (DI) is characterized by the *decreased ability of the kidneys to concentrate urine.*

PATHOPHYSIOLOGY

- Antidiuretic hormone (ADH) is the primary determinant of free water balance
- ADH is produced in posterior pituitary and acts on the V2 receptors of the collecting tubules of the kidney
- ADH alters the permeability of the collecting tubes to control the free water excretion

DI can be due to different distinct *mechanisms* (Figure 117-1).

FIGURE 117-1. Mechanisms of diabetes insipidus

Vasopressinase induced	Nephrogenic
Vasopressinase destroys the native vasopressin but not the synthetic desmopressin	Resistance to ADH activity in the kidney.
Mostly seen in the last trimester of pregnancy or puerperium	**Congenital:** Defective V2 receptors (X-linked) or vasopressin-sensitive water channels in the kidneys called aquaporin 2 (autosomal recessive)
Associated with oligohydramnios, preeclampsia, hepatic insufficiency	**Acquired:** Either due to distortion of the architecture of the kidney (amyloidosis) or chemicals (lithium, demeclocycline)
Primary central	**Secondary central**
No identifiable lesion noted on MRI of the pituitary or hypothalamus.	Due to damage to the hypothalamus or pituitary stalk by tumor, inflammation or injury.
Most of the time due to autoimmunity against hypothalamic arginine vasopressin (AVP) secreting cells.	

(center label: DI)

EPIDEMIOLOGY

- Rare disease with prevalence of 3 per 100,000 population
- No significant sex gender difference

Clinical Presentation	
Symptoms	Clinical findings
Adults–Polyuria, polydipsia, nocturia, and craving for ice water	If thirst mechanism is intact–
	Hydronephrosis and distended bladder due to excessive urinary volume
Children–Anorexia, growth defects, enuresis, sleep disturbance, fatigue, difficulty at school	**If no access to free water or damage to hypothalamic thirst center then–**
Infants–Irritability, chronic dehydration, growth retardation, neurologic disturbance, and hyperthermia	Hypernatremia, dehydration, hypertonic encephalopathy, obtundation, coma, seizure, subarachnoid hemorrhage, and intracerebral hemorrhage

Differential diagnosis

- Diabetes mellitus
- Cushing syndrome
- Lithium
- Psychogenic polydipsia

Diagnosis (Figure 117-2)

- No single diagnostic laboratory test
- 24-hour urine output of less than 2 liters rules out DI
- Hyperuricemia can be seen as urate clearance is reduced due to reduced V1 stimulation
- MRI of the pituitary and hypothalamus should be done to rule out mass lesions
  - In T1-weighted MRI, the normally present bright spot in the sella is lost in most DI patients

FIGURE 117-2. Diagnosis of diabetes insipidus

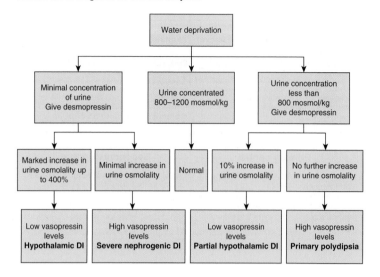

- Water deprivation test is the gold standard for diagnosing DI (see Figure 2)
  ‣ Check baseline Na⁺; do not permit oral intake, measure volume and osmolality of each voided urine sample; weigh patient
  ‣ When two consecutive urine osmolality do not vary by more than 10% and the patient has lost 2% of weight, check Na⁺, urine osmolality and serum vasopressin levels. Then give 2 mg of desmopressin if needed

Treatment
- Goal: to prevent nocturnal enuresis and to control polydipsia
- General: Avoid dehydration by drinking fluids to match the urine output and by providing intravenous fluid replacement with hypo-osmolar fluid

Treatment of Diabetes Insipidus			
Vasopressin	Desmopressin	Diuretics	Other agents
• Has antidiuretic and vasopressor activity • Continuous low-dose infusion preserves organs after brain death • Antivasopressin antibodies can be formed • Caution: can cause myocardial ischemia, therefore concurrent use of nitrates is advisable in susceptible patients	• Synthetic analog of vasopressin • Has markedly reduced pressor activity and is 2000 times more specific for antidiuresis • Only agent for the treatment of DI in pregnancy • Administered IV, PO, or intranasal 2 to 3 times a day • Caution: hyponatremia, emotional changes, erythromelalgia	• Hydrocholorothiazide causes mild hypovolemia→ salt and water retention in proximal nephrons → reduces flow in collecting tubules where ADH acts→ reduce urinary volume • **Amiloride** blocks Na⁺ channels in the collecting duct and prevents lithium absorption • These are the only agents for nephrogenic DI	• **Chlorpropamide** increases renal sensitivity to ADH • **Carbamazepine** promotes ADH release • **Non-steroidal anti-inflammatory drugs** reduce solute load to the urinary collecting tubules and urine output by inhibition of prostaglandin synthesis

PROGNOSIS

DI by itself is an inconvenience but does not alter life expectancy.

REFERENCES

For references, please visit **www.TheAnesthesiaGuide.com.**

CHAPTER 118
Brain Death and Organ Donation

Ronaldo Collo Go, MD and Roopa Kohli-Seth, MD

DIAGNOSIS OF BRAIN DEATH

- Acute CNS catastrophic event excluding acid-base, circulatory, electrolyte, hemodynamic disturbances, and no evidence of poisoning or hypothermia
- Clinical examination: *absent brainstem function*; spinal cord and peripheral nerve reflexes may occur
- Clinical exam *repeated after 6 hours* in patients over 1-year-old
- *Apnea test* performed after second clinical examination
  - Patient disconnected from ventilator and placed on 6 L/min O_2 by T-piece
  - Spontaneous respirations within 8 to 15 minutes = negative apnea test
  - No spontaneous respirations while $PCO_2 \geq 60$ or increase in $PCO_2 \geq 20$ from baseline = positive
- Clinical examination and positive apnea test are sufficient to affirm brain death

Tests	
Confirmatory tests	If clinical exam and apnea test inconclusive
Angiogram	Absence of filling at level of internal carotids or circle of Willis
Electroencephalography	Absence of brain activity for 30 min
Nuclear brain scan	Absence of uptake of isotope
Somatosensory evoked potentials	Absence of response to median nerve
Transcranial Doppler	Small systolic peak without diastolic flow

Incidence and Types of Organ Donation	
54% brain death donor	legal death; causes: cardiovascular accident, trauma, anoxia
40% living donor	preferred for kidney transplant
7 % cardiac death donor	irreversible cessation of respiratory and pulmonary function, which can be controlled (expecting cardiac arrest) or uncontrolled (unexpected cardiac arrest)

FIGURE 118-1. Pathophysiology of increased ICP in the brain-dead patient

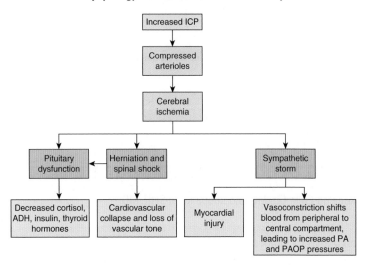

Contraindications to organ donation

- Multiorgan failure secondary to sepsis
- Cancer except skin cancer other than melanoma, certain brain tumors, remote prostate cancer
- Infections: bacterial, viral, fungal, parasitic, prions

Failure of potential donors

- Family refuses consent
- Hemodynamic collapse
- Medically unsuitable according to acceptance criteria

Work-Up and Management of the Potential Organ Donor	
Identify potential donors	Notify local organ donor network, transplant and family coordination services A second brain death examination might be warranted prior to declaration of brain death
Initial labs	Infectious: HIV1, HIV2, HTLV 1, 2; hepatitis panel; CMV IgG and IgM, EBV IgM and IgG, RPR, toxoplasmosis IgG
Routine labs every 6 h	CBC, ABG, AST, Liver Function Test, PT/PTT/INR, Fibrinogen, Troponin, CK, Chem7, Magnesium, Phosphorus, LDH, Amylase, Lipase
Lines	Arterial line (preferably left radial for heart/lung harvest) Central venous catheter (preferably right IJ/subclavian) Pulmonary artery catheter 2 large-bore PVLs
Other	NGT, warming blanket, heater/humidifier on breathing circuit
Monitors	ECG, urine output (Foley), core temperature, thermodilution CO (if PAC)
Optional	Echocardiogram and inotropic support if ejection fraction less than 45% Electrocardiogram Bronchoscopy Cardiac catheterization

DONOR MANAGEMENT

Maintain organ perfusion and oxygenation through fluid, electrolyte, and acid-base management

Maintain temperature between 35.5°C and 38°C

Rule of 100s:
- SBP >100 mm Hg
- U/O >100 mL/h
- PaO_2 >100 mm Hg
- Hemoglobin >100g/L

COMMON PROBLEMS

Hypotension

- Crystalloid versus colloid, depends on the organ (e.g., for lung donors, prefer colloid to minimize pulmonary edema)
- Avoid hydroxyethyl starch due to renal tubular injury and hypernatremia
- If hypervolemic, use an inotrope or vasopressor
  ‣ Dopamine first choice because at <5 µg/kg/min, it vasodilates renal, coronary, and mesenteric vasculature, improving organ perfusion and induces protective enzymes like heme oxygenase-1 that can improve organ survival
    ▪ 10 µg/kg/min upper limit
  ‣ Dobutamine improves organ perfusion by increasing cardiac output
    ▪ Limiting factor: peripheral vasodilator that can cause hypotension; severe tachycardia
  ‣ Epinephrine might be contemplated if dopamine has reached higher limit
  ‣ Vasopressors such as norepinephrine or vasopressin can also be used
    ▪ Norepinephrine can improve coronary and renal perfusion
    ▪ If still insufficient, use vasopressin, effective against diabetes insipidus and that reduces need for catecholamines
  ‣ For refractory hypotension, use hormone replacement therapy

Medications Used for Refractory Hypotension in the Brain-Dead Patient	
Hormone replacement therapy	
Vasopressin	25 units in 250 mL normal saline or D5 Water at 0.5 units/h IV or DDAVP 1–4 µg IV then 1–2 µg every 6 h; in diabetes insipidus; you can give the boluses or infusion at vasopressin infusion at 0.5 unit/h to maximum of 6 unit/h to target urine output of 0.5–3 mL/kg/h and serum sodium 135–145. Sodium measured every 6 h
Methylprednisolone	15 mg/kg IV bolus daily
Insulin	25 units in 250 mL normal saline at 1 unit/h IV (glucose goal 100–140)
Thyroid hormone	First administer 10 units regular insulin with 1 ampule D50 (to prevent hyperkalemia from the T4 bolus), followed by 20 µg T4 IV bolus, then 10 µg/h of T4 IV (200 µg in 500 mL NS), maximum dose 20 µg/h

Arrhythmias
- Follow current guidelines but note that bradycardia may be resistant to atropine

Diabetes insipidus
- Complete or incomplete loss of antidiuretic hormone presenting as massive hypotonic diuresis
- Administer vasopressin as above

Oliguria
- Goal is urine output 1 mL/kg/h
- If fluid resuscitation is not effective, diuretics such as furosemide or low-dose dopamine maybe used

Coagulopathy
- Could be secondary to release of fibrinolytic substances or plasminogen activators from ischemic brain, or other processes
- Administer RBC, FFP, coagulation factors, platelets when deemed appropriate
- Typically aim for TP > 35%; however, for split-liver transplant, PT should be > 60%

Ventilation management
- 6 mL/kg predicted body weight and plateau pressure < 30 cm H_2O (IBW: Males: IBW = 50 + (2.3 × (height in inches − 60); Females: IBW = 45.5 + [2.3 × (height in inches − 60)]
- Beta-agonists should be continued to reduce secretions

ORGAN HARVEST

- Duration: 2 to 5 hours
- Administer NMB and opioids (spinal reflexes typically intact)
- Broad-spectrum antibiotics (institution-specific)
- Continue resuscitation until aortic cross-clamping
- Left radial A-line if heart/lung harvest
- Stop ventilation and resuscitation when heart is explanted

ORGAN DONATION AFTER CARDIAC DEATH

- Rules according to OPTN/UNOS
- Exclusion criteria similar after brain death, consent of next-of-kin needed
- Life-sustaining measures are withdrawn under controlled circumstances in ICU or OR
- Time from the onset of asystole to the declaration of death is generally about 5 minutes, but may be as short as 2 minutes; neither the surgeon who recovers the organs nor any other personnel involved in transplantation can participate in end-of-life care or the declaration of death
- Kidneys and liver but also pancreas, lungs, and, in rare cases, the heart are harvested
- Ischemia or hypoxia of more than 1 hour predicts unusable organs for donation

REFERENCES

For references, please visit **www.TheAnesthesiaGuide.com**.

PART VIII

REGIONAL

CHAPTER 119
Safety in Regional Anesthesia

Erica A. Ash, MD

NEURAXIAL BLOCKS AND HEMOSTASIS

- Rare incidence of neurologic complications due to hematoma formation
- Epidural incidence <1:150,000
- Spinal incidence <1:220,000
- Risk factors:
  - Increased age
  - Spinal cord/spine abnormality
  - Underlying coagulopathy
  - Difficult/traumatic needle placement
  - Indwelling catheter during sustained anticoagulation therapy
  - If treatment with UFH or LMWH >4 days: check platelets prior to neuraxial anesthesia
  - LMWH high dose SC: enoxaparin 1 mg/kg q12 hours, enoxaparin 1.5 mg/kg q day, dalteparin 120 U/kg q12 hours, dalteparin 200 U/kg q day, tinzaparin 175 U/kg q day
- Review medical record to determine concurrent use of medications that affect other components of clotting mechanism
- Traumatic tap in the setting of anticipated full anticoagulation with heparin: delay case for 24 hours

PERIPHERAL NERVE BLOCKS (PNB) AND HEMOSTASIS

- Morbidity of spinal hematoma is due to bleeding into a fixed space. Risk of nerve ischemia may be reduced when there is bleeding into peripheral neurovascular sheath as the sheath is an expandable space
- Twenty-six published cases of significant bleeding after PNB, all of which resulted in neurologic recovery in 6–12 months
- Risk of peripheral technique is not defined, but published cases suggest the greatest risk is blood loss as opposed to neurologic injury
- No definitive recommendations for PNB
- Deep plexus or PNB (paravertebral, psoas compartment, sciatic, possibly infraclavicular): ASRA recommends following neuraxial recommendations; probably too restrictive

ASRA Guidelines for Neuraxial Blocks with Medications Interfering with Coagulation

Drug	Dose	Indication	Time from last dose to wait prior to catheter placement	Time from last dose to wait prior to catheter removal	Time needed to wait to redose after catheter removal
ASA, NSAIDs			No contraindication if only agent and no other concerns (e.g., thrombocytopenia)		
Unfractionated heparin (UFH)	5,000 U SQ q12	Thromboprophylaxis	None	None	None
UFH	5,000 U SQ q8	Thromboprophylaxis		Not recommended	
UFH	Therapeutic IV infusion	DVT/PE treatment	4–6 h Check PTT	2–4 h Check PTT	1 h
UFH	Surgeon-specific	Intraoperative heparinization (vascular surgery)	Catheter placement prior to UFH. Wait 1 h from needle placement to UFH administration	2–4 h Check PTT	1 h
UFH	Full	CPB		Insufficient data	
Low-molecular-weight heparin (LMWH)	Low dose, q day dosing	Thromboprophylaxis	10–12 h	12 h	2 h
LMWH	Low dose, BID dosing	Thromboprophylaxis	Not recommended	Remove catheter prior to initiating LMWH	2 h Wait 24 h postoperatively regardless of anesthetic technique
LMWH	High dose	Thromboembolism treatment	24 h. Ideally catheter removed prior to treatment initiation	24 h	2 h
Warfarin	Therapeutic		4–5 days; check INR: • INR normal if therapeutic • INR <1.5 if only one dose given		

Drug	Dose	Indication			
Clopidogrel (Plavix®)			7 days	Within 24 h of starting dose. If greater than 48 h, wait 7 days	24 h
Ticlopidine (Ticlid®)			14 days	14 days	24 h
Abciximab (ReoPro®)			24–48 h		
Eptifibatide (Integrilin®)			4–8 h		
Tirofiban (Aggrastat®)			4–8 h		
Fondaparinux (Arixtra®) Indirect factor Xa inhibitor	• 2.5 mg SQ q day • 5–10 mg SQ q day	• DVT prophylaxis • DVT/PE therapy	24 h	36 h	12 h
Rivaroxaban (Xarelto®) Direct factor Xa inhibitor	• 10 mg PO q day • 15 mg PO TID × 3 weeks, and then 20 mg PO q day • 20 mg PO q day	• DVT prophylaxis after THA/TKA • DVT/PE therapy (not FDA-approved) • AFib (not FDA-approved)	Not recommended	18 h	6 h
Apixaban (Eliquis®) Direct factor Xa inhibitor	• 2.5 mg PO BID • 5 mg PO BID	• DVT prophylaxis (not FDA-approved) • AFib		Insufficient data	
Dabigatran (Pradaxa®) Direct thrombin inhibitor	• 220 mg PO q day • 150 mg PO BID	• DVT prophylaxis (not FDA-approved) • AFib	Not recommended	Not recommended	4–6 h

http://journals.lww.com/rapm/Fulltext/2010/01000/Regional_Anesthesia_in_the_Patient_Receiving.13.aspx.

LOCAL ANESTHETIC (LA) TOXICITY

Systemic toxicity usually results from inadvertent intravascular injection.

Occasionally secondary to vascular absorption from the periphery:
* *Intravenous > tracheal > intercostal > caudal > paracervical > epidural > brachial plexus > sciatic > subcutaneous*

LA plasma concentration and toxicity determined by:
* Dose injected (maximum doses of LA: see chapter 120)
* Speed of injection
* Site of injection
* Addition of vasoconstrictors
* Arterial versus venous
* CO_2 tension (influences cerebral blood flow)
* pH: acidosis increases intracellular ion trapping and increases the amount of free drug, thereby decreasing seizure threshold

Prevention:
* Slow, fractionated injection with frequent aspiration and patient monitoring to stop injection at first signs suggestive of toxicity
* Increasing evidence to suggest that ultrasound-guided blocks improve safety:
  ‣ Decreased risk of inadvertent intravascular injection
  ‣ Decreased LA dose required

Signs (may present in variable chronological order) (Figure 119-1):

FIGURE 119-1. Systemic toxicity symptoms as function of plasma lidocaine level

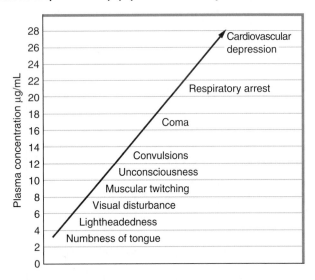

- Early:
  - ‣ Circumoral numbness
  - ‣ Tongue paresthesias
  - ‣ Metallic taste in mouth
  - ‣ Dizziness
  - ‣ Tinnitus
  - ‣ Blurred vision
  - ‣ Agitation
  - ‣ Paranoia
  - ‣ CNS depression
  - ‣ Slurred speech
  - ‣ Unconsciousness
- Late signs:
  - ‣ Muscle twitching
  - ‣ Tonic–clonic seizures
  - ‣ Respiratory arrest
  - ‣ Cardiovascular collapse

Cardiac toxicity:
- Bupivacaine > levobupivacaine > ropivacaine > lidocaine

Mechanism:
- Bupivacaine inhibits the mitochondrial enzyme carnitine-acylcarnitine translocase, effectively preventing state III respiration and the cardiac myocyte's use of fatty acids as fuel
  - ‣ Lipid therapy relies mainly on:
    - ▪ "Lipid sink" with binding of free bupivacaine (lipophilic)
    - ▪ Provision of fatty acids to be used as fuel by the heart
- Bupivacaine: low (compared with lidocaine) dissociation from cardiac sodium channels due to prolonged protein binding

---

ASRA Recommended Treatment for Suspected LA Toxicity

- Call for help
- Airway: hyperventilate with 100% O_2 (reduce $PaCO_2$ to decrease free drug, and to reduce cerebral blood flow); intubate if needed
- Suppress seizures: treat with benzodiazepines (midazolam 2–5 mg), and then with propofol if unsuccessful (avoid propofol if cardiovascular instability)
- Initiate BLS/ACLS as needed; continue resuscitation efforts longer than for another arrest mechanism given mechanism of action of LA
- Reduce individual epinephrine doses to <1 μg/kg
- Avoid vasopressin, calcium channel blockers, beta-blockers, or LA
- Infuse 20% lipid emulsion if signs of cardiac toxicity
  - ‣ Bolus 1.5 mL/kg IBW IV over 1 min (typical adult: 100 mL)
  - ‣ Continuous infusion at 0.25 mL/(kg min) (~18 mL/min)
  - ‣ Repeat bolus 1–2 times if cardiovascular collapse does not improve
  - ‣ Increase infusion to 0.5 mL/(kg min) for persistent hypotension
  - ‣ Continue infusion for a minimum of 10 min after stability is maintained
  - ‣ Recommended maximum 10 mL/kg over the first 30 min
- Cardiopulmonary bypass if above fails
- Prolonged monitoring (>12 h)

PREOPERATIVE NEUROLOGIC EVALUATION

Identify and document cognitive, sensory, motor, and coordination deficits.

Cognition:
• Note baseline mental status—orientation to person, place, and time

Sensory—compare right versus left and degree of asymmetry:
• Sharp versus dull—fragmented tongue depressor versus clean end of tongue depressor
• Temperature—alcohol wipe or ice in glove
• Proprioception—move patient's joint while his or her eyes are closed and query the direction of movement

Dermatomes:
• Area of skin supplied by the dorsal (sensory) root of the spinal nerve
• Overlapping between dermatomes

Motor—compare right versus left and degree of asymmetry:
• Muscle tone—resistance to passive range of motion
• Muscle strength—movement against resistance:
  ‣ 0 = no contraction
  ‣ 1 = trace contraction
  ‣ 2 = active movement without gravity
  ‣ 3 = active movement against gravity
  ‣ 4 = active movement against gravity and resistance
  ‣ 5 = normal

Coordination:
• Finger to nose
• Heel to shin

Preoperative peripheral neuropathy carries increased risk of permanent nerve damage ("double-crush" injury with nerve block). However, this intuitive idea is not supported by evidence.

ASEPTIC TECHNIQUE

No current consensus regarding infection control.

Range of techniques:
• Mask only to full barrier technique (mask, cap, sterile gloves and gown, full drapes)
  ‣ Full barrier technique recommended when placing an indwelling catheter

Most importantly:
• Vigilance and follow-up of site of regional anesthesia
• Catheter site covered with transparent dressing to allow inspection

Chlorhexidine associated with decreased risk of central venous catheter–associated bloodstream infections compared with povidone iodine. Advantage for regional anesthesia/analgesia unclear.

Medication tubing and medication bag changed q96 hours for continuous infusions.

REFERENCES

For references, please visit **www.TheAnesthesiaGuide.com**.

CHAPTER 120
Local Anesthetics and Adjuvants

Robert N. Keddis, MD

- *Weak bases, hydrophilic, tertiary amines* that block *voltage-gated Na+ channels*, preventing depolarization
- *Sensitivity of nerve fibers to blockade*:
  - ▸ *More sensitive*: small diameter and lack of myelin
  - ▸ *Spinal and peripheral nerves*: autonomic > sensory > motor
- *Onset/duration of action*:
  - ▸ *Unionized (uncharged) form*: lipid-soluble, crosses membranes
  - ▸ Increased lipid solubility = decreased onset time, increased duration, increased potency
  - ▸ Increased concentration and total dose = *faster* onset
  - ▸ Site of injection: more vascularized means shorter duration due to systemic uptake
  - ▸ *Note*: Epinephrine is frequently added to increase duration of blockade; however, it is unstable in alkaline conditions:
    - ▪ Bottles containing epinephrine have an acidic pH = *slower onset* than when epinephrine added extemporaneously
- *Systemic vascular absorption (greatest to least)*:
  - ▸ *Intercostal nerve block > caudal > epidural > brachial plexus > sciatic–femoral > subcutaneous*
- *Divided into two groups*:
  - ▸ *Amides* (mnemonic: have two I's in the name):
    - ▪ Metabolized in the liver; liver disease can increase duration and toxicity
  - ▸ *Esters*:
    - ▪ Mostly metabolized by pseudocholinesterase
    - ▪ Pseudocholinesterase deficiency severely prolongs duration; avoid in these patients

Dosage of Local Anesthetics (Also See Chapters 122–123)		Peripheral	Epidural	Spinal	Infiltration	IVRA
Amides						
Bupivacaine	Concentration	0.25–0.5%	0.25–0.75%	0.5–0.75%	n/a	Contraindicated
	Dose	10–40 mL	5–20 mL	1–3 mL	n/a	Contraindicated
	Duration	4–12 h	60–120 min	1–3 h	n/a	Contraindicated
	Onset	Slow	Intermediate	Rapid	n/a	Contraindicated
Lidocaine	Concentration	1–1.5%	1.5–2%	1.5–5%	0.5–1%	0.25–0.5%
	Dose	10–40 mL	20 mL			
	Duration	1–3 h	1.5–2 h	0.5–1.5 h	2–8 h	0.5–1 h
	Onset	Rapid	Rapid	Rapid	Rapid	Rapid

(continued)

Dosage of Local Anesthetics (*continued*)

		Peripheral	Epidural	Spinal	Infiltration	IVRA
Mepivacaine	Concentration	1–1.5%	1.5–2%	2–4%	n/a	n/a
	Dose					
	Duration	2–4 h	1–2 h	1–2 h	n/a	n/a
	Onset	Rapid	Rapid	Rapid	n/a	n/a
Ropivacaine	Concentration	0.5–1%	0.5–1%	0.5–0.75%	0.2–0.5%	n/a
	Dose	10–20 mL				
	Duration	5–8 h	2–3 h	1–3 h	2–5 h	n/a
	Onset	Slow	Intermediate	n/a	Rapid	n/a
Esters						
Benzocaine	Concentration	n/a	n/a	n/a	Topical: maximum 20%	
	Dose					
	Duration	n/a	n/a	n/a	0.5–1 h	
	Onset	n/a	n/a	n/a	Rapid	
Chloroprocaine	Concentration	2%	2–3%	2–3%	1%	
	Dose					
	Duration	0.5–1 h	0.5–1 h	1–2 h	0.5–1 h	
	Onset	Rapid	Rapid	Rapid	Rapid	
Cocaine	Concentration	n/a	n/a	n/a	Topical: 4–10%	
	Dose	n/a	n/a	2–5 mL		
	Duration	n/a	n/a	n/a	0.5–1 h	
	Onset	n/a	n/a	n/a	Rapid	
Procaine	Concentration	n/a	n/a	2%	n/a	
	Dose	n/a	n/a		n/a	
	Duration	n/a	n/a	0.5–1 h	n/a	
	Onset	n/a	n/a	Rapid	n/a	
Tetracaine	Concentration	n/a	n/a	0.5%	Topical: 2%	
	Dose	n/a	n/a	15 mg		
	Duration	n/a	n/a	2–4 h	0.5–1 h	
	Onset	n/a	n/a	Rapid	Rapid	
Prilocaine	Concentration	4%	n/a	2%	4%	0.5%
	Dose	10–15 mL	n/a	80 mg		50 mL
	Duration	n/a	n/a	2–4 h	0.5–1 h	45–90 min
	Onset	Rapid	n/a	Rapid	Rapid	Rapid

Maximum Recommended Doses of Local Anesthetics				
	Maximum recommended dose		Maximum recommended dose with addition of epinephrine	
Medication	mg (adult)	mg/kg	mg (adult)	mg/kg
Lidocaine	300	3–4.5	500	6–7
Mepivacaine	400	4.5	550	7
Bupivacaine	175	2–3	225	2
Levobupivacaine	150	2	No data	2
Ropivacaine	225–300	3	225–300	
Chloroprocaine	800	12	1000	
Procaine	500	12		
Prilocaine		6–8	500	8

Data obtained from different sources; doses in mg and mg/kg do not necessarily match. NB: the evidence supporting these numbers is scant.

SPECIFIC POINTS

- *Mixtures of local anesthetics*:
  - ‣ Commonly used in clinical practice despite no proven advantage; earlier onset usually not clinically significant; duration of blockade significantly shortened
  - ‣ Not recommended
- *Allergic reactions*: true allergic reactions to local anesthetics are rare:
  - ‣ Many patients reporting an allergic reaction to local anesthetic, especially in a dental setting, are likely to have experienced intravascular injection of local anesthetic with epinephrine
  - ‣ True allergic reactions: most commonly the type I anaphylactic and type IV delayed hypersensitivity responses
  - ‣ No cross-reactivity between esters and amides
  - ‣ Ester local anesthetics are associated with a higher incidence of allergic reactions due to one of their metabolites, *para*-aminobenzoic acid (PABA)
- *Chloroprocaine*: avoid in patients with cholinesterase deficiency:
  - ‣ Used in obstetrics due to rapid onset and breakdown and decreased fetal exposure, for top-offs for repairs following vaginal delivery, or for C-sections in parturients who have a labor epidural:
    - ▪ Seems to impede analgesic effect of neuraxial opioids
  - ‣ Preservative-free formulation used off-label for ambulatory spinal anesthesia; short duration, no transient neurologic symptom (TNS) described:
    - ▪ Cauda equina syndromes described in the past with intrathecal administration of larges doses intended for epidural use
    - ▪ Exact mechanism unclear (dose, preservative?)
- *Lidocaine*:
  - ‣ *TNS following spinal anesthesia*:
    - ▪ More common with higher concentration (5%), lithotomy position, knee arthroscopy, early ambulation
    - ▪ Pain usually occurring within 24 hours, resolving within 7 days, in buttocks and lower extremities
    - ▪ No motor or sphincter deficit
    - ▪ Can occur with other local anesthetics (mepivacaine: 6–20%; bupivacaine: rare; chloroprocaine: not described)
    - ▪ Treated with NSAIDs, opioids
  - ‣ *Cauda equina syndrome*:
    - ▪ Associated with continuous lidocaine spinals; described with single-injection of 5%
      - ◆ Varying degrees of urinary and fecal incontinence

- Sensory loss in the perineal area
- Motor weakness in the lower extremities
  - Possible cause can be a direct neurotoxic effect with high concentrations such as 5% being used
  - Can also result from pooling of local anesthetic, even in lower concentrations
- *Bupivacaine*:
  - *Cardiotoxic*: has stronger binding to sodium channels than other local anesthetics; cardiac toxicity often not preceded by seizures (contrary to other local anesthetics):
    - Dissociates very slowly during diastole so that sodium channels do not fully recover, blocking conduction
    - Contraindicated for IV regional blocks
  - Pregnancy, acidosis, hypoxemia increase risk of cardiotoxicity
  - Cardiac resuscitation is difficult, possibly related to its lipid solubility
  - Intralipid 20% may help save patients with bupivacaine-related cardiac arrest (see chapter 119)
- *Benzocaine*:
  - Risk of methemoglobinemia; do not spray on mucosa for >3 seconds

Adjuvants to Local Anesthetics	
Additives	Specific points
HCO₃	• Increases unionized fraction, shortens onset time by a few minutes, often not clinically significant • Decreases burning sensation on injection • Only used with lidocaine and mepivacaine (1:10 ratio); precipitates with bupivacaine
Epinephrine	• Most commonly used adjunct • Vasoconstriction at site resulting in decreased vascular absorption and higher concentration of local anesthetic in proximity of nerve • Alpha-adrenergic stimulation with pain modulation in neuraxium • Epidural: addition can lead to increased duration • Spinal: "epi wash" increases duration of tetracaine and bupivacaine • Peripheral blocks: increases duration by decreasing vascular uptake; concerns about reduced blood flow if preexisting neuropathy
Opioids	• Used as adjuvant to spinal and epidural to prolong surgical block (without significant prolongation of time to block resolution) and faster pain relief when used intrathecally • No longer used for peripheral nerve blocks • Buprenophine (partial mu-opioid receptor agonist) studied in brachial plexus blocks as an additive and shown to improve duration of block, possibly due to its lipophilic properties
Clonidine	• Alpha-2 agonist, modulates pain pathways in neuraxium; prolongs analgesia for peripheral nerve blocks • Initially thought to work by vasoconstriction • Has direct local anesthetic action • Usually used in doses of 30–150 μg • Rare adverse effects: hypotension, sedation, and bradycardia • Most effective when used with intermediate local anesthetics
Dexamethasone	• Used as adjuvant in peripheral nerve blockade • Both motor and sensory block prolonged • Typically 4–8 mg in 20 mL LA • Use only preservative-free formulation • Mechanism of action is still unclear (possibly enhanced neurotoxicity); use not recommended until elucidated

ADVANCES IN DRUG DELIVERY SYSTEMS

- Liposomal delivery systems have been created to prolong the action of local anesthetics without use of catheters, pumps, or adjuvant drugs
- Liposomal bupivacaine (Exparel®) approved for single-dose infiltration into the surgical site
- Still experimental for peripheral nerve blockade

OTHER USES FOR LOCAL ANESTHETICS

- *Tumescent anesthesia*:
  ‣ Local anesthetics used in liposuction procedures
  ‣ Dilute lidocaine (0.05–0.1%) with epinephrine (1:1,000,000) added for hemostasis, buffered with bicarbonate to decrease injection pain
  ‣ Can use total doses as high as 55 mg/kg
  ‣ High doses can be used with rare systemic toxicity, because of high volume, low concentration, and reduced absorption due to epinephrine
- *EMLA cream (5% emulsion containing 2.5% each of lidocaine/prilocaine)*:
  ‣ Topical anesthetic:
    ▪ Used at times in pediatric patients prior to IV placement
    ▪ Melting point of 18°C
  ‣ Case studies have also cited its benefit for pain control and relief of burning sensations in cancer patients, specifically in those with skin tumors such as liposarcoma:
    ▪ Patients experienced relief within 24 hours of application
- *Lidocaine patch*:
  ‣ Topical 5% patch applied for 12 hours to skin (only to be applied to intact skin)
  ‣ Can be used to treat pain of postherpetic neuralgia
  ‣ Adverse reactions can include site reactions; allergies rare
- *Abdominal surgery*:
  ‣ Systemic lidocaine continuous infusion 1 mg/min for 24 hours reduced postoperative pain, shortened duration of ileus and time to discharge compared with placebo
  ‣ Ropivacaine 0.2% at 10 mL/h for 48 hours via a preperitoneal wound catheter decreased diaphragmatic dysfunction versus IV PCA morphine
- *Antimicrobial properties*:
  ‣ Local anesthetics known to inhibit microbial growth in vitro:
    ▪ Bupivacaine was demonstrated to be the most effective against growth against many bacteria
    ▪ Additives frequently used in epidural infusions such as clonidine, epinephrine, and fentanyl showed no additional effect on growth of bacteria
  ‣ No in vivo data
- *Cancer recurrence*:
  ‣ Some studies seem to indicate that regional anesthesia and analgesia might reduce the risk of metastatic recurrence. Still controversial. Mechanism unclear, may be simply by reducing opioid-related immunomodulation

REFERENCES

For references, please visit **www.TheAnesthesiaGuide.com**.

CHAPTER 121
Neuraxial Anesthesia

Toni Torrillo, MD

Contraindications to Neuraxial Anesthesia		
Absolute	Relative	Controversial
• Patient refusal • Infection at injection site • Increased ICP • Coagulopathy (cutoff for PTT, INR, platelet values unclear) • Antiplatelet medications (e.g., clopidogrel [Plavix], ticlopidine [Ticlid]) • Critical aortic or mitral stenosis • Severe spinal deformity or pathology (complete spina bifida, meningocele)	• Uncooperative patient • Sepsis • Preexisting neurological deficits,[1] hydrocephalus, severe convulsive disorders • Complicated surgery (major EBL, potential for respiratory compromise) • Stenotic heart valve—weigh risk/benefit. Consider patient functional status • Severe hypovolemia • Spinal deformity or pathology not at injection site	• Inability to communicate with patient • Demyelinating lesions[1] (multiple sclerosis) • Prior back surgery or fusion • Spinal anesthesia following failed epidural anesthesia

[1]Concern may be more medicolegal than medical.

PREOPERATIVE ASSESSMENT

- Platelets, PTT, INR, platelets, except in ASA 1 patients
- Reassure patients they may have sedation or general anesthesia to supplement neuraxial technique
- Explain risks, benefits, and alternatives
- Adverse effects:
  - ‣ Happen on occasion but not serious:
    - Headache, hypotension, nausea, itching if opioids used, risks of long-acting drugs such as preservative-free morphine, failed attempt, need to try a different level, inability to perform spinal or epidural and need for general anesthesia, difficult/lengthy surgery necessitating conversion to general anesthesia despite working neuraxial technique
  - ‣ Rare but serious:
    - Bleeding, infection, nerve injury, high anesthetic level, respiratory, or cardiovascular compromise

TECHNIQUE

- Anatomy:
  - ‣ Spinal cord from foramen magnum → L1 (adults) or L3 (children)
  - ‣ Dural sac/subarachnoid/subdural space → S2 (adults) or S3 (children)
- Surface landmarks (Figure 121-1)

FIGURE 121-1. Landmarks for neuraxial anesthesia

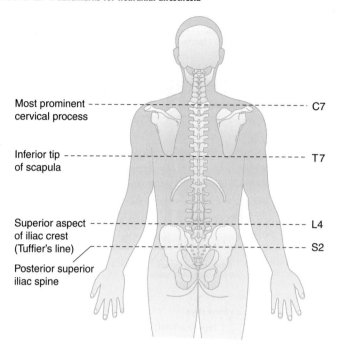

Most prominent cervical process — C7

Inferior tip of scapula — T7

Superior aspect of iliac crest (Tuffier's line) — L4

— S2

Posterior superior iliac spine

- Spine anatomy (Figure 121-2):
  ‣ Ligaments:
    ▪ Supraspinous
    ▪ Interspinous
    ▪ Ligamentum flavum—thickest (3–5 mm) and furthest from meninges (4–6 mm) at midline, thus less likely to get accidental dural puncture with midline approach
- Landmarks for testing level of anesthesia:
  ‣ T4—nipple
  ‣ T7—xiphoid process
  ‣ T10—umbilicus
  ‣ L1—inguinal ligament
- Gentle pinprick (sensory test) or cold alcohol swab (sympathetic):
  ‣ Sympathetic block 2 levels > sensory block 2 levels > motor block
  ‣ Monitor BP q1 minute initially (level stabilizes at 10–15 minutes for short-acting locals and 20-30 minutes for longer-acting locals)
- Positioning:
  ‣ Sitting:
    ▪ Easier to appreciate midline (obese, scoliotic)
    ▪ Chin down, shoulders relaxed, back flexed (angry cat/shrimp)
  ‣ Lateral:
    ▪ Patient on his or her side, chin down, knees flexed (fetal position)
    ▪ Note that males and females have different shoulder/hip width ratios, with the spine typically not horizontal
    ▪ CSF flow typically slower

FIGURE 121-2. Structures to traverse for neuraxial block (A); anatomy of a typical lumbar vertebra (B and C)

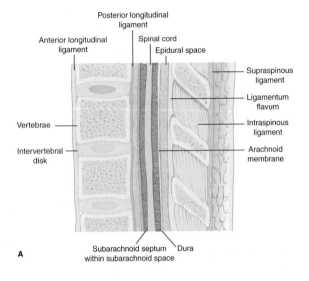

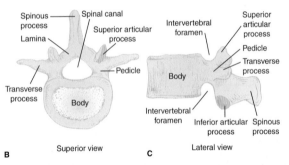

- ▸ Prone:
  - ▪ Spinal anesthesia for anorectal procedures with hypobaric anesthetic and jack-knife position or when fluoroscopic guidance used for neuraxial technique
  - ▪ CSF may not flow freely and may need to be aspirated

FIGURE 121-3. Midline versus paramedian approach

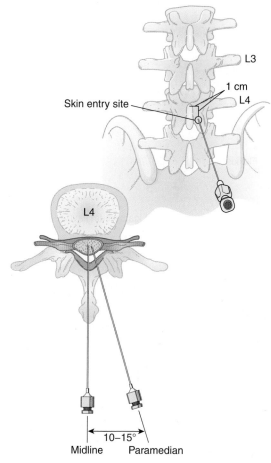

- Approaches (Figure 121-3):
  ▸ Midline:
    ▪ Identify spinous process above and below level to be used
    ▪ Depression between spinous processes is needle entry point
    ▪ Spinous processes course downward; needle direction should aim slightly cephalad for lumbar procedures and fairly acute (30–50°) for thoracic epidural

FIGURE 121-4. Paramedian approach

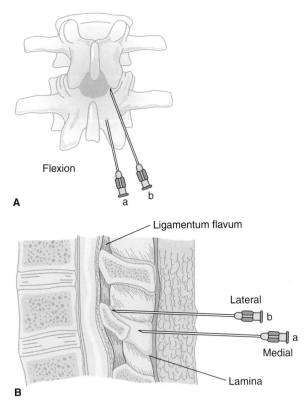

A needle that encounters bone at a shallow depth (a) is usually hitting the medial lamina, whereas one that encounters bone deeply (b) is further lateral from the midline. Posterior view (A). Parasagittal view (B). Reproduced from Morgan GE, Mikhail MS, Murray MJ. *Clinical Anesthesiology.* 4th ed. Figure 16-14. Available at: www.accessmedicine.com. Copyright © The McGraw-Hill Companies, Inc. All rights reserved.

▸ Paramedian (Figure 121-4):
  ▪ Useful in patients who are difficult to position (inability to flex spine) or with calcified interspinous ligaments
  ▪ Identify upper and lower spinous processes at desired level
  ▪ Insert needle 1 cm lateral to the lower spinous process
  ▪ Needle should enter skin at 45° angle cephalad with 15° medial angulation
  ▪ Advance needle into ligamentum flavum
  ▪ Technique bypasses supraspinous and interspinous ligaments
  ▪ More likely to get accidental dural puncture with this approach
  ▪ However, if dura is penetrated with Tuohy, less likely to get spinal headache than if dura penetrated with midline approach

FIGURE 121-5. Taylor approach

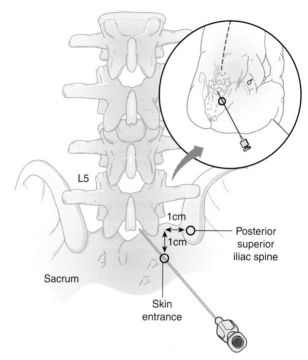

- Taylor approach (Figure 121-5):
  - Modified paramedian approach to L5–S1 interspace
  - Sometimes only available access to the epidural space in patients with ossified ligaments
  - Skin wheal 1 cm medial and 1 cm inferior to the PSIS (Figure 121-5)
  - Needle inserted in a medial and cephalad direction at a 45–55° angle
  - As in classic paramedian, first resistance felt is ligamentum flavum
  - If needle contacts bone (usually sacrum), walk off bone medially and cephalad

Complications of Neuraxial Anesthesia

Complication	Risk factors	Pathophysiology	Treatment
Hypotension	Excessive dose, high spinal level, obesity, pregnancy, older age, hypovolemia	Sympathectomy (arterial and venodilation)	Fluid (consider preloading but avoid overloading), vasopressors (ephedrine, dopamine) phenylephrine may ↓ CO via ↓ HR
Bradycardia Asystole	High block (T1–T4), young age, ASA 1 status, high baseline vagal tone, beta-blockers, hypovolemia	Blockade of cardiac accelerator fibers; decreased venous return and Bezold–Jarisch reflex	Atropine, ephedrine, escalate *rapidly* to epinephrine 5–10 µg (or ACLS dose if necessary)
Total spinal	Excessive dose, unusual sensitivity to local anesthetic, unusual spread of local anesthetic	Hypotension, unconsciousness, apnea; due to sympathetic and medullary hypoperfusion	Supportive care, intubation, fluids, vasopressors. If no response to ephedrine and phenylephrine, use atropine and epinephrine early to prevent cardiac collapse
Anterior spinal artery syndrome	Prolonged severe hypotension	↓ Blood flow to anterior spinal cord	Supportive
Urinary retention	Male, older, prolonged blocks	Blockade of S2–S4 = decreased bladder tone and inhibition of voiding reflex	Time, bladder catheterization, if persistent may indicate neural injury
Postdural puncture headache (see chapter 125)	Large needles, cutting needles, young age, female sex, pregnancy	Breach of dura, leakage of CSF, decreased ICP, traction on vessels	Fluids, caffeine, NSAIDs, blood patch
Backache	Repeated attempts, contact with bone, history of back pain	Tissue trauma, localized inflammatory response	Self-limited, acetaminophen, NSAIDs, rule out abscess/hematoma
Nerve root or spinal cord damage	Needle placed at high level, multiple attempts, failure to remove needle or stop injecting if parasthesia elicited	Direct trauma to nerve root or spinal cord	May resolve spontaneously; early neuro consult if nonresolving or progressive symptoms
Cauda equina syndrome	Continuous small-gauge spinal catheters, lidocaine 5%	Pooling or maldistribution of local anesthetic onto nerve roots causing bowel/bladder dysfunction and leg paresis	Small-gauge catheters no longer available, high-concentration lidocaine no longer recommended, early recognition and neuro consult

(continued)

Complications of Neuraxial Anesthesia (*continued*)			
Complication	Risk factors	Pathophysiology	Treatment
Transient neurological symptoms (TNS)	Only after spinal, not epidural. Ambulatory surgery, lithotomy position, lidocaine (but can occur with all local anesthetics)	Concentration-dependent neurotoxicity of local anesthetics causing back pain radiating to buttocks, no sensory or motor deficits	Self-limited. NSAIDs for pain
Arachnoiditis, Meningitis	Contaminated equipment, patient site infection, nonpreservative free local anesthetic	Introduction of microorganisms or chemical irritants into subarachnoid space	Antibiotics for meningitis, pain management and physical therapy for arachnoiditis
Spinal hematoma	Coagulopathy, thrombocytopenia, platelet dysfunction, fibrinolytic/ thrombolytic therapy, difficult or "bloody" block	Direct pressure injury/ischemia. First symptom may be motor block greater/ longer than expected with local dose	Neurological consultation, MRI/ CT scan, surgical decompression within 8–12 h
Spinal abscess	Contamination of field	Direct pressure injury causing (1) back pain, (2) radicular pain, (3) motor and sensory deficits, (4) paralysis	Suspect if back pain and fever, neuro consult, CT/MRI, antistaphylococcal antibiotics, surgical decompression or percutaneous drainage
Migration of epidural catheter	Can occur in up to one third of patients		Catheter removal if intravascular. Clinician to weigh risk/benefit of leaving intrathecal catheter
Shearing or breaking of epidural catheter	Withdrawing catheter through needle or forceful removal of catheter		Careful observation if remnant deep; surgical removal if remnant superficial, exposed, or neuro symptoms

ANTICOAGULATION AND NEURAXIAL ANESTHESIA

See chapter 119.

REFERENCES

For references, please visit **www.TheAnesthesiaGuide.com**.

CHAPTER 122
Surgical Epidural

Toni Torrillo, MD

FIGURE 122-1. Choice of epidural needle

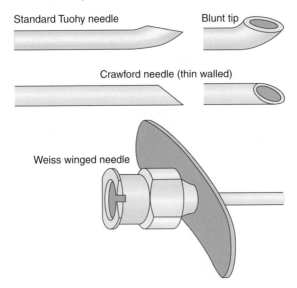

A blunt, curved tip helps push the dura away and avoid inadvertent puncture. Straight needle facilitates catheter insertion but may increase the incidence of dural puncture. Reproduced from Morgan GE, Mikhail MS, Murray MJ. *Clinical Anesthesiology.* 4th ed. Figure 16-18. Available at: www.accessmedicine.com. Copyright © The McGraw-Hill Companies, Inc. All rights reserved.

Choice of Location	
Location of surgery	Level of epidural placement
Thoracic	T4–8
Upper abdomen	T6–8
Middle abdomen	T7–10
Lower abdomen	T8–11
Lower extremity	L2–4

Local Anesthetics

Agent[1]	Concentration (%)	Onset	Sensory block	Motor block
Chloroprocaine	2	Fast[2]	Analgesic	Mild to moderate
	3	Fast	Dense	Dense
Lidocaine	≤1	Intermediate	Analgesic	Minimal
	1.5	Intermediate	Dense	Mild to moderate
	2	Intermediate	Dense	Dense
Mepivacaine	1	Intermediate	Analgesic	Minimal
	2–3	Intermediate	Dense	Dense
Bupivacaine	≤0.25	Slow[3]	Analgesic	Minimal
	0.5	Slow	Dense	Mild to moderate
	0.75	Slow	Dense	Moderate to dense
Ropivacaine	0.2	Slow	Analgesic	Minimal
	0.5	Slow	Dense	Mild to moderate
	0.75–1	Slow	Dense	Moderate to dense

Fast and intermediate agents reach maximum block height in 15–20 minutes. Slow agents can take up to 30 minutes for maximum block height to be achieved.
[1]Always use preservative-free local anesthetic.
[2]Fast is approximately 5–10 minutes.
[3]Slow is approximately 15–20 minutes.

Epidural Adjuvants

Adjuvant[1]	Dose	Onset (min)	Peak (min)	Duration (h)	Comments/side effects
Fentanyl	50–100 µg	5–10	10–20	1–3	Itching; nausea; urinary retention; sedation; ileus; respiratory depression (delayed with morphine—↓ dose with elderly or sleep apnea)
Morphine	2–5 mg	15–30	60–90	4–24	
Hydromorphone	0.75–1.5 mg	20–30	20–30	1–3	
Epinephrine	1:200,000				Prolongs nerve exposure to local anesthetic
Clonidine	150–400 µg				Hypotension; prolonged sensory block
Sodium bicarbonate	1 mEq/10 mL of local anesthetic				Hastens block onset with lidocaine, mepivacaine, chloroprocaine. Will precipitate with bupivacaine

[1]Opioids affect quality more than duration: they prolong the surgical block without significantly delaying recovery. Epinephrine prolongs chloroprocaine, lidocaine, and mepivacaine better than it does bupivacaine and ropivacaine. Peak blood levels of local anesthetic are lower with epinephrine.

TECHNIQUE

Performance:
- LORA/LORS—loss of resistance to air or saline
- Advance needle with stylet through skin into interspinous ligament
- Resistance should be felt
- Remove stylet; attach glass syringe with 2–3 mL air or saline
- Advance millimeter by millimeter until loss of resistance felt
- Thread catheter 3–5 cm into epidural space
  ‣ Deep catheters prone to kinking/coiling
  ‣ Superficial catheters may dislodge

FIGURE 122-2. Angle of epidural needle placement

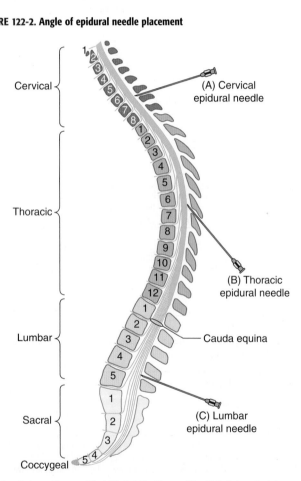

Cervical

(A) Cervical epidural needle

Thoracic

(B) Thoracic epidural needle

Lumbar

Cauda equina

(C) Lumbar epidural needle

Sacral

Coccygeal

- If difficulty finding epidural space, attempt to "walk off" bone or try a different level and/or approach
- If persistent pain or paresthesia on threading catheter or injecting local anesthetic, remove catheter and try a different level. Ask patient which side the pain/paresthesia is and redirect needle in the opposite direction
- Avoid injecting local anesthetic onto nerves or cord!
- One to 2 mL local anesthetic per segment to be blocked (see chapter 162)
- Shorter patient may need 1 mL per segment. Taller patient may need 2 mL
- Elderly/pregnant need less due to smaller/less compliant epidural space
- Gravity (lateral decubitus, Trendelenburg, reverse Trendelenburg) can help achieve desired block

TESTING FOR INTRATHECAL (SUBARACHNOID) AND VASCULAR PLACEMENT

- Aspiration of catheter alone is not sufficient
- No single universal epidural test dose is agreed upon
- 3 mL 1.5% lidocaine + epi 1:200,000 adequate in nonpregnant adult patients. Look for $\uparrow$ SBP ≥15 mm Hg or $\uparrow$ HR ≥10 bpm or increase in T-wave amplitude ≥25%, or spinal block if catheter subarachnoid
- If not adding epinephrine (e.g., 3 mL of 0.25% bupivacaine), look for CNS signs of intravascular injection (tinnitus, metallic taste), or dense block corresponding to intrathecal injection
- 3 mL of air can be used with single-orifice catheter and precordial Doppler
- 100 mcg of fentanyl can test for intravascular placement but not for intrathecal placement

Physiologic Effects of Epidural Anesthesia			
Organ system	Physiology	Pros	Cons
Cardiovascular	Venous pooling, T1–T4 block of cardiac accelerators	Decreased blood loss, lower incidence of DVT	Hypothermia, hypotension, bradycardia
Pulmonary	Impaired intercostal and abdominal muscles	Diaphragm intact, less pain with deep breathing prevents atelectasis, hypoxia, pneumonia, respiratory failure, and decreases postoperative ventilator time	Inability to actively inhale/exhale/cough and clear secretions for patients with limited respiratory reserve
Gastrointestinal	Unopposed vagal tone = small, contracted gut with active peristalsis	Excellent operative conditions for laparoscopic procedures, postoperative epidural hastens return of GI function	Opioids may contribute to ileus
Renal	Loss of autonomic bladder function	Overall renal function not affected	Urinary retention, bladder distension, hypertension
Metabolic/endocrine	Suppression of neuroendocrine stress response	Decreased arrhythmia and ischemia	

PEARLS AND TIPS

- With *disease affecting spine* (neurofibromatosis, metastatic cancer), CT scan or MRI should rule out pathology at the site prior to epidural placement
- Patients *postlaminectomy or spinal fusion*: altered anatomy = paramedian approach may be easier, spinal may be easier than epidural, or choose level above surgical site if possible. Block may be incomplete or anesthetic level achieved unanticipated. Discuss with patient preoperatively
- Preoperative explanation or intraoperative reassurance necessary for patients with high thoracic level of anesthesia and *feeling of dyspnea* due to loss of chest wall proprioceptive sensation
- Factors affecting *level of blockade* are volume, age, height, gravity (although less than for spinal)
- The most important factors determining *density of blockade* are drug, concentration, total dose, level of injection
- *Do not waste too much time* with initial choice of level and approach. If unsuccessful after 5 minutes, try another level and/or approach
- If *unilateral block*, try withdrawing catheter 1–2 cm and reinjecting with patient unblocked side down
- *To block perineum* (avoid sacral sparing) may try loading epidural in sitting position
- Visceral afferents that travel with vagus may not be blocked; may need to supplement with IV opioids or other agents (see chapter 151)
- *Ropivacaine*: less cardiotoxic, less motor block than with bupivacaine
- *Local anesthetic toxicity* from intravascular injection during epidural anesthesia is best avoided with test dose, diligent aspiration prior to any injection, and incremental dosing (typically 5 mL at a time, separated by a few minutes)
- No complications have been reported with epidurals placed in patients with *lumbar tattoos*
- Epidurals in *septic patients* for laparotomy debatable due to potential for epidural abscess, coagulopathy, hemodynamic instability
- Epidurals placed *awake versus asleep* in adult patients controversial. Awake placement recommended. Patient maintains ability to warn of paresthesias and pain on injection, both of which are associated with postoperative neuro deficits

REFERENCES

For references, please visit **www.TheAnesthesiaGuide.com**.

CHAPTER 123
Spinal Anesthesia

Toni Torrillo, MD

SPINAL NEEDLES (FIGURE 123-1)

FIGURE 123-1. Needles used for spinal anesthesia

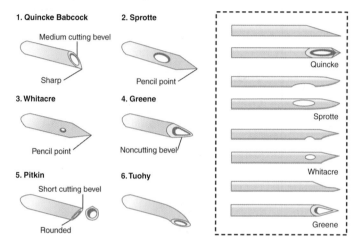

- All have a stylet to avoid tracking epithelial cells into the subarachnoid space
- Quincke is cutting needle with end injection
- Whitacre, Sprotte, Pencan are pencil-point (rounded points and side injection)
- Sprotte has long opening, more vigorous CSF flow but possible failed block if distal part of opening is subarachnoid (with free flow CSF), but proximal part is not past dura and the full dose of medication is not delivered
- Blunt tip (pencil-point) needles and small-gauge needles decrease the incidence of postdural puncture headache

CHOICE OF LOCAL ANESTHETIC

See table on following page.

Dosages, Uses, and Duration of Commonly Used Spinal Anesthetic Agents

Drug	Preparation	Dose (mg)	Procedures	Duration (h) Plain	Epinephrine
2-Chloroprocaine	1%, 2%, 3%	30–60	Ambulatory, T8	1–2	Not recommended (flu-like symptoms)
Lidocaine	2%	40–50	Ambulatory, T8	1–2	Only modest effect, not recommended
Mepivacaine[1]	1.5%	30 (T9)	Ambulatory surgery, knee scope, TURP	1–2	Not recommended
		45 (T6)[2]		1.5–3	
		60 (T5)		2–3.5	
Bupivacaine	0.5%	7.5	Ambulatory lower limb	1–2	
		10	THA, TKA, femur ORIF	2	
		15		3	4–5
Bupivacaine	0.75% in 8.25% dextrose	4–10	Perineum, lower limbs[3]	1.5–2	1.5–2.5
		12–14	Lower abdomen		
		12–18	Upper abdomen		
Ropivacaine	0.5%, 0.75%	15–17.5	T10 level	2–3	Does not prolong block
		18–22.5	T8 level	3–4	
	1% + 10% dextrose (equal volumes D10 and ropivacaine)	18–22.5	T4 level	1.5–2	
Tetracaine	1% + 10% dextrose (0.5% hyperbaric)	4–8	Perineum/lower extremities	1.5–2	3.5–4
		10–12	Lower abdomen		
		10–16	Upper abdomen		

[1]Used as an alternative to lidocaine, but TNS also occurs with mepivacaine.
[2]Each change of 15 mg prolongs or hastens ambulatory milestones by 20–30 minutes. Fentanyl 10 μg extends surgical block but not ambulatory recovery times and should probably be added if using 30 mg dose to ensure adequate duration.
[3]Very low dose (4–5 mg) works well for ambulatory, unilateral, knee surgery. Keep patient lateral, affected side down, for 6 minutes after block.

Common Adjuvants to Spinal Anesthetics			
Adjuvant	Dose (μg)	Duration (h)	Comments/side effects
Fentanyl	10–25	1–2	Itching; nausea; urinary retention; sedation; ileus; respiratory depression (delayed with morphine–↓ dose with elderly or sleep apnea)
Sufentanil	1.25–5	1	
Morphine	125–250	4–24	
Epinephrine	100–200		Prolongs nerve exposure to local anesthetic + alpha-adrenergic modulation
Phenylephrine	1,000–2,000		Hypotension. Prolongs tetracaine but not bupivacaine. Extends tetracaine better than epinephrine does. May cause TNS
Clonidine	15–150		Hypotension. Sedation. Prolongs motor and sensory block

PERFORMANCE

- After sterile prep, drape, and local infiltration of skin:
  - ‣ Advance introducer (not necessary for 22G Quincke needle)
  - ‣ Advance spinal needle through two "pops" (penetration of ligamentum flavum at end of introducer and penetration of dura/subarachnoid membrane)
- Remove stylet, verify free-flowing CSF and inject spinal medication
- If no return of CSF:
  - ‣ Withdraw or advance needle slightly to regain free flow
  - ‣ If no free flow, replace stylet, withdraw spinal needle, and attempt to elicit "pop" into subarachnoid again
- If difficulty getting CSF or finding space, attempt to "walk off" bone or try a different level and/or approach
- If persistent pain or paresthesia when needle "pops" into subarachnoid or on injecting local, withdraw and redirect needle. Ask patient which side the pain/paresthesia is and redirect needle in the opposite direction
- Do not inject into nerves (paresthesia) or spinal cord (interspace above L2–3)

BARICITY AND SPREAD

- The most important factors determining *local anesthetic spread* are baricity, total dose, and patient position during/after injection
- Baricity refers to the density of the injected solution compared with the density of CSF
- The solution can be made hyperbaric by adding dextrose, or hypobaric by adding sterile water. Most local anesthetics without additive are isobaric; chloroprocaine is slightly hyperbaric
- No isobaric solution is FDA-approved for spinal anesthesia, but bupivacaine has been used extensively for years without adverse events
- Hyperbaric solution will follow gravity:
  - ‣ If the patient remains sitting, only the sacral roots will be blocked: *"saddle block" to block perineum* (pilonidal cyst, cerclage, hemorrhoidectomy, etc.). Keep patient sitting for as long as possible after hyperbaric spinal (at least 5 minutes, ideally 15 minutes) to maximize sacral block/minimize cephalad spread/hypotension
  - ‣ If the patient lies down shortly after the injection, the solution will follow the sacral and thoracic curvatures:
    - ▪ A higher level (e.g., T4 with 15 mg hyperbaric bupivacaine) will be reached, allowing abdominal procedures to be performed
    - ▪ Splanchnic vasodilation will cause significantly more hypotension than with isobaric solution
    - ▪ The block is less dense (possible tourniquet pain) and of shorter duration than with isobaric solution
  - ‣ If the patient is kept in lateral decubitus, the dependent side will be blocked

- Hypobaric solution will rise; if the patient is kept in lateral decubitus, the non-dependent side will be blocked (unilateral spinal); this can be useful to minimize hemodynamic changes in elderly, fragile patients
- Position less important for isobaric, although isobaric solution can become slightly hypobaric at body temperature, causing a higher level than expected if patient sitting for too long (e.g., when performing a combined spinal–epidural)

PEARLS AND TIPS

- Spinal cord can end as low as L3 even in adults. Level of iliac crests is also variable. This combined with poor body habitus may contribute to spinal cord injury. *Use lowest interspace possible*
- With *disease affecting spine* (neurofibromatosis, metastatic cancer), CT scan or MRI should rule out pathology at the site prior to spinal placement
- Patients *postlaminectomy or spinal fusion*—altered anatomy = paramedian approach may be easier, spinal may be easier than epidural, or choose level above surgical site if possible. Spinal block may be incomplete or anesthetic level achieved unanticipated. Discuss with patient preoperatively
- Preoperative explanation or intraoperative reassurance necessary for patients with high thoracic spine level of anesthesia and *feeling of dyspnea* due to loss of chest wall sensation
- *Ropivacaine* less cardiotoxic, less motor block than with bupivacaine. Use roughly 1.5× the typical bupivacaine dose
- *Do not waste too much time* with initial choice of level and approach. If unsuccessful after 5 minutes, try another level and/or approach
- *Local anesthetic toxicity* from intravascular injection during spinal anesthesia should not occur, as the dose used is too low
- Incidence of *pruritus* with intrathecal opioids increases with higher doses. If antihistamines (e.g., diphenhydramine [Benadryl] 25 mg IV) unsuccessful, use nalbuphine (Nubain) 5–10 mg IV

REFERENCES

For references, please visit **www.TheAnesthesiaGuide.com**.

CHAPTER 124
Combined Spinal Epidural Anesthesia

Toni Torrillo, MD

The combined spinal epidural technique allows combining:
- Rapid onset and dense block from the spinal anesthesia
- Presence of an epidural catheter to prolong block (if surgery outlasts spinal anesthesia) and/or for postoperative analgesia

NECESSARY EQUIPMENT (NEEDLE-IN-NEEDLE TECHNIQUE)

- Epidural kit
- Spinal needle long enough to exit epidural needle (24–27 gauge pencil-point needle: Whitacre, Sprotte, or Gertie Marx)

Choice of Spinal Local Anesthetic for Inpatient Procedures					
				Duration (h)	
Drug	Preparation	Dose (mg)	Procedures	Plain	Epinephrine
Bupivacaine (isobaric)	0.5%	10	THA, TKA, femur ORIF	2	
		15		3	4–5
Bupivacaine (hyperbaric)	0.75% in 8.25% dextrose	4–10	Perineum, lower limbs	1.5–2	1.5–2.5
		12–14	Lower abdomen		
		12–18	Upper abdomen		
Ropivacaine	0.5%, 0.75%	15–17.5	T10 level	2–3	Does not prolong block
		18–22.5	T8 level	3–4	
	1% + 10% dextrose (equal volumes D10 and ropivacaine)	18–22.5	T4 level	1.5–2	
Tetracaine	1% + 10% dextrose (0.5% hyperbaric)	4–8	Perineum/ lower extremities	1.5–2	3.5–4
		10–12	Lower abdomen		
		10–16	Upper abdomen		

CHOICE OF EPIDURAL LOCAL ANESTHETIC

- Higher concentration to maintain dense block for surgical anesthesia
- Lower concentration for postoperative analgesia

See chapters 122 and 162 for additional information.

PERFORMANCE

- After sterile prep, drape, and local infiltration of skin:
  - ‣ Advance epidural needle into epidural space using loss of resistance technique
  - ‣ Advance spinal needle through epidural needle into subarachnoid space
- Verify free-flowing CSF and inject spinal medication
- If persistent pain or paresthesia when needle "pops" into subarachnoid or on injecting local anesthetic, withdraw and redirect needle. Do not inject local anesthetic onto nerves or cord:
  - ‣ It is useful to ask patient which side the paresthesia was felt and redirect needle in the opposite direction (especially with spine deformities)
- Remove spinal needle
- Thread epidural catheter and secure 3–5 cm into epidural space

PEARLS AND TIPS (SEE ALSO SECTION "PEARLS AND TIPS" IN CHAPTERS 122 AND 123)

- Use of saline to detect epidural space may lead to confusion of saline for CSF when spinal needle placed. Prefer LOR to air
- The risk of threading the epidural catheter into dural hole created by spinal needle is minimal if 25 gauge or smaller spinal needle used
- Epidural drugs should be administered and titrated slowly in small increments because of possible intrathecal injection. Dural hole may increase flux of drugs into CSF and enhance their effects
- Incidence of dural puncture ("wet tap") from epidural needle may be lower with CSE than with epidural technique alone
- Incidence of failed epidural lower with CSE than with epidural alone

REFERENCES

For references, please visit **www.TheAnesthesiaGuide.com**.

CHAPTER 125
Postdural Puncture Headache

Michael Anderson, MD

INCIDENCE

- 22G Quincke = 36%
- 27G Whitacre = 0%
- 16G Tuohy = 70%
- Dural puncture occurs 0–2.6% of the time an epidural is placed for labor analgesia

RISK FACTORS

- Female gender
- Age 20–40
- History of frequent headaches
- Multiple dural punctures during a procedure
- Use of a cutting needle rather than pencil-point

DIAGNOSIS

- Headache usually begins 24–48 hours after spinal or epidural; on occasion later. Headache occurring immediately following dural puncture is typically from pneumocephalus, which usually resolves rapidly
- Headache is usually located in the frontal and occipital regions and often radiates to the neck and shoulders
- The headache is positional, worsened by sitting up and improved with laying supine
- Atypical presentations can include **tinnitus, diplopia, hearing loss, and photophobia without the presence of a headache**. This is from stretching of cranial nerves, and an argument for performing a blood patch early
- Approximately 40% of parturients will experience a headache that is not a PDPH; therefore, one must discern if the headache is from PDPH or from other causes (i.e., tension headache, preeclampsia, migraine, caffeine withdrawal, meningitis)
- Anecdotal evidence of decreased PDPH after wet tap if catheter for 24 hours. Weigh the risk of high spinal if an epidural dose of medication is administered intrathecally by mistake, and of infection, versus the risk of PDPH

TREATMENT

- Most headaches resolve spontaneously. Treatment should be a collaborative process between the anesthesiologist and patient
- Supportive care of fluids, caffeine (500 mg IV or 300 mg oral), and oral analgesics (e.g., APAP/oxycodone) is the first line of treatment

BLOOD PATCH

- Wait 48 hours with conservative treatment before performing blood patch, unless neurologic symptoms are present
- Anticoagulant or antiplatelet therapy should be stopped with a similar time frame as for any epidural (see chapter 119)
- Identify the epidural space (preferably at a lower level than the initial puncture)
- Fifteen to 20 mL of autologous blood is obtained aseptically and then injected into the epidural space
- Injection should be slow and end with the development of back pain/pressure or when 20 mL is reached
- Keep patient supine for about 2 hours following the procedure
- On occasion, a second blood patch is needed
- Complications:
  - ▸ Bradycardia
  - ▸ Abdominal or sciatica pain due to nerve root irritation, typically benign and disappearing after a few days
  - ▸ Low-grade fever common
- If symptoms are still present following two blood patches and the diagnosis is still consistent with PDPH, one should consider specialized consultation and CT imaging to rule out insidious presentation of a subdural hematoma from chronic stretch of the subdural veins
- Prophylactic blood patch remains controversial; risks and benefits of this technique should be weighed as it does not decrease the incidence but can decrease the severity and duration of the PDPH
- Surgery for treatment of a dural tear is the last resort

REFERENCES

For references, please visit **www.TheAnesthesiaGuide.com**.

CHAPTER 126
Principles of Peripheral Nerve Stimulation (PNS)

Caroline Buhay, MD

- Ability to stimulate peripheral nerve or plexus depends on:

Electrical Parameters of Peripheral Nerve Stimulation	
Variable	Clinical significance
Electrical impedance	• Varies with tissue composition • Most stimulators have constant current output generators that automatically compensate for impedance changes
Electrode to nerve distance	• Ability to stimulate nerve at low current flow (<0.5 mA) indicates close proximity to nerve • Target muscle twitch still present at <0.2 mA probably indicates intraneural tip position • Increased current flow and pulse duration increase ability to stimulate nerve at a greater distance from stimulating electrode
Current flow (amperage)	Presence of appropriate muscle twitch at current 0.23–0.5 mA generally results in safe, reliable block
Position of electrodes	• Cathode (negative electrode) is attached to insulated needle and anode (positive electrode) is attached to patient skin via an EKG electrode • Inverting polarities requires four times current to achieve similar response

MATERIALS

- Insulated needle—insulated needle shaft ensures that current dispersion is concentrated at needle tip, allowing specificity of needle tip location
- Nerve stimulator device

Basic Features of Nerve Stimulators		
Feature	Function	Settings
Constant current output	Automatically compensates for changes in impedance of tissues, needles, connecting wires, and grounding electrodes during needle placement to ensure consistent delivery of set current	Present in most modern stimulators
Current meter	• Displays the current being delivered • Make sure it displays in 0.01 mA increments for better accuracy	• PNS: 0.2–1.5 mA • TES: 5 mA
Pulse width/ duration	Short duration (0.05–0.1 ms) targets A-α motor fibers and avoids stimulation of pain fibers at longer duration Pulse duration required to depolarize pain fibers: A-δ (0.17 ms) and C fibers (0.4 ms)	• PNS: 0.1 ms • Diabetic patients with neuropathy may require a longer pulse duration (0.3 or 1ms) to achieve target twitch • TES: 0.2–0.3 ms to achieve motor response at greater distance from nerve
Stimulating frequency	• Determines how quickly pulses are delivered to elicit twitch (pulses/s) • Older models with 1 Hz (1 pulse/s) frequency require slow needle manipulation to avoid missing target twitch	• Usual setting: 2 Hz allows for faster manipulation of needle tip

TECHNIQUE (REFER TO SPECIFIC NERVE BLOCK CHAPTERS FOR MORE DETAIL)

- Identify landmarks, insertion site, direction, target muscle(s) to elicit response:
  - ▸ Due to anatomical variance or large body habitus, the exact course of a nerve can be difficult to identify. In these cases consider doing a surface mapping of the nerve/plexus by transcutaneous electrical stimulation (TES, see below)
- Ensure cathode (negative electrode, black) is attached to insulated needle and anode (positive electrode, red) is attached to patient
- Set starting current to about 1.2–1.4 mA. Much higher current can result in patient discomfort
- Insert needle and advance while observing target muscle group
- Once target muscle twitch is elicited, slowly dial down current while adjusting needle position to optimize muscle response
- If twitch disappears at ≥0.5 mA, turn current up until twitch is again present
- Goal: response present at current 0.2–0.4 mA
- Hold needle securely to ensure it does not move during injection. Ask assistant to ensure patient does not move during injection
- Signs that suggest needle tip is intraneural and needle should be withdrawn slightly:
  - ▸ Twitch still present below 0.2 mA
  - ▸ Paresthesia elicited on needle advancement
  - ▸ High resistance on injection
- Inject 1–2 mL of local anesthetic and observe disappearance of twitch
- Inject remaining local anesthetic with steady constant pressure, with frequent aspirations to ensure needle tip is not intravascular
- Ensure that injection pressure is not elevated (suggestive of intraneural injection)

CAVEAT

- Nerves have motor and sensory components. Muscle response will not be present unless needle tip is in proximity to motor component, which explains why needle tips have been visualized inside nerves by ultrasound with no motor response

TRANSCUTANEOUS ELECTRICAL STIMULATION

Technique of stimulating peripheral nerves transcutaneously to pre-locate needle entry point and nerve course prior to needle insertion. Useful for patients with surface anatomy that is difficult to identify or as "training wheels" when first learning nerve stimulator technique. Nerve stimulator settings for this technique are based on the principle that the farther the stimulating electrode is from the nerve, a higher current, pulse duration, and frequency are needed to achieve depolarization and cause target muscle twitch.

Equipment

- Peripheral nerve stimulator used for neuromuscular blockade monitoring set at 5 mA (small- to average-size patient) or 10 mA (obese patient), 0.2 milliseconds, 2 Hz, single twitch
- Modified EKG lead trimmed circumferentially to about 0.5 cm in diameter, gel intact

Technique

- Anode clamp attached to electrode on patient's skin
- Cathode clamp attached to modified EKG lead
- Ensure peripheral nerve stimulator is working with settings listed above
- Based on patient's anatomy, estimate needle entry point. With current initially set at 5 mA, place cathode electrode at this point and observe for target muscle twitch
- Once twitch elicited, turn down to lowest current with twitch still present. Scan skin with electrode to achieve strongest twitch at lowest current similar to peripheral nerve stimulation (PNS) technique described above. Mark this point as entry point
- Using this same process, the course of the nerve can be mapped to determine the direction of needle advancement

NOTES

- The minimal electrode current with twitch still present will vary among patients and nerve targeted (i.e., femoral versus. interscalene brachial plexus) but will be in the range of 2–3 mA
- If the patient is obese, the skin to nerve distance is farther than an average person; therefore, a higher starting current (10 mA) may be needed before a twitch is appreciated
- Although a pulse duration of 0.2 milliseconds is within the range of stimulating pain fibers, this technique has not been shown to cause a clinically significant increased level of discomfort

Peripheral Nerves with Corresponding Roots, Innervated Muscles, and Expected Responses			
Nerve	Roots	Muscles	Response
Spinal accessory	Cranial	• Trapezius	• Shoulder elevation
Phrenic	C3–C5	• Diaphragm	• Hiccup
Suprascapular	C5–C6	• Supraspinatus • Infraspinatus	• Arm abduction • Arm external rotation
Musculocutaneous	C5–C6	• Biceps • Brachialis	• Elbow flexion

(continued)

Peripheral Nerves with Corresponding Roots, Innervated Muscles, and Expected Responses (continued)

Nerve	Roots	Muscles	Response
Axillary	C5–C6	• Teres major • Deltoid	• Arm adduction
Long thoracic aka thoracodorsal	C6–C8	• Latissimus dorsi	• Arm adduction, internal rotation, extension
Radial	C5–C6	• Brachioradialis	• Forearm flexion and supination
	C5–C6	• Extensor carpi radialis	• Wrist extension, radial deviation
	C6–C8	• Extensor carpi ulnaris	• Wrist extension, ulnar deviation
	C6–C7	• Extensor pollicis longus and brevis	• Thumb extension
	C6–C8	• Extensor digitorum	• Extension of fingers
	C7–C8	• Triceps	• Forearm extension
Median	C6–C7	• Flexor carpi radialis	• Wrist flexion, radial deviation
		• Palmaris longus	• Wrist flexion
		• Opponens, abductor brevis	• Thumb opposition, abduction
	C8–T1	• Flexor digitorum profundus (radial fingers) and superficialis	• Flexion of fingers
		• Flexor pollicis longus	• Thumb flexion
		• Pronator quadratus	• Pronation
Ulnar	C8–T1	• Flexor carpi ulnaris	• Wrist flexion, ulnar deviation
		• Flexor digitorum profundus (ulnar fingers)	• Flexion of ulnar fingers
		• Adductor digiti minimi and flexor digiti minimi brevis	• Fifth finger adduction and flexion
		• Adductor pollicis	• Thumb adduction
		• Interossei	• MP joint flexion
		• Lumbricals	• PIP joint extension
Femoral	L2–L4	• Quadriceps	• Knee extension
	L2–L3	• Sartorius	• Thigh flexion, abduction, and lateral rotation
	L2–L4	• Pectineus	• Thigh adduction and flexion
Obturator	L2–L4	• Adductor longus, brevis, and magnus • Gracilis	• Thigh adduction and external rotation
Sciatic (see branches below)	L5–S2	• Hamstrings	• Hip extension, knee flexion
		• Biceps femoris	• Hip extension, thigh external rotation
Superficial peroneal (branch of sciatic)	L4–S2	• Tibialis anterior	• Foot dorsiflexion and inversion
		• Fibularis longus, brevis, and tertius	• Foot plantar flexion and eversion

(continued)

Peripheral Nerves with Corresponding Roots, Innervated Muscles, and Expected Responses (*continued*)			
Nerve	Roots	Muscles	Response
Deep peroneal (branch of sciatic)	L4–S2	• Tibialis anterior	• Foot dorsiflexion and inversion
		• Extensor digitorum longus • Extensor hallucis longus	• Extension of toes, foot eversion • Extension of great toe, foot eversion
Tibial (branch of sciatic)	L4–S2	• Gastrocnemius • Soleus • Plantaris	• Foot plantar flexion, (knee flexion)
		• Tibialis posterior	• Foot plantar flexion and inversion
		• Flexor digitorum longus	• Flexion of toes
		• Flexor hallucis longus	• Flexion of great toe
		• Plantaris	• Foot plantar flexion

REFERENCES

For references, please visit **www.TheAnesthesiaGuide.com**.

CHAPTER 127
Ultrasound Guidance for Regional Anesthesia

M. Fahad Khan, MD, MHS

Always scan the whole area of interest to locate structures and identify anatomical variations.

ADVANTAGES OF ULTRASOUND GUIDANCE FOR RA

• Visualize nerves or plexus
• Visualize structures to avoid: blood vessels, pleura
• Visualize needle
• Visualize local anesthetic spread:
  ▸ Limit volume, as injection can be stopped when spread deemed adequate
  ▸ Avoid intravascular injection; risk of complication when needle tip in a compressed, poorly visualized vein, and when no spread is seen when injecting as a result
• Confirm position of catheter:
  ▸ Inject fluid, agitated fluid, or air
  ▸ Color Doppler can be used

ASEPTIC TECHNIQUE/PROBE PROTECTION

• Sterile conductive gel and sterile protective cover for ultrasound (US) probe should be used
• Ideally, a telescopic probe cover, fixed in place by an elastic band, should be employed
• After use, probe should be sterilized or disinfected, rinsed, dried, and kept in a clean environment

ULTRASOUND MACHINE AND TRANSDUCER/PROBE

Transducer shape (Figure 127-1):
- Straight (linear) transducers yield an image as wide as the probe
- Curvilinear transducers yield a semicircular picture, allowing visualization of structures not directly underlying the probe
- Probes with special shapes are used to minimize probe "footprint," especially in small patients or children (e.g., "hockey stick" probe)

FIGURE 127-1. Straight, curvilinear, and "hockey stick" probes

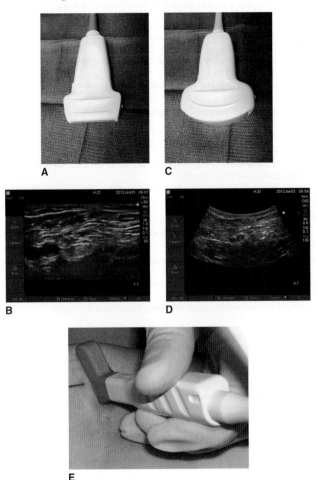

(A and B) Straight probe and ultrasound picture obtained with the probe. (C and D) Curvilinear probe and ultrasound picture obtained with the probe. (E) "Hockey stick" probe. Reproduced with permission from Hadzic A. *The New York School of Regional Anesthesia Textbook of Regional Anesthesia and Acute Pain Management*. New York: McGraw-Hill; 2006. Figure 52-1. Copyright © The McGraw-Hill Companies, Inc. All rights reserved.

Frequency:
- Pick a transducer based on frequency (usually between 3 and 15 MHz)
- High-frequency transducer (8–12 or 15 MHz):
  ‣ Less penetration into deeper structures
  ‣ Best for target depth up to 3–4 cm
  ‣ Higher resolution (picture quality)
- Low-frequency transducer (3–5 MHz):
  ‣ More penetration into deeper structures
  ‣ Best for targets deeper than 5 cm
  ‣ Lower resolution (picture quality)
- After picking the appropriate transducer, fine-tune the frequency of the wave by selecting the upper, mid, or lower frequency range of that specific transducer

Transducer orientation:

Identify which side of transducer corresponds to which side of the image on the US monitor:
- Most transducers have a fixed label (i.e., palpable notch/groove) corresponding to an indicator on the screen
- If in doubt, tap on side of transducer to identify orientation

Gain:
- Affects brightness (hyperechoic) or darkness (hypoechoic) characteristics of the displayed image
- Adjust gain to obtain clear image

Time-gain compensation:
- Affects brightness of US image at specific depths in the field, using either a series of sliding buttons or automatically
- Typically, deeper fields require a higher gain setting due to beam attenuation in deeper tissue planes

Depth:

Adjust depth so that target structures fall within field of view.

Focus:
- Adjusting focus will allow for best lateral resolution, which allows machine to distinguish two objects lying beside each other at the same depth
- The focus arrows should be adjusted to position the focus of the beam at the same level as the target of interest
- Newer machines adjust focus automatically throughout the image

Color Doppler:
- Allows for identification and quantification of blood flow; for regional anesthesia, the goal is to locate blood vessels
- Note that if the beam is exactly perpendicular to the blood flow, no flow will be registered: slightly angle the probe
- Mnemonic = *BART*:
  ‣ *Blue* = *Away* from the transducer
  ‣ *Red* = *Toward* the transducer

Ultrasound Characteristics of Various Tissues	
Tissue	Image characteristics
Nerve root	Hypoechoic
Peripheral nerve	Heterogeneous (hypoechoic fascicles in hyperechoic connective tissue)
Artery	Anechoic and pulsatile, difficult to compress; color Doppler positive
Vein	Anechoic, easily compressible; color Doppler positive
Fat	Hypoechoic, more or less heterogeneous
Muscle	Heterogeneous (hypoechoic with hyperechoic lines)
Tendon	Hyperechoic, more or less heterogeneous; change shape when tracked up/down
Fascia	Hyperechoic
Bone	Strongly hyperechoic (casts hypoechoic shadow)
Local anesthetic, D5W	Hypoechoic; can be hyperechoic and heterogeneous if air bubbles present in the fluid

VISUALIZATION AND NEEDLE GUIDANCE TECHNIQUES (FIG. 127-2)

Short-axis view:

The nerve or vessel is imaged perpendicular to its length.

Long-axis view:

The nerve or vessel is imaged along its length.

In-plane needle approach:
- Needle placed inline with and parallel to transducer
- Full length of needle shaft and tip is visualized
- The transducer should not be moved once an optimal image is obtained, except to slide slightly without tilting in order to better visualize the needle

Out-of-plane needle approach:
- Needle placed perpendicular to transducer
- Needle shaft is visualized as only a hyperechoic dot on monitor
- The probe has to be constantly moved proximally and distally to ascertain the tip position
- Some practitioners insert the needle very close to the probe and almost parallel to the US beam; in that case, the probe should not be moved
- Hydrodissection (see below) can be used if the needle is not well visualized

With both in-plane and out-of-plane techniques, do not aim directly for the nerve, but rather for the margins, in order to avoid nerve injury.

Henpecking
- Rapid to-and-fro motion of the needle by a few millimeters, allowing needle position to be guessed based on tissue motion

Hydrodissection/hydrolocation:
- Small amounts of local anesthetic, or better of D5W (does not impede neurostimulation [NS] if needed), are injected to confirm the needle tip position

Anisotropy:
- Structures are best visualized when the US beam is perpendicular; otherwise most of the US waves are scattered away from the probe
- Need to adjust tilt of probe to obtain best picture
- Especially true for, for example, popliteal sciatic nerve block: the nerve is going from deep to superficial, poorly seen if probe not tilted to be perpendicular to the nerve

DUAL GUIDANCE TECHNIQUE (FIGURE 127-3)

Synergistic concurrent use of NS and US guidance.

Advantage: qualitative anatomical end point (US) plus quantitative functional end point (NS).

FIGURE 127-2. Nerve visualization and needle approach

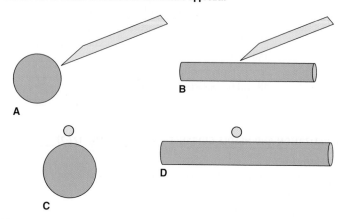

(A) Nerve seen in short axis, needle in-plane. (B) Nerve seen in long axis, needle in-plane. (C) Nerve seen in short axis, needle out-of-plane (only a cross-section of the needle is seen on the ultrasound display as a dot). (D) Nerve seen in long axis, needle out-of-plane (rarely used). The nerve is green and the needle blue.

TROUBLESHOOTING

I can see the nerve but I cannot see the needle:
- Ensure that the needle has been introduced far enough to be under the probe
- Use henpecking motion to have an idea of the needle position
- Slide the probe slightly back and forth, without tilting it, to try to bring the needle into the US beam
- If unsuccessful, retract needle to the skin and assess visually that the path of introduction is parallel to the US beam

I can see the needle but I cannot see the nerve anymore:
- Reposition the probe without moving the needle to find an adequate view of the target structures
- Retract needle to the skin and assess visually that the path of introduction is parallel to the US beam
- If needed, change needle entry point

I can see only part of the needle:
- The needle is introduced at an angle to the US beam
- Retract needle to the skin and assess visually that the path of introduction is parallel to the US beam
- If needed, change needle entry point

I am injecting but I am not seeing any local anesthetic spread:
- Stop injection immediately! Risk of intravascular injection
- Retract needle slightly; release pressure on probe to allow compressed veins to be visualized

I am injecting and the local anesthetic is spreading away from the nerve:
• Stop injection; reposition needle

I am trying to inject but I need to use a very high pressure:
• Stop injection; reassess needle tip position, most likely intraneural
• Reposition needle to have tip close to the nerve but not inside the nerve

FIGURE 127-3. Dual guidance approach

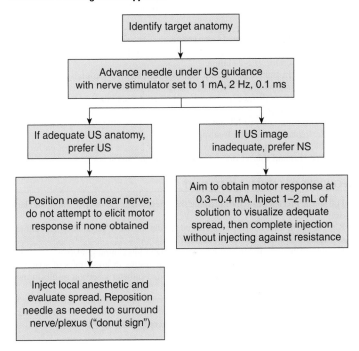

REFERENCES

For references, please visit **www.TheAnesthesiaGuide.com**.

CHAPTER 128
Insertion of Perineural Catheters

Caroline Buhay, MD

Perineural catheters and continuous peripheral nerve blocks (CPNB) are synonymous. Those two terms will be used indifferently in this chapter.

INDICATIONS

- More commonly used for inpatients after surgical procedures expected to cause significant pain for >12–24 hours
- Can be used in ambulatory setting. Appropriate patient selection is paramount
- Help minimize opioid consumption and adverse effects
- Fewer side effects (hemodynamic) than neuraxial analgesia, less interference with thromboprophylaxis
- Sympathectomy and vasodilation to increase perfusion after vascular accident, digit transfer/replantation, or limb salvage
- Possible benefits include increased tolerance of passive range of motion for joint replacements and shorter times to meet discharge criteria

TECHNIQUE OF CATHETER PLACEMENT

- Full sterile precautions (chlorhexidine skin prep, sterile gloves, hat, mask, and large drape)
- Kits on the market contain an insulated needle for nerve stimulation and either a stimulating or a nonstimulating catheter
- If not available, an epidural kit may be used with ultrasound guidance
- Unclear whether using a stimulating catheter results in lower rates of secondary block failure. Some data suggest that US-guided catheter insertion results in more effective postoperative analgesia
- Technique used ultimately dependent on operator preference and time available for procedure. Consider combined use of US and nerve stimulator for deeper nerve blocks (e.g., sciatic, psoas compartment), where US view may be suboptimal

Placement of Stimulating Versus Nonstimulating Catheters Using Neurostimulation	
Nonstimulating catheter	**Stimulating catheter**
1. Clip off hair surrounding block site if needed	• Follow steps 1–6
2. Sterile prep and drape	7. Holding needle steady, inject 5–10 mL D5W (nonconductive) to distend perineural space
3. Set nerve stimulator to 2 Hz, 0.01–0.03 ms, 1.2 mA	8. Attach stimulator to catheter and advance through needle
4. Tuohy needle to elicit appropriate motor response	9. The motor response should be similar to that elicited by needle stimulation
5. Optimize needle position to maintain response at 0.2–0.5 mA	10. Catheter is advanced 2–3 cm beyond the needle tip while maintaining an appropriate motor response
6. Aspirate to rule out intravascular/intrathecal position	11. There is no clear guideline as to what is an acceptable stimulating current to confirm proper catheter placement
7. Hold needle steady in that position and inject desired dose of local anesthetic	12. Remove needle and catheter stylet
8. Catheter is advanced about 2–3 cm past needle tip	13. See the section "Securing Catheter"
9. Remove needle	
10. See the section "Securing Catheter"	

ULTRASOUND GUIDANCE

- Ultrasound can be used in conjunction with nerve stimulator depending on operator preference, but does not necessarily guarantee higher catheter success
- Cover ultrasound transducer with sterile sheath, ensuring there is a generous amount of sterile acoustic gel between the transducer and the inside of sterile sheath
- Once target nerves are visualized on ultrasound, insert Tuohy needle in-plane or out-of-plane depending on operator preference (Figure 128-1). In-plane catheter insertion has similar quality of analgesia as out-of-plane approach and shorter time of insertion

FIGURE 128-1. Techniques of ultrasound-guided perineural catheter insertion

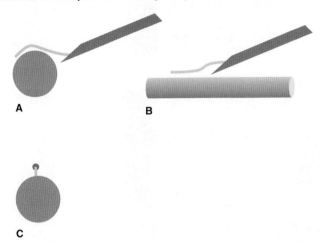

(A) Nerve seen in short axis, needle and catheter in-plane. (B) Nerve seen in long axis, needle and catheter in-plane. (C) Nerve seen in short axis, needle and catheter out-of plane. The nerve is green, the needle blue, and the catheter yellow.

- When Tuohy tip is appropriately positioned, aspirate and inject desired dose of local anesthetic. Alternatively, inject only 3–5 mL of local anesthetic/saline if injecting local anesthetic through catheter
- Put down US, hold needle steady in that position, and insert catheter 1–3 cm past needle tip
- Remove needle
- The catheter tip can be confirmed under US in different ways:
  - ▸ While observing the ultrasound monitor, inject 2–3 mL of air through the catheter and make note of the hyperechoic agitation marking the catheter tip position
  - ▸ Inject the appropriate volume of LA for surgical anesthesia or postoperative bolus through the catheter (instead of the needle) and observe the spread of hypoechoic fluid around the target nerve
- See the section "Securing Catheter."

SECURING CATHETER

This must be done under the same sterile conditions as catheter placement.

FIGURE 128-2

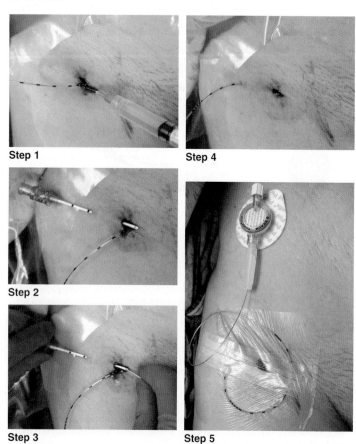

Step 1

Step 2

Step 3

Step 4

Step 5

Tunneling and securing of a perineural catheter. (Step 1) Infiltrate local anesthetic away from catheter insertion site. (Step 2) Tunnel Tuohy needle subcutaneously. (Step 3) Thread catheter into needle. (Step 4) Pull catheter through tunnel, ensuring that the catheter is not kinked. (Step 5) Secure catheter with liquid adhesive (e.g., benzoin, Mastisol®), sterile tape (e.g., Steri-Strips®), and sterile occlusive dressing (e.g., Tegaderm®). Secure catheter–hub connection with either tape or specifically designed devices (e.g., Statlock®).

TABLE 128-1 Surgical Procedures and Corresponding CPNB Sites

Surgical site	Examples of surgical procedure	CPNB site
Shoulder and proximal humerus	Total/hemi shoulder arthroplasty Rotator cuff repair Bankart repair, etc.	Interscalene (occasionally supraclavicular)
Elbow, forearm, and hand	Arthroplasty Fractures	Supraclavicular, infraclavicular
Thorax and breast	Thoracotomy Mastectomy	Paravertebral
Abdomen, iliac crest, and inguinal region	Low abdominal surgery (prostatectomy, appendectomy) Iliac crest bone graft Inguinal hernia repair	Transversus abdominis (TAP) Bilateral catheters can be placed for midline incisions
Hip and thigh	Hip arthroplasty Hip fracture Femoral shaft fracture	Lumbar plexus or femoral
Knee	Knee arthroplasty Supracondylar fracture Tibial plateau fracture (controversial b/o risk of compartment syndrome) ACL/PCL reconstruction	Femoral or lumbar plexus ±Subgluteal sciatic or SI popliteal/tibial
Leg, ankle, and foot	Total ankle arthroplasty Ankle/subtalar arthrodesis	Subgluteal sciatic or popliteal with SI saphenous

SI, single injection.

TABLE 128-2 Potential Complications of Perineural Catheters

Potential complications	Comments
Incorrect catheter placement (secondary block failure)	• If initial bolus of local anesthetic is injected via needle, initial block may be successful but continuous block may fail • The initial bolus can instead be injected through the catheter to ensure correct position • US versus nerve-stimulating catheter discussed above
Catheter dislodgement	• See the section "Securing Catheter" to minimize risk of dislodgement
Vascular puncture/hematoma	• Using US may decrease the risk • ASRA consensus statement on anticoagulation and peripheral blocks notes, "conservatively, the [neuraxial recommendations] … may be applied to plexus and peripheral techniques. However, this may be more restrictive than necessary"
Intravascular injection	• Similar risk as with single-shot injection • Catheter can migrate and erode into vessel. Use test dose (3 mL 1.5% lidocaine with 1:200,000 epi). Always aspirate before injecting or starting an infusion
Nerve injury	• As with single-shot block, nerve injury can result from needle trauma or local anesthetic neurotoxicity • Current evidence suggests incidence of nerve injury from perineural catheters and 0.2% ropivacaine infusion is no higher than single-injection blocks

(continued)

TABLE 128-2	Potential Complications of Perineural Catheters (*continued*)
Potential complications	Comments
Bacterial colonization infection	• Use same sterile precautions as for CVL insertion (chlorhexidine prep, sterile gloves, large drape, hat, and mask) • There is no published limit to how long catheters can remain indwelling; however, keeping it for no more than 3–4 days may reduce this complication. There are reports of catheters kept in place for several weeks (military)
Perineuraxis injection	• It is possible to cannulate the epidural or intrathecal spaces when lumbar plexus or interscalene catheters are placed, especially when a stiff catheter with stylet is used • Use gentle steady pressure when injecting in these sites, as high pressures may hydrodissect into neuraxial spaces
Catheter knotting/ retention	• Avoid advancing catheter more than 5 cm past needle tip
Catheter shearing	• Do not withdraw catheter through the needle

REFERENCES

For references, please visit **www.TheAnesthesiaGuide.com**.

CHAPTER 129
Management of a Neuropathy Following Regional Anesthesia

Arthur Atchabahian, MD

Most neuropathies are of surgical origin. However, postoperative neuropathies seem to have a lower recovery rate when regional anesthesia is associated.

PREVENTION/DOCUMENTATION

• Discuss risk of neuropathy *preoperatively*, especially with patients at risk:
  ‣ DM
  ‣ MS
  ‣ Extremes of body habitus
  ‣ Methotrexate, cisplatin
  ‣ Other preexisting neurologic abnormality
• In these patients:
  ‣ Evaluate risk/benefit ratio of regional anesthesia/analgesia
  ‣ Consider using lower local anesthetic concentration and no epinephrine (decreases nerve blood flow)
• Carefully document *preoperatively* any neurologic finding
• *Document*:
  ‣ Twitch (location, current, disappearance)
  ‣ Negative aspiration
  ‣ Ultrasound use ("no intraneural/intravascular injection")
  ‣ Injection pressure

> ‣ Absence of pain/paresthesia
> ‣ Duration/pressure of tourniquet
> ‣ Positioning

CLINICAL EVALUATION IF POSTOPERATIVE NEUROPATHY

- Document neurologic findings (anesthesiologist, surgeon, neurologist if consulted):
  - ‣ Nerve by nerve and/or dermatome by dermatome
  - ‣ Sensory, motor, and sympathetic (if applicable)
  - ‣ Identify level of lesion if possible
- If neurologic consult requested, clarify that the request is for a *detailed description of deficit* rather than etiologic speculation

ELECTROPHYSIOLOGY

- Ideally electrophysiology ASAP (<72 hours), prior to Wallerian degeneration
- Repeat after 3 weeks
- Bilateral, upper and lower limbs, to elicit subclinical neuropathy
- *EMG* for peripheral neuropathy
- *SSEP* if evaluation for spinal cord and/or sensory root involvement
- *MEP* if evaluation of pyramidal tracts and/or motor root involvement
- Indicate the *severity* of lesion: partial versus complete
- Indicate the *level* of the lesion: spinal cord, root, plexus, branch
- Evaluate for *other lesions* not noted on clinical examination
- The report should include *tracings*

OTHER TESTS

- X-ray, ultrasound, MRI, CT scan as indicated clinically; CT or MRI emergently if suspicion of spinal cord compression

FIGURE 129-1. Management of postoperative neuropathy

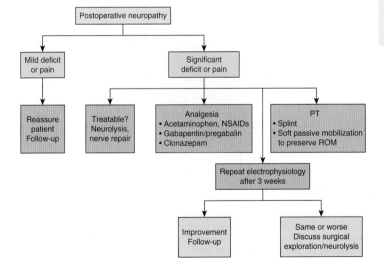

REFERENCES

For references, please visit **www.TheAnesthesiaGuide.com**.

CHAPTER 130
Cervical Plexus Blocks

Michael Anderson, MD

Superficial cervical plexus—skin and superficial structures (see Figures 130-1 and 130-2).

Deep cervical plexus—muscles of the neck, deep structures, and diaphragm (phrenic).

Indications
Thyroid surgery
Tracheostomy
Carotid endarterectomy
Lymph node excision
Superficial neck procedures

FIGURE 130-1. Anatomy of the superficial cervical plexus

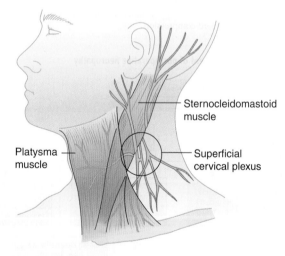

The superficial cervical plexus arises from C1 to C4 and runs between the cervical vertebrae and the sternocleidomastoid muscle. Nerves exit along the posterior border of the sternocleidomastoid coming through the platysma muscle. It provides sensation to the neck, jaw, occiput, and the anterior supraclavicular area. Reproduced from Morgan GE, Mikhail MS, Murray MJ. *Clinical Anesthesiology*. 4th ed. Figure 17-2. Available at: www.accessmedicine.com. Copyright © The McGraw-Hill Companies, Inc. All rights reserved.

FIGURE 130-2. Dermatomal distribution of the superficial cervical plexus

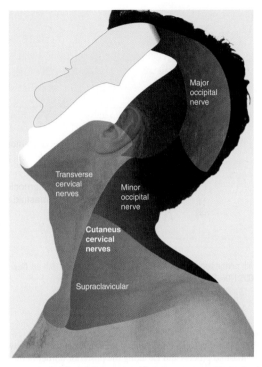

BLOCK PERFORMANCE

Superficial (Figure 130-3):
- Identify the posterior border of the sternocleidomastoid (SCM) muscle
- Find the midpoint of the muscle and inject 5 mL of local anesthesia no deeper than the depth of the SCM
- Infiltrate superficially along the posterior border of the SCM to complete the block
- Ultrasound-guided technique: the injection is made at the level of C6, in the plane under the prevertebral fascia underlying the SCM. In some patients, the nerves of the cervical plexus can be identified in that space (see Fig. 133-4)

FIGURE 130-3. Superficial cervical plexus block

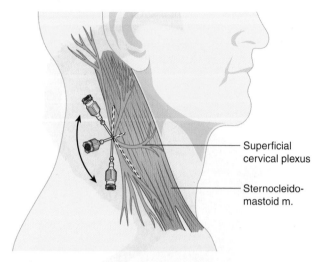

Superficial
cervical plexus

Sternocleido-
mastoid m.

Reproduced with permission from Miller RD, ed. *Miller's Anesthesia*. 6th ed. New York: Churchill Livingstone; 2005:1706. © Elsevier.

Deep (Figure 130-4):
- Identify the mastoid process and the transverse process of C6. Draw a line connecting the mastoid process and C6 along the posterior border of the SCM muscle
- Identify the transverse processes of C2, C3, and C4 on this line; C2 will be the first palpable transverse process inferior to the mastoid process; alternatively, if the transverse processes cannot be palpated, draw the following landmarks:
  ‣ C2 is 1.5 cm posterior to the mastoid–C6 line, and 1.5 cm caudad to the mastoid
  ‣ C3 is 1.5 cm caudad to C2, and 1 cm from the line
  ‣ C4 is 1.5 cm caudad to C3, on the line
- Insert the needle and make contact with the transverse process of C3; withdraw the needle 1–2 mm and inject 5 mL of local anesthesia, and then repeat at C2 and C4
- Conversely, one can also inject 15 mL of local anesthesia at C3 (or C4) alone, in a slow, fractionated fashion, with frequent aspiration
- Ultrasound guidance can be used (Fig 130-5). The transverse processes of C2, C3 and C4 are located, and local anesthetic is injected while the spread is visualized

FIGURE 130-4. Deep cervical plexus block

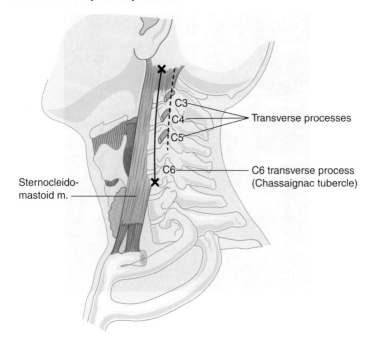

C3
C4
C5
— Transverse processes

C6
Sternocleido-
mastoid m.

C6 transverse process
(Chassaignac tubercle)

Reproduced with permission from Miller RD, ed. *Miller's Anesthesia*. 6th ed. New York: Churchill Livingstone; 2005:1707. © Elsevier.

COMPLICATIONS

- Avoid deep cervical plexus block in patients with severe pulmonary disease; the block of the phrenic nerve could lead to respiratory failure
- Never perform bilateral deep cervical plexus block; this could cause bilateral phrenic nerve palsy
- The deep plexus is near the vertebral artery and the dura; therefore, frequent aspiration is recommended to avoid intravascular or intrathecal injection
- Blocks of vagus and/or hypoglossal nerves possible, especially with higher volumes, causing tachycardia and difficulty swallowing and phonating: monitor patient closely to avoid aspiration

PEARLS

- When using this block for carotid endarterectomy, the surgeon must still inject the carotid body, which is not affected by these blocks. These patients may also be at risk for plaque dislodgement with excessive rotation of the neck

FIGURE 130-5. Ultrasound-guided cervical plexus block

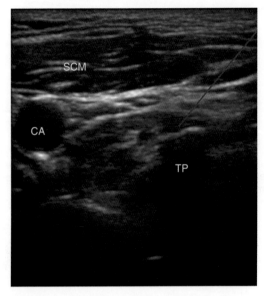

Imaging at the C4 level. SCM, sterno-cleido-mastoid muscle; CA, carotid artery; TP, transverse process. The red line illustrates the needle path. Local anesthetic (3–5 mL) is injected immediately anterior to the TP and spread is visualized.

REFERENCES

For references, please visit **www.TheAnesthesiaGuide.com**.

CHAPTER 131
Brachial Plexus

Denis Jochum, MD

- Two independent layers from the roots to terminal branches:
  - A simple and constant dorsal layer: extensor and supinator muscles
  - A complex and variable ventral layer: flexor and pronator muscles:
    - This explains the variations and the relationships between the median, musculocutaneous, and ulnar nerves
- The brachial plexus can be:
  - "Prefixed" with a contribution from C4 (two thirds of cases), or
  - Normal, or
  - "Postfixed," with the participation of T2
  - Or even spread in both directions:
    - Clinical significance of these variations because motor and sensory distributions are modified

- Origin of the trunks:
  - Upper trunk: confluence of the ventral branches of C5 and C6 (C4 participation, prefixed plexus)
  - Middle trunk: ventral division of C7
  - Lower trunk: confluence of the ventral branches of C8 and T1
- Constitution of the cords (most common configuration):
  - Lateral cord: confluence of ventral divisions of upper and middle trunks (80% of cases)
  - Medial cord: ventral division of lower trunk (95% of cases)
  - Posterior cord: confluence of dorsal divisions of the three trunks (70% of cases)
- Constitution of terminal nerves = branches (at distal edge of the pectoralis minor muscle):
  - Posterior cord: posterior plane of the brachial plexus, with mainly radial and axillary nerves
  - Lateral and medial cords: anterior plane of the brachial plexus with mainly the median nerve, as well as musculocutaneous and ulnar nerves

FIGURE 131-1. Brachial plexus

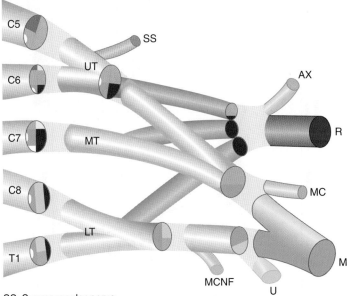

SS: Suprascapular nerve
AX: Axillary nerve
R: Radial nerve
MC: Musculocutaneous nerve
M: Median nerve
U: Ulnar nerve
MCNF: Medial cutaneous nerve of the forearm
UT: Upper trunk
MT: Middle trunk
LT: Lower trunk

FIGURE 131-2. Brachial plexus and muscle innervation

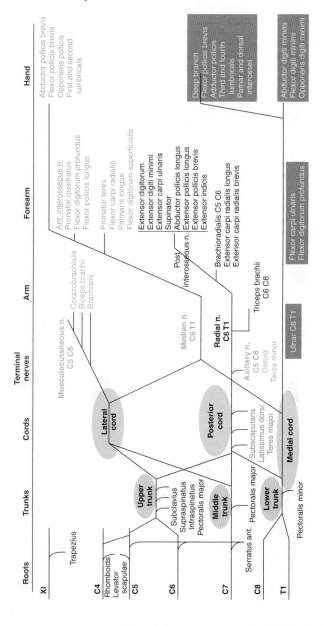

CHAPTER 132
Upper Limb Dermatomes, Myotomes, Sclerotomes

Denis Jochum, MD

FIGURE 132-1. Upper extremity dermatomes, myotomes, and sclerotomes

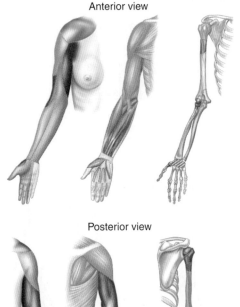

Anterior view

Posterior view

- 🔵 Superficial cervical plexus
- 🔴 Suprascapular nerve
- 🟠 Axillary nerve
- 🟡 Musculocutaneous nerve
- 🟢 Median nerve
- ⚪ Ulnar nerve
- ⚫ Radial nerve
- 🔴 Medial cutaneous nerve of the forearm
- 🟣 Medial cutaneous nerve of the arm

Adapted from Jochum D and Delaunay L, with permission from AstraZeneca France.

DERMATOMES

In the limbs, sensory fibers are distributed to an area further from the axis of the body than the motor fibers of the corresponding root. The skin innervation areas encroach on each other, which justifies the anesthesia of adjacent nerves.

OSTEOTOMES AND JOINT INNERVATION

Bones and joints are the main target for postoperative analgesia.

As a rule, joints receive innervation from the same nerves that innervate the muscles that act on them.

FIGURE 132-2. Shoulder joint innervation

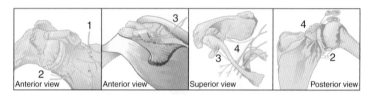

The nerve fibers from C5 and C6 roots are the main ones involved for shoulder surgery.
- For the anterior capsule: branches of subscapular (1), axillary (2), and lateral pectoral nerves (3).
- For the posterior capsule: suprascapular nerve (4) and articular branches of the axillary nerve (2).

FIGURE 132-3. Elbow joint innervation

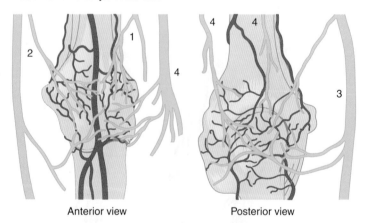

All major branches of the brachial plexus contribute to its innervation.
- The musculocutaneous nerve (1), through the anterior articular nerve of the elbow that comes out from either the main trunk of the nerve or the nerve to the brachialis muscle.
- The median nerve (2), through its articular rami (upper and lower rami, ramus of the nerve to the pronator teres muscle) to the anterior aspect of the joint.
- The ulnar nerve (3), through its articular rami (two to three) to the posterior and medial aspects of the joint.
- The radial nerve (4), through nerves for the medial head of the triceps and to the anconeus muscle, is distributed to the posterior and lateral aspects of the joint.

WRIST JOINT INNERVATION

- Mainly the posterior interosseous nerve (deep branch of radial nerve)
- The anterior interosseous branch of the median nerve, after innervation of the pronator quadratus muscle, pierces the interosseous membrane and anastomoses with the posterior interosseous nerve

CHAPTER 133
Interscalene Block

Arthur Atchabahian, MD

INTERSCALENE BLOCK COVERAGE

Level of blockade	Coverage distribution (Figure 133-1)
Roots/trunks	C5, C6, and C7 C4 and phrenic block quasi-constant by diffusion Inconstantly C8 and T1

FIGURE 133-1. Distribution of blockade after interscalene block

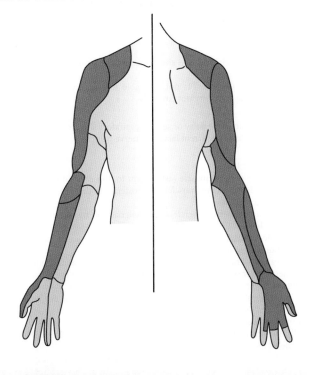

FIGURE 133-2. Schematic anatomy

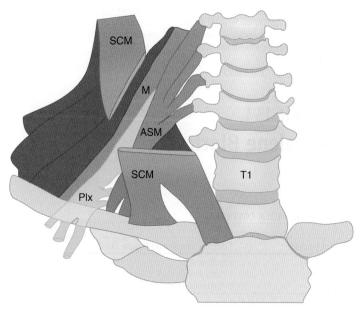

View of the patient's right side. The sternocleidomastoid muscle has been partially cut, exposing the plexus between the anterior and middle scalene muscles. SCM, sternocleidomastoid muscle; ASM, anterior scalene muscle; M, middle scalene muscle; Plx, brachial plexus.

Indications:
- Surgery of the distal clavicle, the shoulder, and the proximal one third of the humerus
- Unreliable block of C8 and T1: not advisable for surgery below midhumerus (medial aspect of the extremity not covered)

Contraindications:
- Contralateral phrenic nerve palsy or severe respiratory disease
- Contralateral vocal cord/recurrent laryngeal nerve palsy

Technique using NS:
- Landmarks (Figure 133-3):
  ‣ Posterior border of SCM muscle (ask patient to lift head if difficult to palpate), anterior and middle scalene muscles just posterior to the SCM, groove between the two scalene muscles
  ‣ Cricoid cartilage, or better tubercle of Chassaignac (i.e., transverse process of C6), to locate the level of C6
- A 5-cm needle is introduced at an angle of about 45° with the long axis of the neck (too perpendicular to the neck, the needle could pass between transverse processes and lead to an epidural or intrathecal injection; aiming too caudad, it increases the risk of pneumothorax). This angle should not change during the procedure. Only the anterior/posterior angle (and the depth) should be altered
- The index finger of the other hand is held on the groove and the needle is aimed at the plane of that groove
- The stimulator is set at 1.2 mA, 2 Hz (0.1 millisecond)
- Typically, the brachial plexus will be encountered after only 1–2 cm. Do not push the needle all the way!

Elicited Motor Responses During Interscalene Block Performance	
Acceptable responses	Unacceptable responses
Deltoid (shoulder abduction/antepulsion)	Trapezius: pull needle back to skin and redirect more anteriorly
Biceps (forearm flexion)	Phrenic (hiccups): pull needle back to skin and redirect more posteriorly
Triceps (forearm extension)	Any response below the elbow: the needle is too deep; pull needle back to skin and reassess landmarks
Pectoralis major (arm internal rotation)	

- Once an acceptable response has been obtained, the current should be decreased while needle position is optimized, until a current of less than 0.4 mA still triggers a motor response. If the response disappears as soon as one decreases the current below 0.5 mA, regardless of needle position changes, this typically means that the needle is outside of the interscalene sheath and needs to be repositioned
- To insert a catheter, the needle insertion point should be about 2 cm more cephalad, with the needle directed more caudad. This will allow the catheter to be more parallel to the plexus

FIGURE 133-3. Landmarks and needle insertion for neurostimulation-guided technique

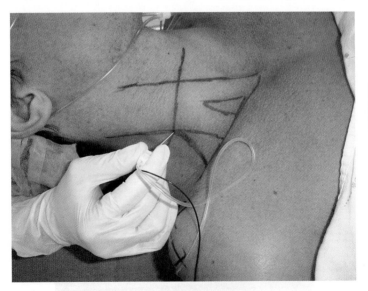

Landmarks include the sternocleidomastoid (SCM) muscle, the clavicle, and either the cricoid cartilage or the tubercle of Chassaignac to determine the level of C6. The interscalene groove can be palpated posterior to, and at an angle with, the posterior border of the SCM. The needle insertion point is at the intersection of the interscalene groove and the line marking C6.

Technique using US:
- The probe is placed on the neck, overlying the SCM muscle, at the approximate level of the cricoid cartilage. The vessels (carotid and internal jugular) are easily seen

- The probe is then moved laterally, allowing visualization of the anterior and middle scalene muscles. The roots of the brachial plexus are visible between the two muscles. Tilting the probe caudad (toward the feet) and moving it up and down helps find the best view, with C5, C6, and C7 lying like "peas in a pod", or a traffic light, between the scalene muscles (Figure 133-4)
- Alternatively, the nerves can be tracked up from the supraclavicular view. Place the probe just above the clavicle, aiming almost toward the feet. Locate the subclavian artery, with the brachial plexus lying immediately lateral and superficial to the artery. Slowly slide the probe cephalad. The plexus will separate into a distal contingent (C8–T1) that will disappear from view, and a proximal contingent (C5–C7) that can be followed until it reaches its typical position between the anterior and middle scalene muscles
- The needle is introduced in-plane, from either the medial (with care to avoid the IJ, and not to "scrape" the anterior aspect of the anterior scalene, with a risk of phrenic nerve injury) or preferably the lateral aspect of the probe, kept in sight in the ultrasound beam, and several injections are performed *between* the nerves, taking care not to penetrate the nerves with the needle. Usually 15–20 mL of local anesthetic will be sufficient for a good coverage
- To insert a catheter, it is easier to insert the needle out-of-plane and attempt to position the tip between the two most superficial nerves (C5 and C6). The position of the tip of the needle in the "sheath" is confirmed by injecting a few milliliters of LA. The catheter is then inserted and advanced 3–4 cm beyond the needle tip. This will usually place the catheter tip in the supraclavicular area. The catheter tip location can be confirmed using US by injecting LA, an agitated solution, or even a small amount of air

FIGURE 133-4. Ultrasound view of the interscalene area

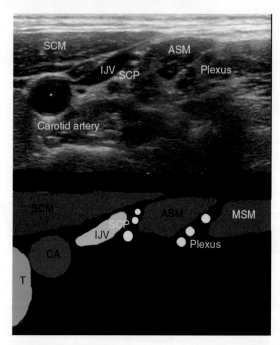

SCM, sternocleidomastoid muscle; ASM, anterior scalene muscle; MSM, middle scalene muscle; T, thyroid gland; CA, carotid artery; IJV, internal jugular vein; SCP, superficial cervical plexus.

Testing:
- Loss of muscle power: the patient can be asked to raise the upper extremity toward the ceiling. This will at first still be possible, with a "dropping" motion when bringing the arm back down, and then will become impossible
- "Money sign" (Figure 133-5): paresthesias will be felt in the three radial fingers, with a typical motion of rubbing the tip of the thumb against the tips of the index and middle fingers
- Pinprick testing can be done over the area covered by the axillary nerve (lateral aspect of shoulder)

FIGURE 133-5. Money sign

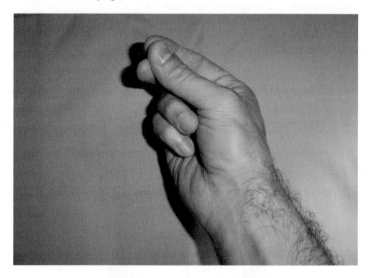

Complications/side effects:
- Constant ipsilateral phrenic nerve palsy (probably less with US guidance and low volume, but still possible): consider risk/benefit ratio in patients with respiratory compromise
- Horner syndrome by diffusion and blockade of the stellate ganglion (cervical sympathetic chain): miosis, ptosis, enophthalmos, hemifacial anhidrosis
- Recurrent nerve blockade with hoarseness: only an issue if contralateral vocal cord palsy
- Pneumothorax: very rare if landmarks respected
- Intravascular injection (essentially vertebral artery leading to seizure), epidural/intrathecal injection (with unconsciousness, apnea, cardiovascular collapse): supportive care

PEARLS

- The innervation of the skin of the top of the shoulder is by the superficial cervical plexus
- The skin overlying the posterior portal for shoulder arthroscopy is typically not covered (innervated by T2): ask the surgeon to inject local anesthetic prior to trocar insertion if surgery done under block + sedation
- Similarly, the skin of the lower part of a deltopectoral incision might not be covered by the block
- The ulnar fingers are usually not blocked: the patient's ability to move some fingers does not signal block failure!

CHAPTER 134
Supraclavicular Block

Arthur Atchabahian, MD

SUPRACLAVICULAR BLOCK COVERAGE

Level of blockade	Coverage distribution (Figure 134-1)
Divisions of the brachial plexus	Whole of the brachial plexus Depending on the volume and the anatomy, theoretical risk of missing the suprascapular nerve (innervating supraspinatus, infraspinatus, and posterior 70% of glenohumeral joint) Depending on volume, possible blockade of phrenic nerve

FIGURE 134-1. Distribution of blockade

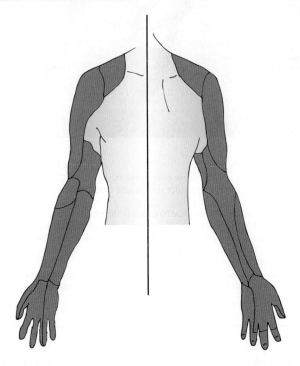

Indications:

Surgery of the whole upper extremity, from clavicle and shoulder to the hand.

Contraindications:
- Contralateral phrenic nerve palsy
- Severe respiratory disease (especially of contralateral lung)
- Contralateral vocal cord/recurrent laryngeal nerve palsy

Technique using NS:
- Not recommended: high risk of pneumothorax

Technique using US (Figures 134-2 to 134-4):
- Position patient with head of bed slightly elevated (in order to lower the shoulder) and head turned to the contralateral side
- Place the probe just above the clavicle, aiming almost toward the feet; locate the subclavian artery, with the brachial plexus lying immediately lateral and superficial to the artery. The plexus can have only a few large nerves, or many smaller ones. Typically, the distal contingent, coming from C8 and T1, lies deeper and closer to the artery, with occasionally nerves between the artery and the first rib. The proximal contingent, coming from C5–6–7, lies more superficial and lateral
- Also identify the pleura (deeper; bright line, mobile with deep inspiration) and the subclavian vein (more medial)
- Use Doppler to identify vessels that can occasionally course between the nerves, such as the cervical transverse artery or the dorsal scapular artery, in order to avoid vascular injury and intravascular injection
- Prep the skin lateral to the probe, and introduce a 100-mm needle in plane. Because of the proximity of the pleura, it is paramount to *keep the needle tip in sight at all times*. The probe can be rocked medially in order to provide more space to maneuver the needle ("heel-up" maneuver)
- Direct the needle into the "corner pocket" of the angle between the subclavian artery and the rib, being careful to *avoid the nerves*. A "pop" is often felt and seen when entering the plexus "sheath." Do not contact the rib (periosteal contact is painful). Aspirate, and then inject local anesthetic solution
- Depending on the case, the needle may need to be repositioned two or three times in order to bathe all the visible nerves. Pay special attention to the nerves covering the area of surgery:
  ‣ Proximal contingent if shoulder/upper humerus
  ‣ Distal contingent if forearm/hand/wrist

FIGURE 134-2. Position of the probe relative to the clavicle and the first rib

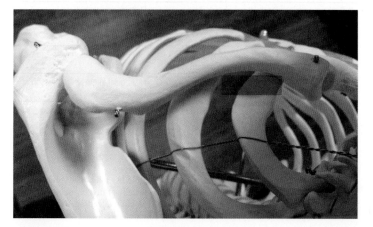

- If nerves are seen between artery and rib, the needle might need to be advanced, after injecting local anesthetic to "open the space," until those nerves are bathed as well
- Typically, 15–20 mL of local anesthetic solution is sufficient

FIGURE 134-3. Position of the probe and needle insertion

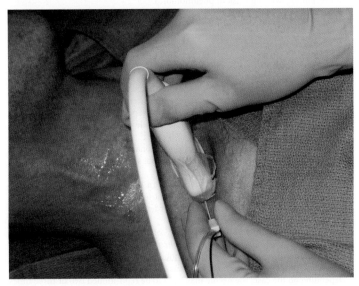

The blue rectangle indicates the position of the probe, just behind the clavicle, straddling the first rib.

Testing:

Nerve	Sensory	Motor
Axillary	Pinch lateral aspect of the shoulder	Deltoid: arm abduction
Musculocutaneous	Pinch lateral aspect of the forearm	Biceps
Radial	Pinch first dorsal web space (between thumb and index)	Triceps, extensor of fingers and wrist
Ulnar	Pinch pulp of fifth finger	First dorsal interossei (abduction of index finger)
Median	Pinch pulp of index finger	Thumb–fifth finger opposition

Complications/side effects:
- Pneumothorax is a risk; *keep needle tip in sight at all times*
- Vascular puncture of the subclavian artery is possible. As long as it is recognized and that intravascular injection is avoided, this is usually of no consequence
- Phrenic nerve palsy can occur even with small volumes, leading to respiratory distress in patients with borderline respiratory function

FIGURE 134-4. Ultrasound image

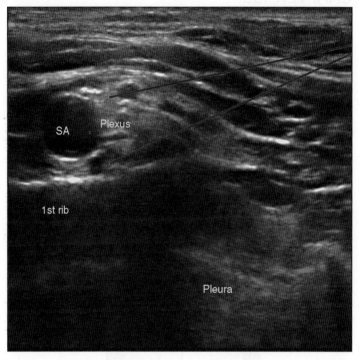

SA, subclavian artery; the red lines shows the paths of the needle to reach the "corner pocket", then to inject local anesthetic near the more superficial part of the plexus for a complete block.

PEARLS

- *Keep needle tip in sight at all times* to avoid pneumothorax
- Catheter insertion can be challenging at this level. Oftentimes, the easiest solution is to insert the catheter out-of-plane in the interscalene area and to thread it down to the supraclavicular level
- In the supraclavicular region, there is a close relationship between the brachial plexus and the subclavian artery, but also some collateral branches. The dorsal artery of the scapula usually takes its origin between the scalene muscles. In its cervical portion, it lies on the brachial plexus and passes either between C6 and C7 or between C7 and C8

CHAPTER 135
Infraclavicular Blocks

Arthur Atchabahian, MD

INFRACLAVICULAR BLOCK COVERAGE

Level of blockade	Coverage distribution (Figure 135-1)
Cords of brachial plexus	Whole upper extremity including axillary nerve Usually not blocked: suprascapular nerve (innervating supraspinatus, infraspinatus, and posterior 70% of glenohumeral joint)

FIGURE 135-1. Area blocked by an infraclavicular block

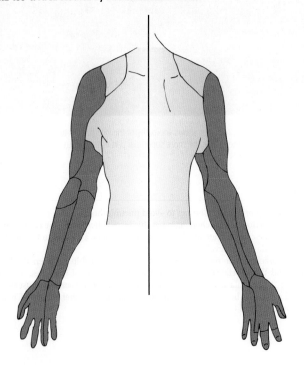

Indications:

Surgery of the upper extremity below the shoulder, as the suprascapular nerve is usually spared.

Contraindications:

Significant coagulopathy, as vessel puncture common (with NS technique), and this is a deep block poorly amenable to compression.

Pacemaker in the area where the block is to be performed.

Technique using NS:
- Paracoracoid approach (Figure 135-2):
  ‣ Patient supine, arm by the body, forearm on patient's chest
  ‣ Locate the coracoid process, caudad to the clavicle and medial to the humeral head
  ‣ From the most salient point of the coracoid, measure 2 cm caudad and 2 cm medial: this is the needle insertion point
  ‣ After prepping and local anesthesia, insert a 100 mm needle (unless patient very thin or small: use a 50 mm needle in that case) vertically toward the floor. Set PNS at 1.2 mA, 2 Hz, 0.1 millisecond
  ‣ *The needle must never be directed medially*: risk of pneumothorax
  ‣ If no response obtained, bring needle back to skin and redirect in 5° increments caudad or cephalad, but *always in a parasagittal plane*
  ‣ Elicit an acceptable response (see below); adjust needle position while decreasing current until response maintained at 0.4 mA
  ‣ If using a short-acting (chloroprocaine) or intermediate-acting (lidocaine, mepivacaine) local anesthetic, aspirate, and then inject the whole volume (40 mL) in a fractionated fashion
  ‣ If using a long-acting (bupivacaine, ropivacaine) local anesthetic, aspirate, and then inject one half of the volume (20 mL) in a fractionated fashion. Retract the needle by 2–3 cm:
    ▪ If an "ulnar" response was obtained, redirect needle cephalad
    ▪ If any other response was obtained, redirect needle caudad
  ‣ Elicit another acceptable response (see below); adjust needle position while decreasing current until response maintained at 0.4 mA; aspirate, and then inject one half of the volume (20 mL) in a fractionated fashion
  ‣ Performing a single injection with a long-acting LA can lead to delayed onset in the areas not covered by the nerve initially stimulated, up to 45 minutes after the injection
- Subclavicular approach:
  ‣ This technique inserts the needle just caudad to the midpoint of the clavicle. It is popular in Europe, and gives good results in experienced hands, but the risk of pneumothorax is higher

FIGURE 135-2. Landmarks for neurostimulation-guided paracoracoid technique

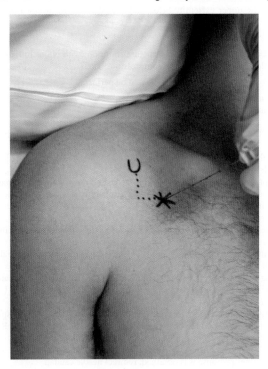

Testing:

Acceptable responses	Unacceptable responses
Any response **below the elbow** Triceps	**Biceps** and **deltoid**, as both musculocutaneous and axillary nerves exit the nerve sheath at a variable level, and could be stimulated outside that sheath

Technique using US (Figures 135-3 and 135-4):
- Patient supine, arm by the patient's body. Abducting the arm raises the clavicle and can facilitate needle insertion
- Place a high-frequency (8–13 MHz) probe in a craniocaudad direction just caudad to the clavicle
- Locate the subclavian artery. The probe might have to be rocked to aim cephalad in order to have a good view, especially in muscular or obese patients
- Slide probe lateral and medial to find the best location. Increase and decrease pressure on probe to locate the veins (typically two) near the artery

- Identify the three cords. Medial and lateral cords are usually well seen; the posterior cord can be masked by the posterior reinforcement artifact of the artery (as US travels unimpeded through a fluid-filled cavity, a hyperechoic artifact is created behind that structure)
- Prep and give local anesthesia to the area between the probe and the clavicle. A 50 or 100 mm (according to patient habitus) needle is introduced in-plane and is usually first brought to 6 o'clock relative to the artery. Local anesthetic is injected and the posterior cord is then better visualized. Often, this injection will spread like a U, surrounding the artery. Assess the spread around the three cords and reposition needle for additional injections if needed. Only rarely is more than one or two additional injections needed
- Typically, 20 mL of local anesthetic will suffice. On occasion, lower or higher volumes are needed for adequate spread
- To insert a catheter, position the Tuohy needle at 6 o'clock; inject LA, and then thread catheter 2–3 cm beyond the needle tip

FIGURE 135-3. Probe and needle position for US-guided block

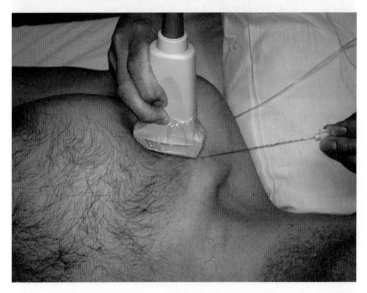

The ultrasound probe is positioned parasagitally under the clavicle, and the needle is introduced between clavicle and probe. A small-footprint probe ("hockey stick") can be useful in small patients. A degree of cephalad "rocking" of the ultrasound probe (i.e., aiming the ultrasound beam more cephalad) might be needed to have a better view of the artery and plexus.

FIGURE 135-4. Ultrasound view for performance of an infraclavicular block

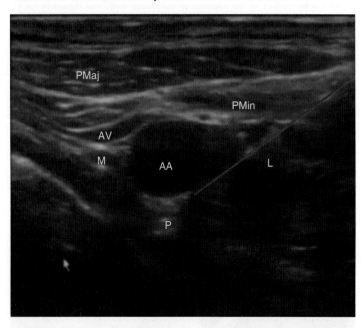

AA, Subclavian/axillary artery; AV, axillary vein (partially compressed); PMaj, pectoralis major muscle; PMin, pectoralis minor muscle; L, lateral cord; P, posterior cord; M, medial cord. The red line shows the path of the needle to the 6 o'clock position deep to the artery. Be careful to avoid injury the lateral cord. *NB*: The posterior cord might be difficult to differentiate from the posterior reinforcement artifact of the artery until after some LA has been injected. Picture courtesy of Dr. Olivier Choquet.

Testing:

Nerve	Sensory	Motor
Axillary	Pinch lateral aspect of the shoulder	Deltoid: arm abduction
Musculocutaneous	Pinch lateral aspect of the forearm	Biceps
Radial	Pinch first dorsal web space (between thumb and index)	Triceps, extensor of fingers and wrist
Ulnar	Pinch pulp of fifth finger	First dorsal interossei (abduction of index finger)
Median	Pinch pulp of index finger	Thumb–fifth finger opposition

Complications/side effects:
- Risk of pneumothorax, low but present
- Risk of vascular puncture (very common with NS technique, usually not an issue unless significant coagulopathy)

PEARLS

- NS technique: *do not aim medially; only redirect needle in a parasagittal plane*
- A single injection with a long-acting LA can lead to a delayed onset in some areas, up to 45 minutes

CHAPTER 136
Axillary Block

Arthur Atchabahian, MD

AXILLARY BLOCK COVERAGE

Level of blockade	Coverage distribution (Figure 136-1)
Branches of the brachial plexus: median, ulnar, and radial nerves + musculocutaneous (outside the "sheath")	Median nerve Ulnar nerve Radial nerve Musculocutaneous nerve (blocked separately)

Board question: which nerve is not blocked by the axillary block? A: the axillary nerve!

And also the musculocutaneous nerve, which has to be blocked separately.

Anatomy:

Typical arrangement of nerves around the axillary artery in the axilla (Figure 136-2).

Variations (Figure 136-3).

Indications:

Upper extremity surgery, preferably below the elbow, as the level of the block is not always adequate for elbow surgery, or for a very proximal tourniquet.

Contraindications:

None besides the usual regional anesthesia contraindications.

Technique using NS:
- Landmarks: the axillary artery pulse *as proximal as possible in the axilla*:
  ‣ On occasion, a Doppler can be necessary to locate the pulse
- Insert needle through the skin overlying the pulse
- Aim first anterior, toward the coracobrachialis muscle if it can be palpated, and elicit a biceps response at 1.2 mA. Decrease current to 0.4 mA (while adjusting needle position to maintain the response) and inject 5–7 mL of local anesthetic
- Pull needle back to skin and locate two out of three of the nerves that are located in the sheath around the artery (see responses below):
  ‣ Typically, the median nerve is anterior to the artery (toward the ceiling when patient supine)
  ‣ Ulnar and radial nerves are posterior to the artery (toward the floor with the patient supine), with the radial being deeper
  ‣ However, anatomic variations are common. Often, one has to insert the needle, and if no response is elicited, pull it back to the skin, slightly change the angle, and reinsert it, thus exploring the tissues surrounding the artery in a fan-like fashion, while avoiding the artery itself

FIGURE 136-1. Distribution of blockade following performance of an axillary block

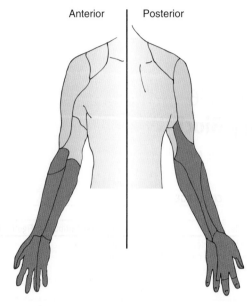

NB: An intercostobrachial block is typically added, which will cover the medial aspect of the elbow and arm.

- Again, start at 1.2 mA and decrease to 0.35 mA, and then inject 10–15 mL of local anesthetic for each nerve located, in a fractionated fashion, with aspiration every 5 mL
- Perform infiltration block of the medial cutaneous nerves of the arm and the forearm ("intercostobrachial") to prevent tourniquet pain: from the same needle entry site, create a posterior (toward the bed) skin wheal with 5–10 mL of 1–2% lidocaine

FIGURE 136-2. Typical arrangement of the nerves around the axillary artery in the axilla

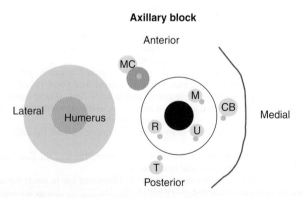

MC, musculocutaneous nerve (in the coracobrachialis muscle); M, median nerve; U, ulnar nerve, R, radial nerve; T, branches to the triceps muscle; CB, intercostobrachial nerves.

FIGURE 136-3. Variations in the position of the nerves

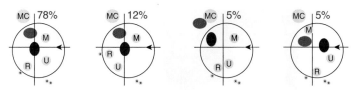

MC, musculocutaneous nerve; M, median nerve; U, ulnar nerve; R, radial nerve; *: branch to the triceps (from radial nerve); **: intercostobrachial nerves; arrowhead: needle insertion from the medial aspect of the arm. Adapted from Partridge BL, Katz J, Benirschke K. Functional anatomy of the brachial plexus sheath: implications for anesthesia. *Anesthesiology*. 1987;66:743–747.

Interpretation of Muscle Responses During Axillary Block	
Acceptable responses	Unacceptable responses
Median nerve: wrist radial flexion, flexion of the radial fingers	Triceps (elbow extension): branches to the triceps can be stimulated outside the sheath
Ulnar nerve: wrist ulnar flexion, flexion of the ulnar fingers	
Radial nerve: extension of elbow, wrist, or fingers	
Musculocutaneous nerve: elbow flexion	

Technique using US:
- Place high frequency (10–12 MHz) over the axillary artery pulse in the axilla
- Locate artery (use color Doppler to confirm if necessary), veins (typically two: release probe pressure to visualize them; it is very important not to inject into them), and nerves (median, ulnar, and radial around the artery, musculocutaneous in the fascial plane between biceps and brachialis muscles) (Figure 136-4)
- *NB*: Do not mistake the posterior reinforcement (artifact) behind the artery for the radial nerve
- Insert needle from anterior side of the probe, in-plane
- Aim first for the musculocutaneous nerve; inject 5–7 mL around the nerve
- Aim then for the other three nerves, one by one, injecting 5–10 mL in order to have a good spread around each nerve
- The absence of visible spread when injecting LA can be a sign of needle position in the vein. Release pressure on probe, pull needle very slightly back, and reassess
- Perform infiltration block of the medial cutaneous nerves of the arm and the forearm ("intercostobrachial") to prevent tourniquet pain: from the same needle entry site, create a posterior (toward the bed) skin wheal with 5–10 mL of 1–2% lidocaine

TESTING THE AXILLARY BLOCK

Nerve	Sensory	Motor
Musculocutaneous	Pinch lateral aspect of the forearm	Biceps
Radial	Pinch first dorsal web space (between thumb and index)	Triceps, extensor of fingers and wrist
Ulnar	Pinch pulp of fifth finger	First dorsal interossei (abduction of index finger)
Median	Pinch pulp of index finger	Thumb–fifth finger opposition

FIGURE 136-4. Technique using US

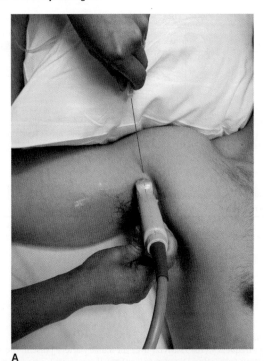

A

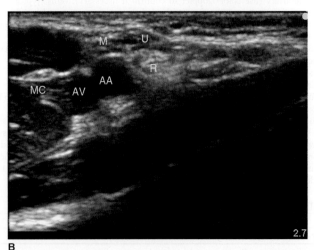

B

(A) Position of probe and needle insertion; (B) ultrasound view. AA, axillary artery; AV, axillary vein; MC, musculocutaneous nerve; M, median nerve; U, ulnar nerve; R, radial nerve. In this patient, all three nerves are located next to each other rather than in opposite corners around the artery (third arrangement in Figure 136-3). Note that the image deep to the artery is a posterior reinforcement artifact.

Complications/side effects:
- Arterial puncture is possible; going through the artery was the mainstay of the old transarterial technique. Very low complication rate if recognized before injection, except for the occasional small hematoma
- Intravascular injection (venous+++ or arterial)

PEARLS

- Avoid the axillary block for surgery proximal to the forearm—prefer supraclavicular or infraclavicular
- Associate with infiltration block of the medial cutaneous nerves of the arm and the forearm to prevent tourniquet pain
- Under ultrasound, the absence of visible spread when injecting LA can be a sign of needle position in the vein. Release pressure on probe, pull needle very slightly back, and reassess
- The two main objectives in an axillary block are the two main nerves of the two layers of the plexus, the radial nerve and the median nerve
- The radial nerve lies between the axillary artery and the tendon of the latissimus dorsi (interest of the US localization of the tendon of the latissimus for axillary block)
- Elbow flexion may be caused by contraction of the brachioradialis. Do not confuse this response (radial nerve) with that of the musculocutaneous nerve
- A merging of the musculocutaneous nerve with the median nerve (specifically the lateral branch of the median nerve) is found in 5% of cases at the axillary level. When performing a NS-guided axillary block, if the musculocutaneous nerve cannot be located, and after administration of local anesthetic in contact with the median nerve, ensure that the musculocutaneous nerve is not already blocked
- At the level of the axilla and proximal half of the arm, it accompanies the neurovascular structures and is located in the ventral side of the axillary vein and the basilic vein. A subcutaneous infiltration in the medial aspect of the arm is not needed to obtain anesthesia of the anterior–medial forearm during an axillary block or a block in the proximal half of the arm
- The median nerve and ulnar nerve are frequently anastomosed in the proximal forearm between the deep and superficial flexor muscles of the fingers (Martin-Gruber anastomosis). Muscle contractions of the flexor carpi radialis and palmaris longus muscles are characteristic of the median nerve stimulation at the axilla or arm. Contractions of the flexor carpi ulnaris are a sign of stimulation of the ulnar nerve at the axilla or in the arm

REFERENCE

For references, please visit **www.TheAnesthesiaGuide.com**.

CHAPTER 137
Branch Blocks at the Elbow and the Wrist

Arthur Atchabahian, MD

AREAS OF BLOCKADE

Level of blockade	Coverage distribution
According to nerve blocked: Median nerve Radial nerve Ulnar nerve	See chapter 132

Indications:

Typically to supplement proximal block when one (or more) branch is not blocked.

Contraindications:

Significant neuropathy (risk of "double-crush" injury with block at two levels).

Technique using NS:
- Median nerve:
  ‣ Elbow: immediately medial to the brachial artery in the elbow crease. Elicit appropriate response (flexor carpi radialis, flexor digitorum, pronator quadratus, opponens, abductor brevis) and inject 5–7 mL of LA (Figure 137-1)
  ‣ Wrist: between tendons of flexor carpi radialis and palmaris longus. Elicit appropriate response (opponens, abductor brevis) and inject 5 mL of LA Median and ulnar nerve blocks at wrist
  ‣ Flexor carpi
  ‣ radialis tendon
  ‣ Flexor
  ‣ carpi ulnaris
  ‣ Ulnar a.
  ‣ Ulnar n.
  ‣ Palmaris
  ‣ longusRadial nerve:
  ‣ Elbow: lateral to the tendon of the biceps in the elbow crease; alternatively, the radial nerve can be located above the elbow joint, on the lateral aspect of the arm, in the crease between biceps and triceps. Elicit appropriate response (brachioradialis, extensor carpi radialis/ulnaris, extensor pollicis, extensor digitorum) and inject 5–7 mL of LA. *NB*: The dorsal aspect of the forearm is typically not anesthetized with the block in the elbow crease, as the posterior cutaneous nerve of the forearm will be missed (Figure 137-1)
  ‣ Wrist: the radial nerve has only sensory rami at this level; they are blocked by infiltrating subcutaneously the skin on the lateral aspect of the wrist (from the midpoint of the dorsum to the midpoint of the volar aspect of the wrist) with 7–10 mL of LA. Pay attention not to lacerate the basilic vein (Figure 137-3)

FIGURE 137-1. Median and radial nerve blocks at the elbow

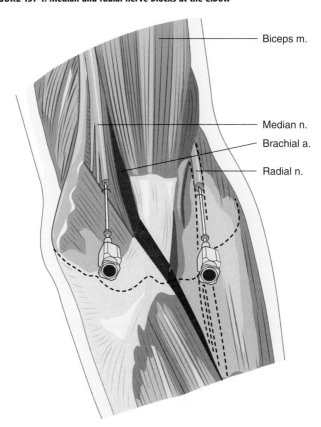

— Biceps m.

— Median n.
— Brachial a.

— Radial n.

- Ulnar nerve:
  - Elbow: the nerve goes through the ulnar groove, posterior to the medial epicondyle. Do not block the nerve in the tunnel, as there is a risk of compression. Locate the nerve slightly more proximal, on the medial aspect of the arm, between biceps and triceps. Elicit appropriate response (flexor carpi ulnaris, hypothenar muscles, adductor pollicis, interossei, and lumbricals) and inject 5–7 mL of LA
  - Wrist: the nerve courses medial to the ulnar artery and deep to the tendon of the flexor carpi ulnaris. Ask the patient to flex the wrist to locate the tendon, and insert needle from the medial side, deep to the tendon. Inject 3–5 mL of LA when an ulnar response is elicited (hypothenar muscles, adductor pollicis, interossei, and lumbricals) (Figure 137-2)

FIGURE 137-2. Median and ulnar nerve blocks at wrist

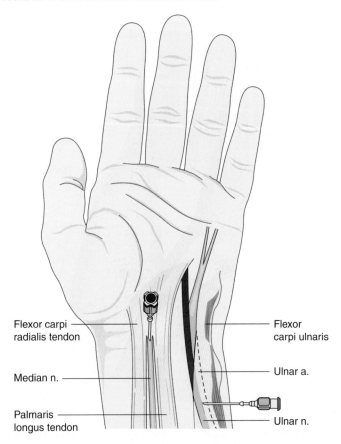

Flexor carpi radialis tendon

Median n.

Palmaris longus tendon

Flexor carpi ulnaris

Ulnar a.

Ulnar n.

Reproduced with permission from Miller RD, ed. *Miller's Anesthesia*. 6th ed. New York: Churchill Livingstone; 2005:1694. © Elsevier.

Technique using US: (NB: once located as described, nerves can be tracked distally using ultrasound and blocked at the desired level)

• Median nerve:
  ‣ Elbow: immediately medial to the brachial artery in the elbow crease. Inject 5–7 mL of LA (Figure 137-4)
  ‣ Wrist: between tendons of flexor carpi radialis and palmaris longus. Inject 5 mL of LA
• Radial nerve:
  ‣ Elbow: lateral to the tendon of the biceps in the elbow crease; alternatively, the radial nerve can be located above the elbow joint, on the lateral aspect of the arm, in the crease between biceps and triceps (Figure 137-5). *NB*: The dorsal aspect of the forearm is typically not anesthetized with the block in the elbow crease, as the posterior cutaneous nerve of the forearm will be missed
  ‣ Wrist: see technique described under NS, as the branches of the radial nerve are too small at the wrist level to be identified by ultrasound

FIGURE 137-3. Radial nerve block at wrist

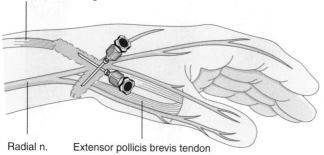

Extensor pollicis longus tendon

Radial n. Extensor pollicis brevis tendon

Reproduced with permission from Miller RD, ed. *Miller's Anesthesia*. 6th ed. New York: Churchill Livingstone; 2005:1694. © Elsevier.

FIGURE 137-4. Ultrasound-guided block of the median nerve at the elbow

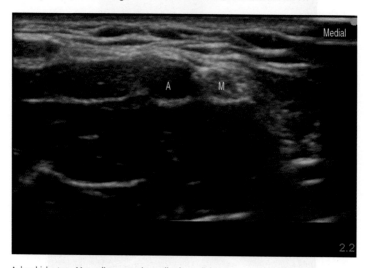

A, brachial artery; M, median nerve, immediately medial to the artery.

- Ulnar nerve:
  ‣ Elbow: the nerve goes through the ulnar groove, posterior to the medial epicondyle. Do not block the nerve in the tunnel, as there is a risk of compression. Locate the nerve slightly more proximal, on the medial aspect of the arm, between biceps and triceps (Figure 137-6). Inject 5–7 mL of LA
  ‣ Wrist: the nerve courses medial to the ulnar artery and deep to the tendon of the flexor carpi ulnaris. Ask the patient to flex the wrist to locate the tendon, and insert needle from the medial side, deep to the tendon. Inject 3–5 mL of LA

FIGURE 137-5. Ultrasound-guided block of the radial nerve at the elbow

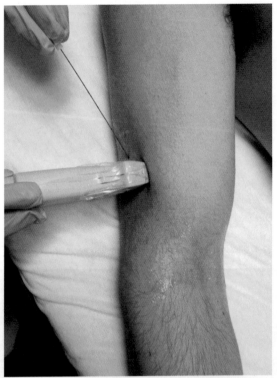

A

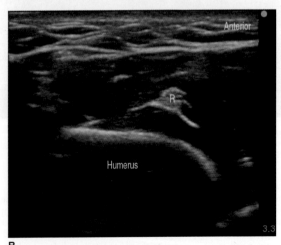

B

(A) Probe placement proximal to the elbow, in the groove between biceps and triceps on the lateral aspect of the arm, needle insertion out-of plane. (B) Ultrasound view; R: radial nerve.

FIGURE 137-6. Ultrasound-guided block of the ulnar nerve at the elbow

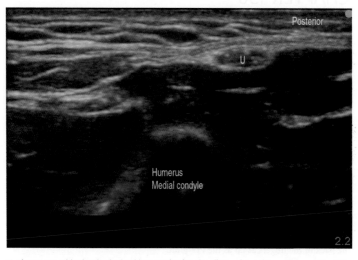

U, ulnar nerve. This view is obtained just proximal to the elbow, above the medial condyle of the humerus on the medial aspect of the arm.

Tests to Confirm Block		
Nerve blocked	Motor	Sensory
Median at elbow	Thumb–index ring	Pulp of index finger
Median at wrist	Thumb adduction (difficult to distinguish from extension)	Pulp of index finger
Radial at elbow	Finger extension	Dorsal first web space
Radial at wrist	N/A	Dorsal first web space
Ulnar at elbow	Thumb adduction; flexor carpi ulnaris	Pulp of fifth finger
Ulnar at wrist	Thumb adduction	Pulp of fifth finger

Complications/side effects:

None specific.

PEARLS

- A block of the radial nerve at the elbow will not anesthetize the dorsal surface of the forearm due to emergence of the proximal posterior cutaneous nerve of the forearm
- In the lateral bicipital groove at the elbow, at a variable level, the radial nerve divides into two terminal branches, an anterior superficial branch and a posterior deep branch, motor, also known as the posterior interosseous nerve
- During venipuncture at the wrist, there is a risk of nerve damage due to the close relationship between the cutaneous branches of the radial nerve and the cephalic vein (the "intern's vein")
- At the wrist, it is conventional to place the median nerve between the flexor carpi radialis laterally and the palmaris longus medially. It is actually the tendon for the index finger of the flexor digitorum superficialis that is the true satellite of the median nerve

CHAPTER 138
Digital Blocks

Arthur Atchabahian, MD

DIGITAL BLOCK COVERAGE

Level of blockade	Coverage distribution
Digital nerves at base of proximal phalanx	Finger

Anatomy:

The common digital nerves are branches of the median and ulnar nerves.

The main digital nerves, accompanied by digital vessels, run on the ventrolateral aspect of the finger immediately lateral to the flexor tendon sheath. Small dorsal digital nerves run on the dorsolateral aspect of the finger and supply innervation to the back of the fingers as far as the PIP joint.

Indications:

Small procedures on the finger.

Contraindications:

Do not use epinephrine-containing local anesthetic.

Technique (Figures 138-1 to 138-2):

FIGURE 138-1. Angle and depth of needle insertion

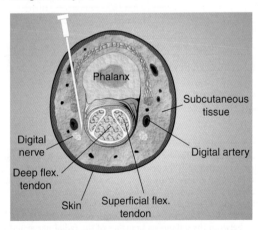

FIGURE 138-2. Needle insertion at the base of the proximal phalanx to block the medial digital nerve

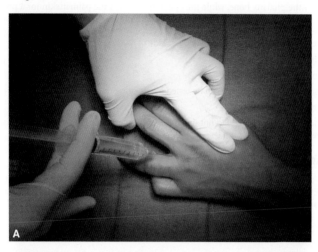

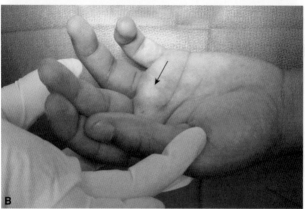

(A) Dorsal view. Reproduced from Hadzic A. *The New York School of Regional Anesthesia Textbook of Regional Anesthesia and Acute Pain Management*. Figure 30-4. Available at: www.accessanesthsiology.com. Copyright © The McGraw-Hill Companies, Inc. All rights reserved. (B) Palmar view. Advancement of the needle is stopped when the needle tip causes a skin bulge on the palmar side. Reproduced from Hadzic A. *The New York School of Regional Anesthesia Textbook of Regional Anesthesia and Acute Pain Management*. Figure 30-5. Available at: www. accessanesthsiology.com. Copyright © The McGraw-Hill Companies, Inc. All rights reserved.

A 25G 1.5 in. needle is inserted at the base of the finger on the dorsolateral aspect, and directed anteriorly toward the base of the phalanx. The needle is advanced adjacent to the phalanx bone, while the operator observes the palmar skin for a protrusion due to the needle. After aspiration, 2–3 mL of local anesthetic is injected, and 2 more mL is injected continuously as the needle is withdrawn back to the skin. The same procedure is repeated on the other side of the finger.

Testing:

No motor block is achieved.

Sensory block of the finger can be tested by pinching or pinprick.

Complications/side effects:

Avoid finger tourniquet. Do not use epinephrine-containing local anesthetic: risk of ischemia.

PEARLS

Another technique is the transthecal block, where 2–3 mL of local anesthetic is injected into the flexor sheath. Success rate is reportedly high. However, there is a risk of infection of the flexor tendon sheath.

CHAPTER 139
Lumbosacral Plexus

Denis Jochum, MD

- The lumbar plexus is usually formed by the ventral rami of the L1–L3 and part of the ventral branch of L4
- The sacral plexus is formed by the lumbosacral trunk (L4, L5), the first sacral ventral ramus, part of the ventral branch of S2, and a small portion of the ventral branch of S3
- Classically, the ventral branch of L4 is the junction between the two plexi; it gives off a branch to the femoral nerve, one to the obturator nerve, and the lumbosacral trunk that becomes part of the sciatic nerve
- There are several varieties of lumbosacral plexus:
  ‣ The most common is a "prefixed" plexus, including all or part of T12
  ‣ A "normal" plexus
  ‣ A "postfixed" plexus
  ‣ Or even a plexus spread in both directions:
    ▪ These anatomical variations can affect regional anesthesia practice because of variations in motor and sensory distributions

FIGURE 139-1. Lumbosacral plexus

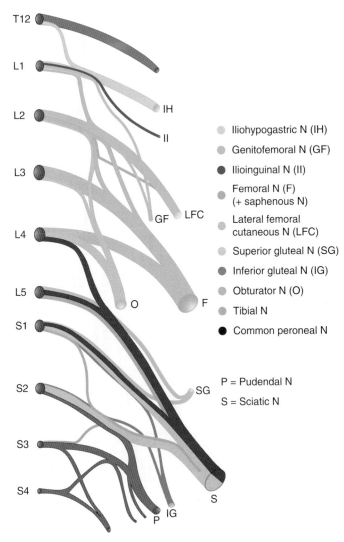

- The division into two planes of the lumbosacral plexus is less clear than for the brachial plexus
- The two terminal branches of the lumbar plexus are the femoral nerve and obturator nerve, which correspond, respectively, to the dorsal and the ventral layers
- For the sacral plexus, the tibial nerve is the ventral layer and the common peroneal nerve the dorsal layer
- The layout of the main nerves of the lumbosacral plexus requires the use of combined blocks for anesthesia of the lower limb

FIGURE 139-2. Lumbosacral plexus and muscle innervation

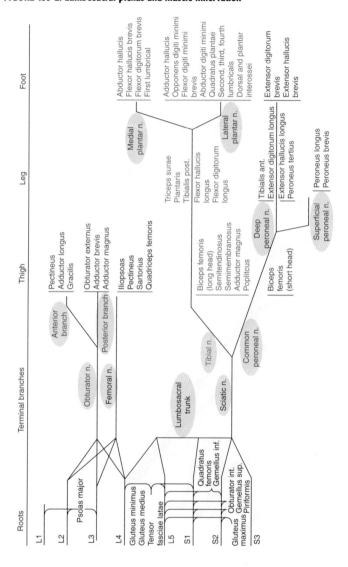

CHAPTER 140
Lower Limb Dermatomes, Myotomes, Sclerotomes

Denis Jochum, MD

FIGURE 140-1. Lower limb dermatomes, myotomes, and sclerotomes

Anterior view

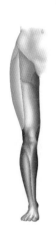
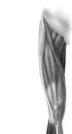
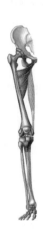

Posterior view

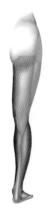
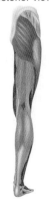
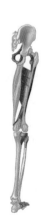

- ○ Iliohypogastric N
- ● Genitofemoral N
- ● Ilioinguinal N
- ● Femoral N (+ saphenous N)
- ● Lateral femoral cutaneous N
- ○ Superior gluteal N
- ● Inferior gluteal N
- ● Obturator N
- ○ Posterior cutaneous N of the thigh
- ● Tibial N
- ● Common peroneal N
- ● Sural N

Adapted from Jochum D and Delaunay L, with permission from AstraZeneca France.

DERMATOMES

In the limbs, sensory fibers are distributed to an area further from the axis of the body than the motor fibers of the corresponding root. The skin innervation areas encroach on each other, which justifies the anesthesia of adjacent nerves.

OSTEOTOMES AND JOINT INNERVATION

Bones and joints are the main target for postoperative analgesia.

As a rule, joints receive innervation from the same nerves that innervate muscles that act on them.

ANKLE JOINT INNERVATION

Anterior aspect: deep peroneal nerve.

Posterior and medial aspects: tibial nerve.

FIGURE 140-2. Hip joint innervation

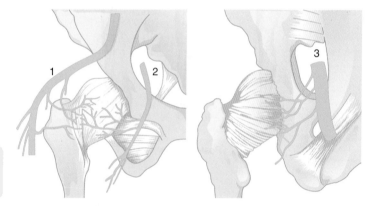

- Anterior portion of the joint capsule: (1) branch of the femoral nerve (L1–L4) along the iliopsoas muscle.
- Anteromedial portion: (2) a branch of the obturator nerve (L1–L4).
- Posterior portion: (3) branches of the sciatic nerve.
- Posteromedial portion: ramus from the nerve of the quadratus femoris muscle (L5–S2).
- Posterolateral portion: rami of the superior gluteal nerve (L4–S1).

FIGURE 140-3. Knee joint innervation

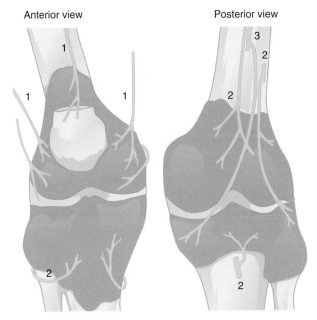

Anterior view   Posterior view

- Anterior and anteromedial aspects: deep branches of the femoral nerve (1).
- Posterior and inferolateral aspects: sciatic nerve (2).
- Posterior aspect: contribution of articular rami of the deep branch of the obturator nerve (3).

CHAPTER 141
Psoas Compartment (Posterior Lumbar Plexus) Block

Arthur Atchabahian, MD

COVERAGE OF THE LUMBAR PLEXUS BLOCK

Level of blockade	Coverage distribution
Lumbar plexus in the psoas muscle, shortly after it exits the spine	*Femoral nerve:* quadriceps muscle, anterior aspect of thigh, medial aspect of lower leg (saphenous nerve), anterior aspect of acetabulum and femur, portion of proximal tibia
	Lateral femoral cutaneous nerve: lateral aspect of hip and thigh
	Obturator nerve: adductor muscles, medial femur
	Ilioinguinal, iliohypogastric, genitofemoral: usually blocked as well

FIGURE 141-1. Distribution of cutaneous anesthesia and analgesia from a lumbar plexus block

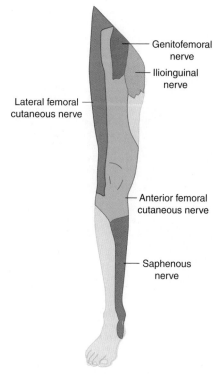

Genitofemoral nerve

Ilioinguinal nerve

Lateral femoral cutaneous nerve

Anterior femoral cutaneous nerve

Saphenous nerve

Anterior

Anatomy:
- The lumbar plexus originates from L1 to L4, with often a contribution from T12. L4 gives off a branch that merges with L5 to form the lumbosacral branch, part of the sacral plexus
- Branches of the lumbar plexus include:
  ‣ Femoral nerve
  ‣ Lateral femoral cutaneous nerve
  ‣ Obturator nerve
  ‣ Ilioinguinal, iliohypogastric, and genitofemoral nerves
- The lumbar plexus courses through the lumbar area and the pelvis in the sheath of the psoas, and then the iliopsoas muscle (Figure 141-2)

Indications:
- Postoperative analgesia of hip or knee surgery (associated or not to a sacral plexus block); probably no advantage over femoral nerve block for knee surgery:
  ‣ Hip arthroscopy
  ‣ Proximal femur ORIF
  ‣ Hip hemiarthroplasty/THA

FIGURE 141-2. Lumbar plexus anatomy

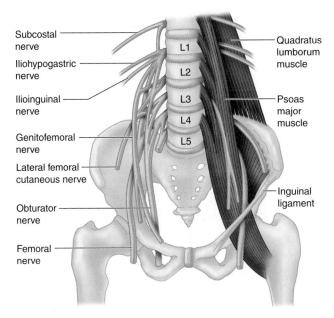

Subcostal nerve
Iliohypogastric nerve
Ilioinguinal nerve
Genitofemoral nerve
Lateral femoral cutaneous nerve
Obturator nerve
Femoral nerve

Quadratus lumborum muscle
Psoas major muscle
Inguinal ligament

L1 L2 L3 L4 L5

- Anesthesia for lower extremity surgery, in association with a sacral plexus block
- The block of the obturator nerve is reliable, contrary to the femoral paravascular block, and the block is more proximal, with theoretically a better coverage of the hip
- When combined with a sciatic block, take into account total dose of local anesthetic
- *This is an advanced block* and should only be performed by experienced practitioners because of potential severe complications

Contraindications:
- Significant coagulopathy; this is a deep block, and a psoas sheath bleeding may go unnoticed, and is not amenable to compression:
  ‣ Single-injection or continuous psoas compartment block should be treated as neuraxial blocks with regards to coagulation issues
- Significant lumbar spine deformity, as the position of the lumbar plexus might be distorted

Technique using NS (Figure 141-3):
- Patient in lateral decubitus, side to be blocked up, nondependent lower extremity slightly flexed; stand behind patient
- Draw Tuffier's line (joining the iliac crests): line A
- Draw a line over the spinous processes (feel for the spine; the median skin fold can sag and not overlie the spine): line B
- Locate the posterior superior iliac spine (PSIS) and draw a line through the PSIS and parallel to the spine: line C
- Divide the portion of line A between lines B and C into three thirds
- The needle insertion point is at the point between lateral one third and medial two thirds

FIGURE 141-3. Landmarks for neurostimulation-guided lumbar plexus block

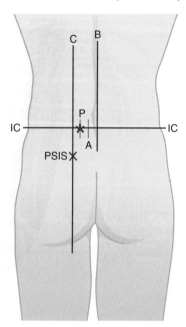

IC, iliac crest; PSIS, posterior superior iliac spine; P, needle insertion point for psoas compartment block.

- Use a 100 or 120 mm needle. After local anesthesia with a 25G needle, insert block needle perpendicular to the patient's back. Avoid especially aiming medially toward the spine, as this could lead to an epidural or intrathecal injection
- Set NS at 1.4 mA, 2 Hz, 0.1 millisecond. When a quadriceps response is obtained, typically around 7–8 cm for an average-sized patient, adjust needle position while decreasing current to 0.4 mA. If a quadriceps response is still present, aspirate and inject slowly, in a fractionated fashion, 20–30 mL of local anesthetic
- Some authors recommend injecting first a test dose of 3 mL of 1.5% lidocaine with 1:200,000 epi to rule out intrathecal or intravascular injection, before injecting the large volume of local anesthetic for the block
- A slow, low-pressure injection decreases the risk of epidural spread
- If the transverse process is encountered, retract needle 2–3 cm while marking the depth. Redirect in a parasagittal plane (*never* medially!) in 5° increments and walk off the transverse process either cephalad or caudad; avoid inserting needle more than 2–3 cm beyond the depth at which the transverse process was contacted
- In order to insert a catheter, use a stimulating 100 or 150 mm Tuohy-type needle. Direct bevel opening caudad to prevent epidural catheter positioning. Thread catheter 5–10 cm beyond needle tip to prevent dislodgment with patient motion. Use test dose with epinephrine

Responses obtained (see Figure 141-4):

Acceptable responses	Unacceptable responses
Quadriceps	Adductors (obturator nerve)
	Hamstrings, lower leg (sciatic nerve)
	Paresthesia in genitalia (genitofemoral nerve)
	Abdominal wall (iliohypogastric nerve)

FIGURE 141-4. Management of response during psoas compartment block performance

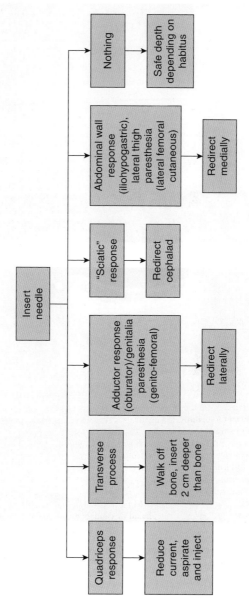

FIGURE 141-5. Ultrasound-guided lumbar plexus block

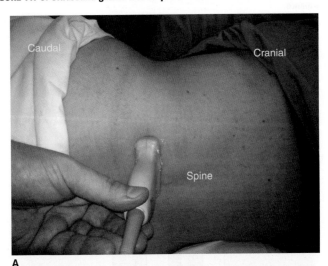

A

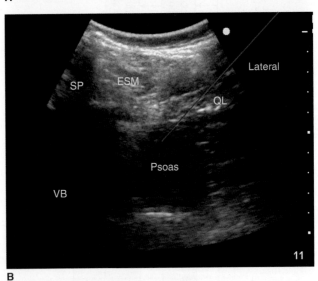

B

(A) Probe placement for transverse imaging. (B) Ultrasound transverse view. SP, spinous process; ESM, erector spinae muscle; QL, quadratus lumborum muscle; TP, transverse process; VB, vertebral body.

FIGURE 141-5. (*continued*)

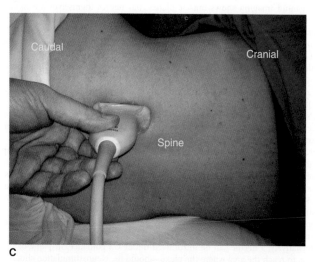

C

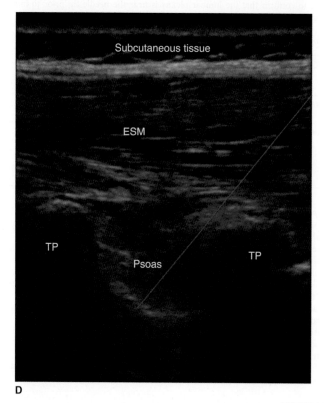

D

(C) Probe placement for parasagittal imaging. (D) Ultrasound parasagittal view. ESM, erector spinae muscle; TP, transverse process. The red line indicates the needle path.

Technique using US (Figure 141-5):
- Ultrasound imaging shows muscle planes, but nerves themselves are rarely distinctly seen
- Use a low-frequency (3–5 MHz) curved probe
- *Transverse imaging* is performed by holding the probe lateral to the spinous process of L4. The transverse process can be seen, as well as the vertebral body
- Slide probe slightly caudad or cephalad until the transverse process disappears. The muscles can then be seen:
  ‣ Erector spinae under the skin, lateral to the spinous process
  ‣ Quadratus lumborum lateral to the transverse process
  ‣ Psoas anterior to the transverse process, lateral to the vertebral body
- The lumbar plexus is located either in the plane between quadratus lumborum and psoas or inside the psoas sheath
- *Parasagittal imaging* is performed by positioning the probe parallel to the spine, slightly lateral, over the insertion site for the NS block
- The transverse processes are seen as bright curved structures with posterior shadows. Superficially, the erector spinae muscle, and deeper, the psoas muscle can be seen. Again, the plane between muscles can be seen, but the plexus is rarely visualized
- Depth measurements can be made, and the block performed using only neurostimulation
- Alternatively, a needle can be introduced under US guidance, in-plane or out-of-plane, to reach the area where the plexus should lie. Neurostimulation should then used to confirm that the lumbar plexus is near the needle tip prior to injecting local anesthetic

Testing:

Femoral nerve	Quadriceps: ask patient to raise leg and keep knee extended Pinch anterior aspect of thigh Saphenous nerve: pinch medial aspect of lower leg
Lateral femoral cutaneous nerve	Pinch lateral aspect of hip/thigh
Obturator nerve	Adductor muscles: ask patient to adduct thigh *NB*: A small portion of adductor power is under femoral and sciatic control; thus, even with a complete obturator nerve block, the patient may have some residual adductor power: compare with contralateral thigh

Complications/side effects:
- Psoas hematoma; this complication has been described even in patients with normal coagulation
- Theoretical risk of peritoneal entry and viscus injury
- Kidney injury (subcapsular hematoma) or ureteral injury: if using ultrasound, scan proximally to locate the lower pole of the kidney
- Risk of epidural spread: bilateral block, hypotension, reduced duration of analgesia; up to 15% of cases; inject slowly under low pressure
- Risk of intrathecal injection: total spinal with loss of consciousness, apnea, and cardiovascular collapse, with lethal risk; some authors recommend injecting a test dose of 3 mL of 1.5% lidocaine with 1:200,000 epi to rule out intrathecal or intravascular injection
- Intravascular injection of local anesthetic with systemic toxicity
- *NB*: Partial loss of sensation in ipsilateral genitalia is possible; reassure patient that this will disappear as block wears off

REFERENCES

For references, please visit **www.TheAnesthesiaGuide.com**.

CHAPTER 142
Femoral Nerve Block, Fascia Iliaca Compartment Block (FICB)

Arthur Atchabahian, MD

FEMORAL NERVE BLOCK COVERAGE

Level of blockade	Coverage distribution (see chapter 140)
• Femoral nerve	• Quadriceps, sartorius muscle, anterior aspect of hip, thigh, and knee, proximal portion of tibia
• Saphenous nerve	• Skin of medial aspect of lower leg
• Lateral femoral cutaneous nerve (LFCN) most often blocked as well	• Skin of lateral aspect of hip and thigh
• *NB*: Obturator nerve only rarely blocked (the "3-in-1 block" is a myth)	

Anatomy:
- Femoral nerve, LFCN, and obturator nerve are branches of the lumbar plexus
- In the inguinal area, femoral nerve separated from femoral vessels by fascia iliaca (fascia of psoas–iliacus muscle). Vessels are superficial to the fascia, but the nerve is deep to it (Figure 142-1). The fascia lata is subcutaneous and superficial to all of these structures
- For the fascia iliaca compartment block (FICB), LA is injected under the fascia iliaca, lateral to the femoral nerve, and allowing it to diffuse to both the femoral nerve and the LFCN

Indications:

Surgery or postoperative analgesia in the coverage distribution of the block:
- Quadriceps tendon repair
- Knee arthroscopy
- Total knee replacement (in association with a sciatic block or spinal/general anesthesia)
- Total hip replacement (less analgesia than psoas compartment block, but lower risk of complication)
- Femoral shaft fracture/ORIF
- Harvest of skin graft from the anterior aspect of the thigh

Contraindications:

Neurostimulation technique best not used if femoral vascular bypass (risk of graft injury).

FIGURE 142-1. Anatomy: transverse cut at the level of the inguinal crease

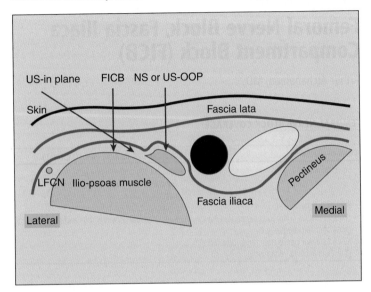

LFCN, Lateral femoral cutaneous nerve (this nerve lies initially under the fascia iliaca; it will then traverse fascia iliaca and fascia lata to become subcutaneous); US-in plane: needle approach for the in-plane ultrasound-guided femoral nerve block; NS or US-OOP: needle approach for the neurostimulation technique or for the out-of-plane ultrasound-guided technique; FICB: needle approach for the fascia iliaca compartment block.

FICB by landmarks (Figure 142-2):
- Patient supine; retract abdominal pannus with tape if needed
- Mark the anterior-superior iliac spine (ASIS) and the femoral pulse in the inguinal crease (these are not the classic landmarks, but they are easier and just as effective)
- Draw a line between the two and mark the center
- Insert needle (either a short-bevel block needle or a spinal needle) perpendicular to the skin, and elicit two "pops" (fascia lata, and then fascia iliaca). Aspirate and inject 20–30 mL of LA, in a fractionated fashion, with aspiration every 5 mL
- This block can be performed using US, but except in the obese patient in whom the pops are poorly felt, there is little advantage, as the beauty of this block lies in its simplicity, and the fact that almost no equipment is needed

Technique using NS (Figure 142-3):
- Patient supine; retract abdominal pannus with tape if needed
- Locate the femoral pulse in the inguinal crease
- Insert needle 1.5 cm lateral, with current set at 1.2 mA
- The stimulator is set at 1.2 mA, 2 Hz (0.1 millisecond). Attempt to elicit a response from rectus femoris (i.e., the central part of the quadriceps) with an elevation of the patella. This results from stimulation of the quadriceps nerve, which is located laterally and deep in the femoral nerve
- Once an acceptable response has been obtained, the current should be decreased while needle position is optimized, until a current of less than 0.4 mA still triggers a motor response
- Inject 20–30 mL of LA, in a fractionated fashion, with aspiration every 5 mL
- For a continuous block, use identical technique and insert catheter 3–4 cm beyond needle tip

FIGURE 142-2. Fascia iliaca compartment block by landmarks

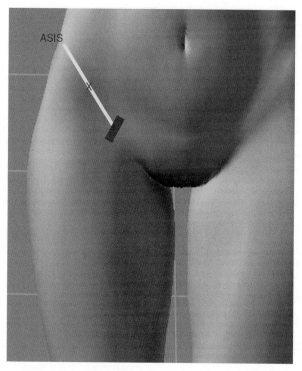

ASIS, anterior-superior iliac spine; the yellow line joins the ASIS and the femoral pulse in the inguinal crease; X, needle insertion point, midway between ASIS and femoral pulse.

FIGURE 142-3. Femoral nerve block using NS

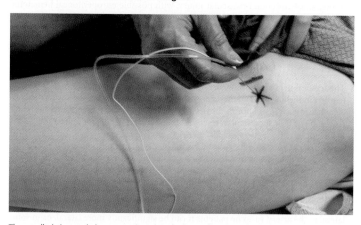

The needle is inserted about 1 cm lateral to the femoral artery pulse in the inguinal crease and directed 45° cephalad.

Responses obtained:

Acceptable responses	Unacceptable responses
Central quadriceps ("patellar tendon")	Any other, especially vastus medialis or lateralis (medial or lateral aspect of the quadriceps), sartorius, local responses

Technique using US (Figure 142-4):
- Patient supine; retract abdominal pannus with tape if needed
- Locate the femoral pulse in the inguinal crease
- Position probe in a short-axis orientation; identify femoral artery and vein (by pressing and releasing the probe: the vein collapses while the artery does not)
- If two arteries are seen (i.e., the femoral profunda has already branched out), slide probe proximally until only one artery is seen
- The femoral nerve is located lateral to the artery. Change tilt to better visualize it, typically hyperechoic with hypoechoic dots. Under the nerve is the psoas muscle
- Prep area lateral to the US probe; insert 100 mm needle about 15 mm away from the probe, in-plane. Aim to position the tip *between* the femoral nerve and the psoas muscle (i.e., *under* the nerve)
- Inject 20–30 mL of LA, in a fractionated fashion, with aspiration every 5 mL. Ensure that LA does not spread superficial to the vessels, which means that the needle tip is *superficial* to the fascia iliaca, as the block would be unsuccessful
- For a continuous block, insert catheter 1–2 cm beyond needle tip. Inject LA and/ or air under US guidance to ensure that the catheter remains close to the nerve. Avoid inserting the catheter too far in, as it will then progress medially, away from the femoral nerve

Testing:

Sensory	Motor
Femoral nerve: medial aspect of middle third of the medial aspect of the thigh Saphenous nerve: anteromedial aspect of the middle third of the lower leg LFCN: lateral aspect of proximal third of thigh	Quadriceps: ask patient to raise lower extremity with the knee extended; hip flexion should be possible, but knee extension paralyzed

Complications/side effects:
- Intravascular injection or vascular injury, with possible retroperitoneal hematoma (rare)
- Block failure if injection superficial to fascia iliaca
- Colonization/infection if continuous block

PEARLS

- The femoral nerve is typically organized in two layers, with the nerve to the rectus femoris in the deep layer; when performing a NS-guided block, if a vastus medialis response is elicited, first push the needle deeper to attempt to obtain a rectus femoris response. If unsuccessful, retract and then redirect needle more laterally
- Following a femoral nerve block, the first area of skin to be anesthetized is the medial aspect of the thigh. Anesthesia of the deep layer of the femoral nerve corresponds to quadriceps motor block associated to sensory block of the saphenous nerve. The many variations between femoral nerve, lateral cutaneous nerve of the thigh, and femoral branch of the genitofemoral nerve account for cases of absence of cutaneous anesthesia of the anterolateral thigh
- Ultrasound shows that, while most of the time the femoral nerve is immediately lateral to the artery, in some patients it can be significantly more lateral, or in some cases deep into the iliacus muscle, near the femur

FIGURE 142-4. Ultrasound-guided femoral nerve block

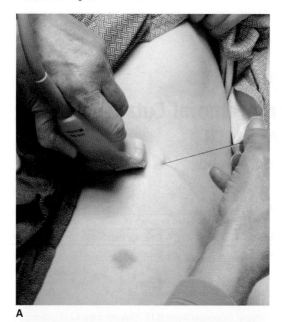

A

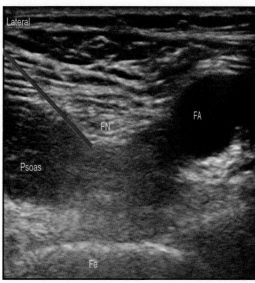

B

(A) The probe is placed at the level of the inguinal crease, perpendicular to the axis of the patient's body. The needle is inserted in-plane from the lateral side. An out-of-plane technique aiming cephalad is also possible. (B) Ultrasound view. FA: femoral artery; Fe: femur; FN: femoral nerve; Psoas: iliopsoas muscle. The needle (red line) is guided in-plane through the fascia iliaca and into the plane between iliopsoas muscle and femoral nerve.

REFERENCE

For references, please visit **www.TheAnesthesiaGuide.com**.

CHAPTER 143
Lateral Femoral Cutaneous Nerve Block

Arthur Atchabahian, MD

LFCN BLOCK COVERAGE

Level of blockade	Coverage distribution
Lateral femoral cutaneous nerve	Skin of lateral aspect of thigh (see chapter 140)

Anatomy:

The lateral femoral cutaneous nerve (LFCN) arises from L2–3. After emerging from the lateral border of the psoas major muscle, it courses inferiorly and laterally toward the anterior superior iliac spine (ASIS). It then passes under the inguinal ligament and over the sartorius muscle into the thigh, where it divides into two branches (anterior and posterior). The LFCN, a small subcutaneous nerve located between the fascia lata and iliaca, provides sensory innervation to the lateral thigh. On occasion, its area of coverage can include the anterior thigh, normally covered by the femoral nerve.

Indications:
- Rare, as the LFCN is usually blocked when performing a femoral nerve block or a psoas compartment block. Rescue block in case of failure of the LFCN to be blocked
- Skin graft harvesting on the lateral aspect of the thigh

Contraindications:

None specific.

Technique using landmarks:
- Patient supine, palpate the ASIS
- Mark a point 1 cm medial and caudal to the ASIS
- After local anesthesia and prepping, insert a short-bevel 50 mm needle until a pop is felt, marking the passage through the fascia lata. The needle is moved fanwise laterally and medially, and 10–15 mL of solution is injected above and below the fascia

Technique using US:
- Small nerve, difficult to visualize
- Place high-frequency probe medial and inferior to the ASIS, parallel to the inguinal ligament
- In that area, the nerve should be between fascia lata and fascia iliaca. On occasion, it can lie deep to the fascia iliaca

Testing:
- Pinch/pinprick of skin of lateral aspect of thigh
- No motor block

Complications/side effects:

None specific.

CHAPTER 144
Obturator Nerve Block

Arthur Atchabahian, MD

OBTURATOR BLOCK COVERAGE

Level of blockade	Coverage distribution
Obturator nerve	• Portion of the hip joint • Most of the adductor muscles • Variable portion of the medial aspect of the femur • Inconstant skin distribution on the medial aspect of the thigh

Anatomy (Figures 144-1 and 144-2):
- Branch of the lumbar plexus (L2–L4)
- Typically emerges from the medial border of the psoas muscle at the level of the pelvic brim, and divides in the obturator canal into anterior and posterior branches, although variations are common with a multiple branching pattern
- The anterior branch gives an articular branch to the hip joint, provides motor innervation of the adductor brevis, adductor longus, gracilis, and occasionally the pectineus (usually femoral nerve), and innervates a variable area of skin; most sources show an area in the medial aspect of the thigh, while others suggest a more distal location at the level of the knee. Sensory testing is thus unreliable
- The posterior branch provides motor innervation to the adductor magnus, obturator externus, and occasionally the adductor brevis (in that case, this muscle is not innervated by the anterior branch), and ends with an articular branch to the knee joint

Indications:
- Supplementation of femoral and sciatic nerve blocks for lower extremity surgery, especially knee surgery
- Prevention of the obturator reflex during transurethral resection of the bladder (TURB). The reflex is due to the stimulation through the bladder of the obturator nerve, resulting in sudden thigh adduction that can cause bladder perforation. Bilateral blocks have to be performed to be effective

Contraindications:

None specific.

FIGURE 144-1. Anatomy of the obturator nerve

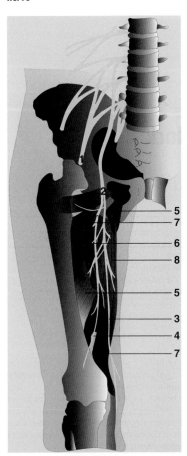

FIGURE 144-2. Sagittal section demonstrating the relationship of the obturator nerve to the adductor muscles

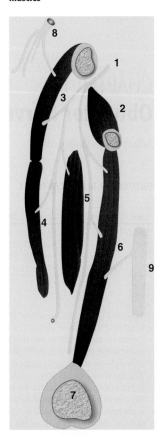

(1) Femoral nerve; (2) obturator nerve; (3) anterior branch; (4) posterior branch; (5) adductor longus; (6) adductor brevis; (7) adductor magnus; (8) gracilis. Reproduced from Hadzic A. *The New York School of Regional Anesthesia Textbook of Regional Anesthesia and Acute Pain Management.* Figure 34-1. Available at: www.accessanesthsiology.com. Copyright © The McGraw-Hill Companies, Inc. All rights reserved.

(1) Obturator nerve passing through the obturator canal; (2) obturator externus; (3) pectineus; (4) adductor longus; (5) adductor brevis; (6) adductor magnus; (7) medial femoral condyle; (8) femoral nerve; (9) sciatic nerve. Reproduced from Hadzic A. *The New York School of Regional Anesthesia Textbook of Regional Anesthesia and Acute Pain Management.* Figure 34-4. Available at: www.accessanesthsiology.com. Copyright © The McGraw-Hill Companies, Inc. All rights reserved.

Technique using NS:
- Labat's original technique is uncomfortable for the patient, as it requires bone contact and multiple redirecting of the needle, and the needle may enter the pelvis if inserted too far
- The technique described by Choquet is preferred (Figure 144-3), as it is more distal and thus minimizes the risk of vascular injury and of entering the pelvis. However, because the nerve is blocked more distally, the branches to the hip joint might not be blocked
- The insertion of the tendon of the adductor longus muscle on the pubic tubercle is identified, using extreme leg abduction
- Draw a line in the inguinal crease from the pulse of the femoral artery to the tendon of the adductor longus muscle. A 100-mm needle is inserted at the midpoint of this line and directed cephalad at a 30° angle
- The PNS is set at 1.2 mA, 2 Hz, 0.1 millisecond
- After 3–5 cm in an average-sized patient, contractions of the long adductor and gracilis muscles can be detected on the posterior and medial aspect of the thigh. After the current is decreased to less than 0.4 mA and the response is preserved, 5–7 mL of local anesthetic is injected after aspiration
- The needle is then redirected slightly laterally and inserted 0.5–1.5 cm deeper until a response from the adductor magnus muscle is obtained on the posteromedial aspect of the thigh. Again, the current is decreased to less than 0.4 mA and 5–7 mL of local anesthetic can be injected
- If no response is obtained, redirect needle medially and laterally in 5° increments until a response is elicited
- Occasionally, the obturator nerve divides more distally, and both motor responses may be observed with a single stimulation. Both branches can then be blocked with a single injection

FIGURE 144-3. Landmarks for neurostimulation-guided obturator nerve block

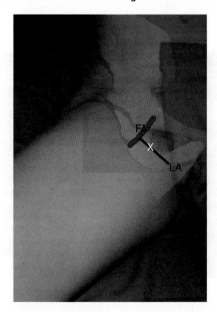

FA, femoral artery; LA, tendon of adductor longus; X, site of needle insertion.

NS-Guided Obturator Nerve Block	
Acceptable responses	Unacceptable responses
• Anterior branch: long adductor and gracilis muscles • Posterior branch: adductor magnus muscle	None

Technique using US (Figure 144-4):
- Patient supine, lower extremity slightly abducted
- A low-frequency (3–5 MHz) ultrasound probe is placed just lateral to the tendon of the adductor longus muscle, perpendicular to the axis of the thigh
- Muscles are identified by scanning between proximal and distal positions. From superficial to deep:
  ‣ Adductor longus, with the pectineus laterally
  ‣ Adductor brevis
  ‣ Adductor magnus (more proximally, the obturator externus muscle)
- The anterior and posterior branches of the obturator nerve have typically a flat and hyperechoic (i.e., white) appearance
- The anterior branch can be found between, superficially, the adductor longus or the pectineus and the adductor brevis
- The posterior branch is found between the adductor brevis and the obturator externus muscle, or, if the probe is positioned more distally, the adductor magnus muscle
- It is useful to track the nerves up and down to confirm that they are indeed continuous structures. Color Doppler can be used to locate the obturator artery or its branches and avoid puncturing it
- The block is often performed using an out-of-plane technique, using a 50 or a 100 mm needle, depending on patient habitus

FIGURE 144-4. Ultrasound view

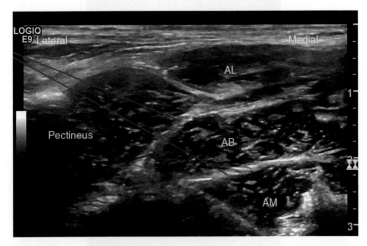

AL, adductor longus muscle; AB, adductor brevis muscle; AM, adductor magnus muscle. The red lines indicate the needle path to block the anterior branch (between pectineus and AB, or between AL and AB more distally) and the posterior branch (between AB and AM). The nerves are often too small to be seen distinctly. Picture courtesy of Dr. Olivier Choquet.

- Careful technique makes the in-plane approach possible, especially if a probe with a small footprint ("hockey stick") is used. A 100 mm needle is often needed to reach the deep branch
- Following aspiration, 5–7 mL of local anesthetic is deposited near both nerves, although some authors recommend injecting 7–10 mL near the superficial branch to block both branches by diffusion

Testing:

Obturator nerve	Adductor power; only about two thirds of the adductors are innervated by the obturator nerve: unless femoral and sciatic blocks associated, adductor power will be reduced but still present

Complications/side effects:
- None reported (besides discomfort on injection), but this block is used relatively infrequently

PEARLS

- The division of the nerve into its two terminal branches happens in the obturator canal in three quarters of cases, but it can happen either above or below the canal
- Skin testing is unreliable for the block of the obturator nerve due to anastomoses between the branches of the femoral nerve and the anterior branch of the obturator nerve
- The absence of contraction of the adductor muscles on the medial aspect of the thigh is the best way to assess the quality of a block of the obturator nerve. However, femoral and sciatic nerves contribute to adduction, and even a complete obturator block will only weaken adduction. Adductor motor strength has been shown to be decreased by about 25% following femoral nerve blockade, and 11% following sciatic nerve blockade

REFERENCES

For references, please visit **www.TheAnesthesiaGuide.com**.

CHAPTER 145
Saphenous Nerve Blocks

Arthur Atchabahian, MD

SAPHENOUS BLOCK COVERAGE

Level of blockade	Coverage distribution (Figure 145-1)
Saphenous nerve at various levels along its route	Anteromedial aspect of the lower leg distal to the level of the blockade, extending more or less down the medial aspect of the ankle and the foot

FIGURE 145-1. Sensory territory of the saphenous nerve block

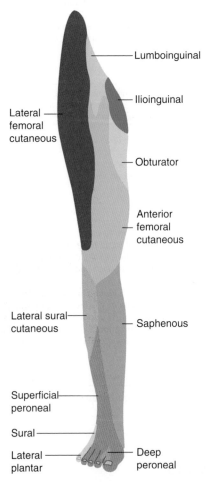

Anatomy (Figure 145-2):

The saphenous nerve is a purely sensory branch of the femoral nerve. It emerges in the inguinal area, travels in the femoral canal, deep to the sartorius muscle, along with the femoral artery and vein and the nerve to the vastus medialis (NVM), which gives branches along the way in the thigh. The saphenous nerve gives off some articular branches to the knee joint. In the lower leg, while traveling in proximity to the greater saphenous vein, it innervates the skin of the anteromedial aspect of the lower leg.

FIGURE 145-2. Anatomy of the saphenous nerve

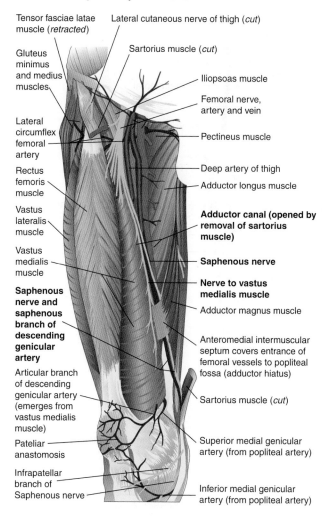

Techniques have been described to block the saphenous nerve at every level along its route (Figure 145-3):

- In the inguinal area (perifemoral)
- In the femoral canal (using a subsartorial or transsartorial approach)
- At the medial femoral condyle
- As a field block below the knee, from the anterior tibial tuberosity to the anterosuperior edge of the muscle belly of the gastrocnemius (Figure 145-4)
- In the lower leg (paravenous approach)
- At the ankle, anterior to the medial malleolus

FIGURE 145-3. Multiple approaches to saphenous nerve blockade

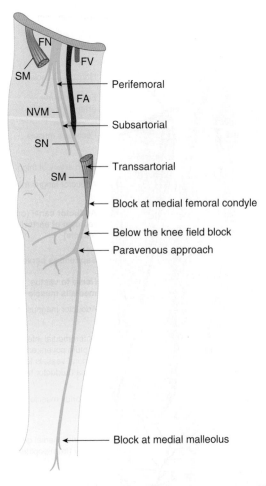

Adapted with permission from Benzon HT, Sharma S, Calimaran A. Comparison of the different approaches to saphenous nerve block. *Anesthesiology*. 2005;102(3):633–638.

FIGURE 145-4. Below-the-knee field block

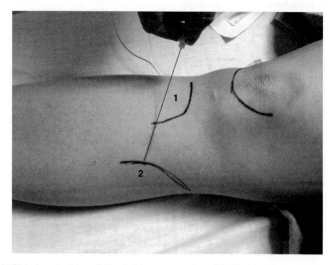

(1) Tibial tuberosity; (2) medial head of the gastrocnemius. A field block is performed by infiltrating the subcutaneous tissues from the tibial tuberosity toward the gastrocnemius. The success rate is poor. Beware not to lacerate the saphenous vein that runs near the anterior aspect of the medial head of the gastrocnemius.

Indications:

Anesthesia or analgesia of the medial aspect of the lower leg or the ankle, in combination with a popliteal sciatic block, for surgery of the lower leg, the ankle, or the foot.

Contraindications:

None specific.

Technique using NS (in the inguinal area):
- Patient positioned supine; locate femoral pulse at the level of the inguinal crease
- Insert a 50-mm stimulating needle about 1 cm lateral to the pulse, aiming 45° cephalad (see chapter 142 for illustration); set nerve stimulator to 1.2 mA, 2 Hz, 0.1 millisecond
- Elicit an isolated response in the vastus medialis. Adjust the needle position to maintain this response while decreasing the current to 0.4 mA
- Inject 5–10 mL of LA
- *NB*: This technique will somewhat reduce the strength of the quadriceps, as the vastus medialis innervation will be blocked
- Differences with femoral nerve block:
  ‣ Elicit medial instead of patellar response
  ‣ Inject *5–10 mL* of local anesthetic instead of 20–30

Tests:

Acceptable responses	Unacceptable responses
Isolated vastus medialis response	Any other, especially rectus femoris ("patellar tendon")

FIGURE 145-5. Probe and needle position for ultrasound-guided saphenous nerve block in the femoral canal (right thigh)

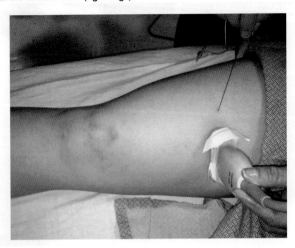

Technique using US:
- In the femoral canal:
  ‣ Using a high-frequency (8–13 MHz) probe positioned perpendicular to the axis of the thigh, follow the femoral vessels from the inguinal area down the thigh (Figure 145-5)
  ‣ The sartorius muscle constitutes the roof of the femoral canal. It is trapezoidal in shape, and is initially slightly lateral to the vessels, and then moves medially, as the femoral canal becomes more medial
  ‣ The NVM and the saphenous nerve accompany the vessels. Typically, the NVM remains lateral, near the quadriceps, while the saphenous nerve, initially next to the NVM, moves to the medial aspect of the femoral canal as it travels distally
  ‣ The nerves are sometimes easily seen on the ultrasound picture, but they are often difficult to identify
  ‣ Around the distal third of the thigh, the vessels dip posteriorly to go through the adductor hiatus to become the popliteal vessels
  ‣ Move the probe back proximally, until the vessels are clearly seen
  ‣ Insert a 100-mm needle anterolateral to the probe, in-plane, aiming to pass in the plane between the sartorius and the quadriceps, to reach the lateral angle of the canal, near the artery (Figure 145-6)
  ‣ Aspirate and inject a few milliliters of LA. The goal is to have LA diffuse to the medial corner of the canal, where the saphenous nerve lies. If necessary, advance the needle in the space opened by the injection, taking care of not entering the artery
  ‣ Typically, 5–7 mL is sufficient
- In the lower leg:
  ‣ Place a venous tourniquet slightly distal to the knee, on the upper part of the lower leg
  ‣ Use the high-frequency probe of the ultrasound to locate the saphenous vein
  ‣ The saphenous nerve lies typically in close proximity, but can be lateral or medial to the vein. If a structure that resembles a nerve is seen, it should be followed up and down to ensure that it is indeed the saphenous nerve. Infiltrate around the nerve, in-plane or out of plane, with 5–7 mL

FIGURE 145-6. US view for ultrasound-guided saphenous nerve block in the femoral canal

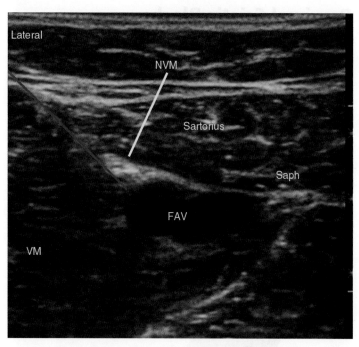

VM, vastus medialis (quadriceps); NVM, nerve to vastus medialis (branch of femoral nerve); FAV, femoral artery and vein; Saph, saphenous nerve. The initial needle approach (from the lateral side) is in red. Once the needle is close to the artery, aspirate, and then inject a few milliliters of local anesthetic. The goal is to have the local anesthetic solution spread to the medial corner of the femoral canal, near the saphenous nerve.

Testing:

Anteromedial aspect of the lower leg.

Complications/side effects:

None specific.

PEARLS

- The cutaneous territory of the saphenous nerve may extend typically down to the base of the first metatarsal. Only in some cases does it reach the medial border of the hallux

CHAPTER 146
Proximal Sciatic Blocks

Arthur Atchabahian, MD

PROXIMAL SCIATIC BLOCK COVERAGE DISTRIBUTION

Level of blockade	Coverage distribution (Figures 146-1 and 140-1)
Posterior cutaneous nerve of the thigh (variable success)	Skin of posterior thigh
Sciatic nerve	Hamstring muscles, posterior aspect of femur Lower leg (motor and sensory) except for skin on medial aspect (saphenous, branch of femoral nerve)

FIGURE 146-1. Sensory innervation provided by the branches of the sciatic nerve

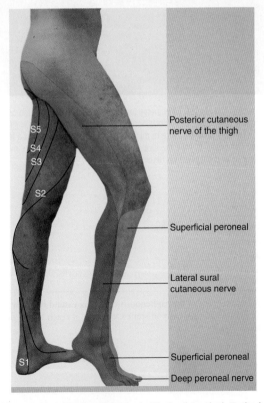

Anatomy (Figure 146-2):

- The sacral plexus is formed by part of the anterior ramus of L4, which with L5 forms the lumbosacral trunk, and S1 to S3
- The roots converge toward the greater sciatic foramen in a triangular sheet to form the sciatic nerve anterior to the piriformis muscle
- The premature division of the nerve in the pelvis or the proximal part of the thigh is fairly common. In the case of a division in the pelvis, the two contingents of the sciatic nerve have different relationships with the piriformis muscle (in most cases, perforation of the piriformis muscle by the common peroneal nerve)
- The posterior cutaneous nerve of the thigh (PCNT) is separate from the sciatic nerve at this level. The more distal the sciatic block, the less constant the block of the PCNT:
  - Parasacral > classic > subgluteal ≈ anterior

Indications:

Anesthesia or analgesia for surgery on the lower extremity, usually in conjunction with a lumbar plexus block (femoral nerve block or psoas compartment block).

FIGURE 146-2. Anatomy of the proximal sciatic nerve

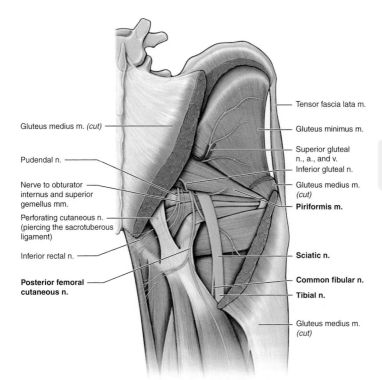

Reproduced with permission from Morton D, Albertine K, Foreman KB. *Gross Anatomy: The Big Picture.* New York: McGraw-Hill; 2011. Figure 35-2B. Copyright © The McGraw-Hill Companies, Inc. All rights reserved.

FIGURE 146-3. Landmarks for classic, parasacral, and subgluteal approaches

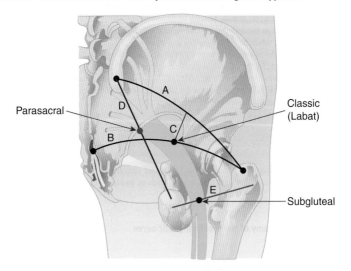

Contraindications:

Depending on the approach used, sciatic blocks are more or less deep; for deep approaches (anterior, parasacral), coagulopathy or anticoagulation is a relative contraindication.

Techniques using NS:

- Classic (Labat) approach (Figure 146-3):
  ▸ Patient prone or in lateral decubitus
  ▸ Draw line A from posterior superior iliac spine (PSIS) to greater trochanter (GT)
  ▸ Draw line B from sacral hiatus (SH) to GT
  ▸ Measure the middle of line A and drop a perpendicular C
  ▸ The intersection of lines B and C is the needle insertion point
  ▸ After prepping and local anesthesia, a 100 mm needle is inserted perpendicular to the skin of the buttock, setting the PNS at 1.4 mA, 2 Hz, 0.1 millisecond
  ▸ Once a hamstring, tibial, or peroneal response is obtained, adjust needle position while decreasing current. If a response is still present at 0.4 mA, aspirate and then inject the local anesthetic (typically 20–30 mL) in a fractionated fashion
  ▸ If no response is obtained on the first pass, the needle is redirected first laterally, and only then medially, in a fan-like fashion
  ▸ Avoid aiming medially, as the vascular bundle lies medial to the sciatic nerve
- Parasacral (Mansour) approach (Figure 146-3):
  ▸ The parasacral block is actually a block of the sacral plexus, under the piriformis muscle
  ▸ Patient prone or in lateral decubitus
  ▸ Draw line D from PSIS to ischial tuberosity (IT), "the bone one sits on."
  ▸ The point on line D 6 cm from the PSIS is the needle insertion point
  ▸ After prepping and local anesthesia, a 100 mm needle is inserted perpendicular to the skin of the buttock, setting the PNS at 1.4 mA, 2 Hz, 0.1 millisecond
  ▸ Once a hamstring, tibial, or peroneal response is obtained, adjust needle position while decreasing current. If a response is still present at 0.4 mA, aspirate and then inject the local anesthetic (typically 20–30 mL) in a fractionated fashion
  ▸ It is preferable to aim slightly medial initially, which can lead to bone contact, and then walk off laterally, as too lateral an aim can lead to needle entry into the pelvis through the greater sciatic foramen

- Subgluteal (Raj) approach (Figures 146-3 and 146-4):
  ‣ This block can be performed with the patient prone or in lateral decubitus, but the typical fashion is with the patient supine, the lower leg elevated so that hip and knee are flexed 90°
  ‣ A line E is drawn between GT and IT
  ‣ The middle point of this line is the needle insertion point
  ‣ After prepping and local anesthesia, a 50 or 100 mm needle, depending on the patient's habitus, is inserted perpendicular to the skin of the buttock, setting the PNS at 1.4 mA, 2 Hz, 0.1 millisecond
  ‣ Once a tibial or peroneal response is obtained, adjust needle position while decreasing current. If a response is still present at 0.4 mA, aspirate and then inject the local anesthetic (typically 20–30 mL) in a fractionated fashion
  ‣ If no response is obtained on the first pass, the needle is redirected first laterally, and only then medially, in a fan-like fashion
  ‣ Avoid aiming medially, as the vascular bundle lies medial to the sciatic nerve
  ‣ There have been claims that the obturator nerve might be blocked as well, but this is rare at best

FIGURE 146-4. Landmarks and needle placement for subgluteal (Raj) approach

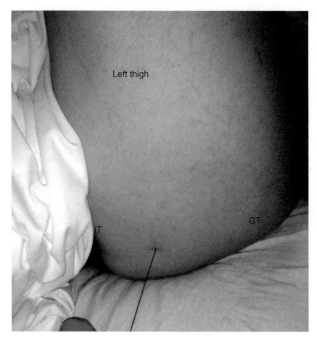

With the patient supine, the leg is raised with hip and knee flexed. The needle insertion point is about halfway between ischial tuberosity (IT) and greater trochanter (GT).

- Anterior (Beck) approach (Figure 146-5):
  ‣ Patient supine
  ‣ A line F is drawn from anterior superior iliac spine (ASIS) to pubic tubercle (PT)
  ‣ A line G parallel to F is drawn through the GT
  ‣ F is divided in thirds, and a perpendicular H is dropped from the medial third
  ‣ The intersection between G and H is the needle insertion point

- An alternative approach (Souron and Delaunay) is to mark the femoral pulse in the inguinal crease, and to measure 6 cm in the direction of the patella, and then 2 cm lateral: that is the needle insertion point
- After prepping and local anesthesia, a 100 or 150 mm needle, depending on the patient's habitus, is inserted perpendicular to the skin of the buttock, setting the PNS at 1.4 mA, 2 Hz, 0.1 millisecond
- Typically, bone will be contacted (the lesser trochanter). The needle will then be retracted by 1–2 cm and walked off the bone medially. Once bone contact is lost, the sciatic nerve is typically contacted 2–3 cm deeper
- Once a tibial or peroneal response is obtained, adjust needle position while decreasing current. If a response is still present at 0.4 mA, aspirate and then inject the local anesthetic (typically 20–30 mL) in a fractionated fashion
- If no response is obtained on the first pass, the maneuver is repeated with an assistant putting the lower extremity in internal rotation
- If still unsuccessful, repeat with the extremity in external rotation
- The last resort is to aim slightly more caudad, or to use a the needle slightly more medial needle insertion point, as the sciatic nerve probably lies posterior to the femur

FIGURE 146-5. Landmarks for anterior approach to the sciatic nerve block

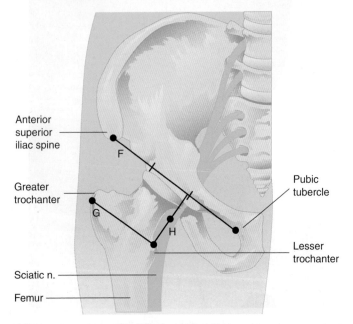

Reproduced with permission from Miller RD, ed. *Miller's Anesthesia*. 6th ed. New York: Churchill Livingstone; 2005:1701. © Elsevier.

NS-Guided Proximal Sciatic Nerve Block

Acceptable responses	Unacceptable responses
Tibial: foot plantar flexion, inversion Peroneal: dorsiflexion, eversion Hamstrings for parasacral or classic blocks	Hamstrings for subgluteal, anterior, or lateral blocks (as direct stimulation of muscular branches cannot be excluded)

Technique using US:

- Subgluteal approach (Figure 146-6):
  ‣ Patient prone or in lateral decubitus
  ‣ Place a high-frequency (8–13 MHz) probe if the patient is thin, or a low-frequency probe (3–5 MHz) if the patient is obese, on a point between the GT and the IT, parallel to the gluteal fold
  ‣ The sciatic nerve can be seen as a flat, ovoid structure between the gluteus maximus and an underlying muscle (usually the quadratus femoris, but variable according to the exact level at which the block is performed)
  ‣ The nerve can be approached either in-plane (preferred for single-injection techniques), using a 100 mm needle, or out-of-plane, usually aiming cephalad, to insert a perineural catheter, with a 50 or 100 mm needle, depending on patient habitus
- Anterior approach (Van der Beek) (Figure 146-7):
  ‣ This is an advanced block, as the nerve is deep and not easily visualized in most patients
  ‣ Patient supine, legs slightly abducted
  ‣ Place a low-frequency (3–5 MHz) curved probe perpendicular to the axis of the thigh, 5–10 cm distal to the inguinal crease

FIGURE 146-6. Typical aspect of the sciatic nerve with the US-guided subgluteal approach

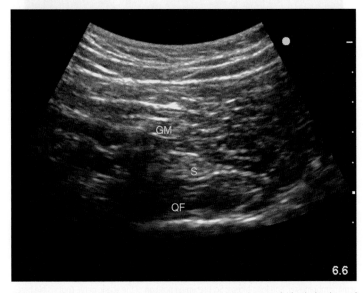

GM, gluteus maximus; S, sciatic nerve; QF, quadratus femoris muscle. Note the lenticular shape of the nerve at that level. It often appears triangular when scanned more distally.

FIGURE 146-7. Probe placement and typical aspect of the sciatic nerve with the US-guided anterior approach

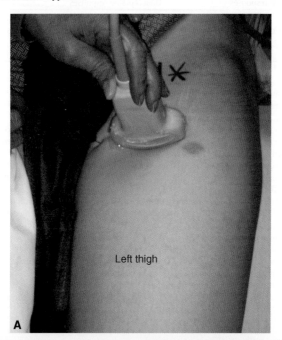

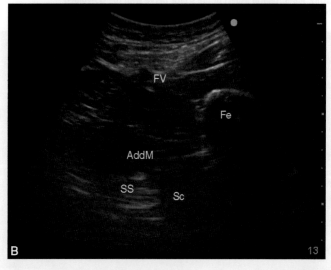

(A) Probe placement, about 6 cm distal to the femoral pulse in the inguinal crease. The needle is inserted from the medial side. (B) Ultrasound view (low-frequency probe, depth 13 cm). FV: femoral vessels; Fe: femur; AddM: adductor magnus muscle; SS: tendons of the semitendinosus, semimembranosus, and long biceps; Sc: presumed position of the sciatic nerve (not visible here).

- ▸ The femoral vessels (much smaller than when performing a FNB, as the scale is different) and the femur can easily be visualized
- ▸ Two different techniques can be used to locate the sciatic nerve:
  - ▪ Drawing an imaginary isosceles triangle with the femur as its apex, the femoral vessels as one corner, the sciatic nerve will lie at the other corner
  - ▪ Locating the small triangular or round muscle mass deep to the adductor magnus. This mass is composed of the semitendinosus, semimembranosus, and the long head of the biceps femoris. The sciatic nerve will lie just lateral to this muscle mass
- ▸ Once the approximate location of the sciatic nerve is determined, a stimulating 100 or 150 mm needle is inserted (after prepping and local anesthesia):
  - ▪ The needle is best visualized when inserted from the medial aspect of the thigh, at a distance from the probe that approximates the depth of the nerve on the screen, as the needle will be perpendicular to the ultrasound beam
  - ▪ Alternatively, the needle can be inserted medial to the US probe
- ▸ The PNS is set at 1.5 mA, 2 Hz, 0.1 millisecond. When a muscle response distal to the knee is elicited, decrease current to 1 mA. If the response is still present, aspirate, and then inject local anesthetic (20–30 mL) in a fractionated fashion
- ▸ Often, the nerve will become more clearly apparent after injection, as it separates from surrounding connective tissue

Testing:

Proximal sciatic	Hamstring muscles: knee flexion strength
Posterior cutaneous nerve of the thigh	Posterior skin of thigh
Tibial nerve	Motor: plantar flexion ("push on the gas pedal") Sensory: posterior aspect of lower leg (medial sural), sole of foot (medial and lateral plantar)
Peroneal nerve	Motor: dorsiflexion Sensory: lateral aspect of lower leg (lateral sural), dorsal aspect of foot (superficial peroneal), first web space (deep peroneal)

Complications/side effects:
- The parasacral approach:
  - ▸ Can theoretically lead to pelvic needle penetration
  - ▸ Usually causes hypoesthesia of the ipsilateral half of the genitalia by blocking the pudendal nerve
- Deep blocks (parasacral, anterior especially, but all sciatic blocks are deep in obese patients) can lead to unrecognized bleeding and hematoma formation

PEARLS

- Complete surgical block can take up to 45 minutes, as the sciatic nerve is large
- Depending on the level of the block, the PCNT might not be blocked. This is usually not a major issue, even when a thigh tourniquet is used, as most of the tourniquet pain is caused by muscle ischemia rather than skin compression
- The cutaneous territory of the PCNT ends most often at the top of the popliteal fossa; however, it sometimes goes down to just above the knee joint, or even down to the heel
- Warn the patient of possible genitalia hypoesthesia with the parasacral approach
- The sacral plexus lies posteriorly on the piriformis muscle, and is covered anteriorly by the fascia of this muscle, making up the pelvic fascia that separates the sacral plexus from the pelvic contents. Thus, with a parasacral sciatic block, the spread of local anesthetic to the obturator nerve is anatomically unlikely
- Take into account total local anesthetic dose when combining sciatic and lumbar plexus blocks

CHAPTER 147
Popliteal Blocks

Arthur Atchabahian, MD

POPLITEAL BLOCK COVERAGE

Level of blockade	Coverage distribution (Figure 147-1 and chapter 140)
Sciatic nerve in the popliteal fossa Alternatively, the tibial or peroneal nerve can be blocked independently	Tibial nerve: • Motor: gastrocnemius and soleus (plantar flexion and inversion) • Sensory: posterior aspect of lower leg • Peroneal nerve: • Motor: anteromedial muscles of the lower leg (dorsiflexion and eversion) • Sensory: lateral aspect of lower leg • Sciatic nerve: combination of both

FIGURE 147-1. Coverage distribution of the popliteal block

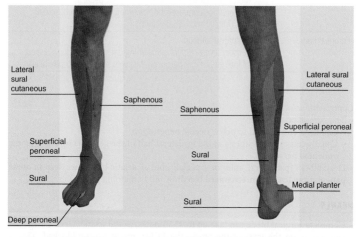

Anatomy (Figure 147-2):

The sciatic nerve divides into tibial and peroneal nerves at a variable level, typically 7–10 cm above the flexion crease, but occasionally as high as the buttock, or below the knee joint.

It emerges in the popliteal fossa between the biceps femoris laterally, and the semi-tendinosus/semimembranosus medially.

FIGURE 147-2. Anatomy of the popliteal fossa

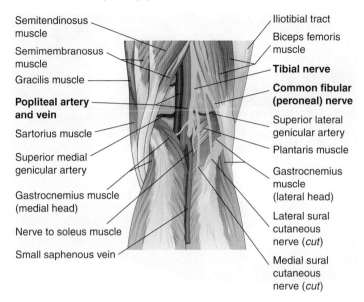

Semitendinosus muscle

Semimembranosus muscle

Gracilis muscle

Popliteal artery and vein

Sartorius muscle

Superior medial genicular artery

Gastrocnemius muscle (medial head)

Nerve to soleus muscle

Small saphenous vein

Iliotibial tract

Biceps femoris muscle

Tibial nerve

Common fibular (peroneal) nerve

Superior lateral genicular artery

Plantaris muscle

Gastrocnemius muscle (lateral head)

Lateral sural cutaneous nerve (*cut*)

Medial sural cutaneous nerve (*cut*)

Indications:
- Surgery of the lower leg, ankle, and foot (in combination with a saphenous block if the skin of the anteromedial aspect of the lower leg or the medial aspect of the ankle or foot is involved)
- Isolated tibial nerve block for postoperative analgesia after knee surgery (in combination with a continuous femoral block, and GA/spinal for anesthesia, especially if a thigh tourniquet is to be used)

Contraindications:

None specific.

Technique using NS:
- Posterior approach:
  ‣ Patient prone or in lateral decubitus, lying on the nonoperative side
  ‣ Mark the flexion crease and the muscles on each side (biceps femoris laterally, semitendinosus and semimembranosus medially)
  ‣ Draw a perpendicular extending cephalad, about 1 cm lateral to the center of the flexion crease line. The needle insertion point is 7 cm cephalad to the flexion crease
  ‣ Insert a 50 mm needle aiming 45° cephalad, setting the PNS at 1.2 mA, 2 Hz, 0.1 millisecond, and elicit a response in the tibial or peroneal innervation territory
  ‣ If a tibial response is obtained, adjust needle position while decreasing current. If a response is still present at 0.4 mA, aspirate and then inject one half of the local anesthetic (typically 10–15 mL) in a fractionated fashion, and redirect needle laterally to obtain a peroneal response. In a similar fashion, inject 10–15 mL of local anesthetic
  ‣ If a peroneal response is obtained initially, redirect needle medially after injection
- Lateral approach (Figures 147-4 and 147-5):
  ‣ Patient supine, rolled sheet under thigh to slightly flex the knee (15°)
  ‣ Locate the groove on the lateral aspect of the thigh between vastus lateralis (quadriceps) and biceps femoris

FIGURE 147-3. Landmarks for posterior approach using NS

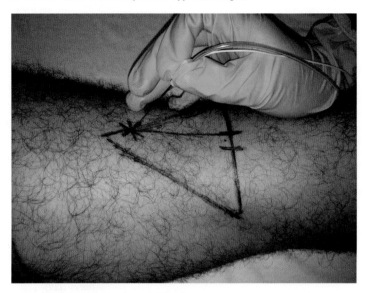

The needle insertion point is 7 cm cephalad to the flexion crease, about 1 cm lateral to the center of the flexion crease line.

FIGURE 147-4. Anatomy for lateral approach using NS

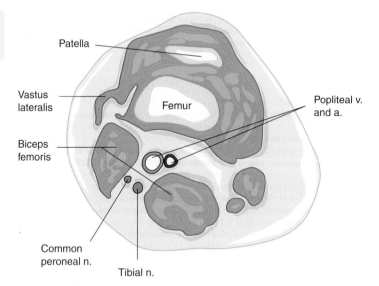

Reproduced with permission from Miller RD, ed. *Miller's Anesthesia*. 6th ed. New York: Churchill Livingstone; 2005:1702. © Elsevier.

FIGURE 147-5. Landmarks for lateral approach using NS

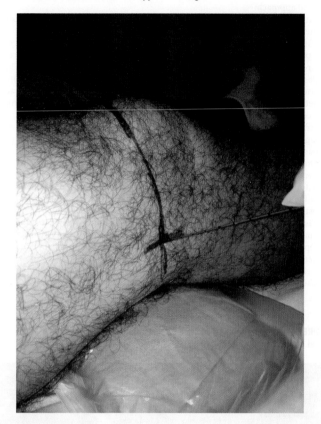

- ‣ Draw a line extending laterally from the proximal pole of the patella
- ‣ After local anesthesia, insert 100 mm needle with a 30° angle toward the floor, perpendicular to the axis of the thigh, setting the PNS at 1.2 mA, 2 Hz, 0.1 millisecond
- ‣ If a tibial response is obtained, adjust needle position while decreasing current. If a response is still present at 0.4 mA, aspirate, and then inject one half of the local anesthetic (typically 10–15 mL) in a fractionated fashion, and redirect needle laterally (i.e., at a sharper angle toward the floor) to obtain a peroneal response. In a similar fashion, inject 10–15 mL of local anesthetic
- ‣ If a peroneal response is obtained initially, redirect needle medially after injection

NS-Guided Popliteal Block	
Acceptable responses	Unacceptable responses
Tibial nerve: plantar flexion, inversion	None
Peroneal nerve: dorsiflexion, eversion	

Technique using US:
- Lateral approach:
  ‣ Patient prone or in lateral decubitus; occasionally supine with leg elevated so that the popliteal fossa is at least 15 cm from the bed:
    ▪ If patient in lateral decubitus, it is more comfortable to stand in front of the patient, facing the patella, with the US machine on the other side, in order to rest one's wrist on the patient's thigh while performing the block (Figure 147-6)
  ‣ Position high-frequency (8–13 MHz) probe in the joint crease. Locate popliteal artery and vein. The tibial nerve is typically superficial and lateral to the artery, heterogeneous with dark fascicles in white connective tissue. Tilting the probe in a cephalad direction can help to better visualize the nerve
  ‣ Follow the tibial nerve cephalad (add gel) until the peroneal nerve is seen merging with the tibial nerve (Figures 147-6 and 147-7). The peroneal nerve typically has one large fascicle (dark)
  ‣ Once the nerves have merged, going further cephalad will only make the sciatic nerve deeper
  ‣ Estimate depth of the nerve using the scale on the screen. Prep the lateral aspect of the thigh, infiltrate with local anesthetic, and then insert a 100 mm needle in-plane at approximately the same depth as the nerve
  ‣ Visualize the needle under US, advance needle, not aiming straight at the nerve, but just deep to the nerve, aspirate, and inject local anesthetic. Visualize spread; reposition needle as needed to obtain a "donut" of local anesthetic around the nerve
  ‣ Keep vessels in sight to avoid puncturing them
  ‣ Usually 15–20 mL of solution is sufficient (Figure 147-8)

FIGURE 147-6. Probe position and needle insertion site for US-guided lateral approach

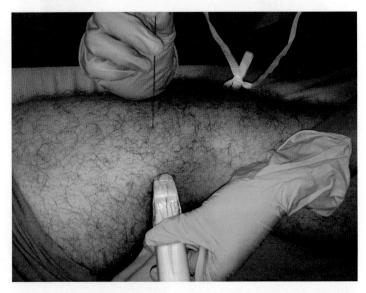

The patient is in lateral decubitus, the side to be blocked up. The anesthesiologist stands on the side of the patella.

FIGURE 147-7. Tibial and peroneal nerves low in the popliteal fossa

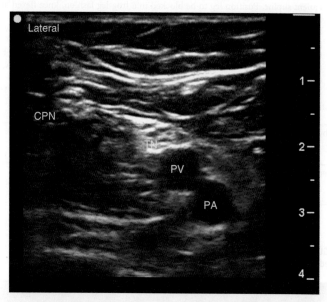

TN, tibial nerve; CPN, common peroneal nerve; PV, popliteal vein; PA, popliteal artery. Picture courtesy of Dr. Eryk Eisenberg.

FIGURE 147-8. Merged tibial and peroneal nerves constituting the sciatic nerve in a more cephalad position

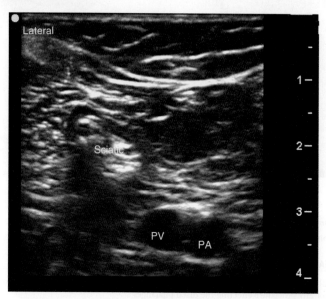

Sciatic, sciatic nerve; PV, popliteal vein; PA, popliteal artery. Picture courtesy of Dr. Eryk Eisenberg.

- Medial approach (Figure 147-9):
  ▸ Patient supine. Position leg to be blocked in a frog-leg fashion, knee flexed and sole of foot against contralateral calf
  ▸ Similarly, visualize tibial nerve at the crease level; track it up until merged with peroneal nerve
  ▸ Insert needle in-plane from medial aspect of thigh. The distance to reach the nerve is longer, making this approach slightly more difficult than the lateral approach. Avoid this approach in very obese patients
  ▸ Similarly, local anesthetic is injected until spread is visualized around the nerve

Testing of the popliteal block:

Tibial nerve	Motor: plantar flexion ("push on the gas pedal") Sensory: posterior aspect of lower leg (medial sural), sole of foot (medial and lateral plantar)
Peroneal nerve	Motor: dorsiflexion Sensory: lateral aspect of lower leg (lateral sural), dorsal aspect of foot (superficial peroneal), first web space (deep peroneal)

FIGURE 147-9. Probe position and needle insertion site for US-guided medial approach

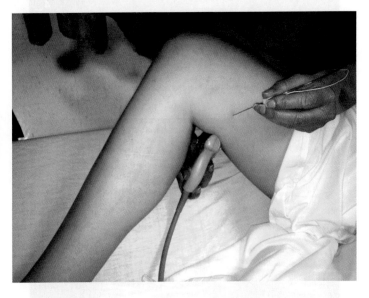

Complications/side effects:

None specific.

PEARLS

- Blocking the tibial nerve is essential not only for bone surgery of the foot but also for any procedure affecting the distal phalanges

CHAPTER 148
Ankle Block

Arthur Atchabahian, MD

ANKLE BLOCK COVERAGE

Level of blockade	Coverage distribution
Terminal branches of sciatic nerve at the level of the ankle + saphenous nerve (a branch of the femoral nerve)	Foot below the ankle (Figures 140-1 and 148-1)

FIGURE 148-1. Distribution of blockade

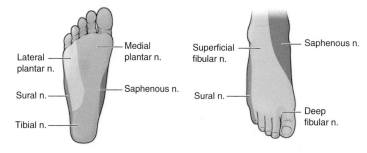

Neurovascular supply cutaneous innervation of the right foot, showing the plantar (A) and dorsal (B) surfaces. Lateral and medial plantar Nn. are terminal branches of the tibial nerve. Reproduced from Morton D, ed. *Gross Anatomy: The Big Picture.* Figure 38-3, p. 447. McGraw-Hill. Copyright © The McGraw-Hill Companies, Inc. All rights reserved.

Indications:
- Any surgery on the foot (but consider tourniquet use; ideally no thigh tourniquet; Esmarch band above the ankle OK if not too >1 hour)
- *Not* effective for ankle surgery (e.g., popliteal + saphenous block should be used, although this would not cover a thigh tourniquet; in that case, use sciatic + femoral, or a spinal if blocks are only for postoperative pain)

Contraindications:
- Infection/rash on injection site
- Severe peripheral vascular disease with risk of local necrosis
- Three of the five blocks are subcutaneous infiltrations, and two are in close proximity to blood vessels, with a risk of local anesthetic toxicity; prefer ropivacaine to bupivacaine; avoid bilateral blocks because of the increased total dose

Technique using landmarks:
- Blocks done just proximal to the level of the malleoli, above the ankle joint (Figure 148-2):
  - Deep peroneal nerve block (Figure 148-3):
    - Located next to the DP pulse and/or the extensor hallucis longus tendon; insert needle straight down to the bone, pull back 3–4 mm, aspirate, and infiltrate with 5–7 mL of LA

FIGURE 148-2. Schematic position of the nerves to be blocked at the level of the right ankle

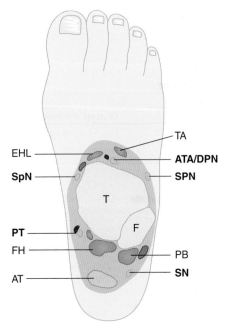

T, tibia; F, fibula; EHL, extensor hallucis longus tendon; ATA/DPN, anterior tibial artery/deep peroneal nerve; SPN, superficial peroneal nerve; PB, peroneus brevis tendon; SN, sural nerve; AT, Achilles tendon; FH, flexor hallucis tendon; PT, posterior tibial nerve and artery; SpN, saphenous nerve (and vein); TA, tibialis anterior tendon.

- Superficial peroneal nerve block (Figure 148-3):
  - Create a skin wheal from the needle insertion point for the deep peroneal block to the lateral malleolus (5–7 mL)
- Saphenous nerve block (Figure 148-3):
  - Create a skin wheal from the needle insertion point for the deep peroneal block to the medial malleolus (5–7 mL)
- Posterior tibial nerve block (Figure 148-4):
  - Locate PT pulse in the posterior aspect of the medial malleolus; if not felt, aim for the area of the tendon "pulley" behind the malleolus. Insert needle in a posterior to anterior fashion, contact bone, pull back 2–3 mm, and infiltrate with 7–10 mL
- Sural nerve block (Figure 148-4):
  - Create a skin wheal from the Achilles tendon to the lateral malleolus (5–7 mL)

FIGURE 148-3. Deep peroneal, superficial peroneal, and saphenous nerve blocks

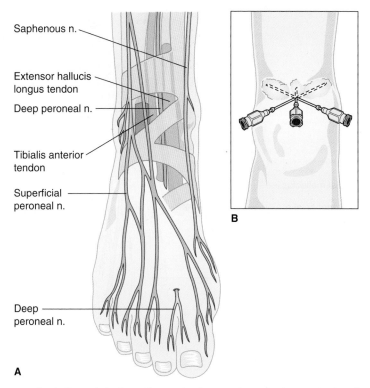

Saphenous n.

Extensor hallucis longus tendon

Deep peroneal n.

Tibialis anterior tendon

Superficial peroneal n.

Deep peroneal n.

B

A

Reproduced with permission from Miller RD, ed. *Miller's Anesthesia*. 6th ed. New York: Churchill Livingstone; 2005:1704. © Elsevier.

Technique using US:

The deep peroneal and posterior tibial blocks can be performed using ultrasound guidance.
- Deep peroneal nerve block:
  ‣ Located near the DP artery (Figure 148-5)
- Posterior tibial nerve block:
  ‣ Located near the PT artery (Figure 148-6)

FIGURE 148-4. Posterior tibial and sural nerve blocks

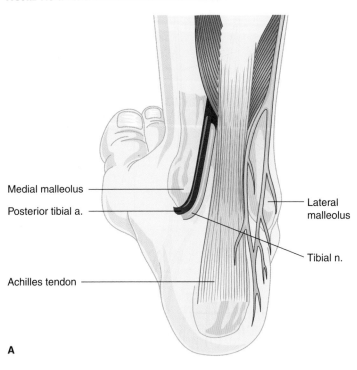

Medial malleolus

Posterior tibial a.

Achilles tendon

Lateral malleolus

Tibial n.

A

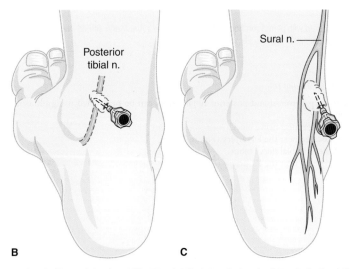

Posterior tibial n.

Sural n.

B

C

FIGURE 148-5. Ultrasound-guided deep peroneal nerve block

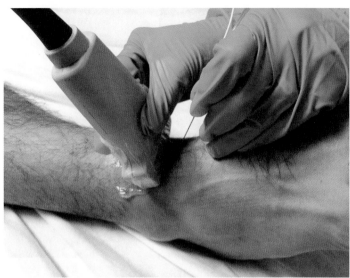

A

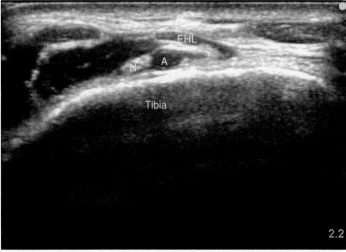

B

(A) Probe placement, out-of-plane needle insertion; (B) ultrasound image. N, deep peroneal nerve; A, deep peroneal artery; EHL, tendon of extensor hallucis longus.

FIGURE 148-6. Ultrasound-guided posterior tibial nerve block

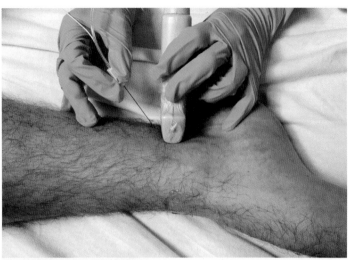

A

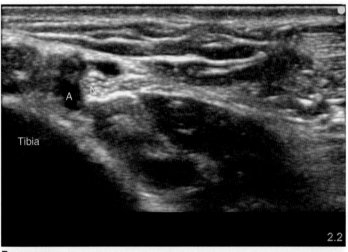

B

(A) Probe placement, out-of-plane needle insertion; (B) ultrasound image. N, posterior tibial nerve; A, posterior tibial artery.

Testing of an Ankle Block	
Deep peroneal nerve block	Pinch first web space
Superficial peroneal nerve block	Pinch pulp of great toe
Saphenous nerve block	Pinch skin of medial dorsum of foot
Posterior tibial nerve block	Pinch pulp of fifth toe
Sural nerve block	Pinch skin of lateral aspect of foot

Complications/side effects:

Risk of local anesthetic toxicity.

PEARLS

- The deep blocks, especially the PT, are the most difficult
- The territory of cutaneous innervation of the sural nerve is classically limited to the lateral edge of the fifth ray; actually, it often extends medially to the lateral edge of the third ray of the dorsum of the foot

CHAPTER 149
Thoracic Paravertebral Blocks

Jan Boublik, MD, PhD

INDICATIONS

Surgical procedure	Levels to be blocked
Thoracotomy	T4–T9
Thoracoscopy	T4–T9
Rib fractures	Level of fracture with one level above and below
Cardiac surgery	T2–T6 bilaterally
Mastectomy, breast surgery	T2–T6
Mastectomy with axillary dissection	T1–T6 with superficial cervical plexus block
Breast biopsy	Level of lesion with one level above and below
Inguinal hernia repair	T10–L2
Umbilical hernia repair	T9–T11 bilaterally
Incisional hernia repair	According to level of repair
Ileostomy closure	T8–T12
Nephrectomy	T8–T12
Cholecystectomy	T6–T10
Appendectomy	T10–T12
Adjunct for shoulder surgery (subdeltoid incision)	T1–T2
Adjunct for hip surgery	T11–T12 with lumbar plexus block ± parasacral sciatic block
Bone marrow aspiration	T11–L2 bilaterally
Iliac crest bone harvesting	T11–L1

FIGURE 149-1. Landmarks for thoracic paravertebral blocks

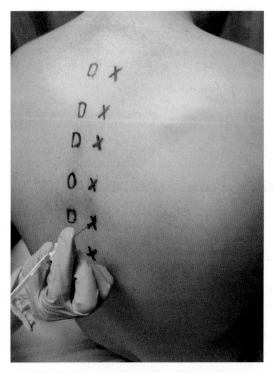

The rectangles are drawn over the spinous processes, the X 2.5 cm lateral, overlying the transverse process of the vertebra one level down from the spinous process.

Contraindications	
Absolute	Patient refusal
	Skin infections/empyema/paravertebral tumor at injection site
	Local anesthetic allergy
	Severe hemodynamic instability
Relative	Coagulopathy
	Severe chest deformity
	Prior thoracotomy

Advantages of Paravertebral Block

- Dense sensory, motor, and sympathetic nerve block (*"complete" abolition of evoked potentials at the level of the paravertebral injection in 100% of patients*, rare with epidural)
- Unilateral or bilateral segmental block
- Wide application for various surgical procedures
- Decreased stress response to surgery
- Postoperative analgesia similar or better than epidural
- Low postoperative opioid requirements

- Infrequent opioid-related side effects (nausea, vomiting, sedation)
- Hemodynamic stability
- Preservation of pulmonary function
- Preservation of lower-extremity motor strength
- Preservation of bladder function
- Enhanced perioperative efficiency

Complications/Side Effects

Complication	Reported incidence (%)
Block failure (no surgical anesthesia)	6.1 (multiple injections) to 10.7 (single injection)
Inadvertent vascular puncture	3.8–6.8
Hypotension	4.0–5.0 (usually mild)
Localized hematoma	2.4
Localized pain	1.3
Pleural puncture	0.8–0.9
Pneumothorax	0.3–0.5
Epidural spread	1.0–1.1
Pulmonary hemorrhage Intrathecal spread Dural puncture headache Brachial plexus block Horner syndrome Local anesthetic toxicity Nerve injury Infection	Case reports

Local anesthetic regimen for paravertebral nerve blocks

- Bupivacaine 0.25–0.5% and ropivacaine 0.2–0.5% most frequently used agents; duration of analgesia is similar to brachial plexus anesthesia
- Epinephrine frequently added to indicate intravascular injection; reduce the peak local anesthetic blood level (25% reduction) and to improve analgesia

Single-level injection	Adults: 10–20 mL local anesthetic (e.g., 0.5% ropivacaine with epinephrine 1:400,000) Children: 0.5 mL/kg up to 20 mL local anesthetic
Multiple-level injections	3–5 mL local anesthetic per segment
Continuous infusion	0.1–0.2 mL/kg/h (8–10 mL/h for standard adult) local anesthetic (e.g., 0.2% ropivacaine, 0.06% bupivacaine, 0.25% lidocaine)

ANATOMY (SEE FIGURES 149-2, 149-6, AND 149-7)

FIGURE 149-2. Figure showing orientation of the ultrasound transducer

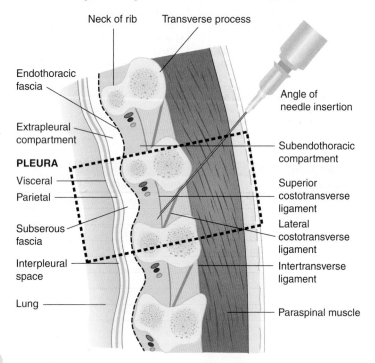

The injection has to be made in the subendothoracic compartment, between the superior costotransverse ligament and the endothoracic fascia (see on left side of picture). The black box shows the angle and direction of the ultrasound beam. Reproduced with permission from Hadzic A. *The New York School of Regional Anesthesia Textbook of Regional Anesthesia and Acute Pain Management.* New York: McGraw-Hill; 2006. Figure 43-3. Copyright © The McGraw-Hill Companies, Inc. All rights reserved.

- Wedge-shaped space:
  - Anterolateral border: parietal pleura; medial: vertebral body/intervertebral disc
  - Posterior border: transverse process of vertebra, costotransverse ligament
- Two fascias:
  - Endothoracic fascia: fibroelastic, between superior costotransverse ligament (posterior) and parietal pleura anteriorly; endothoracic fascia thus divides the thoracic paravertebral space (TPVS) into two potential fascial compartments:
    - The anterior *extrapleural paravertebral compartment*
    - The posterior *subendothoracic paravertebral compartment*
  - Subserous fascia: layer of loose areolar connective tissue
- Two potential compartments in TPVS:
  - anterior/extrapleural
  - posterior/subendothoracic
- Medial communication with epidural space, lateral with intercostal space, cranial extension (controversial whether this is a continuous space)
- Because of the sharp angulation of the spinous processes in the thoracic area, the spinous process is at the same level as the transverse process of the underlying vertebra

Mechanism of Block and Distribution of Anesthesia

- Ipsilateral somatic and sympathetic block (direct effect)
- Often bilateral and more extensive than level injected (epidural spread in about 70% of patients, more common with medial direction of needle or large volume injected)
- Single-level paravertebral injection of 10–15 mL of local anesthetic in adults and 0.5 mL/kg in children; **on average sensory block of four to five dermatomes, *independent of age, height, weight, or gender*; sympathetic block on average eight dermatomes**
- *Solution spread more caudad than cephalad.* Multilevel, small volume preferable to single-level, large-volume injection. (Theoretical) potential advantage of a single-needle insertion reduction in the incidence of side effects such as pleural puncture or pneumothorax versus multiple injections (small volume of local anesthetic at each level injected, theoretical advantage of more extensive and complete anesthesia of the desired dermatomes)

Block Techniques

General aspects
- Patient sitting—better surface anatomy and more comfortable
- 22G blunt-tip needle (single shot) or epidural set with 18G Tuohy needle (catheter technique)
- Mark skin 2.5 cm lateral to spinous process (needle insertion site)
- Routine monitoring, supplemental O_2, sedation 2–3 mg midazolam, and 50–100 µg fentanyl

Thoracic technique using landmarks (Figure 149-1)
- **LOR technique**
  1. Skin and underlying tissues infiltrated with 1% lidocaine
  2. Insert needle perpendicular to skin plane
  3. Depth of transverse process varies (3–4 cm) with level of needle insertion (deepest T1 and lumbar). To avoid pleural puncture, do not insert needle deeper than 4 cm in an average-sized patient
  4. No bone contact; needle is between two transverse processes; back to skin level and angle cephalad (first) or caudad about 10° to same maximal depth
  5. If still no bone contact, repeat process 0.5 cm deeper
  6. Once bone encountered, walk needle off **caudad** and advance gradually until LOR encountered (*much more subtle than epidural space!*); loss best appreciated with glass syringe filled with air
- **Predetermined distance technique**
  ‣ 1–5. See above
  ‣ Advance needle 1 cm (*no more than 1.5 cm!*) past depth of bone contact

Tips/pearls
- "Loss of resistance" as needle traverses the **superior costotransverse ligament (SCL)**, usually within 1.5–2 cm from the transverse process. *Occasionally a subtle pop* is felt; unlike epidural space location, the loss of resistance felt as the needle enters the TPVS is subjective and indefinite. *Usually change of resistance* rather than a definite give
- Bone contact deep to the transverse process → likely rib; further advancement of needle can result in pleural puncture and pneumothorax. Risk can be minimized when needle redirected caudally after initial bony contact
- If the rib unintentionally contacted first, caudal redirection will bring the block needle in contact with the transverse process at a shallower depth

(continued)

Block Techniques (*continued*)

Technique using ultrasound
- *Basics*
  - ▸ Perform preview scan first
  - ▸ Axis for the scan or the intervention matter of individual preference and experience. Transverse approach has a higher risk of epidural or intrathecal injection, and theoretically more discomfort given longer needle path compared with approach with traditional technique
  - ▸ Transducer used depends on patient habitus, typically low-frequency (2–5 MHz) probe for sagittal and intermediate (5–8 MHz) for transverse approach
- *Paramedian sagittal oblique technique (Figures 149-3 to 149-5)*
  - ▸ Transducer positioned 2–3 cm lateral to the midline with orientation marker directed cranially
  - ▸ *Tilt transducer aiming slightly lateral* for better visibility of the superior costotransverse ligament (not easily seen), the paravertebral space, and the parietal pleura (PP). See Figures 149-4 and 149-5
  - ▸ Prep and anesthetize skin at insertion site
  - ▸ Position midpoint of transducer midway between two contiguous transverse processes. Block needle inserted in-plane cranially from transducer and aimed craniocaudally. Often challenging to visualize given acute angle needle (**Figures 149-4 and 149-5**)
  - ▸ Advance needle to contact the lower edge of the TP; walk off bone caudally, and then advance a further 1–1.5 cm
  - ▸ Aspirate; inject 3–5 mL NS: turbulence at the level of the injection, forward displacement of the parietal pleura, increased echogenicity of the pleura suggest the tip of the needle is in the TPVS
  - ▸ The calculated dose of local anesthetic is then injected in a fractionated fashion, with frequent aspiration

Tips/pearls
- Local anesthetic spread will be difficult to view because of the overlying bones
- Transverse approaches to thoracic paravertebral space
  - ▸ *Transverse scan of the thoracic paravertebral region (Figures 149-6 and 149-8)*:
    - ▪ Transducer positioned transverse, lateral to the spinous process
    - ▪ Paraspinal muscles clearly delineated, superficial to the transverse process; transverse process (TP) seen as hyperechoic structure, acoustic shadow completely obscures TPVS (Figure 149-6)–lateral to the TP, hyperechoic pleura moves with respiration, "lung sliding sign"
    - ▪ Slide the transducer slightly cranially or caudally for transverse scan of the paravertebral region between two transverse processes
      - ◆ Superior costotransverse ligament (posterior border of the TPVS) visible (not easily seen), blending laterally with the internal intercostal membrane (posterior border of the posterior intercostal space)
  - ▸ *Transverse scan with out-of-plane needle insertion (technique A) (Figure 149-7)*:
    - ▪ Determine depth of transverse process and pleura
    - ▪ Direction of needle insertion similar to TPVB using surface anatomical landmarks (needle visualized only as a hyperechoic [bright] spot; the aim of this approach is to guide the needle to the TP)
    - ▪ Once the TP is contacted, the needle is slightly withdrawn and readvanced by a further 1.5 cm caudally under the transverse process into the TPVS
    - ▪ After negative aspiration, local anesthetic is injected
    - ▪ Observe for widening of the apex of the TPVS and anterior displacement of the pleura. LA may also spread to the posterior intercostal space laterally. Widening of the contiguous paravertebral spaces by the injected local anesthetic can also be visualized on a sagittal scan

(continued)

Block Techniques (continued)

▸ *Transverse scan with in-plane needle insertion (intercostal approach) (technique B)*
  (Figures 149-6, 149-7, and 149-8):
  Advanced technique for experienced practitioners
  Risk of intrathecal and epidural injection!
  ▪ Position transducer as above, and identify ribs and pleura (ask patient to take deep
    breath–visible movement pleura/lung)
  ▪ Rotate probe until oriented immediately over the long axis of the rib. Tilting the probe
    identifies the intercostal muscles deep and inferior to the rib
  ▪ Advance 18G Tuohy needle to contact with the rib **8 cm** lateral to the midline, in-plane at
    the lateral end of the probe
  ▪ Orientation of the tip of needle should be about at an angle 45° cephalad and 60°
    medial to the sagittal plane (transducer 45° cephalad) with the bevel directed medially
    (may reduce likelihood of pleural puncture by presenting the needle's rounded
    "shoulder" against the pleura and easier catheter advancement toward the paravertebral
    space in desired tissue plane)
  ▪ Advance needle in increments aiming at the space between the internal and innermost
    intercostal muscles. After each advance, inject normal saline until the fascial plane
    between the muscles is dilated and anterior displacement of the pleura is seen
  ▪ Ask patient to breathe deeply to exclude accidental pleural puncture
  ▪ After a negative aspiration test, inject LA in a fractionated fashion:
    • 5 mL per level for single-shot blocks
    • 10 mL of LA at catheter level if placing catheter (to "open" space)

Tips/pearls
• Best visualization of block needle as it is an in-plane approach
• However, **advanced** technique, since the needle inserted toward the intervertebral
  foramen, with higher risk of epidural or intrathecal injection
• Greatest amount of discomfort, as needle traverses the greatest amount of soft tissue

Continuous PVBs
• See either traditional or ultrasound-based technique for needle placement
• Consider using single-injection 22-gauge 10-cm Tuohy needle initially to estimate the
  depth of transverse process and paravertebral space
• Use larger-bore (e.g., 18G) Tuohy needle capable of accommodating a 20-gauge epidural
  catheter
• A syringe is attached to the needle to create a closed circuit and mitigate entrainment
  of air if the pleura is punctured
• The catheter is threaded approximately 5–7 cm into the paravertebral space to minimize
  the risk of migration. Consequently, a catheter with a single distal orifice is used to reduce
  leakage of local anesthetic solution outside of the paravertebral space

FIGURE 149-3. Position of US probe and needle insertion for the paramedian sagittal approach

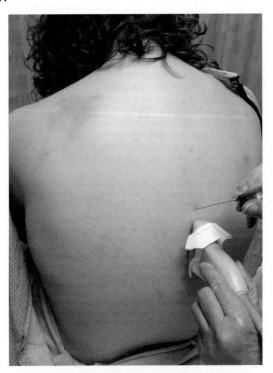

FIGURE 149-4. Ultrasound-guided thoracic paravertebral block (TPVB) using a paramedian oblique sagittal scan (unmarked)

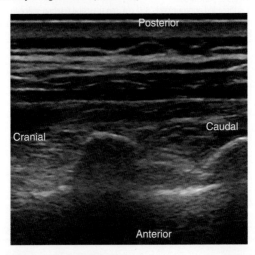

Transducer to be tilted slightly laterally (outwards) during scan (courtesy of Dr Jean-Louis Horn).

FIGURE 149-5. Paramedian oblique sagittal sonogram of the thoracic paravertebral region

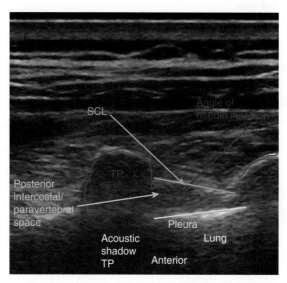

Note the pleura, superior costotransverse ligament, and the TPVS are clearly delineated. TP, transverse process; SCL, superior costotransverse ligament (courtesy of Dr Jean-Louis Horn).

FIGURE 149-6. Figure showing the orientation of the ultrasound transducer (black rectangle) and the direction of the ultrasound beam during a transverse scan of the thoracic paravertebral region

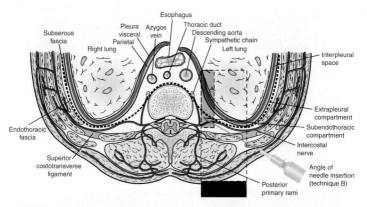

Depending on the level, the transverse process can cast an acoustic shadow (represented in gray) obscuring the ultrasound visibility of the thoracic paravertebral space. The probe should then be moved slightly cephalad or caudad to reach the space between transverse processes. The injection has to be made in the subendothoracic compartment, between the superior costotransverse ligament and the endothoracic fascia (see on left side of picture). Modified with permission from Karmaker MK. Thoracic paravertebral block. *Anesthesiology*. 2001;95:771.

FIGURE 149-7. Anatomy of the thoracic paravertebral region showing the various paravertebral ligaments and their anatomical relations to the thoracic paravertebral space

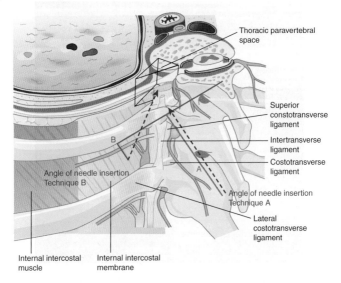

Line A delineates the approach for the paramedian sagittal in-plane approach, Line B the transverse, oblique in-plane approach. Modified with permission from Karmaker MK. Ultrasound-guided thoracic paravertebral block. *Tech Reg Anesth Pain Manag*. 2009;13:142. © Elsevier.

FIGURE 149-8. Transverse sonogram of the thoracic paravertebral region with the ultrasound beam lateral from midline, overlying the transverse process

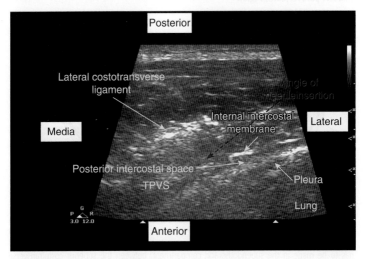

The hypoechoic space between the parietal pleura and the lateral costotransverse ligament and internal intercostal membrane laterally represents the apex of the TPVS or the medial limit of the posterior intercostal space. (Courtesy of Dr Jean-Louis Horn.)

FIGURE 149-9. Transverse sonogram of the thoracic paravertebral region with the ultrasound beam at the spinous process

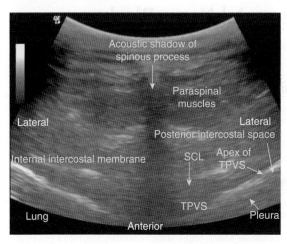

Parts of the TPVS and the anteromedial reflection of the pleura are now visible. The superior costotransverse ligament that forms the posterior border of the TPVS is also visible. The communication between the TPVS and the posterior intercostal space is also clearly seen. SCL, superior costotransverse ligament; TPVS, thoracic paravertebral space.

PEARLS/TIPS

- Anticoagulation concerns same as epidural (deep, noncompressible space, and communication with epidural space)
- Graduate from single injections to continuous infusions; catheter harder to thread than in epidural space
- Unintentional pleural puncture can result from deep insertion of the nerve block needle. Early warning signs include coughing during needle insertion. (Aspiration of air only if lung punctured or if air introduced into the pleural cavity by the needle.)
- Systemic absorption of local anesthetic with resulting toxicity is rare

REFERENCES

For references, please visit **www.TheAnesthesiaGuide.com**.

CHAPTER 150
Intercostal Nerve Blocks

Michael Anderson, MD

INDICATIONS

- Thoracic surgery
- Rib fractures
- Open cholecystectomy
- Gastrectomy
- Mastectomy

ANATOMY (FIGURE 150-1)

- Nerve runs in a neurovascular bundle just inferiorly to the rib; the nerve is the most inferior structure in this bundle
- Nerve runs between the internal intercostal and the innermost intercostal muscles
- Lateral cutaneous branch begins at the midaxillary line; therefore, one should block proximally to this point
- The block should be done lateral to the beginning of the angle of the rib; the intercostal groove is largest here; therefore, theoretically safer

FIGURE 150-1. Anatomy of the intercostal space

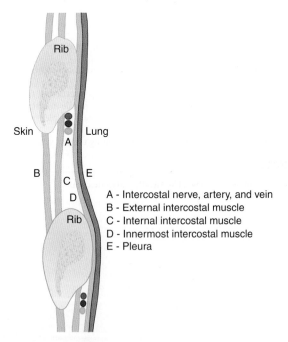

A - Intercostal nerve, artery, and vein
B - External intercostal muscle
C - Internal intercostal muscle
D - Innermost intercostal muscle
E - Pleura

(A) Intercostal nerve, artery, and vein; (B) external intercostal muscle; (C) internal intercostal muscle; (D) innermost intercostal muscle; (E) pleura.

COVERAGE

- Both sensory and motor at the level blocked; only ipsilateral side effected
- Skin, muscle, and parietal peritoneum, if being used for upper abdominal surgery postoperative analgesia, then additional coverage required for visceral pain
- Appropriate for thoracic and upper abdominal procedures
- Bupivacaine or lidocaine with epinephrine provides a block lasting an average of 12 hours

COMPLICATIONS

- Pneumothorax (<1%)
- Local anesthetic toxicity (this block has a high absorption of local anesthetic; consider the use of epinephrine in the local anesthesia to decrease systemic absorption)
- Hematoma
- Spinal or epidural anesthesia

LANDMARKS FOR BLOCK

- Put the patient in a sitting position (lateral and prone are also possible)
- Palpate and identify the appropriate level of intercostal spaces
- Identify the angle of the rib, usually about 7 cm from midline. The block can be performed anywhere proximal to the midaxillary line
- Lift the skin from the intercostal groove up over the rib
- Insert a 22G, 50-mm needle at a 20° cephalad angle; the needle should come in contact with the rib within about 1 cm (Figure 150-2)
- Walk the needle off of the rib inferiorly, but keep the 20° cephalad angle of the needle
- The nerve generally lies less than 3 mm deeper than the depth of the rib; a pop is often felt with a short bevel needle
- Inject 5 mL of local anesthesia at each level necessary; do not exceed the maximum dose for the chosen local anesthetic

FIGURE 150-2. Intercostal block technique ("blind" technique)

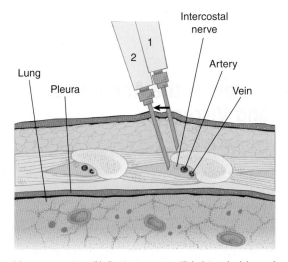

ULTRASOUND-GUIDED BLOCK (FIGURE 150-3)

- Ultrasound imaging can be used to identify the intercostal spaces. Especially helpful in obese patients or patients with challenging anatomy
- Similar to a landmark-based technique for positioning, a high-frequency linear probe can be placed vertically on the patients back to visualize the rib, intercostal space, and pleura
- The needle is inserted in an in-plane or out-of-plane technique paying close attention to the depth identified on the ultrasound image. Small frequent boluses of local anesthesia can be used for hydrodissection and needle guidance
- Once in the correct location, the local anesthesia is injected and one can visualize the spread of local anesthesia pushing the pleura away

FIGURE 150-3. Ultrasound-guided intercostal block

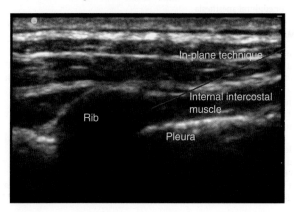

REFERENCES

For references, please visit **www.TheAnesthesiaGuide.com**.

CHAPTER 151
Innervation of the Abdominal Wall and Viscera

Marc Beaussier, MD, PhD

GENERAL CONSIDERATIONS

- Recent findings emphasize the "two-wound model" after abdominal surgery:
  ▸ The *somatic wound* corresponds to the abdominal wall
  ▸ The *autonomic wound* corresponds to the peritoneal layer and visceral component
- Pain after abdominal surgery arises *predominantly from parietal somatic afferents*, making parietal blocks very effective
- Peritoneal and visceral sensory innervation is provided by visceral afferents running along the *sympathetic nerves* and joining the dorsal horn at the higher thoracic levels. However, a significant part of these afferents may reach the central nervous system by the *vagus nerve, and will not be blocked even by an epidural block*

ANATOMY (FIGURES 151-1 TO 151-4)

- The abdominal wall is innervated by intercostal nerves (arising from T6 to T12) and ilioinguinal/iliohypogastric nerves (arising from L1). These nerves are easily blocked throughout their course between the abdominal muscles
- After emerging from the paravertebral space, intercostal nerves lie between the *transversus* and the *obliquus internus abdominis* muscles in the so-called transversus abdominis plane (TAP) (Figure 151-4)
- Approximately at the level of the midaxillary line, intercostal nerves give out perforating branches innervating the lateral abdominal wall (Figures 151-1 and 151-2)
- Segmental nerves T6–T9 emerge from the anterior costal margin between the midline and the anterior axillary line
- At the level of the *rectus abdominis* muscle, intercostal nerves enter the muscle sheath and give out perforating musculocutaneous branches that provide the sensitive innervation of the anteromedial abdominal wall (Figures 151-1 and 151-2)
- Near the anterior superior iliac spine, ilioinguinal and iliohypogastric nerves, previously located in the TAP, move to the space between *obliquus internus* and *obliquus externus* muscles (Figure 151-3). They provide the sensory innervation to the inguinal territory and the area just above the pubic symphysis (where Pfannenstiel incisions are performed)

FIGURE 151-1. Abdominal wall innervation

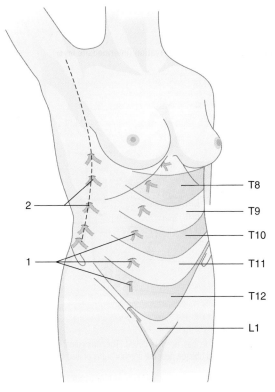

(1) Perforating musculocutaneous branches exiting the rectus abdominis sheath; (2) perforating cutaneous branches from the intercostal nerves exiting at the level of the midaxillary line.

FIGURE 151-2. Abdominal wall innervation (superficial layer)

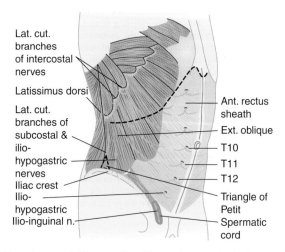

Superficial layer: the external oblique muscle and the anterior rectus sheath. Cutaneous branches of the intercostal nerves and of the iliohypogastric nerves, and perforating branches from the rectus sheath, innervate the skin.

FIGURE 151-3. Abdominal wall innervation (intermediate layer)

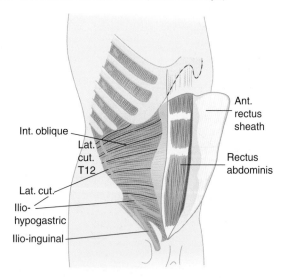

The external oblique muscle has been removed. The ilioinguinal and iliohypogastric nerves emerge through the internal oblique near the anterior superior iliac spine.

FIGURE 151-4. Abdominal wall innervation (deep layer)

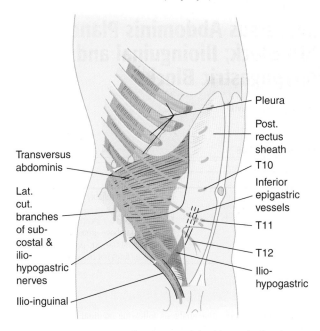

The external and internal oblique, as well as the rectus abdominis muscles, have been removed. The intercostal, ilioinguinal, and iliohypogastric nerves course in the transverse abdominis plane, superficial to the transverse abdominis muscle and deep to the internal oblique.

REFERENCES

For references, please visit **www.TheAnesthesiaGuide.com**.

CHAPTER 152
Transversus Abdominis Plane (TAP) Block; Ilioinguinal and Iliohypogastric Blocks

Michael Anderson, MD

TAP BLOCK COVERAGE

Nerves	Level blocked
Subcostal nerves (T9–L1) Ilioinguinal/iliohypogastric nerves (T12–L1)	**T10–L1 blocked reliably** T9 blocked 50% T4–T8 described but inconsistently blocked: **No analgesia above umbilicus** Covers skin, muscle, and parietal peritoneum Visceral structures not blocked

Indications:
• Unilateral block: postoperative analgesia following inguinal hernia repair, appendectomy, renal transplant, anterior iliac crest bone harvest
• Bilateral block: median laparotomy, radical prostatectomy, hysterectomy, various laparoscopic procedures, C-section; typically performed preoperatively, except for C-section

Anatomy:
See chapter 151.

Landmarks "blind" technique:
• Patient supine, arm abducted to allow access to lateral abdomen
• Identify the triangle of Petit (delimited by latissimus dorsi, iliac crest, and external oblique):
  ‣ Can be very difficult in obese patients
• Needle inserted perpendicular to the skin
• "Double pop" felt as needle inserted (blunt needle gives more obvious pops):
  ‣ First pop—fascia between external and internal oblique muscles
  ‣ Second pop—fascia between internal oblique and transverse abdominis muscles
• Twenty milliliters of local anesthesia is injected

Ultrasound technique (Figure 152-1):
• Landmarks: between costal margin and iliac crest in midaxillary line
• Muscle planes are identified with a high-frequency (8–13 MHz) probe
• Muscles are hypoechoic (dark); fascia is hyperechoic (bright)
• A 100-mm short-bevel needle inserted in-plane, anterior to posterior (i.e., from the medial side). An out-of-plane approach is also possible but requires more experience
• Inject a few milliliters of saline to ascertain correct position of needle tip
• Local deposition in the fascial layer between the internal oblique and transverse abdominis muscles; typically 15–20 mL of 0.25% bupivacaine or ropivacaine
• Oblique subcostal approach has been tried to increase block height: probe placed parallel along the costal margin, needle inserted in an in-plane technique from lateral to medial

FIGURE 152-1. Probe and needle placement

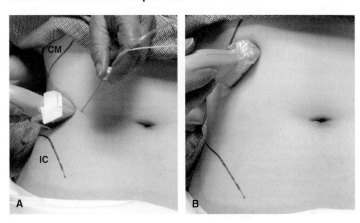

(A) "Traditional" TAP block. The needle can be introduced from the medial or the lateral side in-plane, or it can be placed out-of-plane. IC: iliac crest; CM: costal margin. (B) Oblique subcostal approach: probe parallel to the costal margin. The needle is typically inserted in-plane from the lateral side (not shown).

FIGURE 152-2. Ultrasound target for the TAP block

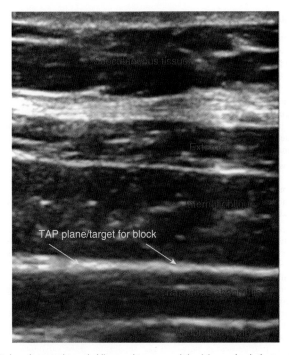

The TAP plane, between internal oblique and transverse abdominis muscles, is the target for the local anesthetic injection.

Testing:
- Pinprick testing can be performed to assess block level
- Block is most commonly done for postoperative analgesia after induction of general anesthesia
- Block is dependent on volume, not concentration; 20 mL of 0.25% bupivacaine routinely gives 18–24 hours of analgesia

Side effects/complications:

Low-risk analgesic block:
- General risks:
  - Needle trauma
  - Intravascular injection
  - Local anesthetic toxicity
  - Poor/failed block
- Specific side effects:
  - Flank bulge sign (relaxed abdominal muscles)
- Specific complications:
  - Peritoneal perforation (significance is unclear)
  - Liver hematoma (one case report with blind technique)

PEARLS

- If you are unsure which layer is the correct plane, scan to the rectus abdominis muscle; the lateral edge of the muscle points to the correct fascial line
- This block will provide good analgesia but it is *not* superior to an epidural—especially as it does not cover the viscera
- On occasion, vessels can be seen in the transversus abdominis plane (TAP) plane. Avoid injecting near or into them

ILIOINGUINAL/ILIOHYPOGASTRIC BLOCKS

Indications:
- Inguinal hernia repair
- Orchiopexy
- Pfannenstiel incisions
- Lower abdominal surgery

Anatomy (Figure 152-3; also see chapter 151):
- Ilioinguinal and iliohypogastric nerves are branches of L1
- At the level of the block, nerves run between the transverse abdominis and internal oblique, or between internal and external oblique muscles
- Landmarks—ASIS and umbilicus

Block coverage:
- Lower abdominal wall
- Skin, muscle, and parietal peritoneum
- Does not cover visceral peritoneum: for complete anesthesia of a hernia, the hernia sac must also be injected

Landmark ("blind") technique:
- Identify an imaginary line between the ASIS and umbilicus
- Approximately 2 cm medially and 2 cm superior to the ASIS is the needle insertion site. Approximately 15 mL of local anesthesia is injected between this point and the ASIS
- Further infiltration of the skin in a fan-like pattern from the umbilicus and ASIS branching off the imaginary line provides a larger field of anesthesia
- Significant volumes of local anesthesia often required for the landmark technique (40–60 mL); therefore, to decrease the possibility of local anesthetic toxicity, consider using an ultrasound technique

FIGURE 152-3. Relevant anatomy for the ilioinguinal and iliohypogastric blocks

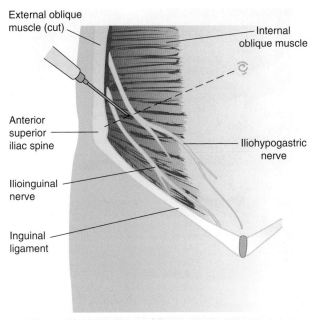

External oblique
muscle (cut)

Internal
oblique muscle

Anterior
superior
iliac spine

Iliohypogastric
nerve

Ilioinguinal
nerve

Inguinal
ligament

The nerves are shown here in the plane between internal and external oblique muscles. Reproduced from Morgan GE, Mikhail MS, Murray MJ. *Clinical Anesthesiology*. 4th ed. Figure 17-35. Available at: www.accessmedicine.com. Copyright © The McGraw-Hill Companies, Inc. All rights reserved.

Ultrasound-guided block (Figure 152-4):
- Identify the ASIS and umbilicus; imagine a line connecting the two structures
- Place a linear high-frequency ultrasound probe longitudinally on this line, adjacent to the ASIS
- Identify the muscle layers; the small nerves can often be seen between the internal oblique and transverse abdominis muscles
- Using an in-plane or out-of-plane approach, insert a blunt block needle near the ASIS trying to appreciate the two pops
- Deposit local anesthetic (10–20 mL) between the internal oblique and transverse abdominis muscles. The nerves run with two small arteries; deposit the local anesthetic near these vessels if unable to identify the nerves directly
- On occasion, the nerves, or some of their branches/divisions, already lie in the more superficial plane, between internal and external oblique muscles. One should therefore *systematically infiltrate both planes* to ensure complete blockade

Complications:
- Femoral nerve block by diffusion—occurs up to 5% of the time
- Bowel perforation (rare)
- Pelvic hematoma (rare)

PEARLS

- If unsure about the anatomy or if surgeon concerned about hydrodissection in area of the block, then move laterally and perform a TAP block; this will give a larger area of anesthesia

FIGURE 152-4. Ultrasound-guided ilioinguinal and iliohypogastric nerve blocks

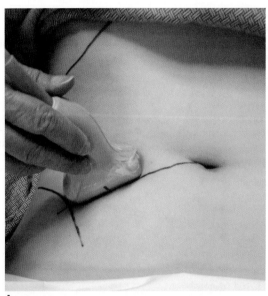

A

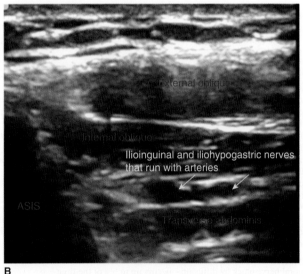

B

(A) Ultrasound probe position, on a line between umbilicus and anterior superior iliac spine (ASIS), straddling the ASIS. (B) Ultrasound view. ASIS: anterior superior iliac spine. *NB*: In this case, the nerves are seen between transverse abdominis and internal oblique muscles. Depending on the level and the patient, they can lie in this plane or between internal and external obliques. The nerves are usually not as large as in this patient. One should systematically infiltrate both planes (between transverse abdominis and internal oblique, and between internal and external obliques) to ensure a complete block of all branches and divisions.

- Perform block as proximal as is convenient, as cutaneous branches if the iliohypogastric nerve might not be blocked with a more distal block
- The iliohypogastric and ilioinguinal nerves give a number of branches and can run between transverse abdominis and internal oblique and/or between internal and external obliques. Thus, one should infiltrate the spaces between the transverse and internal oblique muscles of the abdomen *and* between the two oblique muscles of the abdomen
- An injection posterior to the transversus abdominis muscle may explain the spread to the lumbar plexus and especially to the femoral nerve with a risk of fall if unrecognized
- In children, consider a caudal that appears about as effective for hernia repair

REFERENCES

For references, please visit **www.TheAnesthesiaGuide.com**.

CHAPTER 153
Regional Analgesia for Abdominal Surgery

Marc Beaussier, MD, PhD

A comprehensive approach of analgesia after abdominal surgery is based on the understanding of parietal and visceral innervation (see chapter 151).

VARIOUS REGIONAL TECHNIQUES ARE AVAILABLE

Intercostal, ilioinguinal, and iliohypogastric nerves can be blocked at different levels, from proximal to distal.

Epidural analgesia (EDA):
- Remains the gold standard for pain relief after open abdominal surgery
- Low thoracic catheter for at least 48 hours after surgery
- Mixture of local anesthetics and opioids
- Patient-controlled administration
- Risk–benefit ratio questionable after laparoscopic surgery

Intrathecal morphine (ITM):
- Small dose of PF morphine (100–500 µg) in the lumbar area
- Limited duration of action
- No demonstrated benefit on postoperative rehabilitation
- Need for prolonged monitoring (risk of delayed respiratory depression)
- Interest of ITM is questionable as better regional techniques available

Transversus abdominis plane block (TAP block):
- TAP block consists of blocking intercostal nerves at the level of lateral abdominal wall *between internal oblique and transverse abdominis muscles*
- Variable success rate, probably improved by ultrasound guidance
- Subcostal TAP block must be considered for incisions on dermatome higher than T10
- Must be performed bilaterally in order to cover a midline incision
- Duration of action (using long-lasting local anesthetics) after a single injection: up to 24 hours
- No clear benefit demonstrated on postoperative rehabilitation

Ilioinguinal/iliohypogastric block (IIB):
- Actually a variant of the TAP block, with the injection being more specifically oriented toward these nerves (i.e., more anterior in the abdominal wall)
- At this level, nerves to be blocked are *between the internal and external oblique muscles*
- Usually indicated for anesthesia and analgesia after inguinal hernia repair. But also highly effective for pain relief after abdominal gynecological procedure as well as for C-section (bilateral blocks)
- Keep in mind that a genitofemoral block must be associated with an IIB in order to provide optimal analgesia during inguinal hernia repair. Moreover, nerves coming from the contralateral intercostal nerves have to be blocked by a local infiltration at the medial side of the incision

Rectus sheath block:
- Consists of injecting the local anesthetic directly into the *rectus abdominis* muscle at the level where intercostal nerves enter the muscle
- Only intended for midline incision (usually for umbilical hernia repair)
- Very easy to perform. Ultrasound-guided techniques could improve success and safety (look out for the epigastric artery, which is very close to the injection point)
- Usually 10 mL of long-acting local anesthetic on each side
- Multiple injections should be performed to block more than one dermatome level

Wound infiltration:
- Consists of injecting local anesthetic directly into the wound
- Should be used as a component of a multimodal analgesic regimen
- Duration of action after a single bolus injection is usually too limited to provide clinically significant benefit
- A multiperforated catheter can be inserted into the wound by the surgeon at the end of the procedure in order to prolong the effect with a continuous infusion (CWI)
- Factors associated with optimal efficacy of CWI (for abdominal surgery) are:
  ‣ Catheter length of fenestration closely adapted to the length of the incision
  ‣ High flow rate of local anesthetic (>5 mL/h)
  ‣ Catheter placement in deep abdominal wall layer:
    • Subcutaneous placement: no significant benefit
    • Placement deep to the musculoaponeurosis layer (preperitoneal location) seems to be the most effective
- Continuous preperitoneal infusion of 10 mL/h of ropivacaine 0.2% for 48 hours reduces morphine consumption, improves pain relief (both at rest and at mobilization), and has beneficial effect on recovery course (faster transit resumption and shorter hospital LOS). Furthermore, by improving pain and blocking parietal afferents, CWI could be able to reduce the diaphragmatic dysfunction induced by abdominal surgery
- CWI is very simple, devoid of side effects, and could be used in almost all patients
- CWI is indicated for all abdominal incisions, including digestive, liver surgery, gynecological procedures, or C-section
- After laparoscopic surgery, the benefit to locally infiltrate trocar sites is demonstrated

Intra-abdominal instillation:
- The administration of local anesthetics directly into the abdominal cavity should be considered for pain relief after laparoscopic cholecystectomy
- May be considered in association with other "parietal" techniques in order to block peritoneal afferents running into the vagus nerve
- Usually 20 mL of long-duration local anesthetic, half directly on the surgical bed, half on the interhepatodiaphragmatic space
- Beware of the rapid systemic absorption of the local anesthetic: risk of toxicity

Characteristics of different blocks:

	EDA	ITM	TAP block–IIB	RSB	CWI
Analgesia at rest	Yes	Yes	Yes	Yes	Yes
Analgesia at mobilization	Yes	No	Yes	Unclear	Yes
Opioid-sparing effect	Yes	Yes	Yes	Yes	Yes
Ability to prolong analgesia (>24 h)	Yes	No	Unclear	Yes	No
Blockade of visceral afferents	Yes	Yes	No	No	Yes[1]
Occurrence of failures	Yes	No	Yes[2]	Unclear	No
Applicable in almost all patients	No	No	Yes	Yes	Yes
Beneficial effect on gastric ileus resumption	Yes	No	Unclear	Unclear	Yes
Beneficial effect on postoperative rehabilitation	Yes	No	Unclear	Unclear	Yes
General side effects	Yes	Yes[3]	No	No	No
Need specific postoperative monitoring	Yes	Yes	No	No	No

EDA, epidural analgesia; ITM, intrathecal morphine; IIB, ilioinguinal and iliohypogastric block; RSB, rectus sheath block; CWI, continuous wound infiltration.
[1]Peritoneal afferents could be blocked if wound catheter is placed in preperitoneal position.
[2]May be reduced by the use of ultrasound guidance.
[3]High risk of respiratory depression (OR = 7.8 in comparison with parenteral morphine).

REFERENCES

For references, please visit **www.TheAnesthesiaGuide.com**.

CHAPTER 154
Infiltration Analgesia for Lower Limb Arthroplasty

Nicholas B. Scott, FRCS(Ed), FRCA

NB: This is a relatively new technique but it is getting increasingly popular. We asked a very experienced practitioner to describe his "recipe." Keep in mind that success seems to be surgeon-dependent.

BASICS

- Early mobilization reduces both the incidence of DVT and PE, and the hospital LOS
- Pain is only one of a number of issues that prevent a patient getting out of bed in the early postoperative period. Other factors include patient personality, motivation, fear, staff attitudes, hypotension, motor block, stiffness, dizziness, PONV, surgical morbidity, etc

- Complete analgesia is no longer necessary or desirable for lower limb arthroplasty. Preoperative conditioning and the combination of an intraoperative spinal with intra-articular catheters appears to provide the "ideal" balance between good analgesia and the ability to mobilize early for these procedures
- Avoiding perioperative systemic and intrathecal opioids via multimodal nonopioid analgesia (MMA) reduces the incidence of urine retention and PONV
- Wound infiltration alone *without* a postoperative wound catheter appears to be all that is required for THA, while a postoperative catheter for 24–48 hours is needed for TKA
- In an ongoing prospective series beginning in January 2007 of over 7,000 patients undergoing THA and TKA using wound infiltration in an enhanced recovery program in Scotland, the success rate for the technique is 94%. A total of 96% of patients can be mobilized within 24 hours of surgery with median pain scores less than 3. Postoperative IV fluids are only required in 5% of patients and only 7% require urinary catheterization. The median PONV score is zero and median postoperative stay has been reduced from 6.5 to 3.7 days. Notably, joint infection remains low at 0.9% and the need for blood transfusion is very low—2% for THR and 0.6% for TKR compared with the national (UK) average of 20%

PREOPERATIVE

- *Assessment in outpatient clinic*:
  - ‣ Within 2 weeks of planned day of surgery
  - ‣ Multidisciplinary approach from all perioperative specialties
  - ‣ Patient education regarding: pain, mobilization, rehabilitation, etc
  - ‣ Target a realistic day for discharge based on local data
  - ‣ Address individual expectations, hopes, and fears
  - ‣ Ensure Hb level >12 g/L. If Hb level <12 g/L, initiate appropriate treatment (iron, folate, EPO) and postpone surgery if needed
  - ‣ Optimize comorbidities, especially cardiovascular disease and hypertension
- *On admission*:
  - ‣ Liberal oral fluids ± hypocaloric drinks up to 2 hours before surgery
- *Premedication*:
  - ‣ Avoid strong sedatives that delay getting out of bed
  - ‣ Multimodal analgesia:
    - ▪ Dexamethasone 0.1–0.2 mg/kg orally:
      - ♦ Antiemetic and analgesic
      - ♦ No problems of wound healing or infection with short course
    - ▪ Gabapentin 600 mg orally
    - ▪ Oxycontin 10 mg orally
    - ▪ Acetaminophen 1 g orally
    - ▪ Ibuprofen 400 mg orally

INTRAOPERATIVE

- 2.5–5 g IV tranexamic acid before incision
- *Low-dose spinal anesthesia*:
  - ‣ For example, 6–7.5 mg levobupivacaine or bupivacaine
  - ‣ Advantages:
    - ▪ No need for full GA—only sedation required; see below
    - ▪ Avoids systemic opioids in early postoperative period
    - ▪ Reduced blood loss
    - ▪ Reduced thromboembolism
    - ▪ Reduced PONV
    - ▪ Reduced surgical site infection
  - ‣ *A unilateral spinal anesthetic (USA)* can be achieved by having patient lying on side with *operating side up*, that is, in same position as for surgery. Adding 1 mL

of sterile water (not saline) to isobaric bupivacaine, ropivacaine, or levobupivacaine results in a *hypobaric* solution. *Inject slowly over 2 minutes to avoid excessive spread*
  - USA minimizes motor block and need for urinary catheterization. Wait at least 15 minutes before turning supine if TKA. Foot and ankle are often spared. Block usually effective for 2–2.5 hours
  - *NB*: However, slow surgeons may dictate higher dose of LA!!
- Consider:
  - 2% prilocaine or 3% PF chloroprocaine (off-label) as a shorter-acting alternative to hasten recovery. *NB*: Only if surgeon fast and cooperative!
  - Low-dose alpha-agonist to increase duration of analgesia, for example, 15–20 μg clonidine
- *Do not add intrathecal opioid* as these increase the need for urinary catheterization independent of the dose or choice of opioid
- Minimal IV fluids—restrict to 1000–1500 mL of hetastarch plus overt losses to maintain intravascular volume. Avoid crystalloids, since these only remain in intravascular compartment for 1–2 hours. Remember you want your patients to get out of bed—not to be shackled to a drip stand
- Music via headphones
- Ketorolac 30 mg *or* diclofenac 75 mg IV
- Propofol to provide sedation/anesthesia and early postoperative antiemesis, ideally via target-controlled pump
- Supplementary low-dose ketamine 0.1–0.3 mg/kg provides early postoperative analgesia, reduced opioid use, *without* hallucinatory side effects
- *Wound infiltration*:
  - 300 to 400 mg loading dose of either 0.2% ropivacaine or 0.125% bupivacaine or levobupivacaine
  - Performed immediately prior to insertion of prosthesis
  - *NB*: *Must be performed meticulously with special attention to capsule* using a systematic technique to ensure uniform delivery of the local anesthetic to all tissue that has been incised or instrumented during the procedure
  - Avoid sloppy technique or "wound sloshing."
  - Avoid epinephrine that may cause skin necrosis without added analgesia
  - Avoid ketorolac; if desired, give systemically as above
- *Hip infiltration*:
  - *Total volume 170 mL of 0.2% ropivacaine or equivalent*
  - 50 mL injected in the periacetabular tissues immediately prior to insertion of the acetabular cup
  - 50 mL injected intramuscularly after insertion of femoral prosthesis
  - *NB*: Postoperative pain is frequently *above* the incision, so pay close attention to gluteal and rotator muscles and the lateral thigh muscles
  - If desired, place an epidural catheter (16 or 18G) several centimeters distal to the incision and tunneled into the hip joint with the tip near the femoral head
  - 20 mL injected into the joint (or catheter)
  - 50 mL injected fanwise into the subcutaneous layers. (*NB*: Do not use epinephrine for skin.)
- *Knee infiltration (Figures 154-1 to 154-4)*:
  - *Total volume 170 mL of 0.2% ropivacaine or equivalent*
  - 50 mL infiltrated through posterior capsule and femur
  - 80 mL infiltrated into anterior capsule, quads, collaterals, and anterior femur
  - 50 mL into subcutaneous tissues
  - 20 mL after closure into joint through catheter
  - Following infiltration, *for knees* an intra-articular catheter is placed into posterior aspect of joint
- The above volumes may approach or exceed the recommended maximum doses in the literature. However, the capsule and ligaments of the hip and knee are relatively avascular, and the use of a tourniquet for knee arthroplasty allows for "tissue binding." Data in the literature show plasma levels following intra-articular instillation and reinfusion drains to be well below toxic levels

POSTOPERATIVE

- *NB: Primary aim of LIA is to have patients walking "as soon as possible." If surgical protocols enforce bed rest, the main advantage of this technique is lost*
- Patient can eat and drink immediately
- No surgical drains—totally unnecessary, increased risk of infection and transfusion requirements
- Cryocuff for up to 24 hours—reduces postoperative pain, swelling, and analgesic requirements
- Tourniquet, if used, should be released *after* closure of wound
- Thromboembolic prophylaxis per surgeon/institution
- Mobilization as able—30–50% of patients can mobilize on day of surgery
- *Avoid bed rest*—leads to increased risk of sepsis and thromboembolism
- *"No" routine postoperative IV fluids: avoid the need for the drip stand! NB:* Patients are elderly, frail, arthritic, recovering from major surgery, and unsteady on their feet. A drip stand makes such patients dependent and unwilling to get out of bed
- *Multimodal analgesia as follows:*
  - *Gabapentin:* a single further dose of 600 mg on the night of surgery is sufficient as it is both analgesic and sedative. However, if patient has chronic pain issues or is opioid tolerant, continue for 5 days and review
  - Oxycontin 10 mg q12 hours × three doses
  - Acetaminophen 1 g four times per day for 5 days
  - Ibuprofen 400 mg three times per day (if able)
  - Intra-articular infiltration through catheter (0.2% ropivacaine):
    - *Either* continuous infiltration via elastomeric pump at 10 mL/h
    - *Or* 40 mL boluses 3×/24 hours
    - *Rescue:*
  - Oxycodone 10 mg 3 hourly PRN
  - Additional intra-articular boluses as above (maximum of two in any hour)
- *NB:* If the above is deemed ineffective, femoral nerve blockade or lumbar epidural may be necessary in 5–10% of patients

FIGURE 154-1. Step 1—infiltration of posterior capsule after bone cuts

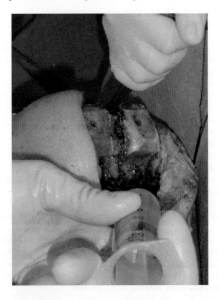

FIGURE 154-2. Step 2–infiltration of soft tissues

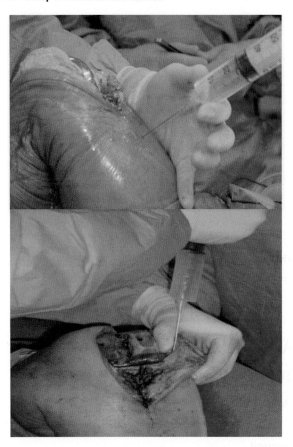

FIGURE 154-3. Step 3–catheter placement once implant in place

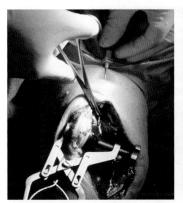
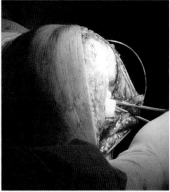

FIGURE 154-4. Step 4—skin infiltration during closure

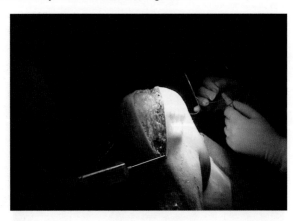

REFERENCES

For references, please visit **www.TheAnesthesiaGuide.com**.

CHAPTER 155
Superficial Blocks of the Face

Lucie Beylacq, MD

INTRODUCTION

- Currently underused because the technique is not widely known and taught
- Ultrasound may make these blocks easier and more effective

SUPERFICIAL TRIGEMINAL NERVE BRANCHES (FIGURE 155-1)

- The sensory nerve of the face, part of the ear, the orbit, nasal fossae, and oral cavity is the trigeminal nerve (fifth cranial pair)
- It has three branches: the ophthalmic (V1), the maxillary (V2), and the mandibular (V3)
- It is also the motor nerve of mastication
- Each branch divides in terminal branches, which emerge with a small artery from their respective foramina:
  - The frontal and supratrochlear nerves (branches of V1) emerge from the supraorbital foramen
  - The infraorbital nerve (branch of V2) emerges from the infraorbital foramen
  - The mental nerve (branch of V3) emerges from the mental foramen
- The three foramina are (theoretically) in line with the pupil, at 2.5 cm from the midline in most patients
- For the blocks, the patient is in supine position with the head on a pillow

FIGURE 155-1. Skin innervation, landmarks, and ultrasound probe position for superficial blocks of the face

Dermatomes	Anatomical landmarks	Probe position
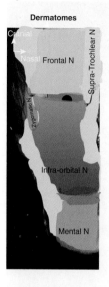	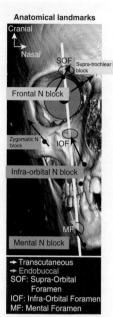	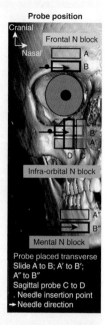

FRONTAL (FIGURE 155-2) AND SUPRATROCHLEAR NERVE BLOCKS

- Frontal and supratrochlear nerves supply cutaneous sensation to the forehead from the upper eyelid up to the coronal suture of the skull
- Indications are upper blepharoplasty or surgery performed on the scalp, including craniotomies and anterior dermoid cyst excisions
- The main landmark is the supraorbital foramen, usually easy to find by palpating the roof of the orbital rim, in line with the pupil
- Keep the finger above the foramen. Insert a 25G needle under the finger and, after aspiration, inject 3 mL of local anesthetic toward the foramen, without entering it
- The needle is then redirected toward the angle of the upper nasal bone and the orbit, to block the supratrochlear nerve with 1 mL of local anesthetic
- Very rare complications have been described, such as hematoma, intravascular or intraneural injection, or transient eyelid paresis

INFRAORBITAL NERVE BLOCK

- The infraorbital nerve exits through the infraorbital foramen, with the infraorbital artery and vein
- It supplies sensation to the lower eyelid, the skin of the nose, the cheek, and the upper lip
- Block indications are lower blepharoplasty, dermoid cyst excisions, or wounds of the cheek or the upper lip, and, especially in children, cleft lip surgery or transsphenoidal pituitary surgery
- The landmark is the infraorbital foramen. It is palpated at 8 mm from the floor of the orbital rim, approximately 3.4 cm from the midline (not really in line with the pupil)
- Transcutaneous approach: with a finger on the foramen, a 25G needle is inserted below the foramen and directed toward it; avoid intraneural injection or penetration in the orbit

FIGURE 155-2. Supraorbital foramen and technique for frontal nerve block

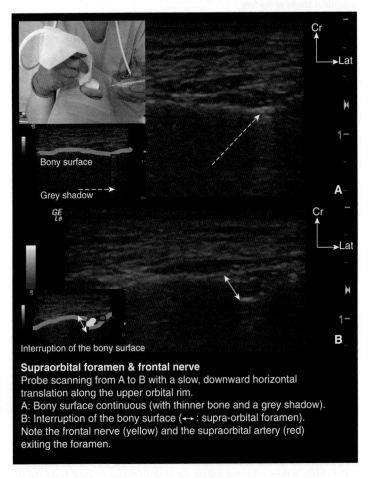

Bony surface

Grey shadow

Interruption of the bony surface

Supraorbital foramen & frontal nerve
Probe scanning from A to B with a slow, downward horizontal translation along the upper orbital rim.
A: Bony surface continuous (with thinner bone and a grey shadow).
B: Interruption of the bony surface (↔ : supra-orbital foramen).
Note the frontal nerve (yellow) and the supraorbital artery (red) exiting the foramen.

- Oral approach especially used for children: the needle is inserted through the buccal mucosa, at the level of the first premolar and directed toward the foramen. With this approach, the dental nerve is more often blocked as well. After aspiration, 3 mL of local anesthetic is injected
- Rare complications such as hematoma, intravascular or intraneural injection, eyelid edema, diplopia, or eyeball injury have been described

MENTAL NERVE BLOCK

- The mental nerve emerges from the mental foramen and supplies cutaneous sensation to the chin and the lower lip
- Like for the infraorbital nerve, two approaches can be used
- The mental foramen is easily palpated, in line with the pupil and the first premolar. The needle can be inserted transcutaneously toward the foramen, or after eversion of the lip at the level of the first premolar into the buccal mucosa. After aspiration, 2 mL of local anesthetic is injected. Complications are rare: hematoma, intravascular or intraneural injection

ULTRASOUND IMAGING TO LOCALIZE FACE FORAMINA

- Palpation of the foramina is sometimes difficult because they are not on line with the pupil, or they consist only of a notch or are absent (10%)
- Ultrasound can help identify the foramen or the small satellite artery
- High-frequency linear probe (>12 MHz) placed on the expected foramen location
- Bone appears as a hyperechoic linear edge with an anechoic shadow
- Just next to the foramen, the bone is less thick and appears less hyperechoic with a gray shadow
- The foramen appears as a bony surface break: a disruption of the hyperechoic line
- Position probe transverse for all three blocks
- The infraorbital foramen can also be located by scanning in a sagittal plane, medial to lateral, along the lower orbital rim
- Color Doppler can help locate the small satellite artery; note that the mental artery is really difficult to visualize
- On occasion, the nerve can be identified before the injection
- Needle insertion is in plane from lateral to medial
- Visualizing the needle avoids vascular entry and allows injection just outside of the foramina
- The spread of local anesthetic can be seen around the nerve, avoiding ineffective superficial injection and intraneural or intravascular injection

REFERENCES

For references, please visit **www.TheAnesthesiaGuide.com**.

PART IX

ACUTE PAIN (POSTOPERATIVE)

CHAPTER 156
Multimodal Postoperative Analgesia

Lisa Doan, MD

DEFINITION

Multimodal analgesia consists of using various modalities to reduce pain, thus providing more effective analgesia while reducing doses and side effects.
- *Use regional techniques when possible*:
  - ‣ Continuous or single-injection peripheral nerve blocks (see chapter 163)
  - ‣ Epidural infusions (see chapter 162)
- *Nonopioid analgesics* (see chapter 157)
- *Opioid analgesics* (see chapter 159):
  - ‣ IV PCA (see chapter 158)
- *Adjuvant medications* (see also chapters 160 and 161):

Adjuvant Medications Used for Multimodal Analgesia			
Drug	Dosing	Common side effects	Comments
Gabapentin (Neurontin)	Start at 300 mg qhs, can be titrated to 2,400 mg per day divided in three doses	Dizziness, somnolence, peripheral edema	Adjust doses in patients with renal insufficiency. Doses should be tapered when discontinuing therapy
Pregabalin (Lyrica)	Start at 50 mg qhs, can be titrated to 300 mg per day divided three times daily	Confusion, dizziness, somnolence, edema, weight gain	Similar mechanism of action as gabapentin. Doses should be adjusted in patients with renal insufficiency. Doses should be tapered when discontinuing therapy
Ketamine	0.1–0.5 mg/kg/h IV	Hallucinations, vivid dreams, drowsiness	Especially useful in opioid-tolerant patients

These medications, while not FDA-approved to treat acute pain, are commonly used off-label for that purpose.

REFERENCES

For references, please visit **www.TheAnesthesiaGuide.com**.

CHAPTER 157
Nonsteroidal Anti-Inflammatory Drugs (NSAIDs)

Naum Shaparin, MD

MECHANISM OF ACTION

Inhibition of the enzyme cyclooxygenase preventing synthesis of prostaglandin and thromboxane.

INDICATIONS

Mild to moderate pain, inflammation, and fever.

Adverse Effects and Contraindications	
System	Adverse effects
Cardiovascular	Hypertension, can exacerbate or induce heart failure, thrombotic events, possible increased risk of thrombotic/cardiovascular events with long-term use (use with caution in patients with preexisting disease; more likely with Cox2 inhibitors)
Respiratory	Nasal polyps, rhinitis, dyspnea, bronchospasm, angioedema, may exacerbate asthma
Hepatic	Hepatitis
Gastrointestinal	Gastropathy (can be asymptomatic), gastric bleeding, esophageal disease, pancreatitis
Hematological	Increased intraoperative bleeding due to platelet inhibition/dysfunction (coxibs do not affect platelet function), will potentiate anticoagulation effect
Dermatological	Urticaria, erythema multiforme, rash
Genitourinary	Renal insufficiency (use with caution in patients with preexisting renal disease), sodium/fluid retention, papillary necrosis, interstitial nephritis
Central nervous system	Headache, aseptic meningitis, hearing disturbances
Skeletal	Potential to inhibit bone growth/healing/formation
Pharmacologic interactions	NSAIDs displace albumin-bound drugs and can potentiate their effects (e.g., warfarin)

NEURAXIAL ANESTHESIA CONSIDERATIONS

ASRA consensus guidelines: nonsteroidal anti-inflammatory drugs (NSAIDs) alone should not interfere with the performance of neuraxial blocks or the timing of neuraxial catheter removal.

INTRAOPERATIVE SURGICAL CONSIDERATIONS

At many institutions, it is customary for the anesthesiology team to verbally confirm adequate hemostasis (and surgeon's agreement) prior to administering IV NSAIDs.

DRUG CLASS

Nonselective COX-1 and COX-2 inhibitors and selective COX-2 inhibitors:

Subclasses	Drug
Salicylate	Salsate, diflunisal, and choline magnesium trisalicylate
Proprionic	Ibuprofen, ketoprofen, naproxen, fenoprofen
Indole	Indomethacin, sulindac, tolmetin
Fenamate	Mefenamic, meclofenamate
Mixed	Piroxicam, ketorolac, diclofenac
Coxib (only selective COX-2 inhibitor)	Celecoxib (rofecoxib/valdecoxib removed from market)

Drug (PO—adult usage)	Starting dose	Maximum dose
Aspirin (Bayer)	325 mg q6 h	975 mg q6 h
Celecoxib (Celebrex)	100 mg q12 h	200 mg q12 h
Diclofenac potassium (Cataflam)	50 mg q12 h	50 mg q8 h
Diclofenac sodium (Voltaren)	50 mg q12 h	50 mg q8 h
Etodolac (Lodine)	200 mg q8 h	400 q8 h
Fenoprofen calcium (Nalfon)	200 mg q6 h	800 mg q6 h
Flurbiprofen (Ansaid)	50 mg q8 h	100 mg q8 h
Ibuprofen (Advil, Motrin)	200 mg q6 h	800 mg q6 h
Indomethacin (Indocin)	25 mg q12 h	50 mg q8 h
Ketoprofen (Orudis, Oruvail)	25 mg q8 h	75 mg q6 h
Meloxicam (Mobic)	7.5 mg q day	15 mg q day
Nabumetone (Relafen)	1,000 mg q day	2,000 mg q day
Naproxen (Naprosyn, Naprelan)	250 mg q8 h	500 mg q8 h
Naproxen sodium (Aleve, Anaprox)	275 mg q8 h	550 mg q8 h
Oxaprozin (Daypro)	600 mg q day	1,200 mg q day
Piroxicam (Feldene)	10 mg q day	20 mg q day
Salsalate (Amigesic, Anaflex)	1,000 mg q8 h	1,000 mg q8 h
Sulindac (Clinoril)	150 mg q12 h	200 mg q12 h

Drug (IV)—adult usage	Starting dose	Maximum dose
Ketorolac (Toradol)	15 mg q6 h	30 mg q6 h (for 5 days maximum)
Ibuprofen (Caldolor)	400 mg q6 h	800 mg q6 h

- Ibuprofen seems to have less effect on platelet function than ketorolac
- There is no maximum duration of treatment for ibuprofen as there is for ketorolac
- Ibuprofen can be converted to PO using the same dose (PO ketorolac not commonly used)

ACETAMINOPHEN (ADULT USAGE)

Mechanism: unknown (not an NSAID).
Indications: mild to moderate pain and fever (limited anti-inflammatory effect).
Contraindications: avoid with hepatic dysfunction.

Drug (IV)—adult usage	Starting dose	Maximum dose
Acetaminophen (Tylenol) (PO)	325 mg q6 h	1,000 mg q6 h
Acetaminophen (Ofirmev) (IV)	1,000 mg q6 h (15 mg/kg in children)	1,000 mg q6 h

CHAPTER 158
IV PCA (Intravenous Patient-Controlled Analgesia)

Vickie Verea, MD, Christopher Gharibo, MD, and Lisa Doan, MD

INDICATIONS

Management of moderate to severe pain when inadequate analgesia would result from oral pain medications or intermittent intravenous opioid boluses.

Typically started after initial opioid titration to comfort in the PACU.

CONTRAINDICATIONS

- Patients who do not have the cognitive ability to understand how to use a patient-controlled analgesia (PCA) device
- Patients physically incapable of activating the PCA demand function

PROGRAMMING THE PCA DEVICE

The PCA device may be programmed to deliver a demand dose with or without a basal rate. PCA order must include the following elements:
- Selected opioid and its concentration (often, this will be institutionally standardized)
- Demand (bolus) dose
- Lockout time interval of the demand dose in minutes

Optional parameters include:
- Loading dose (administered when initiating the PCA)
- Basal (continuous) infusion hourly rate
- Clinician dose (extra doses that can be administered by the RN in case of breakthrough pain; this should prompt a call to the pain service, but will ensure timely treatment)

Patient-Controlled Analgesia (PCA) Recommendations for the Average Adult			
Drug	Bolus	Lockout interval (min)	Optional basal rate (opioid-naïve patient)
Morphine	0.5–3 mg	5–20	0–1 mg/h
Fentanyl (Sublimaze)	10–25 µg	5–20	0–10 µg/h
Hydromorphone (Dilaudid)	0.05–0.3 mg	5–20	0–0.2 mg/h

Loading dose is encouraged on PCA initiation (and during significant PCA dose increases) to give the patient prompt analgesia. Omitting the loading dose can cause the patient to be undertreated, to over-rely on the demand doses in an attempt to get prompt analgesia, and to declare the PCA modality ineffective.

Use of a *basal infusion* is controversial:
- Not shown to improve pain outcomes
- Associated with higher incidence of side effects and respiratory depression
- May be needed in patients who are on high dose of daily opioids and those who have significant opioid physiological dependence

Increasing the demand dose is preferable to a basal infusion rate.

PATIENT EDUCATION AND EXPECTATIONS

Patient and family education prior to the start of PCA are critical. Discuss how much pain can be expected despite optimal PCA use.

Discuss dangers of someone other than the patient pressing the button for a bolus dose (especially for pediatric patients).

BENEFITS

- Higher patient satisfaction—personal control aspect of PCA and rapid onset of pain relief
- Improved postoperative analgesia when compared with PRN analgesic regimens
- Improvements in postoperative morbidity such as postoperative pulmonary function and earlier postoperative mobilization
- Better continuous incremental titration compared with intermittent PRN analgesic dosing
- Not more cost effective
- No decrease in LOS

SIDE EFFECTS

Nausea and vomiting, pruritus, ileus, sedation, and confusion. More pruritus with morphine. If unresponsive to treatment, change to another opioid (hydromorphone or fentanyl).

Consider use of a multimodal analgesic regimen to reduce opioid requirements and opioid-induced side effects.

FIGURE 158-1. Management of IV PCA

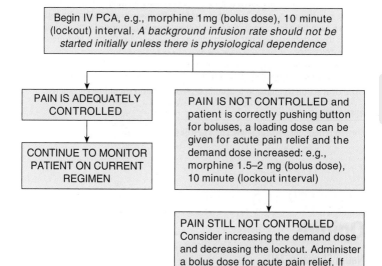

RISKS

- Respiratory depression—associated more frequently with the following factors:
  - ▸ Advanced age
  - ▸ History of obstructive sleep apnea—use of basal infusion is particularly discouraged in this population
  - ▸ Basal infusion
  - ▸ Programming errors on PCA pump (commonly an error when inputting concentration of medication)
  - ▸ Patients who have renal impairment may be unable to excrete active metabolites of morphine (morphine-6-glucuronide). In these patients, the use of a drug with no active metabolites, such as hydromorphone or fentanyl, would be preferred
- Operator-related problems, drug errors, and equipment malfunctions may affect efficacy and patient safety. Operator errors include entering an incorrect bolus dose, incorrect drug concentration, incorrect basal infusion rates, and programming a basal infusion rate when not indicated

TRANSITIONING TO PO OPIOIDS

Once pain is well controlled on a PCA and the patient is able to take PO medications, IV opioids may be transitioned to PO form.
- Determine the total amount of opioid administered over the last 24 hours
- Calculate the equianalgesic amount of the desired PO opioid (see chapter 159, Opioid Dose Equivalence Table)
  - ▸ Depending on the calculated amount of opioid (and the patient's level of pain), 1/2 to 2/3 of the daily opioid requirement may be given as a long-acting opioid
  - ▸ The remaining one half to one third can be given as a short-acting opioid for breakthrough pain
- Divide the PO opioid amount into the appropriate frequency for a 24-hour period

Notes:
- When switching from one route to another (e.g., IV to oral morphine), a dose reduction may be considered due to the greater bioavailability of the IV route. It is more prudent to start at a lower dose and titrate upward rather than the converse
- When switching from one opioid to another, dose reductions of 50% or more may need to be done to account for variations in patient metabolism and incomplete cross-tolerance
- Fentanyl patches are generally not recommended for the management of postoperative pain due to slow onset of action and length of time necessary for dose titrations

Dose conversion to methadone is complex; consultation should be considered.

REFERENCES

For references, please visit **www.TheAnesthesiaGuide.com**.

CHAPTER 159
Opioids

Naum Shaparin, MD

Bind to opioid receptors; specifically, analgesia takes place at the mu receptor.
Indications: moderate to severe pain.

ADVERSE EFFECTS AND CONTRAINDICATIONS

Opioid receptor–specific agonists (see below for meperidine, methadone, and tramadol):

System	Effects
Cardiovascular	• HR and BP decrease usually due to decreased sympathetic tone with pain relief • Dose-dependent increase in vagal tone may cause bradycardia • Histamine release from morphine may cause hypotension and resultant tachycardia • Minimal effect on contractility • May enhance myocardial depressant effects of other medications
Respiratory	• Decrease in RR due to decreased response to CO_2 • Increased tidal volume • Decreased minute ventilation • Suppression of cough reflex • Muscle rigidity with large IV boluses that can make ventilation difficult without paralysis (may be prevented with benzodiazepine premedication)
Ophthamological	• Miosis via stimulation of the Edinger–Westphal nucleus
Gastrointestinal	• Nausea/vomiting from direct stimulation of chemoreceptor trigger zone (usually happens at initiation of therapy or with dose changes) • Gastric stasis (may also be cause of nausea/vomiting) • Constipation; most patients never become tolerant to constipation (thus requiring laxatives and stool softeners) • Spasm of sphincter of Oddi
Endocrine	• May block stress response at high doses • Decrease testosterone levels with long-term use at high doses (to the point that supplementation is needed to treat sexual dysfunction)
Obstetrical/neonatal	• Neonatal CNS and respiratory depression (cross placenta)
Genitourinary	• Urinary retention due to increased ureter tone (can be reversed with atropine)
Central nervous system	• Analgesia • Sedation • Euphoria, dysphoria, or agitation • Unreliable amnesia (at high doses) • Decreased CBF and metabolic rate • Increased ICP (if opioid-induced hypoventilation is uncontrolled) • Withdrawal symptoms may occur with abrupt discontinuation • Addiction
Skin	• Histamine release (from morphine and meperidine) • May cause pruritus, redness, and hives at injection site

Meperidine (in addition to those listed above for opioid receptor–specific agonists):

System	Effects
Cardiovascular	• Myocardial depressant • May cause increased HR and contractility due to anticholinergic effect • Histamine release may cause hypotension and resultant tachycardia
Gastrointestinal	• Sphincter of Oddi spasm may be decreased compared with other opioids
Central nervous system	• Seizures may result from accumulation of the metabolite normeperidine
Skin	• Histamine release • May cause pruritus, redness, and hives at injection site

Methadone (in addition to those listed above for opioid receptor–specific agonists):

System	Effects
Cardiovascular	• QT prolongation usually above 100 mg daily dose • Review EKG if increasing dose over 100 mg per day
Respiratory	• Unexpected and delayed respiratory depression due to prolonged biphasic elimination • Especially with rapid dose increases causing accumulation
Central nervous system	• Unexpected and delayed sedation due to prolonged biphasic elimination (especially with rapid dose increases causing accumulation) • May have a role in the treatment of neuropathic pain due to NMDA receptor antagonist activity • Thought to cause less tolerance than other opioids • Useful in opioid maintenance therapy and detoxification due to long duration of action

Tramadol (in addition to those listed above for opioid receptor–specific agonists):

System	Effects
Respiratory	• Decreased risk for respiratory depression compared with other opioids
Central nervous system	• Can cause dizziness and vertigo

Tapentadol (in addition to those listed above for opioid receptor–specific agonists):

System	Effects
Renal/hepatic	• Not recommended with severe renal impairment • Reduce dosing with moderate to severe liver impairment
Respiratory	• Use with caution if COPD/respiratory compromise • Critical respiratory depression may occur even at therapeutic doses
Central nervous system	• Additive toxicity may occur with concurrent use of CNS depressants • Do not administer with MAOIs and avoid with tramadol/SSRIs • Rare risk of serotonin syndrome • Dizziness/somnolence common side effects

DRUG INTERACTIONS

Opioids potentiate the effects of other sedative and hypnotic agents.

Meperidine and MAOI/COMT can cause hyperthermia and/or delirium.

Methadone has multiple drug interactions and should be used with caution in patients with complicated medical problems, specifically those on antivirals and antibiotics (such as fluoroquinolones).

RENAL FAILURE/DIALYSIS PATIENTS

Metabolites may accumulate; therefore, consider using fentanyl or methadone as first choice opiate.

RECTAL OPIOIDS

Available for use in rare circumstances. Morphine, hydromorphone, and oxymorphone suppositories are commercially available.

OPIOIDS AND GASTRIC TUBE

No extended-release opioid recommended via GT tube due to immediate release and absorption.

OPIOID-INDUCED CONSTIPATION

Recommend use of stool softeners/mild peristaltic stimulants for chronic opioid patients.

For refractory constipation consider methylnaltrexone 8 mg q other day (weight 38–62 kg) and do not exceed 8 mg/24 h. Available IV (12 mg/0.6 mL). Contraindication: bowel obstruction.

Opioid Dose Equivalence Table				
Drug	mg PO (equipotent)	mg IV (equipotent)	Half-life (h)	Duration (h)
Morphine	30	10	2–3	3–4
MS Contin	30	–	2–3	8–12
Oxycodone	20	–	2–3	3–4
Oxycontin	20	–	2–3	8–12
Hydrocodone	30	–	3–4	4
Hydromorphone	7.5	1.5	2–3	2–4
Methadone	2 24 h oral morphine/ methadone ratio <30 mg 2:1 31–99 mg 4:1 100–299 mg 8:1 300–499 mg 12:1 500–999 mg 15:1 1,000–1,200 mg 20:1 >1,200 mg; *consider consult*	1.5 oral dose 2 mg methadone PO = 1 mg methadone IV	12–100	4–12
Fentanyl	–	100 µg single dose IM/IV PO below 80 µg buccal 24 h oral morphine dose/patch 30–59 mg = 12.5 µg/h 60–134 mg = 25 µg/h 135–224 mg = 50 µg/h 225–314 mg = 75 µg/h 315–404 mg = 100 µg/h	3–4	48–72 per patch
Oxymorphone	10	1	3–14	4–24
Tapentadol	100	–	4	4–6
Tramadol	200	–	5.5–7	6–8
Buprenorphine	0.4 (sublingual only)	0.3	20–70	

Opioid Medications, Doses, Precautions, Onset, and Duration of Action

| Medication | Usual starting dose (opioid naive >50 kg) | | Onset of action | Duration of action |
	IM/IV	PO		
Morphine	2.5–5 SC/IV q3–4 h (1.25–2.5 mg†) PCA Loading bolus 1.5 mg (usual 2 mg) Intermittent dose (PCA) 0.5–3 mg (usual 1 mg) Lockout interval 6–8 min Continuous 0.5–2 mg/h Usual concentration 1 mg/mL	5–15 mg q3–4 h (IR/oral) (2.5–7.5 mg†) *Availability:* MS IR 15, 30 mg, tablets q4 h MS IR oral solution 10 or 20 mg/mL solutions MS Contin ER in 15, 30, 60, 100, 200 mg tablets q12 h Kadian ER daily or q12 h in 10, 20, 30, 40, 50, 60, 80, 100, 200 mg capsule; Avinza ER (once daily) in 30, 45, 60, 75, 90, 120 capsules Oramorph ER 15, 30, 60, 100 mg q12 h Available rectally	PO 60 min IV 5–10 min IM 10–20 min	PO 8–12 h IV 3–4 h IM 3–4 h
Oxycodone	NA	5–10 mg q3–4 h (2.5 mg†) *Availability:* Oxycontin ER as 10, 15, 20, 30, 40, 60, 80 q8–12 h Oxy IR 5 mg q4–6 h Combinations such as Percocet (oxycodone with Tylenol) 5/325, 7.5/325, 7.5/500, 10/325, 10/650; and Percodan (with aspirin) 4.835S/325	10–15 min	3–4 h
Hydromorphone	0.2–0.6 mg SC/IV q2–3 h (0.2 mg†) PCA Bolus 0.1–0.5 mg Intermittent dose 0.05–0.5 mg Lockout 6–8 min (range up to 15 min) Continuous 0.1–0.5 mg/h Usual concentration 0.2 mg/mL	1–2 mg q3–4 h (0.5–1 mg†) *Availability:* PO IR in 2, 4, 8 mg tablets q4–6 h and liquid 5 mg/mL (brand as Dilaudid) IV 10 mg/mL Exalgo ER 8, 12, 16 mg (daily) Available rectally 3 mg q6–8 h	PO 15–30 min IV 5 min IM 10–20 min	PO 12 h IV 3–4 h IM 3–4 h

Drug	Parenteral dose	Availability / oral	Onset	Duration
Hydrocodone	NA	5 mg q3–4 h (2.5 mg†) *Availability: hydrocodone is not available in single entity form. Combination preparations are with acetaminophen or ibuprofen. Common APAP combination preparations are: Vicodin 5/500, Vicodin ES 7.5/750, Vicodin 10/660, Lorcet 10/650, Lortab 7.5/500, Lortab 10/500, Norco 10/325. Ibuprofen with hydrocodone marketed as Vicoprofen 7.5/200*	30–60 min	4–6 h
Codeine	15–30 mg SC/IM q4 h (7.5–15 mg†) No IV	PO 15, 30, and 60 mg q3–4 h, IV available as 15 mg/mL	30–45 min	4–6 h
Meperidine	75 mg SC/IM q2–3 h (25–50 mg†) Generally not recommended	Not recommended Available PO 50, 100 mg q3–4 h, and syrup 50 mg/5 mL	PO 30–60 min IV 5–10 min IM 10–20 min	PO 2–4 h IV 3–4 h IM 2–4 h
Fentanyl	25–50 µg IM/IV q1–3 h (12.5–25 µg†) PCA IV: intermittent dose (demand): range 10–50 µg (usually 10) Lockout interval 6–8 min Continuous (basal) 10–60 µg/h Usual concentration 10–50 µg/mL	Transdermal patch 12.5 µg/h q72 h Oral transmucosal has relatively rapid effect onset since significantly more vascular. Intent to be absorbed by saliva and absorbed through mucosal surface. Fentanyl as Actiq or OTFC available in 200, 400, 600, 800, 1,200, 1,600 µg. No biting/chewing. Stick lollipop should be swirled around oral mucosa. Conversion between Actiq and Fentora requires dosage conversion. Oral prep has immediate release (15–20 min) *Availability: patch as 12, 25, 50, 75, 100 µg/h. Also marketed as Duragesic. Fentora buccal tablets as 100, 200, 400, 600, 800 µg*	Patch 12–24 h IV 1–2 min Oral transmucoral 5–15 min	Patch 48–72 h IV 3–4 h Oral transmucoral 1–2 h
Methadone	2.5–5 mg q8 h (1.25 mg†)	2.5–5 mg q8 h (1.25–2.5 mg)	PO 30–60 min IV 10 min IM 10–20 min	PO 4–8 h IV 4–8 h IM 4–8 h

(continued)

Opioid Medications, Doses, Precautions, Onset, and Duration of Action (*continued*)

| Medication | Usual starting dose (opioid naïve >50 kg) | | Onset of action | Duration of action |
	IM/IV	PO		
Tapentadol	NA	50–100 bid; up to maximum 600 mg daily Nucynta brand name *Availability:* Available as 50, 75, 100 mg tablets	1.25–1.5 h	4–6 h
Oxymorphone	10 mg	5–10 mg q12 h Give 1/2 total daily dose if Opana ER *Availability:* Opana SA 5, 10 mg and ER 5, 7.5, 10, 15, 20, 30, 40 mg. Food can increase plasma concentration, so take on empty stomach Available rectally	IV 5–10 min IM 10–20 min Rectal 15–30 min PO 30–45 min	3–6 h
Tramadol	NA	50–100 daily to maximum 300 mg Available as Ultram ER or Ryzolt 100, 200, 300 mg or with Tylenol Ultracet 37.5/375 2q4–6 h (IR)	60 min	5–9 h
Pentazocine (Talwin)	IM/IV 30–60 mg q3–4 h Renal impairment Creat.¹ Clear 10–15 mL/min; give 75% dose Creat. Clear <10; give 50% of normal dose	Caution with liver disease High incidence CNS adverse effects. May precipitate withdrawal in narcotic-dependent patient Talwin available 30 mg/mL; Talwin + APAP 25/650 mg and Talwin + naloxone 50/0.5 q3–4 h	PO 15–30 min IV 5 min IM 15–20 min	3–4 h
Nalbuphine (Nubain)	Surgical anesthesia 0.3–3 mg/kg over 10–15 min and maintenance 0.25–0.5 mg/kg Pain management 10 mg/70 kg q3–6 h Maximum daily dose 160 mg Opioid-induced pruritus IV 2.5–5 mg	May precipitate withdrawal in narcotic-dependent patient Available 10 or 20 mg/mL q3–6 h	IV 5 min IM <15 min	4–6 h

Butorphanol (Stadol)	Preoperative 2 mg 60–90 min prior to surgery IM initial 2 mg; may repeat 3–4 h IV 1 mg; may repeat 3–4 h Intranasal (for HA) one spray in one nostril and may repeat after 1 h	Produces generalized CNS depression IV 1, 2 mg/mL Also available as nasal spray 10 mg/mL q3–4 h	IV 5 min IM 10–20 min	3–4 h
Buprenorphine (Buprenex)	IM/IV 0.3 mg and may be repeated once in 30–60 min Transdermal patch; if patient takes <30 mg PO morphine, use 5 µg/h patch for 1 week. If 30–80 mg PO morphine, then 10 µg/h patch for 1 week duration	Not recommended with liver disease May precipitate withdrawal in narcotic-dependent patient IV 0.3 mg/mL Patch 5, 10, 20 µg/h Sublingual 2, 8 mg (Subutex)	IV 5 min IM 10–20 min	IV 3–4 h IM 3–6 h
Remifentanil	0.5–1 µg/kg/min except if intubation occurs in <8 min, and then an initial dose of 1 µg/kg/min may be given over 30–60 s. Supplemental bolus 1 µg/kg q2–5 min prn. See PDR for dosage administration with other anesthetics	Slightly more potent than fentanyl. Rapid infusion may result in skeletal muscle/chest wall rigidity, impaired ventilation. Minimally affected by renal/hepatic function Available for reconstitution 1, 2, 5 mg	IV 1–3 min	Half-life 10–20 min; continuous infusion recommended 5 min s/p initial dose
Sufentanil (Sufenta)	IV 1–2 µg/kg with nitrous oxide maintenance; epidural 10–15 µg with 10 mL bupivacaine 0.125%	Most potent of the fentanils Available 50 µg/mL (1, 2, 5 mL)	IV 1–3 min Epidural 10 min	IV 1 h Epidural 1.7 h
Alfentanil (Alfenta, Rapifen)	Induction period <30 min, and then 8–20 µg/kg Induction period 30–60 min, and then 20–50 µg/kg Continuous infusion >45 min, and then 50–75 µg/kg	Least potent of fentanils; 1/40 as potent as fentanyl. Recommended for ESRD if need for opioid analgesia; caution if h/o bradyarrhythmias, respiratory conditions, head trauma Available 500 µg/mL (2, 5, 10, 20 mL)	Rapid	30–60 min

¹One half dose if elderly/renal impairment/liver impairment.

REVERSAL

Naloxone (Narcan) should only be used in emergencies; dilute naloxone 0.4 mg with 9 mL NS. Give 1 mL (40 µg) IVP, may repeat once or twice after waiting at least 3–5 minutes until desired effect (patient still somnolent but breathing). Avoid excessive doses that can lead to severe pain, agitation, myocardial ischemia, and pulmonary edema. May need to repeat in 30–60 minutes or start an infusion (0.4 mg/h; typically 2 mg in 500 mL) as half-life is 20–30 minutes.

REFERENCES

For references, please visit **www.TheAnesthesiaGuide.com**.

CHAPTER 160
Antidepressants and Anticonvulsants Used in Pain Management

Lucia Daiana Voiculescu, MD and Chaturani Ranasinghe, MD

Antidepressants Used for Pain Management				
Drug/principal mechanism of action	Pain indications	Common dosing[1]	Common side effects	Special considerations
Amitriptyline Tertiary amine TCA Serotonin and norepinephrine reuptake inhibitor	• Chronic pain • Neuropathic pain[2] • Headache: treatment and prophylaxis • Postherpetic neuralgia: treatment and prophylaxis	25 mg QHS to maximum 100 mg/day	Dry mouth, orthostatic hypotension, urinary retention, constipation, sedation, weight gain	**Black box warning**: increased risk of suicidality in patients younger than 24 years Caution in the elderly, patients with CAD, after acute MI, seizure disorder, angle-closure glaucoma Cardiac conduction effects. Prolonged QT if combined with cisapride Increased drug levels with other CYP 450-2D6 inhibitors.[3] Fatal in overdose Serotonin syndrome when combined with SSRIs or MAOIs **Pregnancy Class C**

(continued)

Antidepressants Used for Pain Management (*continued*)				
Drug/principal mechanism of action	Pain indications	Common dosing[1]	Common side effects	Special considerations
Nortriptyline Secondary amine TCA Serotonin and norepinephrine reuptake inhibitor	• Chronic pain[2] • Neuropathic pain[2] • Myofascial pain[2] • Burning mouth syndrome[2]	25 mg QHS to maximum 150 mg/day	Dry mouth, orthostatic hypotension, urinary retention, constipation, sedation, weight gain,[4] etc.	**Black box warning:** increased risk of suicidality in patients younger than 24 years Caution in the elderly, patients with CAD. Cardiac conduction effects including prolonged QT Drug interactions with other CYP 450-2D6 inhibitor drugs.[3] Fatal in overdose Serotonin syndrome **Pregnancy Class C**
Duloxetine • Serotonin and norepinephrine reuptake inhibitor • Weak inhibitor of dopamine reuptake	• Diabetic neuropathy[5] • Fibromyalgia[5] • Chronic musculoskeletal pain[5]	Start at 30 mg/day Maximum 60 mg/day (for pain)	Nausea, xerostomia, constipation, insomnia, somnolence, fatigue, etc.	**Black box warning:** increased risk of suicidality in patients younger than 24 years Duloxetine is not FDA approved for use in children Withdrawal syndrome Serotonin syndrome **Pregnancy Class C**
Venlafaxine • Serotonin and norepinephrine reuptake inhibitor • Weak inhibitor of dopamine reuptake	• Neuropathic pain[5] • Tension-type headache: prophylaxis[5]	37.5 mg q day or BID Maximum 225 mg/day	Somnolence, dizziness, nervousness, headache, nausea, sweating, etc.	**Black box warning:** increased risk of suicidality in patients younger than 24 years Withdrawal syndrome Caution in patients with seizure history, elderly, CV risk factors,[6] etc. Serotonin syndrome **Pregnancy Class C**

Note: SSRIs and other SNRIs not found to be effective for neuropathic pain; therefore, not included in this table.

[1] Starting at low doses and slow titration were found to reduce most adverse effects and common side effects of antidepressants used in pain management.

[2] Off-label usage.

[3] Drugs such as methadone, protease inhibitors, cimetidine, cocaine, fluoxetine, paroxetine, sertraline, bupropion can cause increased levels of TCAs.

[4] Secondary amine tricyclics have fewer reported adverse effects, such as anticholinergic side effects, compared with tertiary amine tricyclic antidepressants.

[5] FDA approved.

[6] Less commonly, cardiac conduction abnormalities and hypertension have been reported.

Anticonvulsants Used for Pain Management

Drug/principal mechanism of action	Pain indications	Common dosing[1]	Common side effects	Special considerations
Carbamazepine Sodium channel blockade	• Trigeminal neuralgia[2] • Glossopharyngeal neuralgia[2] • Neurogenic pain[4] • Pain[4] • Restless legs syndrome[4]	Start at 100 mg BID Gradual increase to 400 mg BID	Drowsiness, unsteadiness, nausea and vomiting, fatigue, suicidal ideation	**Black box warnings:** serious skin rashes such as Stevens–Johnson syndrome and toxic epidermal necrolysis.[3] Rarely aplastic anemia, agranulocytosis, and other blood dyscrasias reported (perform baseline and then q3–6 months hematologic testing) **Pregnancy Class D**
Oxcarbamazapine Sodium channel blockade	• Neuropathic pain[4] • Trigeminal neuralgia[4]	150 mg QHS to 1,200 mg BID maximum	Dizziness, somnolence, headache, abnormal gait, nausea, hyponatremia	**Black box warnings:** serious skin rashes such as Stevens–Johnson syndrome and toxic epidermal necrolysis.[3] Rarely aplastic anemia, agranulocytosis, and other blood dyscrasias reported (perform baseline and then q3–6 months hematologic testing) Lower dose in patients with renal insufficiency Liver enzyme P450 CYP3A4 inducer[5] Contraindicated with MAOIs. Risk of serotonin syndrome in combination with SSRIs, TCAs etc. **Pregnancy Class C**
Lamotrigine • Sodium channel blockade • Weak inhibitory effect on the 5-HT$_3$ receptor	• Neuropathic pain[4] • Trigeminal neuralgia[4] • Migraine[4]	Start at 25 mg q day Gradual increase to 400 mg/day	Dizziness, diplopia, nausea, risk of suicidality, rash	**Black box warnings:** serious skin rashes (Stevens–Johnson, rare toxic epidermal necrolysis, and rash-related deaths).[3] Age is the only risk factor identified (not indicated in patients younger than 16 years) Avoid abrupt withdrawal Adjust dose if renal insufficiency **Pregnancy Class C**

Drug / Mechanism	Uses	Dosing	Side effects	Comments
Topiramate • Na, Ca channel blockade • NMDA antagonist • Weak inhibitor of carbonic anhydrase	• Migraine prophylaxis[2] • Neuropathic pain[4]	Start at 25 mg q day; titrate gradually to 200 mg BID	Somnolence, dizziness, confusion, weight loss	Metabolic acidosis, acute myopia associated with secondary angle-closure glaucoma, nephrolithiasis, leucopenia, and osteoporosis have been reported CYP3A4 inducer[5] Increased risk of suicidal thoughts/behavior Adjust dose if renal insufficiency Do not discontinue therapy abruptly **Pregnancy Class C**
Pregabalin • Calcium channel alpha(2)-delta site ligand	• Diabetic neuropathy[2] • Postherpetic neuralgia (PHN)[2] • Fibromyalgia[2] • Postoperative pain[4] • Central pain[4]	Start at 50 mg TID or 75 mg BID Gradual increase to 600 mg/day	Dizziness, sedation, weight gain	Rarely; angioedema, rhabdomyolysis, serious skin rashes, suicidality have been reported Not metabolized by hepatic enzymes. Adjust dose if renal insufficiency Avoid abrupt withdrawal **Pregnancy Class C**
Gabapentin Unknown	• Postherpetic neuralgia[2] • Neuropathic pain[4] • Diabetic peripheral neuropathy[4] • Postoperative pain: preemptive therapy[4] • Fibromyalgia[4] • Migraine prophylaxis[4]	Start at 100–300 mg QHS Gradual increase to 3,600 mg/day	Dizziness, sedation, weight gain, peripheral edema, ataxia	Not metabolized by hepatic enzymes. Adjust dose if renal insufficiency Increased risk of suicidal thoughts/behavior Tumorigenic potential (in rats) Avoid abrupt withdrawal **Pregnancy Class C**

Note: Due to the sedative side effects of anticonvulsants, caution is advised when combining with other CNS depressants and alcohol.

[1] Starting at low doses and slow titration were found to reduce most adverse effects and common side effects of antiepileptics used to treat neuropathic pain.

[2] FDA approved.

[3] Total incidence of rash is 10% and severe rash is 3 in 1,000. Nearly all cases associated with first 2–8 weeks after initiation of therapy. If rash develops, discontinue medication.

[4] Off-label usage.

[5] May decrease efficacy of medications such as oral contraceptives, plavix, protease inhibitors, tramadol, etc.

CHAPTER 161
Other Adjuvant Agents Commonly Used in Pain Management

Lucia Daiana Voiculescu, MD and Amit Poonia, MD

Various Adjuvant Agents Used for Pain Management				
Drug/principal mechanism of action	Pain indications	Common dosing[1]	Common side effects	Special considerations
Tramadol Dual mechanism: serotonin/ norepinephrine reuptake inhibition Weak mu-opioid receptor agonism	• Acute and chronic pain: moderate– severe[1] • Postoperative pain[2] • Neuropathic pain[2]	50–100 mg po q6–8 h	Nausea, vomiting, constipation, dizziness, headaches Serious reactions: seizures, serotonin syndrome	Caution if history/risk of seizure Avoid abrupt cessation Risk of suicidality **Pregnancy Class C**
Clonidine Central alpha-2 adrenergic agonist	• Peripheral neuropathy[2] • Postherpetic neuralgia[2] • Cancer pain[2] • CRPS[2] • Postoperative pain[2] • Adjuvant in neuraxial and peripheral nerve blocks[2] • Opioid withdrawal[2]	0.1 mg po q12 h weekly titration up to 2.4 mg/day 0.1 mg/day transdermal Up to 0.6 mg/ day 30 μg/h epidural infusion	Hypotension, bradycardia, AV block, dry mouth, drowsiness, sedation fatigue, depression, fever	Avoid abrupt withdrawal, risk of rebound hypertension **Pregnancy Class C**
Ketamine NMDA receptor antagonism	• Intraoperative and postoperative pain[2] • Burn pain[2] • Cancer pain[2] • Neuropathic pain[2] • Opioid- induced hyperalgesia[2]	IV infusion Transdermal SQ infusion	In analgesic doses: hypersalivation, anorexia, nausea, elevated BP, hallucinations, withdrawal syndrome (long-term use)	**Black box warnings:** emergence reactions— various degrees of psychologic manifestations from pleasant dream-like states to irrational behavior and emergence delirium. The 100 mg/ mL concentration of ketamine hydrochloride injection should not be injected intravenously without proper dilution **Pregnancy Class D**

(continued)

Various Adjuvant Agents Used for Pain Management (*continued*)				
Drug/principal mechanism of action	Pain indications	Common dosing[1]	Common side effects	Special considerations
Lidocaine • Blocks sodium channels • Decreases ionic flux through the neuronal membrane	• Postherpetic neuralgia[1] • Local anesthesia, postoperative pain[1] • Neuropathic pain[2] • Burn pain[2]	Topical: transdermal maximum three patches/ 24 h IV: various protocols		**Pregnancy Class C**

[1]FDA approved.
[2]Off-label usage for neuropathic pain.

Muscle Relaxant Agents Commonly Used in Pain Management				
Drug/principal mechanism of action	Pain indications	Common dosing[1]	Common side effects	Special considerations
Baclofen GABA-B agonist	• Spasticity[2] • Myofascial pain[3] • Trigeminal neuralgia[3] • GERD[3]	Oral: start at 5 mg TID Maximum 80 mg/day Intrathecal: for severe spasticity	Drowsiness, weakness, fatigue, hypotension, constipation, nausea	**Black box warnings (for the intrathecal administration):** avoid abrupt cessation–high fever, altered mental status, exaggerated rebound spasticity, and muscle rigidity after abrupt D/C **Pregnancy Class C**
Benzodiazepines: Diazepam Clonazepam GABA-B agonist	• Diazepam: • Muscle spasm • Acute postoperative myofascial pain[3] • Clonazepam: • Neuralgia • Periodic leg movement • Spasticity[3]	Diazepam: 2–10 mg po q6–8 h 5–10 mg IM/ IV[4] q3–4 h prn Clonazepam: 0.5–4 mg po q8 h	Drowsiness, dizziness, impaired coordination, amnesia, confusion, somnolence, irritability	Significant dependence, abuse and addiction potential associated with chronic benzodiazepine administration **Pregnancy Class D**
Tizanidine Central alpha-2 adrenergic agonist	• Spasticity[2] • Muscle spasm and pain[3] • Acute pain[3] • Chronic headache[3]	2–8 mg TID	Drowsiness, dry mouth, somnolence, asthenia, hypotension, bradycardia	Additive effects with alcohol and other CNS depressants Reduced clearance with oral contraceptives **Pregnancy Class C**

(*continued*)

Muscle Relaxant Agents Commonly Used in Pain Management (*continued*)				
Drug/principal mechanism of action	Pain indications	Common dosing[1]	Common side effects	Special considerations
Cyclobenzaprine Centrally acting muscle relaxant	• Muscle spasm and pain[2] • Fibromyalgia[3] • TMJ disorder[3]	5–10 mg po TID	Drowsiness, dry mouth, nervousness, irritability, nausea, heartburns	Pregnancy Class B
Orphenadrine Not fully identified	• Musculoskeletal pain[2]	100 mg po q12 h 60 mg IM/IV[4] q12 h	Dry mouth, tachycardia, blurred vision, urinary hesitancy, weakness	Pregnancy Class C

[1]Starting at low doses and slow titration were found to reduce most adverse effects and common side effects.
[2]FDA approved.
[3]Off-label usage.
[4]The injectable form can be useful in the immediate postoperative period.

CHAPTER 162
Epidural Analgesia

Frantzces Alabre, FNP-C, DNP and Christopher Gharibo, MD

BENEFITS OF EPIDURAL PATIENT-CONTROLLED ANALGESIA (EPCA)

- Superior pain relief when compared with IV PCA, subcutaneous and oral analgesics
- Superior static and dynamic (mechanical) analgesia and hence improved mechanical DVT prophylaxis
- Improved mobilization and physical rehabilitation
- Improved pulmonary function
- Earlier return of postoperative bowel function
- Increased extremity perfusion due to vasodilatation and reduced platelet aggregation
- Reduced risk of complications related to immobility
- No evidence of decreased cognitive dysfunction in elderly patients

CONTRAINDICATIONS

- Coagulopathy: functional platelet abnormalities; platelets <80,000; elevated PT, PTT, and INR. Antiplatelet medications. See chapter 119 for more information
- Sepsis, local, or systemic infection
- Surgeons often request no regional analgesia when there is a concern of possible compartment syndrome (e.g., tibial plateau fracture). However, there is no evidence in the literature to support the claim that diagnosis could be delayed by regional analgesia

CHECKING PLACEMENT OF EPIDURAL CATHETER

- Check all connections, tubing, and pump function
- Check catheter insertion and measurement at the skin (a transparent dressing makes this easier). Determine if catheter has pulled out of the epidural space
- Aspirate the epidural catheter for blood or cerebrospinal fluid (CSF)
  - ‣ If blood return, the epidural catheter can be pulled back 0.5–1 cm and reaspirated
  - ‣ If CSF return, remove epidural and consider epidural catheter replacement
- Consider rebolusing the epidural after the catheter has been pulled back and aspirate is negative

Test dose with 3 mL 1.5% lidocaine with epinephrine 1:200,000

- If there is an increase in heart rate (≥10 bpm) or blood pressure (SBP increase by ≥15 mm Hg), or an increase in T-wave amplitude by more than 25%, the catheter is likely intravascular
- If there is profound sensory or motor block in the abdomen and extremities within 5 minutes, the catheter is in the subarachnoid space
- If there is an abdominal sensory level (for a lumbar placement), the catheter is in the epidural space. That is not always obtained with such a small dose
- Please note: subarachnoid and epidural placements are often associated with a drop in blood pressure following test dose administration

EPIDURAL INFUSION ANALGESICS

The more hydrophilic the opioid, the more cephalad spread will be seen, with the risk of respiratory depression.

Opioids		
Fentanyl	Lipophilic	2–5 µg/mL
Hydromorphone	Intermediate	10–30 µg/mL
Morphine	Hydrophilic	–

Local Anesthetics	
Bupivacaine	0.0625–0.125–0.25%
Ropivacaine	0.125–0.2–0.25%

MOST COMMONLY USED COMBINATION OF OPIOIDS AND LOCAL ANESTHETICS

Fentanyl/bupivacaine:

Fentanyl 2 µg/bupivacaine 0.125%	Fentanyl 5 µg/bupivacaine 0.125%
Fentanyl 2 µg/bupivacaine 0.0625%	Fentanyl 5 µg/bupivacaine 0.0625%

Fentanyl/ropivacaine:

Fentanyl 2 µg/ropivacaine 0.125%	Fentanyl 5 µg/ropivacaine 0.125%
Fentanyl 2 µg/ropivacaine 0.25%	Fentanyl 5 µg/ropivacaine 0.25%

INITIAL LOAD

- Spread depends on volume; typically the volume that will block 1 lumbar dermatome will block only 0.7 thoracic dermatome and 2 cervical dermatomes: 1L = 0.7T = 2C
- A rule of thumb to determine the needed volume (lumbar placement):
  - One milliliter per dermatome (counting from S5) for 150 cm of height + 0.1 mL per dermatome for each 5 cm above 150 cm
  - For example, to reach T8 (i.e., 15 dermatomes from S5) in a 170-cm patient, one should inject $(15 \times 1) + (15 \times 0.1 \times 4) = 21$ mL (fractionated, 5 mL at a time)
  - Decrease this dose by about 30% in the elderly and in pregnant women
- For CSE, once spinal is wearing off, load with a reduced dose (typically 4–8 mL) and initiate infusion

TYPICAL INITIAL INFUSION RATES

Basal 3–6 mL/h; bolus 3–4 mL q15–30 minutes.

INITIAL TITRATION OF DOSAGE

- If persistent pain and stable vital signs: one may give 4–5 mL loading dose of the infusion mixture
- Initial dosing and titration are related to the need for mobilization
  - For example, 4 mL/h, bolus 3 mL q15 minutes for patient with minimal mobilization
  - Use higher basal and/or bolus for, for example, total knee replacement on CPM machine
- Start at low volumes and reassess and titrate if needed q30–60 minutes
- If no pain relief after 30–60 minutes and vital signs are stable, reevaluate; determine abdominal sensory level with alcohol swab; check epidural placement for possible catheter migration. If indeterminate, one may also use a test dose with lidocaine and epinephrine (see above)

Side effects and complications:
- Hypotension
- Excessive numbness/weakness of lower limbs—some degree of sensory or motor block may be acceptable
- Excessive block on one side of the body
- Sedation
- Pruritus (related to the opioids)
- Urinary retention
- Respiratory depression—much less common with epidural opioids than IV opioids
- Local anesthetic toxicity—metallic taste in the mouth, confusion, dizziness, hypotension, seizures
- Epidural technique and catheter-related complications: "wet tap," postdural puncture headache
- Catheter migration
- Infection (1:100,000)
- Epidural hematoma (1:100,000)/abscess:
  - Cardinal signs: progressive diffuse back pain, progressive neurological deficits, cauda equina syndrome, bowel and bladder incontinence
  - If spinal compression is suspected, obtain prompt neurosurgical or neurology consultation and STAT CT or MRI. Time is of the essence to perform a laminectomy and allow return of neurological function

SIDE EFFECTS MANAGEMENT

- *Opioid-related side effects:*
  - Consider decreasing basal and/or demand dose. Consider switching to a lower concentration of opioid or switching to a pure local anesthetic solution

- In low doses (40–200 μg/h), intravenous naloxone will minimize the unpleasant side effects associated with epidural opioids without decreasing the analgesic effect. It is indicated for treatment of generalized itching and nausea/vomiting. Higher doses are necessary when treating respiratory depression or oversedation
  - When naloxone is utilized in the treatment of epidural analgesia, it *must be administered via intravenous or intramuscular route* and may not be given epidurally
  - Side effect management with naloxone must always be infused by a pump for a continuously regulated infusion. Naloxone infusion may be required for approximately 24 hours for treatment of side effects of epidural opioids
  - Prepare a 10 μg/mL naloxone NS solution. Initial bolus is 80–120 μg (8–12 mL). Naloxone rate is 1–3 μg/kg/h for pruritus; therefore, a starting dose for a 70-kg person is 7 mL/h with a PCA bolus of 3 mL with a lockout of 6 minutes
- *For respiratory depression, do not use naloxone PCA*
  - Support ventilation, administer oxygen
  - Stop opioid administration
  - Administer naloxone bolus. Dilute 0.4 mg naloxone in 10 mL and administer 1–2 mL at a time to reverse the opioid effect
  - Large doses may reverse analgesia or induce cardiopulmonary failure
  - If necessary, begin naloxone infusion 5–10 μg/kg/h until effects of opioid overdose have dissipated. Patients should be in a monitored setting
- *Numbness and weakness*: A mild degree of numbness or weakness that does not impair standing and ambulation may be acceptable. Reinforce fall precautions during the entire period that epidural analgesics are in effect
- *Hypotension*:
  - Immediately stop the infusion if clinically significant
  - Consider IV and/or PO hydration, or vasopressors if fluid administration must be limited (lung surgery)
  - Consider switching to a lower concentration of local anesthetic or to a pure opioid solution
- *One-sided numbness*: Reposition patient on unaffected side if permissible and/or pull back epidural catheter by 1 cm, retape, and consider giving the patient a syringe bolus
- *Pruritus*: Diphenhydramine (Benadryl) 25–50 mg IV q4 hours prn or Vistaril 25 mg IM q4 hours prn or nalbuphine 5–10 mg IV q6 hours prn. All have some sedative effect
- *Nausea/vomiting*: Refer to chapter 69

DVT PROPHYLAXIS AND EPIDURAL ANALGESIA

See chapter 119.

CONSIDERATION FOR ORAL ANALGESICS AFTER EPIDURAL REMOVAL

- Short-acting analgesic choices: oxycodone hydromorphone (Dilaudid); hydrocodone with or without acetaminophen
- Long-acting analgesics: MS Contin 15 mg po q12 hours or Oxycontin 10 mg po q12 hours
- Neuropathic pain agents: pregabalin (Lyrica) 50 mg bid or gabapentin (Neurontin) 300 mg tid
- Skeletal muscle relaxant: tizanidine (Zanaflex) 2–6 mg qHS or bid
- NSAIDs: celecoxib (Celebrex) 100–200 mg q12 hours, meloxicam (Mobic) 7.5 mg bid

REFERENCES

For references, please visit **www.TheAnesthesiaGuide.com**.

CHAPTER 163
Management of Continuous Peripheral Nerve Blocks

Lisa Doan, MD

Operative site	Catheter location	Typical settings using 0.125–0.2% ropivacaine: basal rate (mL/h)/ bolus (mL)/lockout (min)
Shoulder, proximal humerus	Interscalene	4/3/15
Distal humerus, elbow, forearm, wrist, hand	Supraclavicular, infraclavicular, axillary	4/3/15
Thorax, breast, abdomen	Paravertebral	6/4/15
Hip	Lumbar plexus	4–6/4/15
Thigh, knee	Lumbar plexus or femoral ± sciatic	4/3/15
Ankle, foot	Popliteal sciatic	4/3/15

Typical Settings for Continuous Peripheral Nerve Block Infusions

Catheter infusions often use 0.125% bupivacaine or 0.2% ropivacaine (less motor block), although some practitioners use higher or lower concentrations.

Infusion rates should be adjusted for optimal analgesia and to limit motor block that can interfere with physical therapy.

MANAGEMENT OF COMMON ISSUES

- Inadequate analgesia:
  - ‣ Intravenous or oral analgesics may be needed for pain in areas not covered by the block. Typically, brachial plexus blocks should cover the full area of the surgery, while lower extremity blocks might not (e.g., lumbar plexus block for THA or femoral block for TKA will not cover areas innervated by the sciatic nerve)
  - ‣ Assess for catheter dislodgement or disconnection
  - ‣ Give a 5–15 mL bolus of local anesthetic (fractionated). Reassess after 15–20 minutes
  - ‣ Consider replacing the catheter or using alternative forms of analgesia
- Dislodgement:
  - ‣ Methods to secure catheters include the following:
    - ▪ Benzoin or other topical adhesive is placed around the catheter entry site. Skin adhesive strips and a clear occlusive dressing are placed on the adhesive
    - ▪ A stabilization device may be used
    - ▪ Tunneling or suturing may be considered
- Leakage at insertion site:
  - ‣ There may be some minimal leakage at the insertion site as local anesthetic can track along the catheter. The dressing can be reinforced
  - ‣ Leakage may also occur if there is dislodgement of the catheter
- Blood in/around catheter:
  - ‣ Assess for intravascular catheter migration. Monitor the patient for signs and symptoms of local anesthetic systemic toxicity

- Excessive numbness/motor block:
  - Reduce the infusion rate and reassess the patient within an hour
  - If pain control is inadequate with lower infusions, discuss with patient alternative forms of analgesia versus increasing infusion rate again
  - If numbness or motor block is persistent, consider nerve injury and/or hematoma (see the section "Complications")

CONTINUOUS PERIPHERAL NERVE BLOCKS AND ANTICOAGULATION

- There are no clear recommendations
- Current ASRA guidelines recommend for deep plexus or peripheral block using the same guidelines for neuraxial anesthesia (Grade 1C recommendation): see chapter 119
- Retrospective studies suggest these guidelines may be too strict, but further studies are needed

COMPLICATIONS

- Bleeding:
  - Pain, neurological deficit, drop in hematocrit
  - Imaging such as CT
  - Supportive therapy, surgical consultation
- Neurological injury (see chapter 129):
  - Symptoms normally noted after block recedes: numbness, weakness, pain, paresthesias
  - Rule out bleeding or vascular injury. If bleeding, surgical consultation and supportive therapy
  - For minor deficits, schedule follow-up. If deficit does not resolve, consult neurology
  - For major deficits, consult neurology (possible EMG/NCS). Supportive therapy such as PT/OT
- Infection:
  - Risk factors:
    - ICU stay
    - Catheter in place >48 hours (but with impeccable care, catheters have been kept in place for weeks, e.g., in combat casualty patients who need multiple surgeries)
    - Femoral or axillary catheter
  - Management:
    - Remove the catheter
    - Administer antibiotics
    - Consider consultation with infectious disease specialist
    - Deep tissue infections may require imaging and surgical consultation
- Falls (lower extremity catheters):
  - Patient and PT education is paramount. Loss of proprioception might be more important than motor block
  - Literature data are conflicting as to whether falls are more common in patients with perineural catheters

AMBULATORY CATHETERS

- Patient selection:
  - Patients may require a caretaker the day of the procedure or longer and possibly for removal of the catheter
  - Avoid in patients with renal or hepatic insufficiency to avoid local anesthetic toxicity
- Various infusion pumps are available with varying reservoir volumes and varying basal infusion and/or bolus dose capabilities
- Patient education:
  - Patients should be educated on signs of infection and local anesthetic toxicity
  - Instruction on the infusion pump and on catheter site care should be discussed
  - Oral analgesics may be needed
  - Limb protection and fall precautions should be discussed
  - Instructions should be given verbally and in writing, including contact information for a health care provider

- Catheter removal options:
  - ‣ Written instruction for patient or caretaker
  - ‣ Telephone instruction for patient or caretaker
  - ‣ Health care provider removal

REFERENCES

For references, please visit **www.TheAnesthesiaGuide.com**.

CHAPTER 164
Pain and Sedation Scales in Adults

Lisa Doan, MD

PAIN SCALES

Numerical Rating Pain Scale: 0 (no pain) to 10 (most severe pain) scale.

FIGURE 164-1. Visual Analog Scale (VAS)

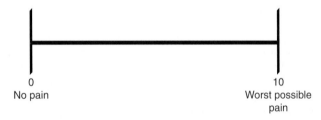

0
No pain

10
Worst possible
pain

It is a horizontal line with no pain on the left and severe pain on the right. Patients mark along the line to represent their level of pain, which is then measured in mm. A 10 cm long line is recommended.

FIGURE 164-2. Wong–Baker FACES Pain Rating Scale

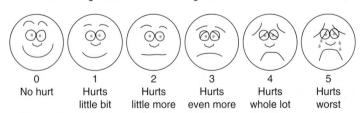

0	1	2	3	4	5
No hurt	Hurts little bit	Hurts little more	Hurts even more	Hurts whole lot	Hurts worst

This scale uses six drawings of facial features ranging from smiling (no pain) to crying (severe pain). It has been validated for use in children over 3 years of age. Reprinted with permission from Hockenberry M, Wilson D, Winkelstein ML. *Wong's Essentials of Pediatric Nursing*, 8th ed. Copyright © 2009, Mosby, St. Louis.

SEDATION SCALES

The following are commonly used scales to monitor sedation in patients receiving opioids; monitoring sedation during PCA use is especially critical.

Pasero Opioid-Induced Sedation Scale	
Score	Level of sedation
S	Sleep, easy to arouse
1	Awake and alert
2	Slightly drowsy, easily aroused
3	Frequently drowsy, arousable
4	Somnolent, hard to arouse

Ramsay Sedation Scale	
Score	Level of sedation
1	Anxious and agitated or restless, or both
2	Cooperative, oriented, and tranquil
3	Responds to commands only
4	Brisk response to light glabellar tap or loud auditory stimulus
5	Sluggish response to light glabellar tap or loud auditory stimulus
6	No response to a light glabellar tap or loud auditory stimulus

Richmond Agitation–Sedation Scale		
Score	Level of agitation or sedation	Description
+4	Combative	Combative or violent
+3	Very agitated	Attempts to remove tubes or catheters or is aggressive toward staff
+2	Agitated	Nonpurposeful movement or ventilator dyssynchrony
+1	Restless	Anxious but nonaggressive or nonvigorous movements
0	Alert and calm	
−1	Drowsy	Not fully alert but with >10 s awakening with eye contact to voice
−2	Light sedation	<10 s awakening with eye contact to voice
−3	Moderate sedation	Any movement other than eye contact to voice
−4	Deep sedation	Not responsive to voice but moves with physical stimulation
−5	Unarousable	Not responsive to voice or physical stimulation

REFERENCES

For references, please visit **www.TheAnesthesiaGuide.com**.

CHAPTER 165
Pediatric Postoperative Analgesia

F. Wickham Kraemer III, MD

FACTORS IN DETERMINING POSTOPERATIVE PAIN TREATMENT PLAN

- *Severity of pain*:
  - ‣ Minor or outpatient procedures require oral opioids or NSAIDs to complement any regional anesthesia block
  - ‣ Major surgery requires regional anesthesia, if applicable, and scheduled or continuous opiate administration with NSAIDs, benzodiazepines, or other pain medications as indicated
- *Type of surgery*:
  - ‣ Abdominal: regional, opioids, NSAIDs, multimodal
  - ‣ Thoracic: regional strongly recommended, opioids, NSAIDs, multimodal
  - ‣ Laparoscopic: opioids, NSAIDs, local infiltration
  - ‣ Neurosurgical: opioids, infiltration regional (less loss of motor function in neurologic exam), avoid sedation, generally avoid NSAIDs
  - ‣ ENT: opioids, avoid sedation in airway compromise, avoid NSAIDs in T&A
  - ‣ Orthopedic: regional anesthesia, benzodiazepines and antispasmodics, opioids, NSAIDs
  - ‣ Plastic: opioids, NSAIDS for minor surgery—avoid in reconstructive surgery, local infiltration
  - ‣ Ophthalmologic: opioids, topical local anesthetics, NSAIDs
  - ‣ Urologic: regional anesthesia—caudals, opioids, NSAIDs, antispasmodics (bladder)
  - ‣ Cardiac: opioids, NSAIDs, regional anesthesia (neuraxial based on postoperative coagulation plan)
- *Age and size of child*:
  - ‣ Weight-based dosing regimens to account for various sizes of children, ideal weight-based dosing for obese adolescents
  - ‣ Neonates:
    - ▪ Require higher monitoring due to generally narrower therapeutic range
    - ▪ Require continuous or scheduled delivery of pain medications due to inability to communicate
  - ‣ Infants have similar needs based on decreased communication. Frequent pain evaluation with developmentally appropriate rating scales prevents inadequate treatment of pain
  - ‣ By age 4, can communicate differing intensities of pain
  - ‣ Age 6 or 7: can self-administer medications through patient-controlled analgesia (PCA) and patient-controlled epidural analgesia (PCEA) systems; if they can play a video game, they should cognitively be able to press a button for pain
- *Use of regional anesthesia/analgesia*:
  - ‣ Parents agree to regional anesthesia by experienced provider
  - ‣ Contraindications: local infection, sepsis, preexisting neurologic condition, allergy or hypersensitivity, coagulation issues per ASRA guidelines for neuraxial anesthesia
- *Comorbidities*:
  - ‣ Spina bifida and previous spine surgery (myelomeningocele, hardware) and coagulopathy are relative contraindications to neuraxial regional anesthesia
  - ‣ Liver dysfunction requires dosing adjustments for opioids, benzodiazepines
  - ‣ Renal dysfunction requires dosing adjustments for opioids, NSAIDs

- ‣ Respiratory dysfunction including OSA requires dosing adjustment for opioids, benzodiazepines; special consideration with NSAIDs and asthmatic patients
- ‣ Neurologic dysfunction, central or peripheral deficits are relative contraindications to regional anesthesia

TIPS

- Multimodal pain treatment is guided by using different medications at moderate doses to decrease the risk of side effects or toxicity from any one therapy
- Be flexible and adaptive in treating children's (and parents') pain, as all pain is perceived differently—some have more emotional pain; others have more sensory pain

PHARMACOLOGY: OPIOIDS, LOCAL ANESTHETICS, NSAIDS, AND THE REST

- Opioids can be delivered through many routes: PO, nasal, IV through PCA, continuous infusion and intermittently, epidural and intrathecal
- IM and SQ injections should be avoided as young patients have more fear of the delivery method than of the pain itself
- Local anesthetics can be delivered through peripheral injections, peripherally placed catheters, epidural catheters and caudal injections, as well as intrathecal placement. Topical gels and patches are contraindicated on incisions
- Additional treatment medications: NSAIDs, benzodiazepines, NMDA antagonists, alpha-2 antagonists

Typical Settings for IV Patient-Controlled Analgesia				
Drug	Demand dose (μg/kg)	Lockout interval (min)	Basal infusion (μg/kg/h)	One-hour limit (μg/kg)
Morphine	20	8–10	0–20	100
Hydromorphone	4	8–10	0–4	20
Fentanyl	0.5	6–8	0–0.5	2.5
Nalbuphine	20	8–10	0–20	100

Typical Doses of Opioids		
Opioid	Route	Dose and interval
Morphine	Oral	0.3 mg/kg q3–4 h
	IV	25–100 μg/kg q3–4 h
	Infusion	10–30 μg/kg/h
Hydromorphone	Oral	40–80 μg/kg q4 h
	IV	10–20 μg/kg q3–4 h
	Infusion	3–4 μg/kg/h
Fentanyl	IV	0.5–1 μg/kg q2 h
	Infusion	0.25–1 μg/kg/h
Nalbuphine	IV	25–100 μg/kg q4 h
Methadone	Oral	0.05–0.1 mg/kg q6–12 h
	IV	0.025–0.1 mg/kg q6–12 h
Oxycodone	Oral	0.05–0.15 mg/kg q4 h
Hydrocodone	Oral	0.05–0.1 mg/kg q4 h

Local Anesthesia Dosing					
Drug (mg/kg)	Spinal	Epidural	Infusion (h)	Peripheral	Infiltration
Chloroprocaine	NR	10–30	30	8–10	8–10
Lidocaine	1–2.5	5–7	2–3	5–7	5–7
Bupivacaine	0.3–0.5	2–3	0.4	2–3	2–3
Neonates			0.25		
Ropivacaine	NR	2.5–4	0.4–0.5	2.5–4	2.5–4
Neonates			0.25		

NR: not recommended. Neonatal dosing is lower due to immature liver function and decreased protein binding capacity.

Peripheral Nerve Blocks		
Body area	Blocks	Surgical location
Upper extremity blocks	Interscalene	Shoulder/proximal humerus
	Supraclavicular	Shoulder to hand
	Infraclavicular	Elbow/forearm/hand
	Axillary	Forearm/hand
	Wrist	Hand
Lower extremity blocks	Lumbar plexus	Hip/anterior thigh/knee
	Femoral; 3-in-1; fascia iliaca	Anterior thigh/knee
	Sciatic	Ankle/foot
	Ankle block	Foot
Abdominal, genital, head blocks	Ilioinguinal/iliohypogastric	Inguinal hernia/orchidopexy
	Pararectus sheath block	Umbilical hernia
	Penile block	Circumcision/hypospadias
	Supraorbital/supratrochlear	Scalp incision/headaches
	Infraorbital	Cleft lip/sinus surgery
	Greater auricular	Otoplasty/tympanoplasty
	Occipital	Occipital incision/headaches

Nonsteroidal Anti-Inflammatory Drugs and Acetaminophen			
Drug	Dose	Interval (h)	Daily maximum
Aspirin	10–15 mg/kg (PO)	4–6	90 mg/kg/d
Acetaminophen	10–15 mg/kg (PO)	4–6	40–75 mg/kg/d (up to 4 g)
	15–20 mg/kg (PR)	6–8*	
	10–15 mg/kg (IV)	6–8	
Ibuprofen	6–10 mg/kg (PO)	4–6	40 mg/kg/d (up to 2.4 g)
Naproxen	5–10 mg/kg (PO)	12	20 mg/kg/d
Ketorolac	0.5 mg/kg, maximum 30 mg (IV) Not for neonates	6	2 mg/kg/d (up to 120 mg)

Neonatal dosing denoted with "*".

ADJUVANT THERAPY

- Diazepam: treatment of painful muscle spasm and anxiety; 0.05 mg/kg IV and 0.1 mg/kg PO every 6–8 hours; patients with spasticity or tolerance to benzodiazepines may require larger dose or more frequent interval

- Ketamine: powerful analgesia in subanesthetic doses for opioid-tolerant patients or refractory pain, that is, neuropathic or palliative; continuous infusion 0.1–0.2 mg/kg/h to start up to 1 mg/kg/h titrated while patient is highly monitored, usually critical care setting. Oral dosing should be done by chronic pain expert
- Clonidine: used in combination with opioids; provides sedation; 2–4 µg/kg PO every 12 hours with transdermal dosing of 0.1 mg for children weighing more than 25 kg; 1 µg/kg added to local anesthesia for peripheral nerve blocks can prolong the sensory and motor block by a few hours

NONPHARMACOLOGIC THERAPY

- Infants: swaddling, pacifier, sucrose drops, rocking, holding, music
- Children: comfort toy/blanket, music, video games, parental presence, gentle reassurance, and guidance
- Adolescents: guided imagery, hypnosis, deep breathing, music, biofeedback, acupuncture

REFERENCES

For references, please visit **www.TheAnesthesiaGuide.com**.

CHAPTER 166
Acute Pain Management of the Chronic Pain Patient

Vickie Verea, MD and Christopher Gharibo, MD

Higher postoperative opioid requirements due to chronic opioid and other adjuvant pain medication use.

OPIOID TOLERANCE

Many patients have opioid tolerance and dependence; difficulty in managing acute pain.
- *Tolerance*: increasing amounts of opioids needed to provide comparable pain relief
- *Physical dependence*: withdrawal symptoms on abrupt cessation of the opioid
- *Addiction*: behavioral condition with recreational use of a substance in spite of harmful effects
- *Pseudoaddiction*: iatrogenic phenomenon in which patients are *perceived* by health care workers as displaying addictive behavior due to their increasing requests for pain medications in the setting of mistreatment or undertreatment of their pain

PREOPERATIVE PERIOD

- *Identify* the patient on chronic opioid therapy *early*, preferably prior to the day of the surgery (e.g., during *preadmission testing*)
- Detailed history and thorough assessment including a *detailed analgesic history* of current medications, dosages, past favorable and adverse reactions to analgesics
- Would patients benefit from *"medical optimization" by their pain medicine physician* and/or by receiving preoperative nerve blocks or spinal injections to decrease their chronic pain? (For example, a patient with complex regional pain syndrome undergoing orthopedic surgery may benefit from preoperative sympathetic nerve

blocks; a patient with lumbosacral radiculopathy may benefit from epidural steroid injections prior to joint surgery.)

- Develop a *multimodal analgesic plan* for the postoperative period in coordination with the pain service. Educate patient with respect to the multimodal analgesic plan of care, what to do in case of pain, expectations, and limitations. Ideally, include continuous regional anesthetic or epidural technique as well as a selective use of combination of NSAIDs, anticonvulsants, anxiolytics, antispasmodics, and antidepressants
- Do not underestimate the *psychological* dimension of pain. Psychological/psychiatric support might be useful
- Patients should *continue all analgesics into the preoperative period including the day of surgery, unless contraindicated.* Otherwise, the patient will have considerable rebound pain and withdrawal discomfort and pain due to absence of his or her routine analgesics
- *Preemptive treatment with NSAIDs and anticonvulsants* can be implemented the morning of the surgery to decrease postoperative opioid requirements and enhance analgesia. Examples:
  ‣ Gabapentin 300 mg PO before surgery, and then 300 mg PO q8 hours × 48 hours
  ‣ Celecoxib (Celebrex®) 400 mg PO before surgery, and then 200 mg PO q12 hours × 48 hours
  ‣ Acetaminophen 1,000 mg PO/IV before surgery, and then 1,000 mg PO q6–8 hours × 48 hours
- Anticonvulsants may reduce postoperative opioid requirements by up to 60% Mechanisms include:
  ‣ Stabilization of the neuronal membrane by blockage of pathologically active voltage-sensitive Na^+ channels (carbamazepine, phenytoin, lamotrigine, topiramate)
  ‣ Blockage of voltage-dependent calcium channels (gabapentin, pregabalin)
  ‣ Inhibition of presynaptic release of excitatory neurotransmitters (gabapentin, lamotrigine)
  ‣ Enhancement of the activity of GABA receptors (topiramate)

INTRAOPERATIVE PERIOD

- Implement *regional part* of multimodal analgesic plan: continuous perineural or epidural analgesia, neuraxial opioids
- Ensure patient has received *adequate intraoperative doses* of opioids, local anesthetics, and other adjuvant pain medications. Adjust doses to compensate for the patient's opioid dependence
- Optimize the patient's pain relief prior to leaving OR
- Consider administering 1 g of intravenous *acetaminophen* 30–60 minutes prior to arrival in PACU (if not given preoperatively). *Ketorolac* (15–60 mg IV) can also be considered, if not contraindicated
- Ask the surgeon to infiltrate the wound with 0.25–0.50% bupivacaine

POSTOPERATIVE PERIOD

- *Communicate* with patient, *nurses, and the surgical team* the postoperative multimodal analgesic plan
- *Equianalgesic doses of opioids are reduced by 50% or more* based on patient's medical condition and the opioid-sparing effects of the multimodal plan
- When initiating an intravenous opioid PCA, the patient's *current* condition determines how much opioid the patient can get. Do not assume the patient should, at a minimum, receive his or her outpatient dose orally or through the IV PCA. Often a *continuous (background) infusion* rate is programmed (along with a demand bolus and lockout interval) to provide the patient's daily maintenance opioid dose at home if the patient cannot take PO medications in the immediate postoperative period

- *Pain scores are evaluated every 1–4 hours and the plan adjusted accordingly.* Treatment decisions should be based on vital signs, respiratory rate, mental status, ability to ambulate, as well as patients' self-reported pain scores
- Distinguish between nociception and poor coping. Antidepressants or even psychiatry or social work consult may be warranted
- Avoid benzodiazepines because of their synergistic respiratory depressant effects:
  ▸ Consider anticonvulsants if a mood stabilizer is indicated
  ▸ Consider muscle relaxants such as baclofen or tizanidine for muscle spasms
- Continue to work with the pain management service to *develop an appropriate home medication regimen* in advance of the patient being discharged from the hospital
- Continue nonopioid analgesics

REFERENCE

For references, please visit **www.TheAnesthesiaGuide.com**.

PART X

PEDIATRICS

CHAPTER 167
Drug Dosages for Pediatric Anesthesia

Philipp J. Houck, MD and Leila Mei Pang, MD

Drugs and dosage are intended as general guidelines *only*. Adjust dosages based on clinical situation: hepatorenal function, cardiopulmonary bypass, ECMO, etc.

RESUSCITATION MEDICATIONS

- Atropine: 0.01–0.03 mg/kg IM, IV, ET, IC, IO
- Sodium bicarbonate: 1–2 mEq/kg ($0.3 \times$ kg $\times$ BE) IV, IC, IO
- Calcium chloride 10–30 mg/kg IV, IC slowly (maximum 1 g/dose)
- Calcium gluconate 60–100 mg/kg IV, IC (maximum 2 g/dose)
- Dextrose 0.5–1 g/kg IV = 1–2 mL/kg D_{50}; or 2–4 mL/kg D_{25}W or 5–10 mL/kg D_{10}W or 10–20 mL/kg D_5NS
- Diltiazem (Cardizem): 0.25 mg/kg over 2 minutes; may repeat in 15 minutes at 0.35 mg/kg over 2 minutes
- Ephedrine: 0.2–0.3 mg/kg/dose
- Epinephrine 10 µg/kg IV, IC, IO; ET = 100 µg/kg
- Lidocaine: 1 mg/kg IV, IC, ET, IO
- Lipid emulsion (Intralipid) 20%, 1.5 mL/kg over 1 minute $\times$ 3 prn, 0.25 mL/kg/min, and then 0.5 mL/kg/min if hypotensive
- Dantrolene: 2.5 mg/kg IV load; repeat until signs of MH are reversed; up to 30 mg/kg may be necessary; maintenance: 1.2 mg/kg IV q6 hours as needed

DEFIBRILLATION/CARDIOVERSION

- V-fib: 2 J/kg, and then 4 J/kg (defibrillation = unsynchronized) using the largest paddles that fit
- Synchronized cardioversion: 0.5–1 J/kg, and then 2 J/kg
- Adenosine: 0.1 mg/kg IV push (maximum 6 mg); repeat 0.2 mg/kg (maximum 12 mg)

CARDIAC

- Amiodarone: V-fib—5 mg/kg IV load over 30 seconds (maximum 300 mg); SVT: 5 mg/kg over 10 minutes $\times$ 5 doses; non-PVC container
- Digoxin: initial load 4–25 µg/kg IV:
  ‣ Maintenance 5–10 µg/kg/dose BID
  ‣ IV dose = 2/3 PO dose

- Diltiazem: 0.25 mg/kg over 2 minutes; may repeat in 15 minutes at 0.35 mg/kg over 2 minutes
- Dopamine, dobutamine: 2–20 µg/kg/min
- Ephedrine: 0.2–0.3 mg/kg/dose
- Epinephrine, isoproterenol, norepinephrine: 0.05–1 µg/kg/min
- Esmolol: 0.5 mg/kg bolus over 1 minute; maintenance: 50–300 µg/kg/min
- Lidocaine: 1–2 mg/kg/dose IV; 20–50 µg/kg/min (adult dose 1–4 mg/min)
- Magnesium sulfate for torsades de pointes: 25–50 mg/kg (maximum 2 g) over 10–20 minutes
- Milrinone: 20–50 µg/kg load; maintenance: 0.3–0.7 µg/kg/min
- Nitroglycerin: 0.5–5 µg/kg/min
- Nitroprusside: 0.5–10 µg/kg/min
- PGE_1 (alprostadil): 0.05–0.1 µg/kg/min
- Phenylephrine: 0.1–0.5 µg/kg/min; 1 µg/kg bolus
- Procainamide: 3–6 mg/kg (maximum 100 mg each dose) over 5 minutes × 3 q5–10 minutes; maintenance: 20–80 µg/kg/min (adult 1–4 mg/min)
- Propranolol: 0.05–0.15 mg/kg IV slowly (maximum 5 mg)
- Vasopressin: mix 10 U in 50 mL, so 1 mL = 0.2 U
  ‣ Hypotension: 0.0005–0.002 U/kg/min
  ‣ GI bleed: 0.002–0.005 U/kg/min
- Verapamil: 0.05–0.2 mg/kg IV over 2 minutes (maximum 5 mg)

MUSCLE RELAXANTS

- Cisatracurium: 0.1–0.2 mg/kg/dose IV; lasts 15–45 minutes
- Pancuronium: 0.1 mg/kg/dose IV; lasts 1–2 hours
- Rocuronium: 0.4–1.0 mg/kg/dose IV; 0.6 mg/kg/h
- Succinylcholine: 1–2 mg/kg IV; 4 mg/kg IM; consider giving atropine first
- Vecuronium: 0.1 mg/kg/dose IV; lasts 30 minutes

SEDATIVE/IV ANESTHETICS

- Chloral hydrate: 30–80 mg/kg/dose PO, PR
- Clonidine: 0.004 mg/kg PO (maximum 0.1 mg)
- Dexmedetomidine: load with 1 µg/kg IV over 5 minutes, and then 0.2–1 µg/kg/h
- Diphenhydramine: 0.2–2 mg/kg/dose IV q4–6 hours; or 1.25 mg/kg/dose q6 hours (maximum 400 mg per day)
- Etomidate: 0.3 mg/kg IV
- Haloperidol: 1–3 mg IM for patient >6 years
- Ketamine: 1–2 mg/kg IV; 3–6 mg/kg PO; 6–10 mg/kg PR; 3 mg/kg intranasal
- Methohexital: 1–2 mg/kg/dose IV; 30–40 mg/kg PR
- Midazolam: 0.05–0.3 mg/kg IV, IM:
  ‣ Infusion: 0.4 µg/kg/min
  ‣ PO: 0.5–0.75 mg/kg
  ‣ PR: 0.5–1 mg/kg
  ‣ Intranasal: 0.2 mg/kg
- Pentobarbital: 2 mg/kg IM, IV, PO
- Propofol: 2–3 mg/kg IV; maintenance: 50–300 µg/kg/min
- Thiopental: 3–7 mg/kg IV; PR: 20–40 mg/kg

ANALGESICS

NSAID:
- Acetaminophen: PO 10–15 mg/kg q4 hours:
  ‣ PR (first dose only) 30–40 mg/kg, next PO dose 6 hours later
  ‣ Maximum 30 mg/kg per day in newborns
  ‣ Maximum 60 mg/kg per day in infants
  ‣ Maximum 90 mg/kg per day in children
  ‣ Maximum 4 g per day in adults

- Ibuprofen: 10 mg/kg PO q6 hours
- Ketorolac: 0.5 mg/kg IV q6 hours (maximum 30 mg) normal renal function and no bleeding diathesis; maximum 120 mg per day; maximum 5 days

Opioids:
- Codeine: 0.5–1.0 mg/kg PO q4 hours
- Tylenol #1: acetaminophen 300 mg + codeine 7.5 mg
- Tylenol #2: acetaminophen 300 mg + codeine 15 mg
- Tylenol #3: acetaminophen 300 mg + codeine 30 mg
- Tylenol #4: acetaminophen 300 mg + codeine 60 mg
- Fentanyl: 0.5–1 µg/kg/dose IV q1 hour prn
- Hydrocodone/oxycodone: 0.05–0.15 mg/kg PO q4 hours (usual start dose 0.1 mg/kg)
- Hydromorphone: 0.03 mg/kg PO q4 hours; 0.015 mg/kg IV q2–4 hours prn
- Meperidine: for shivering or rigors (blood products, Amphotericin B, etc.) 0.1 mg/kg IV once
- Methadone: sliding scale:
  ‣ Mild pain: 25 µg/kg IV q4 hours prn
  ‣ Moderate pain: 50 µg/kg IV q4 hours prn
  ‣ Severe pain: 75 µg/kg IV q4 hours prn or as a long-acting opioid 0.1 mg/kg q8–12 hours (beware of cumulative effects after 48–72 hours)
- Morphine: 0.05–0.15 mg/kg IV q2–4 hours prn; 0.3–0.5 mg/kg/dose PO q4 hours
- Remifentanil: 0.1–0.5 µg/kg/min, 1–4 µg/kg bolus
- Sufentanil: 10–25 µg/kg induction

REVERSALS

- Neostigmine 0.05 mg/kg with glycopyrrolate 0.01 mg/kg
- Edrophonium:
  ‣ For myasthenia—0.2 mg/kg IV
  ‣ NMB reversal—1 mg/kg IV with atropine 0.014 mg/kg
- Flumazenil:
  ‣ Sedation reversal—0.01 mg/kg IV q1 minute:
  ‣ Overdose: 0.01 mg/kg q1 minute or 0.005–0.01 mg/kg/h (maximum 0.2 mg/dose; cumulative maximum 1 mg)
- Naloxone: 0.01–0.1 mg/kg/dose IV, ET; lasts 20 minutes
- Physostigmine: 0.01 mg/kg slowly IV (adult dose 2 mg) with atropine 0.01–0.02 mg/kg

FLUIDS/ELECTROLYTES/DIURETICS

- Maintenance: 4 mL/kg/h for first 10 kg + 2 mL/kg/h for second 10 kg + 1 mL/kg/h for every kg >20 kg
- Calcium: 200–300 mEq/kg per day
- Furosemide: 0.5–1 mg/kg PO, IV; 0.06–0.24 mg/kg/h
- Glucose: 8 mg/kg/min
- Hyperkalemia: dextrose 1 g/kg IV over 15 minutes with 0.2 U regular insulin/g dextrose
- Ca^{2+} = 4–5 mg/kg IV over 5–10 minutes
- Kayexalate: 1–2 g/kg PO, PR (with 20% sorbitol)
- Insulin: 0.02–0.1 U/kg/h
- Magnesium sulfate: 25–50 mg/kg (maximum 2 g) over 10 minutes; maintenance: 16 mg/kg/h to achieve plasma levels of 0.8–1.2 mmol/L (maximum 2 g)
- Mannitol: 0.25–1 g/kg IV
- Potassium: 2–3 mEq/kg per day
- Shock: 10–20 mL/kg of NS, RL or 5% albumin
- Sodium bicarbonate ($NaHCO_3$): 1–2 mEq/kg
- Vasopressin for diabetes insipidus: 0.0005 U/kg/h; double as needed based on urine output q30 minutes up to 0.01 U/kg/h, dilute to 0.04 U/mL

ANTIBIOTICS

- Ampicillin: 25–50 mg/kg q4–6 hours (maximum 2 g)
- Cefazolin: 30 mg/kg IV q4 hours (maximum 2 g)
- Cefoxitin: 30 mg/kg IV q4 hours (maximum 2 g)
- Clindamycin: 10 mg/kg q6 hours (maximum 900 mg) over 30 minutes
- Gentamicin: 2 mg/kg (maximum 80 mg) over 30 minutes, no redose
- Metronidazole: 7.5 mg/kg IV q6 hours over 30 minutes (maximum 500 mg)
- Tobramycin: 2.5 mg/kg (maximum 200 mg) over 30 minutes q8 hours
- Unasyn: 75 mg/kg IV over 30 minutes q4 hours
- Vancomycin: 15 mg/kg over 60 minutes q6–8 hours
- Zosyn:
  ‣ <9 months: 240 mg/kg per day; divide q6–8 hours
  ‣ >9 months: 300 mg/kg per day; divide q6–8 hours

ANTIHYPERTENSIVES

- Esmolol: 0.5 mg/kg bolus over 1 minute; maintenance: 50–300 µg/kg/min
- Hydralazine: 0.1–0.2 mg/kg IM, IV q4–6 hours
- Labetalol: 0.25 mg/kg IV q1–2 hours
- Nifedipine: 0.01–0.02 mg/kg IV or 1–2 mg/kg per day PO, SL (adult dose 10–30 mg PO)
- Phentolamine: 0.1 mg/kg/dose IV
- Propranolol: 0.01–0.15 mg/kg IV slowly

ANTIEMETICS/H$_2$ BLOCKERS

- Granisetron: 10 µg/kg/dose IV/PO q12 hours
- Metoclopramide (Reglan): 0.1 mg/kg IV/PO q6 hours (caution regarding extrapyramidal signs)
- Esomeprazole (Nexium): 1 mg/kg IV q day (maximum 40 mg)
- Ondansetron: 0.15 mg/kg IV/SL/PO q8 hours slowly (maximum 8 mg/dose; 32 mg per day)
- Prochlorperazine (Compazine): >2 years 0.1 mg/kg/dose IV/PO q8 hours (caution regarding extrapyramidal signs)
- Ranitidine (Zantac): 1–2 mg/kg/dose BID PO, IV (maximum 150 mg BID)

STEROIDS

- Dexamethasone: 0.3–1 mg/kg IV (for ENT 0.5 mg/kg, maximum 10 mg)
- Hydrocortisone (Solu-Cortef): 0.2–1 mg/kg q6 hours (anti-inflammatory); status asthmaticus: load 4–8 mg/kg, and then 2–4 mg/kg q4–6 hours
- Methylprednisolone (Solu-Medrol): 0.04–0.2 mg/kg q6 hours (anti-inflammatory); status asthmaticus: load 2 mg/kg, and then 0.5–1 mg/kg/dose q4–6 hours
  ‣ Spinal shock: 30 mg/kg IV over 1 hour, and then 5.4 mg/kg/h × 23 hours
  ‣ Liver transplantation: 20 mg/kg

ANTIPRURITICS

- Diphenhydramine: 0.5 mg/kg/dose PO/IV q6 hours
- Hydroxyzine: 0.5 mg/kg/dose PO/IV q6 hours
- Nalbuphine: 0.1 mg/kg/dose q6 hours IV over 20 minutes (maximum 5 mg)

BRONCHODILATORS

- Albuterol nebulizer (0.5% solution): 0.01 mL/kg/2.5 mL NS (maximum 0.5 mL = 2.5 mg)
- Aminophylline: 7 mg/kg slowly over 30 minutes IV; maintenance: 0.5–1.5 mg/kg/h
- Epinephrine (1:1,000): 10 µg/kg SC (maximum 400 µg)
- Racemic epinephrine: 0.25–0.5 mL in 5 mL NS nebulized
- Isoproterenol: 0.05 µg/kg/min increasing by 0.1 µg/kg/min to effect
- Metaproterenol nebulizer (5% solution): 0.01 mL/kg/2.5 mL NS (maximum dose 0.3 mL = 15 mg)
- Terbutaline 10 µg/kg SC (maximum 250 µg)

PCA

- Hydromorphone (0.2 mg/mL):
  - Demand: 0.003 mg/kg/dose q10 minutes
  - Continuous infusion (optional): 0.003 mg/kg/h
  - Clinician boluses: 0.006 mg/kg q20 minutes up to three times q4 hours
- Morphine (1 mg/mL); if under 10 kg (0.5 mg/mL):
  - Demand: 0.015 mg/kg q10 minutes
  - Continuous infusion (optional): 0.015 mg/kg/h
  - Clinician boluses: 0.03 mg/kg q20 minutes up to three times q4 hours

EPIDURAL

- Bupivacaine 0.1% (1 mg/mL ± fentanyl 1–2 µg/mL ± clonidine 0.1 µg/mL): 0.1–0.4 mL/kg/h

Do not exceed:
- Neonates 0.2 mg/kg/h of bupivacaine, no longer than 48 hours
- Older children 0.4 mg/kg/h of bupivacaine
- Caudal (single shot): 0.25% bupivacaine (±epinephrine premixed) 0.75–1 mL/kg ± clonidine 1 µg/kg

BLOOD PRODUCTS/COAGULATION

- Aminocaproic acid:
  - Cardiac: 200 mg/kg, and then 16.7 mg/kg/h, maximum 18 g/m^2 per day
  - Orthopedic: 100–150 mg/kg, and then 10–15 mg/kg/h, maximum 18/m^2 per day
- Heparin: 50–100 U/kg IV bolus, and then 10–20 U/kg/h; cardiopulmonary bypass: 300 U/kg IV
- Factor VIIa: 40 µg/kg IV, redose 90 minutes later with 90 µg/kg IV, and then redose 2 hours later with 90 µg/kg
- PRBC: 10 mL/kg will raise Hb by 1 g
- Platelets: 5–10 mL/kg will raise count 50–100 × 10^9/L; for >10-kg patient 1 U/10 kg

Note: ET, endotracheal; IC, intracardiac; IM, intramuscular; IO, intraosseous; IV, intravenous; PO, oral; PR, rectal; SC, subcutaneous.

CHAPTER 168
Newborn Resuscitation

Wanda A. Chin, MD

RESUSCITATION (FIGURE 168-1)

- Start *stabilization* (dry, warm, position, assess the airway, stimulate to breathe):
  - ‣ Routine intrapartum oropharyngeal and nasopharyngeal suctioning for infants born with clear or meconium-stained amniotic fluid is no longer recommended
  - ‣ Cord clamping should be delayed for at least 1 minute in babies who do not require resuscitation. Evidence is insufficient to recommend a time for clamping in those who require resuscitation
  - ‣ Evaluate heart rate and respirations to determine next step in resuscitation
- *Ventilation*—spontaneously breathing preterm infants who have respiratory distress may be supported with CPAP or intubation and mechanical ventilation
  - ‣ Assisted ventilation rates of 40–60 bpm have been used, although efficacy has not been reviewed. Adequate ventilation is assessed by prompt improvement of heart rate
  - ‣ Use pulse oximetry to evaluate oxygenation because assessment of color is unreliable
  - ‣ Supplementary oxygen should be regulated by blending oxygen and air, and the concentration delivered should be guided by oximetry
  - ‣ The available evidence does not support or refute the routine endotracheal suctioning of infants born through meconium-stained amniotic fluid, even when the newborn is depressed
- *Chest compressions* (Figure 168-2)—if HR <60, start chest compressions:
  - ‣ 3:1 compression to ventilation ratio
  - ‣ Two thumb-encircling hands method
  - ‣ Centered over the lower third of the sternum
  - ‣ Compression depth one third the anterior–posterior diameter
- *Medications*—*naloxone* is not recommended as part of the initial resuscitation for newborns with respiratory depression in the delivery room
- *Volume expansion*—early volume replacement with crystalloid or red cells is indicated for babies with blood loss who are not responding to resuscitation. While volume administration in the infant with no blood loss who is refractory to conventional resuscitation is not routinely performed, a trial of volume administration may be considered in these babies because blood loss may be occult
- *Therapeutic hypothermia* should be considered for infants born at term or near term with evolving moderate to severe hypoxic-ischemic encephalopathy, with protocol and follow-up coordinated through a regional perinatal system
- It is appropriate to *consider discontinuing resuscitation* if there has been no detectable heart rate for 10 minutes. Multiple factors should be taken into account to decide whether to continue beyond 10 minutes

FIGURE 168-1. Resuscitation of the neonate

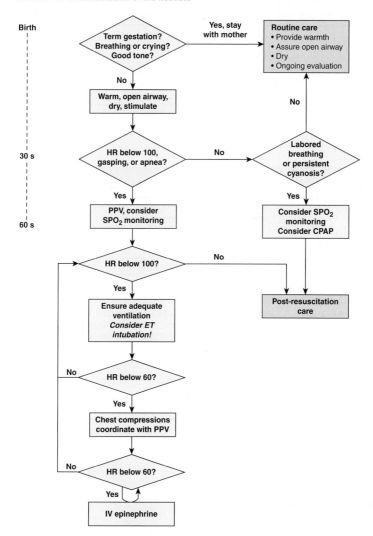

NB: Epinephrine dose: 0.01–0.03 mg/kg IV. Adapted with permission from Perlman JM, Wyllie J, Kattwinkel J, et al. Part 11: neonatal resuscitation: 2010 international consensus on cardiopulmonary resuscitation and emergency cardiovascular care science with treatment recommendations. *Circulation*. 2010;122(suppl 2):S516–S538.

Target Preductal SpO₂ after Birth	
Time after birth (min)	Target preductal SpO₂ (%)
1	60–65
2	65–70
3	70–75
4	75–80
5	80–85
10	85–95

Apgar Score			
Parameter	0	1	2
Color	Blue, pale	Body pink, extremities blue	Pink
Muscle tone	None, limp	Slight flexion	Active, good flexion
HR	0	<100	>100
Respiration	Absent	Slow, irregular	Strong, regular
Reflex irritability (response to nasal catheter)	None	Some grimace	Good grimace, crying

Normally assessed at 1 and 5 minutes. If 5-minute Apgar <7, repeat every 5 minutes up to 20 minutes. Any score <3 indicates moderate to severe asphyxia; start aggressive resuscitation. *NB*: Apgar score *not used* to guide resuscitation. *Do not delay* resuscitation in order to perform Apgar score.

FIGURE 168-2. Proper chest compression technique in the neonate

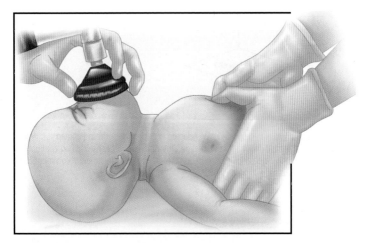

Reproduced with permission from Strange G, Ahrens W, Lelyveld S, Schafermeyer R, eds. *Pediatric Emergency Medicine: A Comprehensive Study Guide*. 3rd ed. New York: McGraw-Hill; 2009. Figure 27-4. Copyright © The McGraw-Hill Companies, Inc. All rights reserved.

REFERENCES

For references, please visit **www.TheAnesthesiaGuide.com**.

CHAPTER 169
Pediatric Difficult Airway

Wanda A. Chin, MD

Initial Airway Assessment		
History	Does this child have a history of airway distress or difficult airway management?	Evaluate for Hx of stridor, dyspnea, FTT, previous anesthetics, OSA
Physical exam	Is there current active airway distress? Does the patient have any dysmorphic features?	Note level of airway distress and features such as micrognathia, high arched palate, choanal atresia, decreased mouth opening
Special studies	Will further workup help to formulate a plan?	CT scans, laryngoscopies, sleep studies
Patient maturity	Can patient cooperate with airway management?	Emotionally, psychologically, or intellectually
Surgical procedure	What is needed for this procedure?	Regional versus general Mask versus LMA versus ETT versus surgical airway

DIFFERENCE IN AIRWAY FOR INFANTS AND CHILDREN

- Larynx higher in neck
- Narrowest part of airway is cricoid
- Epiglottis stiffer, larger, and more posterior
- Tongue disproportionately larger
- Short neck
- Head/occiput larger relative to body size

PEDIATRIC DIFFICULT AIRWAY ALGORITHM (FIGURE 169-1)

- Assess the likelihood of management problems:
  ‣ Difficult ventilation
  ‣ Difficult intubation
  ‣ Difficult patient cooperation
  ‣ Difficult surgical airway
- Provide supplemental oxygen
- Consider basic management choices:
  ‣ Surgical airway versus noninvasive airway
  ‣ Awake intubation versus intubation after induction: Most pediatric patients will lack the maturity to cooperate for awake intubation and intubation attempts are performed after induction of general anesthesia
  ‣ Spontaneous ventilation versus ablation of spontaneous ventilation: Due to the limited respiratory reserve in small pediatric patients, it is often safer to maintain spontaneous ventilation while attempting intubation

FIGURE 169-1. Pediatric difficult airway flow diagram

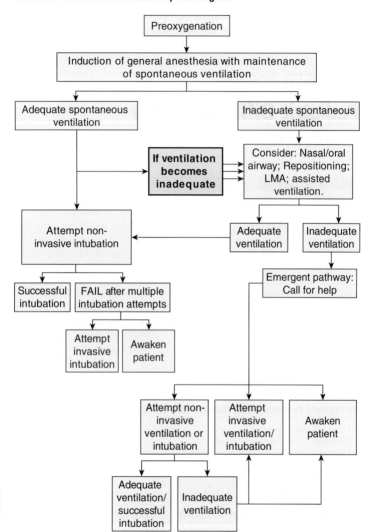

Suggested Equipment for Pediatric Difficult Airway Cart	
Equipment	Size
Oral and nasopharyngeal airways	Various sizes
ETT	Pediatric and adult
Laryngeal mask airway	Sizes 1, 1.5, 2, 2.5, 3, 4, 5
Combitube (small adult size)	
Fastrach LMA	Sizes 3, 4, 5
Laryngoscope handles	Short and long handles
Laryngoscopy blades	Mac 0, 1, 2, 3, 4
	Miller 0, 1, 2, 3, 4
	Oxyscope (with port built-in for blow-by oxygen)
Batteries for handles	
Magill forceps	Pediatric and adult
IV catheters	
Syringes	
Intubation guides	Stylets
	Tube exchangers
	Elastic bougies
Tracheostomy kit	
Percutaneous needle cricothyrotomy kit	
Swivel adapters	
No. 3 straight connectors	
Suction catheters	6, 8, 10, and 14 Fr
Yankauer suction tip	Pediatric and adult
Surgical lubricant	
2% and 4% lidocaine for topicalization	
Atomizer	
Face masks	Size 1, 2, 3, 4, 5
Ambu bag	Pediatric and adult
Advanced airway equipment	Flexible fiber-optic bronchoscope
	Rigid bronchoscope
	Retrograde intubation kit with guidewire
	Lighted stylets

REFERENCES

For references, please visit **www.TheAnesthesiaGuide.com**.

CHAPTER 170
Pediatric Vital Signs

Wanda A. Chin, MD

Age	Weight (kg)	Pulse (bpm)	RR (bpm)	SBP (mm Hg)	DBP (mm Hg)	Minute ventilation (L/min; mL/min/kg)	VC (mL; mL/kg)	Hct (%)
Pediatric Vital Signs								
Premature	1	130–150	40–60	42–52	21 ± 8			35–65
Premature	1–2	125–150	40–60	50–60	28 ± 8			35–65
Newborn	2–4	120–150	40–60	60–70	37 ± 8	1.05; 200–260	120; 40	45–65
1 month	4–7	100–140	24–35	80–96	46 ± 16			
6 months	7–10	100–140	24–35	89–105	60 ± 10	1.35; 140–190		33–36
1 year	10–12	95–130	20–30	96–110	66 ± 25	1.78; 150–180	450; 45	35
2–3 years	12–14	85–125	18–25	99–115	64 ± 25	2.46; 175–200	870; 60	38
4–5 years	16–18	80–115	18–25	99–115	65 ± 20	5.5	1,160; 60	
6–9 years	20–26	70–110	14–25	100–120	65 ± 15	6.2	1,500; 60	40
10–12 years	32–42	65–95	12–20	112–125	68 ± 15	6.2	3,100; 60	
>14 years	>50	65–90	12–18	115–130	75 ± 15	6.4; 90	4,000; 60	40–50

RR, respiratory rate; SBP, systolic blood pressure; DBP, diastolic blood pressure; VC, vital capacity; Hct, hematocrit.

Age-Based Estimates of Body Water Compartments					
Age	Premature	Neonate	1 year	10 years	Adult
TBW (%)	85	75	70	55	50
ICF (%)	35	40	40	30	30
ECF (%)	50	35	30	25	20

TBW, total body water; ICF, intracellular fluid; ECF, extracellular fluid.

PEARLS

- Normal pediatric vital signs include higher heart rates and lower blood pressures than adults
- Infants are heart rate dependent for their cardiac output because of a fixed stroke volume
- Children have a higher oxygen consumption per kilogram than adults
- Pediatric patients may respond to stress, such as hypoxia, by becoming bradycardic, and therefore decreasing CO
- Tidal volume (7 mL/kg) and dead space (2 mL/kg) are equivalent to adults on a per kilogram basis
- FRC is decreased under anesthesia, leading to increased atelectasis
- Until 4–5 months, limited urine concentration capacity
- Neonates have a low blood protein content with a high free drug fraction for many drugs; they are also at risk for hypoglycemia and hypocalcemia

- Peak for thrombosis risk: birth (deficit in ATIII, Pt C and S) and around puberty
- PT physiologically prolonged by 8–10 seconds in neonates and breastfed infants because of vitamin K deficit

REFERENCES

For references, please visit **www.TheAnesthesiaGuide.com**.

CHAPTER 171
Pediatric Sizing Chart

Philipp J. Houck, MD

Age- and Weight-Based Sizing Chart										
Age (or weight)	Uncuffed ETT	Cuffed ETT	Laryngoscope blade	DL ETT	CVL	A-line	LMA	Foley	Chest tube	Salem Sump
1 kg	2.5		Miller 00		5 Fr	24 G	1	5 Fr	8 Fr	
2 kg	3		Miller 00		5 Fr	24 G	1	5 Fr	10 Fr	10 Fr
3 kg	3		Miller 0		5 Fr	24 G	1	5 Fr	12 Fr	10 Fr
Term newborn	3.5		Miller 1		5 Fr	24 G	1	5 Fr	12 Fr	10 Fr
5 kg	3.5		Miller 1		5 Fr	24 G	1.5	5 Fr	12 Fr	10 Fr
1 year	4		Miller 1		5 Fr	24 G	1.5	5 Fr	16 Fr	10 Fr
2 years	4.5		Miller/Mac 2		5 Fr	24 G	2	8 Fr	16 Fr	14 Fr
3 years	4.5		Miller/Mac 2		5 Fr	22 G	2	8 Fr	20 Fr	14 Fr
4 years	5		Miller/Mac 2		5 Fr	22 G	2	8 Fr	20 Fr	14 Fr
5 years		5	Miller/Mac 2		5 Fr	22 G	2	8 Fr	20 Fr	14 Fr
6 years		5	Miller/Mac 2		7 Fr	22 G	2.5	8 Fr	20 Fr	14 Fr
7 years		5	Miller/Mac 2		7 Fr	22 G	2.5	8 Fr	20 Fr	14 Fr
8 years		5.5	Miller/Mac 2	26 Fr	7 Fr	22 G	2.5	8 Fr	20 Fr	14 Fr
9 years		5.5	Miller/Mac 2	26 Fr	7 Fr	22 G	2.5	10 Fr	20 Fr	14 Fr
10 years		6	Miller/Mac 3	28 Fr	7 Fr	20 G	2.5	10 Fr	20 Fr	14 Fr
11 years		6	Miller/Mac 3	28 Fr	7 Fr	20 G	3	10 Fr	24 Fr	14 Fr
12 years		6	Miller/Mac 3	28 Fr	7 Fr	20 G	3	10 Fr	24 Fr	14 Fr
13 years		6	Miller/Mac 3	32 Fr	9 Fr	20 G	3	12 Fr	24 Fr	16 Fr
14 years		7	Miller/Mac 3	32 Fr	9 Fr	20 G	3	12 Fr	32 Fr	16 Fr
15 years		7	Miller/Mac 3	35 Fr	9 Fr	20 G	4	12 Fr	32 Fr	16 Fr
16 years		7	Miller/Mac 3	35 Fr	9 Fr	20 G	4	12 Fr	32 Fr	16 Fr
17 years		7	Miller/Mac 3	35 Fr	9 Fr	20 G	4	12 Fr	36 Fr	16 Fr
18 years		7	Miller/Mac 3	35 Fr	9 Fr	20 G	4	12 Fr	36 Fr	16 Fr

ETT, endotracheal tube; DL, double-lumen; LMA, laryngeal mask airway; Fr, French; G, gauge.

ETT depth (cm) = three times ETT size (mm ID).
ETT size (mm ID) = (age [in years])/4 + 4.

CHAPTER 172
Gastroschisis/Omphalocele

Wanda A. Chin, MD

BASICS

Differences Between Omphalocele and Gastroschisis		
	Omphalocele	Gastroschisis
Etiology	Failure of gut migration from yolk sac into abdomen	Occlusion of omphalomesenteric artery with ischemia to the right periumbilical area
Location	Within umbilical cord	Periumbilical
Prenatal diagnosis by U/S	Yes	Yes
Incidence	1:6,000, M >F	1:15,000, M >F
Peritoneal covering	Yes	No
Location	Central through umbilicus	Lateral to umbilicus
Associated anomalies	High incidence	Low incidence
	Cardiac	GI–intestinal atresia
	GI–Meckel's diverticulum, malrotation	
	GU–bladder extrophy	
	Metabolic–Beckwith–Wiedemann (congenital disorder associated with macrosomia, macroglossia, organomegaly, and hypoglycemia)	
	Chromosomal abnormalities (trisomy 21), congenital diaphragmatic hernia	
Survival rate	70–95%	>90%

PREOPERATIVE

- Broad-spectrum antibiotics to prevent contamination of the peritoneal cavity preoperatively
- Similar preoperative management of neonates: preventing infection and minimizing fluid and heat loss
- Covering the exposed viscera or membranous sac with sterile saline-soaked dressings and plastic wrap immediately after delivery decreases evaporative fluid and heat loss
- Surgical correction of an omphalocele or gastroschisis is urgent but can be delayed until full anesthesia workup and resuscitation
- Rule out associated anomalies; may need echocardiogram, renal U/S
- Correct fluid and electrolyte abnormalities
  ‣ Because of significant ongoing fluid losses with an open abdominal wall defect, administer an IV fluid bolus (20 mL/kg lactated Ringer's solution or normal saline), followed by 10% dextrose in 1/4 normal sodium chloride solution at two to three times the baby's maintenance fluid rate
- Decompress stomach with OGT

MONITORING

- Standard ASA monitors with temperature + urine output
- Individualized for patient needs
- A-line helpful for monitoring pH and guiding fluid therapy:
  ‣ Also useful if concomitant cardiac defects present
- A pulse oximeter probe on the lower extremity will detect a decrease in oxygen saturation that could be caused by congestion of the lower extremities due to obstruction of venous return
- Measurement of intragastric pressure, CVP, or cardiac index can aid in determining whether primary closure is appropriate

INDUCTION

- GETA + RSI. May also do awake intubation. Avoid N_2O because of possibility of gastric distention
- Maximal muscle relaxation mandatory

MAINTENANCE

- Anesthetic management involves volume resuscitation (~50–100 mL/kg of isotonic fluids during the case) and the prevention of hypothermia
- Major complications from increased intra-abdominal pressure when replacing viscera into abdomen:
  ‣ Ventilatory compromise:
    ▪ Watch for increased peak airway pressures and decreased tidal volumes
  ‣ Decreased organ perfusion
  ‣ Bowel edema
  ‣ Anuria
  ‣ Hypotension
- If inspiratory pressure is >25–30 cm H_2O or intragastric pressure >20 cm H_2O, primary closure is not recommended

POSTOPERATIVE

- Postoperative management depends on the type of repair and whether or not the child has associated anomalies
- Fluid resuscitation should continue postoperatively because fluid loss through the viscera continues, especially in a staged repair, where the viscera are left extraperitoneally
- Parenteral nutrition can be needed, especially if prolonged ileus
- Most children remains intubated for 24–48 hours to monitor airway pressures postoperatively

REFERENCES

For references, please visit **www.TheAnesthesiaGuide.com**.

CHAPTER 173
Tracheoesophageal Fistula (TEF)
Wanda A. Chin, MD

BASICS (FIGURE 173-1)

- Approximately 1 in 3,000 babies is born with tracheoesophageal fistula (TEF)
- Thirty to 40% neonates are premature
- Associated anomalies such as cardiac, gastrointestinal, genitourinary, musculoskeletal, or craniofacial anomalies are present in 30–50% of newborns with esophageal atresia and TEFs
  - VATER (i.e., vertebral and vascular anomalies, imperforate anus, TEF, radial aplasia, and renal abnormalities)
  - VACTERL (i.e., vertebral anomalies, imperforate anus, cardiac anomalies, TEF, renal abnormalities, radial limb aplasia) association
- Most common abnormality is blind upper esophageal pouch with distal fistulous tract between the trachea and distal esophagus (Type IIIB), observed in 90% of cases

FIGURE 173-1. The five types of TEF

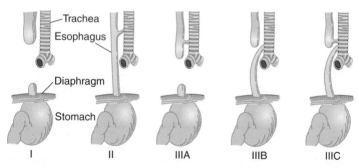

I   II   IIIA   IIIB   IIIC

Type IIIB represents 90% of cases. Reproduced from Morgan GE, Mikhail MS, Murray MJ. *Clinical Anesthesiology*. 4th ed. Figure 44-3. Available at: http://www.accessmedicine.com. Copyright © The McGraw-Hill Companies, Inc. All rights reserved.

PREOPERATIVE

- Prenatal diagnosis by ultrasound; associated with polyhydramnios (decreased fluid swallowing)
- Confirmed postnatally by failure to pass orogastric tube into newborn's stomach
- Neonatal symptoms: coughing and choking with first feeding:
  - Recurrent pneumonias associated with feeding
- Radiographic confirmation: tip of radio-opaque catheter in esophagus:
  - Air in stomach if fistula present
- Occasionally TEF diagnosis not made until later in the child's life
- Morbidity and mortality associated with pulmonary and cardiac complications. Ascertain position of the aorta to decide on side of thoracotomy

- Minimize risk of aspiration pneumonitis by placing neonate in semirecumbent position and inserting oroesophageal catheter to decrease accumulation of secretions
- All feeds are held as these patients are at high risk of aspiration. Patients are often started on a dextrose intravenous solution, TPN or PPN
- Antibiotics may be necessary for treatment of pneumonia
- Emergency gastrostomy under local anesthesia may be necessary to relieve gastric distension and improve ventilation before the definitive surgery 48–72 hours later
- The Waterson classification was used extensively in the past. However, patients currently are individually categorized based on clinical status

Waterson Classification for Neonates with TEF		
A	Birthweight over 2.5 kg and healthy	95% survival
B	Birthweight between 1.8 and 2.5 kg and healthy, or weight >2.5 kg with moderate pneumonia or other congenital anomalies	68% survival
C	Birthweight under 1.8 kg or weight >1.8 kg with severe pneumonia or severe congenital anomalies	6% survival

Spitz Classification for Neonates with TEF		
I	Birthweight greater than 1.5 kg and no congenital heart defect	99% survival
II	Birthweight less than 1.5 kg or congenital heart defect	82% survival
III	Birthweight less than 1.5 kg and presence of congenital heart defect	50% survival

- With improved ICU care, respiratory status has become a smaller factor in survival
- In general, whatever classification system is used, infants who have stable cardiac and respiratory status undergo expedition thoracotomy and repair. High-risk infants, especially those who are premature (<1,000 g) and have severe respiratory ailments or congestive heart failure, may require delay in therapy and may be treated initially with an emergency gastrostomy along with distal esophageal Fogarty balloon obstruction under local anesthesia
- Atropine generally is the only premedication of infants with esophageal atresia and TEF. It is given to decrease the risk of bradycardia from vagal stimulation during intubation, and to maintain cardiac output during the induction of anesthesia

MONITORING

- Routine monitors including temperature
- NIBP—A-line if cardiac issues or right thoracotomy for correction
- Precordial stethoscope placed on the left chest under the axilla (heart and breath sounds)

INDUCTION

- GETA ± rapid sequence induction versus inhalational induction with maintenance of spontaneous ventilation:
  ‣ If difficult airway anticipated, maintain spontaneous ventilation through awake intubation versus inhalational induction ($2 \times$ MAC)
  ‣ Benefit of maintenance of spontaneous ventilation is minimization of gastric distension from positive pressure ventilation through fistula
- Placing the ETT into a mainstem bronchus and withdrawing it until breath sounds are equal may prevent ventilation of the fistula, because the TEF is generally located on the posterior aspect of the trachea and just proximal to the carina

- Rotating the ETT during intubation so the bevel faces posteriorly may prevent intubation of the fistula
- A gastrostomy may make ventilation difficult if the volume of gas flowing through the fistula is high. A balloon Fogarty catheter placed in the fistula through a bronchoscope, or inserted under fluoroscopic guidance, will occlude the fistula and allow for easier ventilation of the child

MAINTENANCE

- Once the fistula is ligated, positive pressure can be implemented
- Balanced anesthetic technique is often used
- Airway obstruction can occur if the trachea is compressed, secretions become inspissated, or a blood clot forms in the airway
- Compression of the right lung during surgical dissection, fistula ligation, and esophageal anastomosis can cause atelectasis, desaturation, and hypoventilation
- Differential diagnosis of acute desaturation:
  ‣ Gastric distension
  ‣ ETT obstruction (clot)
  ‣ Right mainstem intubation
  ‣ Tracheal compression by the surgeon
  ‣ ETT through the fistula
  ‣ Reversal to fetal circulation
  ‣ Bronchospasm

SURGICAL TECHNIQUE

- The open surgery is performed through a right posterolateral, extrapleural thoracotomy, unless the aortic arch is on the right side
- The distal esophageal fistula usually lies immediately beneath the azygous vein. An extrapleural dissection is performed to the thoracic inlet and azygous vein. The pleura and lung are then retracted medially
- The fistula is divided, taking care not to remove any tracheal wall
- The proximal and distal esophageal ends are mobilized and anastomosed

POSTOPERATIVE

- Infants may be extubated if they are awake and are not at risk for postoperative respiratory problems
  ‣ Many patients have preexisting pulmonary compromise from prematurity or preoperative aspiration
  ‣ Ensure ETT is suctioned prior to extubation
- Regional anesthesia, specifically caudal catheters threaded up to the thoracic level, have decreased postoperative pain and aided in early extubation
- Those who are at risk for respiratory problems (e.g., postanesthetic apnea) should remain intubated until they demonstrate that they can sustain adequate ventilation postoperatively
- Neonates with TEF frequently have tracheomalacia. Dynamic collapse of the trachea during inspiration may be increased with increased respiratory efforts postoperatively
- Premature extubation also may be dangerous in these babies because the recently closed fistula may be ruptured on reintubation
- Anastomotic leak in 15% of cases
- GERD and esophageal dysmotility occur commonly

REFERENCES

For references, please visit **www.TheAnesthesiaGuide.com**.

CHAPTER 174
Pyloric Stenosis

Wanda A. Chin, MD

BASICS

- Incidence 2–4:1,000 live births
- Male to female 4:1
- Usual age of presentation is 2 weeks to 2 months
- Symptoms:
  ‣ Persistent nonbilious "projectile" vomiting with feeds
  ‣ Dehydration and electrolyte abnormalities:
    ▪ Hypokalemia, hypochloremia, metabolic alkalosis
    ▪ If dehydration is severe, may see mixed metabolic acidosis
    ▪ If patient is still alkalotic postoperatively, hypoxia can occur as the baby attempts to correct the alkalotic state by hypoventilating
  ‣ "Olive" palpable in hypogastric area on exam
  ‣ Not often associated with other abnormalities

PREOPERATIVE

- Medical emergency, *not* surgical emergency
- Make sure patient is normovolemic and electrolyte abnormalities have been corrected. Serum values of bicarbonate, chloride, and potassium should be within normal limits. However, the most useful measure of adequate resuscitation is the clinical assessment—adequate urine output (minimum of 1 mL/kg/h), skin turgor, heart rate, etc
- Children with severe dehydration should receive deficit fluid therapy with isotonic crystalloid solution (10–20 mL/kg) initially. However, ongoing resuscitation should be performed with 0.45% NaCl in D5W at a rate of approximately 1.5–2.0× maintenance to prevent rapid changes in volume and electrolyte levels, which can result in seizures
- When urine output has been demonstrated, potassium chloride (10–20 mEq/L) can be added to the fluids
- Resuscitation may take 48–72 hours, depending on degree of dehydration
- Vitamin K given if needed

MONITORING

- Standard monitors: NIBP, EKG, SpO_2, temperature

ANESTHETIC OPTIONS–GA VERSUS REGIONAL

- GA most common, but regional (spinal, epidural, and caudal) has been used with success
- Perceived advantage is the minimization of respiratory depressant use and risk of apnea postoperatively
- Required analgesic level for pyloromyotomy is between T4 and T10 for open cases, depending on incision location (see "Surgical approach" below in the Maintenance section)
- *Epidural*:
  ‣ Single-shot epidural in left lateral position at T10–11
  ‣ Use 20G, 50 mm Tuohy needle with LOR to saline (to minimize risk of air embolization). A catheter can also be threaded if needed
  ‣ Ropivacaine 0.75% (0.75 mL/kg)

- *Caudal*:
  ‣ Caudal blockade with bupivacaine 0.25%
  ‣ Difficult to obtain a sufficient thoracic level from a caudal
  ‣ 1.6 mL/kg for pyloromyotomy achieved a success rate of 96% in one study
- *Spinal*:
  ‣ 25G (0.6 × 30 mm) or 23G (0.50 × 51 mm) neonatal LP needle
  ‣ Isobaric bupivacaine (5 mg/mL), 0.7–0.8 mg/kg, without epinephrine is injected using a 1-mL syringe
  ‣ Adequacy of SA determined by the presence of profound motor block in the lower extremities, inability to move feet, knees, and legs, and the absence of a skin prick response at the level of the surgical incision
  ‣ IV sedation (midazolam 0.1 mg/kg) can be used before or during the operation if the child is crying/restless in the presence of adequate SA
  ‣ However, patient remains at high risk for aspiration; sedation should be used either sparingly or not at all
  ‣ Surgical time is often limited to <90 minutes, as the duration of spinal blockade in this patient population is less than that observed in adults

INDUCTION

- High aspiration risk
- RSI versus awake intubation
- Prior to induction, stomach is emptied with orogastric/nasogastric tube. Patient is positioned supine, right lateral and left lateral during suctioning to ensure optimal evacuation of stomach secretions

MAINTENANCE

- Procedure is stimulating but fairly short (about 20 minutes)
- Increased sensitivity to anesthetics (physiology of neonates/young infants + recent acid/base abnormalities) may prolong the anesthetic
- Isotonic crystalloid (up to 10 mL/kg/h) used intraoperatively to replace any fluid deficit, loss, or maintenance
- Dextrose solutions are reserved for premature patients and patients on chronic dextrose infusions such as PPN or TPN, who may not have sufficient glycogen stores to maintain serum glucose levels
- Use short-acting anesthetics and titrate narcotics slowly, if at all
- Local anesthetic injected by surgeon to minimize incisional pain
- Reverse NMB at the end of the case
- Acetaminophen (15–40 mg/kg PR or 15 mg/kg IV) can be used to decrease narcotic requirement postoperatively
- *Surgical approach*:
  ‣ The patient is positioned supine
  ‣ The surgery can be performed open or laparoscopically
  ‣ Open procedures:
    ▪ Incision horizontally in the RUQ or supraumbilically
    ▪ Pylorus identified and delivered through the wound
    ▪ A 1–2 cm longitudinal incision through the avascular portion of the anterior wall (along the plane of the pylorus) is made
    ▪ The incision is taken down through the serosal and muscle layers until the mucosa is exposed, taking great care not to incise the mucosa
    ▪ Depending on surgeon preference, the integrity of the mucosa is tested by observing either air or methylene blue injected through an orogastric tube at the pyloric incision
    ▪ Incision closed in a multilayered fashion
  ‣ The laparoscopic approach has the benefit of faster recovery, although the open approach may have higher efficacy rates and fewer complications

POSTOPERATIVE

- Patients are usually extubated unless conditions do not support it
- Usually NGT/OGT removed, unless the gastric or duodenal mucosa was breached, in which case the patient will be kept NPO for 48 hours
- If the operative course is uncomplicated, the patient is started on feeds as per the surgeon either immediately postoperatively when the patient is alert enough to take PO or after several hours of NPO. Initially dilute, intermittent feeds and advanced as tolerated until full feeds
- Crystalloid resuscitation is continued postoperatively until the patient returns to full feeding
- Infants with pyloric stenosis have an increased incidence of postoperative apnea and bradycardia. These infants should be placed on an apnea and cardiac monitor for 24 hours following the operation
- Postoperative pain can be controlled by gentle titration of fentanyl (0.5 µg/kg) or morphine (0.05 mg/kg)
- Patient is recovered in PACU unless comorbidities dictate a PICU admission
- Monitor glucose for 3–4 hours postoperatively

REFERENCES

For references, please visit **www.TheAnesthesiaGuide.com**.

CHAPTER 175
Necrotizing Enterocolitis

Philipp J. Houck, MD

BASICS

- Disease of the premature infant: bowel ischemia leads to intestinal mucosal injury
- Mortality up to 30%
- Presentation:
  ‣ Abdominal distension
  ‣ Bilious vomiting
  ‣ Bloody stools
  ‣ Poor feeding, vomiting
  ‣ Temperature instability
  ‣ Hyperglycemia
  ‣ Toxic appearance
  ‣ In severe cases: hypotension, DIC, and metabolic acidosis
  ‣ Free air may be seen on abdominal x-ray once perforated; this is an urgent indication for a surgical intervention
- Medical management will avoid surgery in 85% of cases:
  ‣ Cessation of feeding with NG suction
  ‣ TPN, IV fluids
  ‣ Antibiotics
  ‣ PRBC and platelet transfusions
- Indications for surgery:
  ‣ Perforation
  ‣ Obstruction
  ‣ Peritonitis
  ‣ Worsening acidosis

PREOPERATIVE

- Typically only the sickest patients fail medical therapy: critically ill
- Correct as much as possible hypovolemia, metabolic acidosis, coagulopathy, hypocalcemia, thrombocytopenia

MONITORING

- Standard ASA monitoring in addition to a peripheral arterial line
- Adequate venous access is mandatory due to the high fluid requirements

ANESTHESIA

- Most infants are already intubated; otherwise an awake intubation or a modified rapid sequence is indicated. Risk of intracranial hemorrhage from awake intubation, but it may be the safest technique given the absence of respiratory reserve
- Induction: succinylcholine or rocuronium; if hemodynamically tolerated, fentanyl with or without sevoflurane
- Maintenance of anesthesia consists of fentanyl, muscle relaxants, and minimal concentrations of volatile anesthetics, if tolerated
- Nitrous oxide is avoided because of the already distended bowels
- Use air/oxygen mixture to maintain SpO_2 around 90% (PaO_2 50–70 mm Hg)
- Have PRBC, FFP, and platelets available
- A dopamine infusion may be necessary to maintain cardiac output, especially in sepsis
- Expect very high fluid requirements because of extreme third space losses; give up to 100 mL/kg/h of crystalloids
- Prevent hypothermia aggressively:
  - Increase room temperature
  - Radiant heat lamps
  - Warming blanket
  - Warmed and humidified gases
  - Wrap extremities and head in plastic wrap

POSTOPERATIVE

- Ventilation in the NICU. Transport in warmed isolette with full monitoring
- Intraoperative opioids usually make any further analgesia or sedation unnecessary for the first day
- Prolonged ileus. Place CVL for TPN if not already in place

PEARLS

- Remove umbilical artery catheters if possible to improve mesenteric blood flow
- Dramatic fluid requirements once abdomen is open

REFERENCES

For references, please visit **www.TheAnesthesiaGuide.com**.

CHAPTER 176
Pediatric Inguinal Hernia Repair
Philipp J. Houck, MD

BASICS

- Inguinal hernia: protrusion of intestinal organs through an open processus vaginalis
- Incarcerated hernia: content does not slide back into the abdominal cavity
- Strangulated hernia: vascular supply becomes insufficient

INTRAOPERATIVE

- Depending on associated morbidity and surgical requirements, neuraxial anesthesia, GETA, LMA, or a mask airway is appropriate
- A wide variety of regional anesthesia techniques can be used for inguinal hernia repair, either as an anesthetic or for analgesia
  ‣ Caudal blocks can be used, more often as an adjunct to general anesthesia
  ‣ In older patients, ilioinguinal and iliohypogastric nerve blocks can be performed either preoperatively percutaneously or during the procedure by the surgeon
- Spinal anesthesia for infants:
  ‣ Not demonstrated to reduce risk of postoperative apnea
  ‣ Experienced helper who positions and holds patient, keeps head in neutral position to avoid airway obstruction
  ‣ Skin infiltration with 1% lidocaine
  ‣ 22G 1.5-in styletted needle L4/5 or L5/S1
  ‣ One-milliliter syringe with 0.8 mg/kg 1% tetracaine in D5W, may add epinephrine wash
  ‣ Slow injection of anesthetic to avoid total spinal, maintain patient horizontal after injection to avoid cephalad spread
  ‣ Airway obstruction or apnea indicates a total spinal, which requires immediate endotracheal intubation

POSTOPERATIVE

- Postoperative apnea in 20–30% of otherwise healthy former preterm infants undergoing inguinal hernia repair
- Risk of postoperative apnea decreases with the postconceptional age of the infant
- Spinal anesthesia often chosen for these patients, although not shown to reduce incidence of apnea and bradycardia
- Admit for observation overnight to monitor for apnea:
  ‣ Ex-preemies (patients born at 36 weeks or earlier) <60 weeks postconception
  ‣ Patients born full term (37 weeks or later) <45 weeks postconception

PEARLS

- Laryngospasm may occur during surgical manipulation of the hernia sac, if anesthesia is too light
- Most common surgical procedure in children
- Higher incidence in premature babies
- Often bilateral, debate about need to explore contralateral side
- In ex-preemies, surgery usually performed prior to discharge from NICU
- Laparoscopic inguinal hernia repair usually requires endotracheal intubation. However, a brief insertion of a laparoscopic camera in the contralateral hernia sac after an open repair of the other side does not require a change in the anesthetic technique

REFERENCES

For references, please visit **www.TheAnesthesiaGuide.com**.

CHAPTER 177
The Hypotonic Child

Philipp J. Houck, MD

PATHOPHYSIOLOGY

Patients with undiagnosed neuromuscular disorder and hypotonia frequently present for a muscle biopsy. Most patients present because they do not carry a diagnosis yet. Hence, there is always uncertainty about the underlying pathophysiology. The toddler with an undiagnosed hypotonia could have a mitochondrial myopathy or a muscular dystrophy, which would require a different anesthetic management.

PREOPERATIVE

Review of the patient's extensive workup is essential. The neurologist's note could be helpful. Review lactate levels, cardiac workup, and family history. Look for signs and symptoms of a cardiomyopathy and pulmonary aspiration.

ANESTHESIA

Muscular dystrophy:
- Succinylcholine is contraindicated: risk of hyperkalemia and MH
- Avoid volatile anesthetics because of concerns for MH (only Evans myopathy, King syndrome, and central core disease are truly associated with MH, but in doubt, better to avoid any triggering agents)

Mitochondrial myopathy:
- Avoid propofol. (The long-chain fatty acids interfere with fatty acid oxidation and the mitochondrial respiratory chain. A clinical picture similar to propofol infusion syndrome may result.)

If the patient does not clearly fall in one of the above categories, a trigger-free, propofol-free technique should be considered:
- Midazolam 0.5–0.7 mg/kg po + N_2O + remifentanil 0.1–0.3 µg/kg/min
- Mask airway
- Supplemented with IV midazolam or ketamine boluses
- Use NS; avoid LR, since patients may have lactic acidosis. Avoid hypoglycemia
- Consider a lateral femoral cutaneous nerve block

POSTOPERATIVE

Most patients can be treated as outpatients. Acetaminophen is usually sufficient to control postoperative pain. Patients who are on noninvasive ventilation support at home should continue this support immediately postoperatively in the ICU or PACU.

PEARLS AND TIPS

In cases where an additional skin biopsy is needed, avoid infiltration with local anesthetic that will destroy the sample.

REFERENCES

For references, please visit **www.TheAnesthesiaGuide.com**.

CHAPTER 178
Pediatric Regional Anesthesia

Clara Lobo, MD

NB: Also refer to chapters 119–155.

GENERAL ASPECTS

Key Points
Performance under deep sedation/general anesthesia (GA) not contraindicated in children
Awake regional anesthesia (RA) remains popular in ex-premature neonates, children susceptible to malignant hyperthermia and/or with muscular diseases
Never exceed local anesthetic (LA) maximum dose, especially in small children (mg/kg) and with a repeated bolus or continuous infusion (mg/kg/h) technique
Prefer long-acting LAs. Adequate analgesia achieved with concentrations of 0.2–0.25% (bupivacaine/levobupivacaine/ropivacaine) for PNB and 0.1% for central neuraxial blocks (CNB)
Single dose: minor surgery or short postoperative pain Continuous infusion: prolonged surgery, expected severe postoperative pain, painful physical therapy, or complex regional pain syndrome
Nerve localization techniques: peripheral nerve stimulators (PNS) (if GA, do not use NMB), ultrasound guidance, or both
Children have a better "acoustic window" than adults Ultrasound-guided (UG) blocks have faster onset time and increased success rate and use lower LA doses High-frequency (linear) transducers are more suitable (especially small-footprint "hockey stick" probes) for small children
Epinephrine test dose can help signal IV injection
Obtain consent for RA from parents (preferentially in a written form) and child (if mature enough). Explain that the anesthetized region will "feel" different; discuss possible complications (severity and rate) and an alternate plan if block failure
Complication rate and severity is lower than in adults

Anatomy and Physiology of Children Relevant to Regional Anesthesia				
Anatomic structure	Children		Adults	Comments
	Birth	1 year – 8 years		
Conus medullaris	L3	L1	L1	Higher risk of spinal cord injury in small children
Tuffier's/ intercrestal line	L5–S1	L5	L4; L4–L5	For spinal, do not place the needle above this line
Dural sac	S3	S2	S2	Increased risk of dural puncture in smaller children during performance of caudal block
Sacral hiatus	More cephalad position when compared with adults			

(continued)

Anatomy and Physiology of Children Relevant to Regional Anesthesia (*continued*)

Anatomic structure	Children Birth	1 year – 8 years Adults	Comments
Sacrum	Not ossified Flatter and narrower	Completes ossification	Better "acoustic window" for UG blocks in smaller children; caudal block is more difficult in older children (>8 years)
Lumbar lordosis	No	Yes	Allows easy catheter advancement from caudal to higher levels (lumbar and thoracic)
CSF	4 mL/kg	2 mL/kg	Shorter duration of intrathecal anesthesia/analgesia in children (60–90 min)
Response to sympathetic block	Little or none	Hypotension	High block levels better tolerated hemodynamically
Connective tissue	Looser connective tissue around neuraxial structures and peripheral nerves ("sheaths") when compared with adults	Improved LA spread in children. Easier advancement of catheters	
Nerves	Small diameter, thin myelin sheath, short internodal distances than in adults	Lower concentrations of LA produce an adequate surgical block in infants and younger children	

Local Anesthetic Pharmacology in Children

LAs most commonly used are amino amides (lidocaine, bupivacaine, ropivacaine, and levobupivacaine)

Ropivacaine and levobupivacaine have a safer cardiovascular profile than bupivacaine

Amino esters (chloroprocaine) metabolized by serum esterases and very fast clearance (Cl) (even for neonates)

Amino amide bound to serum proteins (mainly alpha-1-acid glycoprotein [AAG]) and metabolized by hepatic enzymes
Serum concentration of AAG at birth is low (reach adult levels at 1 year) and increases in the postoperative period
Ropivacaine and bupivacaine metabolisms follow similar patterns (low at birth and increases in the first year). Ropivacaine's metabolism only reaches maturity by 3–5 years, although it is still safe to use in younger patients
Increased risk of higher free fraction of LA and systemic toxicity for smaller children

Children have higher Vd

Vd for ropivacaine < Vd for bupivacaine in children <1 year

LA clearance increases with increasing age

Bupivacaine and ropivacaine have similar total body clearance after single-dose administration (low at birth and increases during the first year)

(*continued*)

Local Anesthetic Pharmacology in Children (*continued*)

During prolonged non-IVLA administration, total clearance decreases with time and total concentrations measured in serum can be higher than after a single dose

Single dose: levobupivacaine better than ropivacaine

Continuous infusion: ropivacaine better than levobupivacaine
Lidocaine is not recommended for continuous infusion or when repeated doses are necessary

After epidural injection, bupivacaine t_{max} is similar between adults (~20 min) and children and infants (~30 min); ropivacaine t_{max} is different between infants (115 min) > children (60 min) > adults (~26 min)

Smaller children have a higher risk of toxic reactions (main contributing factors: low intrinsic clearance of LA and decreased serum protein binding; acidosis significantly decreases protein binding.)

t_{max}: time to maximum serum concentration.

Adjuvants to Local Anesthetics

	Dose or concentration/ type of block	Other effects	Comments
Epinephrine	1/400,000 (2.5 mg/L)/ epidural	Prolongs duration of LA effect	Use with caudal bupivacaine
	1/200,000 (5 mg/L)/PNB	Prolongs analgesia (alpha effect) for CNB	Do not exceed 2.5 μg/ mL (1/400,000) in children <1 year
	Test dose: *lidocaine 1% with 0.5 μg/kg epinephrine*	Decreases systemic absorption	for caudal/lumbar epidural (higher risk of permanent neurological complications)
		Marker of inadvertent IV injection	
Clonidine	2 μg/kg (single-shot dose); 3 μg/kg/24 h (continuous infusion)/ epidural or PNB	Increases sedation	Use with LA Best for continuous epidural infusion Respiratory depression has been reported
Ketamine	0.25–0.5 mg/kg/epidural block	No side effects in this dose range	Use preservative-free formulation Use with LA Best for single-injection caudal use
Midazolam	0.25–0.5 μg/kg/caudal epidural	No sedation with this dose	Safety concerns of neurotoxicity
Morphine	4–5 μg/kg/spinal 30 μg/kg every 8 h/ epidural	Nausea/vomiting (32%) Pruritus (37%) Urinary retention (6%)	Risk of severe respiratory depression not increased with low-dose morphine Spinal and epidural morphine not recommended for preterm and term neonates

Most common adjuvants: ketamine (32%) and clonidine (26.9%). Still not enough evidence supporting routine use of additives in outpatient surgery. Dexamethasone not recommended because of neurotoxicity concerns.

Monitoring and Prevention of Local Anesthetic Toxicity		
Criteria for positive test dose in anesthetized children		Recommendations to prevent systemic LA toxicity
HR increase >10 beats/min[1] Systolic blood pressure (BP) increase >15 mm Hg Increase in T-wave amplitude >25% in lead II[2] If any of these criteria is observed, stop the injection immediately	IV injection	Closely monitor the EKG, BP, and respiratory rate Incremental injection of LA, frequent and gentle aspirations during injection PNS: make sure motor twitches disappear after injection of 1 mL of the LA solution UG: observe LA spread with injection; if no spread visualized, possible IV injection: reassess
	Systemic absorption	Respect maximum LA dose Add epinephrine to LA solution

[1]Monitoring only for HR changes during inhalation anesthesia will miss 25% of IV injections.
[2]ST segment changes will detect 97% of the cases. During propofol/remifentanil anesthesia, look for BP changes, because T-wave morphology has poor sensitivity.

LA Maximum Recommended Doses			
LA	Single bolus maximum dose (mg/kg)	Continuous infusion (mg/kg/h)	
		Neonates and infants	Older children
Ropivacaine	3	0.2	0.4
Bupivacaine	2.5–4	0.2	0.4
Levobupivacaine	2–4	0.2	0.4
Lidocaine	7 (10 with epinephrine)	Not recommended	
	3–5 (if IV regional anesthesia)		
2-Chloroprocaine	20	Not recommended	

BLOCK EQUIPMENT AND MONITORING

Needles and catheters:

Use the shortest needle possible, with clear depth markings.

For epidural block LOR technique, saline should be used for children.

For caudal block, IV cannula is useful for single dose. Blunt cannula is associated with less venous/dural puncture, intraosseous injection, and neural damage.

Infusion devices:

Elastomeric pumps are easy to handle and appropriate for pediatric population. Be sure to choose one with appropriate flow rate.

BLOCK TECHNIQUES

NB: The figures are block demonstrations for didactic purposes, rather than actual procedures. Hence, for better visibility, sterility precautions such as gloves, transducer cover, skin preparation, and sterile draping were omitted.

Mastering a few techniques can help you to manage most cases in the pediatric population: head and neck blocks, anterior abdominal wall blocks, penile block, neuraxial blocks (spinal, epidural, and caudal), and axillary, femoral and sciatic blocks.

HEAD AND NECK BLOCKS

Most of these blocks are sensory nerve blocks, easy to perform (field blocks).

Use low volume of LA solution, usually 0.25% bupivacaine with epinephrine.

Head and Neck Blocks (Also See Chapter 155)

Nerve	Indications	Technique	LA mL	Complications
Trigeminal nerve (V1 division)				
Supraorbital	Anterior scalp lesions	Supine position; identify the supraorbital foramen/notch at the orbital rim at the level of the pupil; make a subcutaneous injection with a 30G needle. Remove the needle and apply firm pressure to prevent hematoma	1	Hematoma, IV injection, eye lesions (rare)
Supratrochlear		Use the same approach as for the supraorbital nerve; redirect the needle 0.5 cm more medially	0.5	
Trigeminal nerve (V2 division)				
Infraorbital (four sensory branches—inferior palpebral, external and internal nasal, and superior labial nerves)	Cleft lip repair Endoscopic sinus surgery Nasal septum repair (bilateral block) Transsphenoidal hypophysectomy	Supine position **Extraoral approach:** palpate orbital rim floor and identify infraorbital foramen (intersection of a vertical line through the pupil and a horizontal line through the alanasae). Introduce needle perpendicular to skin (not cephalad) and enter the foramen; inject after a negative aspiration test. Remove the needle and apply firm pressure **Intraoral approach:** palpate infraorbital foramen; use a 45° bent needle and insert it into the buccal mucosa in the subsulcal groove at the level of the canine or the first premolar. Advance the needle cephalad, until it reaches the foramen. The finger placed externally will feel the LA spread and prevent further cephalad advancement of needle	0.5–2	IV injection, hematoma, eye lesions (rare) Inform patient/parent that the upper lip will be numb as the child could bite it and it may interfere with feeding
Greater palatine	Cleft palate repairs	Supine position, with mouth open **Intraoral approach:** the palatine foramen is medial and anterior to the first molar. Use a 27-G needle to inject LA in the mucosa over the palate, after negative aspiration	1	IV injection, intraneural injection

(*continued*)

Head and Neck Blocks (*continued*)

Nerve	Indications	Technique	LA mL	Complications
Trigeminal nerve (V3 division)				
Mental nerve	Surgery involving lower lip Cutaneous surgery of the lower front teeth, skin of the chin	Supine position **Intraoral approach:** evert lower lip and inject LA into the mucosa in the subsulcal groove, between the canine and first premolar	1	IV injection, hematoma, and intraneural injection
Superficial cervical plexus (four branches: lesser occipital, great auricular, transverse cervical, and supraclavicular nerves)	Tympanomastoid surgery Cochlear implant Otoplasty One-sided block—procedures at the lateral aspect of the neck Bilateral block–procedures at the midline of the neck Clavicular fracture reduction	Supine position, head turned to the opposite side Draw a line from the cricoid cartilage to intersect the posterior border of the clavicular head of SCM. At that point make a subcutaneous injection of LA after careful negative aspiration (proximity to the external jugular vein)	2–3	IV injection, hematoma, deep cervical plexus block with associated adverse effects (phrenic nerve blockade)
Greater occipital nerve	Posterior fossa craniotomy Shunt revisions Chronic occipital neuralgia	Lateral or prone position Identify the pulse of occipital artery lateral-inferior to the posterior occipital protuberance and insert a 27-G needle lateral and cephalad to the pulsating artery along the superior nuchal line. Inject the LA using a "fanning" technique	3	Rare
Nerve of Arnold (vagus nerve auricular branch)	Myringotomy	Supine position, head turned to the opposite side Apply gentle retraction of the tragus and insert a 27-G needle to the posterior aspect of the tragus	0.2	Hematoma

LA mL, local anesthetic dose in milliliters; SCM, sternocleidomastoid muscle.

ANTERIOR ABDOMINAL WALL BLOCKS (SEE CHAPTERS 151 AND 153)

Rectus Sheath Block	
Indications	Umbilical hernia Linea alba hernia (perform at the hernia level)
Contraindications	Absolute: exomphalos, laparoschisis
Nerves involved	9th to 11th intercostal nerves (periumbilical area)
Landmarks	Umbilicus. Lateral border of rectus abdominis muscle (RAM) or linea semilunaris
Blind technique	Insert the needle with a 60° angle toward the umbilicus, at the intersection point (circle) between a horizontal line (dashed line) through umbilicus midline and the lateral border of RAM (straight line) (Figure 178-1)
UG	Transducer over the linea semilunaris at the umbilicus level (and above the arcuate line) (Figure 178-2) Identify the anterior and posterior sheaths of RAM (Figure 178-3). Introduce the needle until the posterior sheath. LA is deposited between RAM's posterior muscle wall and RAM's posterior sheath
Complications	Bowel perforation Intraperitoneal injection Hematoma
LA solution	Ropivacaine 0.2–0.5% or levobupivacaine 0.25–0.5%
LA dose	Single dose: 0.1–0.2 mL/kg
Comments	UG increases safety and efficacy Hydrolocation can be used to confirm the correct needle position

FIGURE 178-1. Blind technique landmarks for rectus sheath block

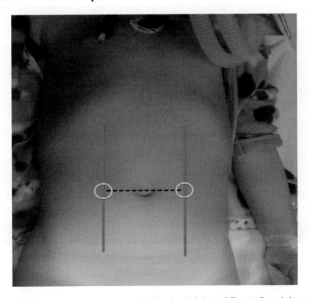

Red lines: lateral edges of rectus muscles. Black line: level of the umbilicus. Yellow circles: needle insertion point.

FIGURE 178-2. Ultrasound-guided rectus sheath block

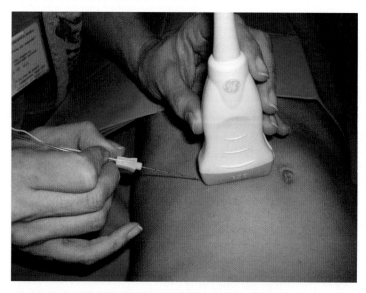

Transducer over linea semilunaris. Needle introduced in-plane from the lateral side.

FIGURE 178-3. US view showing the sheath of the rectus abdominis and the umbilicus

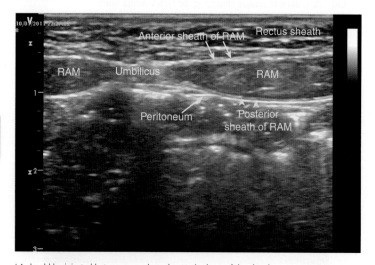

LA should be injected between muscle and posterior layer of the sheath.

Transversus Abdominis Plane (TAP) Block (See Chapter 152)	
Indications	Laparotomy Appendectomy Major abdominal wall surgery Colostomy placement and closures
Nerves involved	T10 to L1 thoracolumbar nerves run between the internal oblique (IO) and transversus abdominis (TA) muscle (the transversus abdominis plane)
Landmarks	Iliac crest. Anterior axillary line
Patient position	Dorsal decubitus
Blind technique	There is no distinctly palpable triangle of Petit in children Not recommended
UG	Transducer–lateral to the umbilicus and slide it laterally above the iliac crest, until the anterior axillary line (Figure 178-4) Identify the three anterior abdominal wall muscles (Figure 178-5) Insert the needle in-plane, and position it in the TAP plane, that is, between internal oblique and transverse abdominis LA injection expands the TAP plane, moving the TA muscle posteriorly *NB*: Some authors recommend performing two injections–one between EO and IO, and another between IO and TA–as there are anatomic variations and some nerves can travel in the more superficial plane
Complications	Bowel perforation Hepatic puncture Intraperitoneal injection
LA solution	Ropivacaine 0.2–0.5% Levobupivacaine 0.25–0.5%
LA dose	Single dose: 0.1–0.2 mL/kg
Comments	UG increases safety and efficacy Hydrodissection can be used to confirm correct spread of LA

FIGURE 178-4. Position of the US probe for TAP block

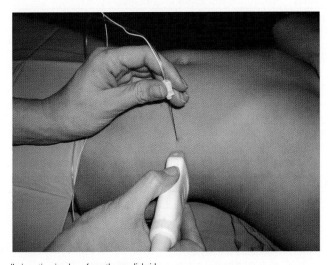

Needle insertion in-plane from the medial side.

FIGURE 178-5. Ultrasound view showing the muscle planes

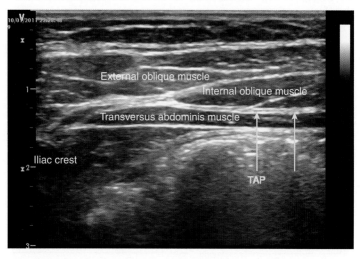

TAP: plane between transverse abdominis and internal oblique.

Ilioinguinal/Iliohypogastric Nerve Blocks (See Chapter 152)	
Indications	Inguinal hernia Orchidopexy (if low scrotal incision, make local infiltration) Varicocele ligation Hydrocele
Nerves involved	Both nerves are terminal branches of L1 spinal nerve The iliohypogastric runs cephalad to the ilioinguinal nerve in the TAP compartment
Landmarks	Umbilicus. Anterior superior iliac spine (ASIS)
Blind technique	Needle introduced 5–10 mm medial and inferior to ASIS or 2.5 mm medial along a line between ASIS and the umbilicus (Figure 178-6). The needle is introduced perpendicular to the skin, and injection starts after a single fascial click
UG	Transducer medial to the ASIS (Figure 178-7). Identify the three layers of abdominal muscles (Figure 178-8). Insert the needle and advance it to the plane between the IO and TA muscles *NB*: Some authors recommend performing two injections—one between EO and IO, and another between IO and TA—as there are anatomic variations and some nerves can travel in the more superficial plane
Complications	Bowel perforation Intraperitoneal injection Pelvic hematoma Femoral nerve block by spread (11% patients)
LA solution	Ropivacaine 0.2–0.5% or levobupivacaine 0.25–0.5%
LA dose	Single dose: 0.1–0.2 mL/kg
Comments	UG increases safety and efficacy The genital branch of the genitofemoral (GF) nerve also supplies the inguinal canal and is not blocked with this approach 30% failure with blind technique Hydrodissection can be used to confirm correct spread of LA

FIGURE 178-6. Needle insertion point for blind technique for the ilioinguinal and iliohypogastric blocks

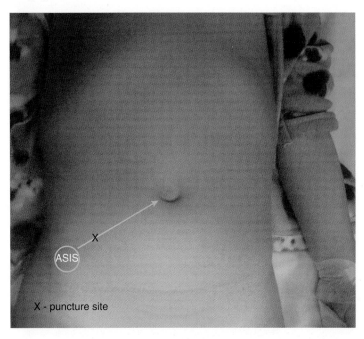

X - puncture site

FIGURE 178-7. Ultrasound-guided technique for the ilioinguinal and iliohypogastric blocks

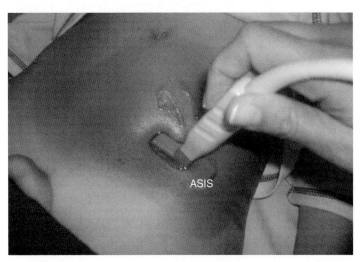

Ultrasound probe positioned on a line from umbilicus to ASIS, straddling the ASIS.

FIGURE 178-8. Ilioinguinal and iliohypogastric nerves in the planes between IO and TA

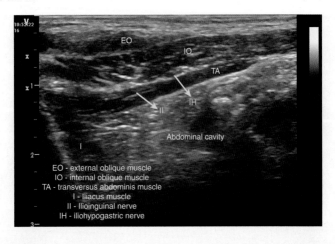

EO - external oblique muscle
IO - internal oblique muscle
TA - transversus abdominis muscle
I - Iliacus muscle
II - Ilioinguinal nerve
IH - iliohypogastric nerve

Penile Block	
Indications	Circumcision
Contraindications	Absolute: LA solutions containing epinephrine
Nerves involved	Dorsal penile nerves run at 10 and 2 o'clock positions in the penile shaft Ventral penile nerves run midline, subcutaneously in the penile–scrotal junction
Landmarks	Ring block: base of the penis Subpubic block: pubic symphysis, midline
Patient position	Dorsal decubitus
Blind technique	Ring block: needle introduced subcutaneously around the base of the penis Subpubic block: needle inserted midline, under pubic symphysis with a posterior direction and 10° caudal and 20° lateral angles, both sides. Feel two "pop" (superficial and Scarpa fascia). Success rate improved by blocking the ventral penile nerves, with a subcutaneous wheal of LA midline in the penile–scrotal junction
Complications	Ring block: superficial hematoma Subpubic block: deep hematoma with potential vascular compromise and ischemia
LA solution	Levobupivacaine 0.25–0.5%
LA dose	Ring block: 1–2 mL Subpubic block: single injection–0.1 mL/kg (maximum 5 mL) per side

UPPER EXTREMITY BLOCKS

Axillary block (see chapter 136 for figures):

Axillary Block	
Indications	Forearm, wrist, and hand surgery
Nerves involved	Terminal nerves of the BP surround the AA: radial nerve is midline and deep to the artery; ulnar nerve is medial and superficial; median nerve is superficial and lateral to the artery. Musculocutaneous nerve is out of the brachial sheath, between coracobrachialis and biceps muscle
Patient position	Dorsal decubitus, the head turned slightly to the contralateral side. Position the arm with 90° abduction, elbow flexion
PNS	Insert the needle with a cephalad orientation over the pulse of the artery. Advance the needle under the artery, and inject LA after radial nerve stimulation; redirect needle and inject LA after ulnar nerve stimulation. Redraw the needle and pass it above the pulse; inject after median nerve response and advance further the needle until musculocutaneous response
UG	Transducer axial to the humerus, as proximal as possible with slight pressure to avoid vessels to collapse—use Color Doppler. Insert the needle in-plane. Nerve structures are very superficial and surround the artery. Look for musculocutaneous between biceps and coracobrachialis muscles. Inject LA in order to surround the nerves
Complications	IV injection Intraneural injection Hematoma
LA solution	Ropivacaine 0.2–0.5% Levobupivacaine 0.25–0.5% Add epinephrine 1:200,000 for inadvertent IV injection detection
LA dose	Single dose: 0.2–0.3 mL/kg
Comments	Continuous technique not very popular at this level

LOWER LIMB BLOCKS

Femoral nerve block (see chapter 142 for figures):

Femoral Nerve Block	
Indications	Femoral shaft, hip, and knee surgery Surgery of the anterior aspect of the thigh, medial aspect of calf and ankle
PNS	Puncture site 1 cm lateral to the FA pulse at femoral crease. Introduce needle with a 30° angle cephalad orientation. Surface mapping can also be used to locate the nerve. The puncture of the fascia iliaca is felt ("pop"). With 0.5 mA/0.1 ms current, look for quadriceps muscle response (patella twitch), and then reduce to 0.4 mA and inject the local anesthetic. If sartorius muscle twitches, redraw the needle and redirect it 30° laterally
UG	High-frequency transducer, parallel and inferior to inguinal ligament. Advance needle in-plane from lateral end of the transducer and insert inside the fascia iliaca. Visualize the spread of the LA surrounding the nerve

(continued)

Femoral Nerve Block (*continued*)	
Continuous technique	Can be performed with combined PNS–UG technique. The puncture site is the same, but the out-of-plane technique is more suitable if UG is used. The needle should be angled 10–20° rostrally to allow threading of catheter. Insert 2–3 cm of catheter
Complications	IV injection Arterial puncture and hematoma Intraneural injection
LA solution	Ropivacaine 0.2–0.5% or levobupivacaine 0.25–0.5% Lidocaine 1% with 1/400,000 epinephrine
LA dose	Single dose: 0.2–0.4 mL/kg (maximum 15 mL) Continuous infusion: 0.2–0.4 mg/kg/h

Sciatic nerve block (see chapters 146 and 147 for figures):

Sciatic Nerve Block	
Indications	Surgery of the posterior aspect of the thigh, lateral aspect of lower leg, ankle, and whole foot
Contraindications	Absolute: none specific Relative: risk of compartment syndrome of lower extremity
Nerves involved	Sciatic nerve (Sc) and its branches (tibial and common peroneal nerves)
Landmarks	Subgluteal approach: ischial tuberosity (IT) and greater trochanter (GT) Popliteal posterior approach: medial aspect–tendon of semitendinous (ST) and semimembranous (SM) muscles; lateral aspect–tendon of biceps femoris (BF) muscle; popliteal skin crease (PP) and popliteal artery pulse Popliteal lateral approach: groove between vastus lateralis (VL) muscle and BF; PP
Patient position	Subgluteal approach: prone, lateral, or supine with hip and knee flexion Popliteal posterior approach: prone or lateral decubitus position Popliteal lateral approach: supine position
PNS	Subgluteal approach: insert the needle perpendicular to the skin at the midpoint between IT and GT. Inject LA with a foot response (plantar or dorsiflexion) to 0.4–0.5 mA/0.1 ms current Popliteal posterior approach: draw the popliteal skin crease with the midline of the popliteal fossa and the medial and lateral muscular borders Puncture point distance from the PP: <1 year = 1 cm; 1 year = 3.2 cm; 2–4 years = 4–5.3 cm; 5–8 years = 5.8–7.3 cm; 9–14 years = 7.7–9.7 cm Insert the needle with cephalad orientation, 45° to the skin Inject LA with 0.5–0.4 mA/0.1 ms current foot twitch response Popliteal lateral approach: identify the groove between VL and BF. Insert the needle (puncture site calculated from the above reference) with a 30° posterior angle to the skin

(*continued*)

Sciatic Nerve Block (*continued*)	
UG	Subgluteal approach: with the patient in the supine position, insert the needle proximal to the high-frequency transducer or if in the prone position, insert the needle in-plane. Identify the sciatic nerve close to the surface and inject the LA
	Popliteal posterior approach: place a high-frequency transducer cephalad to the PP; identify the nerve lateral and superficial to the popliteal artery and the point at which the nerve furcates into its two branches. Insert the needle in-plane or out-of-plane and surround the nerve with LA
	Popliteal lateral approach: place the lower limb over a foot support and place the transducer at the posterior aspect of the thigh. Insert the needle in-plane after identifying the depth of the nerve
Continuous technique	Any of the approaches described is suitable for a continuous catheter. Insert the needle parallel to the nerve, with a 30–45° angle to better thread the catheter. Introduce 2–3 cm catheter
Complications	IV injection Neuropathy
LA solution	Ropivacaine 0.2–0.5% or levobupivacaine 0.25–0.5% Avoid solutions containing epinephrine
LA dose	Single dose: 0.3–0.5 mL/kg (maximum volume 20 mL) Continuous infusion: 0.2–0.4 mg/kg/h
Comments	Combine with saphenous nerve block to block lower limb below the knee

NEURAXIAL BLOCKS

Spinal (Subarachnoid) Block		
Indications	Medical conditions	Preterm infant <52 weeks postconceptual age for inguinal hernia repair–most common indication
		Conditions that increase risk of GA: muscular or neuromuscular diseases, severe asthma, laryngomalacia, macroglossia, micrognathia, congenital heart disease, Down syndrome, adrenogenital syndrome, failure to thrive, arthrogryposis, Gordon syndrome
	Surgical procedures	Abdominal Perineal Lower limb Meningomyelocele repair Cardiac (for morphine administration in patients who will be ventilated postoperatively)
Contraindications	Absolute: increased ICP, VP shunt, hemodynamic instability, poorly controlled seizures and procedures expected to last more than 60 min (unless epidural block performed simultaneously) Relative: neuromuscular diseases (central core or congenital) and spine deformities	

(*continued*)

Spinal (Subarachnoid) Block (*continued*)	
Landmarks	Tuffier's line, typically interspace L4–L5 or L5–S1; dorsal midline (spinal processes)
Patient position	Lateral or sitting position Avoid flexing the neck and causing airway obstruction
Technique	Prefer a midline approach at the interspace L4–L5 or L5–S1, below *conus medullaris* (lower in children) Apply EMLA cream preoperatively or make local infiltration if awake or sedated children Use short needles (22-G or 25-G, too thin needles are unhelpful) and advance carefully (*ligamentum flavum* is soft, so a distinctive "pop" may not be perceived when dura mater is penetrated) Once CSF flow is seen, inject the LA with no barbotage If a hyperbaric LA solution is used, do not elevate lower limbs of the patient or a total spinal can occur (placement of electrocautery return electrode or Trendelenburg position)
Block assessment	The speed of onset in neonates is very fast, but its assessment can be difficult in small children. The response to cold solutions or pinprick can be helpful In older children (>2 years) use Bromage scale: free movement of legs and feet–no block (0%); just able to flex knees with free movement of feet–partial (33%); unable to flex knees, but with free movement of feet–almost complete (66%); unable to move legs or feet–complete (100%)
Complications	Hypotension and bradycardia (rare) Postoperative apnea (4.9%) in preterm infants Postdural puncture headache (PDPH) (1–8%) Transient radicular symptoms Failure (1.6–20%)
LA solution	Ropivacaine 0.5%: 0.5–1.08 mg/kg (mean duration–60 min) Levobupivacaine 0.5%: 0.5–1 mg/kg (mean duration–80 min) Bupivacaine 0.5% hyperbaric: 0.5–1 mg/kg (mean duration–77 min) Tetracaine 0.5–1 mg/kg (mean duration–86 min)
Adjuvants	Epinephrine wash Clonidine 1–2 μg/kg Morphine 10 μg/kg (only for cardiac surgery)
Comments	RA decreases but does not eliminate postoperative apnea in preterm infants, so maintain the same postoperative monitoring as for GA. Sedation increases risk of postoperative apnea in that group Considerations for difficult airway and spinal block: ability of practitioner to manage the airway, nature of surgical procedure (site, duration, and patient position), and age (if sedation is considered, as in preschool and school-age child, it has its own set of risks) PDPH is rare in neonates, but irritability and other behavior changes should raise the suspicion. High incidence of PDPH in older children. Consider it if symptoms of dizziness, nausea, and hearing loss. Conservative treatment includes rest, hydration, analgesics, and caffeine. If that fails, consider epidural blood patch (0.3 mL/kg of blood, aseptically taken); associated side effects are back stiffness, paresthesia, and subdural hematoma

Caudal Block	
Indications	Lower abdomen, pelvic and lower limb surgery
Contraindications	Relative: abnormal sacral anatomy (skin pigmentation, dimples, hair patches can be associated with spinal dysraphism or tethered spinal cord—confirm normal neuroanatomy before attempting the block)
Landmarks	PSIS; sacral cornua (SC); body of S4; sacral hiatus (SH) roofed by the sacrococcygeal membrane (SM); coccyx
Patient position	Lateral decubitus with hips and knees flexed 90°
Blind technique	Use styletted needles or IV cannula (author's preference), 25-G for neonates or 20-G for older children. A practical way to identify the SH is by squeezing the gluteus muscles and the SH is at the end of the intergluteal fold (Figure 178-9). Insert the needle midline, at the SH with a 45° angle to the sacrum, and advance through the SM until a LOR is felt; do not introduce more than 2–3 mm into the epidural space (ES). After penetrating the SM, remove the needle and advance the plastic cannula into the ES (Figure 178-10). Leave the cannula open to air for a few seconds (to detect blood/CSF leakage) and inject LA dose after a negative aspiration test
Tests for correct needle placement	*Aspiration/test dose*: negative aspiration is not reliable to exclude IV or intrathecal injection; EKG changes (>25% increase in T wave) could signal an IV epinephrine test-dose injection *Fluoroscopy with contrast agent injection*: "gold standard" to define tip of catheter location, but exposes to ionizing radiation and contrast agent, more expense *Epidural stimulation test*: used to confirm and guide catheter position in the ES, stimulating spinal nerves with a low-amplitude electrical current conducted through normal saline via a catheter that has a metal element disposed within its lumen (a special adapter is needed). Correct catheter position is shown by a motor response elicited with a current between 1 and 10 mA; responses with lower current (<1 mA) suggest intrathecal or subdural position, or placement very close to a nerve root. Inappropriate after MR/LA injection. The safety of this test is not known *Pediatric epidural stimulation catheter*: the styletted catheter advancement is monitored transmitting low current through a conducting fluid injected in the ES, causing muscle twitches from the lower limbs to the intercostal nerves. Inappropriate after MR/LA injection *Epidural EKG test*: using the epidural EKG monitoring lead, the anatomic position of the epidural catheter is determined by comparing the EKG signal from the tip of the catheter with a signal from a surface electrode positioned at the "target" segmental level. Still valid after MR/LA injection, but it cannot warn about intrathecal, subdural, or IV catheter placement *UG*: real-time visualization may be used for catheter placement and advancement; LA spread and anatomy scan. Limited value in older children *"Woosh" test*: confirmation of caudal ES successfully cannulated by injecting air while auscultating over the thoracolumbar spine. Not recommended (risks of patchy block, venous air embolus, or possibly neurological damage) *"Swoosh" test*: injecting LA or saline instead of air and listening for a "swoosh" sound over the lower lumbar spine *Anal sphincter tone*: relaxed sphincter is a positive predictor of successful caudal blockade

(*continued*)

Caudal Block (*continued*)	
UG	Scan the region rotating the transducer from a transverse (Figures 178-11 and 178-12) to sagittal (or parasagittal in older children) plane (Figures 178-13 and 178-14). Insert the needle in either plane (transverse to view LA spread, sagittal to view the needle) through the SH into the ES
Continuous technique	Very similar to the single-shot technique. Use the IV cannula to thread the epidural catheter. The appropriate length of epidural catheter is measured against the patient's back (from sacral to target level). Advance the catheter carefully and then confirm its localization with an objective test (described above). The catheter introduced reaches thoracic levels in 85% of premature neonates and 95% of term infants
Complications	Failure (increase with age) Urinary retention Motor block Dural puncture and intrathecal injection IV injection Subdural block High risk of catheter colonization, but infections are rare with short-term use (<72 h)
LA solution	Ropivacaine 0.2% or levobupivacaine 0.125–0.25%
LA dose	Single dose—Armitage formula (maximum of 20 mL): 0.5 mL/kg–sacral nerve roots 1.0 mL/kg–lower thoracic and upper lumbar nerve roots 1.25 mL/kg–midthoracic (T6) nerve roots Continuous infusion: 0.2–0.4 mg/kg/h
Comments	Mongolian blue spots are no contraindication to caudal block

FIGURE 178-9. Palpation of the sacral hiatus

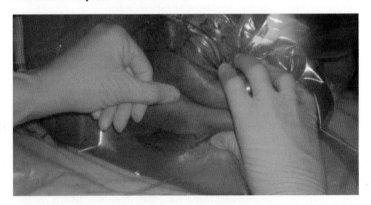

Squeeze the cheeks, and the sacral hiatus can be palpated at the end of the fold.

FIGURE 178-10. Cannula placement for caudal block

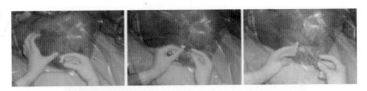

FIGURE 178-11. Position of the US probe for US-guided caudal block (transverse view)

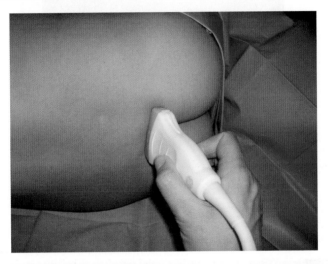

FIGURE 178-12. Transverse view of the sacral hiatus

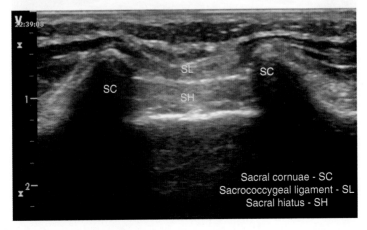

Sacral cornuae - SC
Sacrococcygeal ligament - SL
Sacral hiatus - SH

FIGURE 178-13. Position of the US probe for US-guided caudal block (sagittal view)

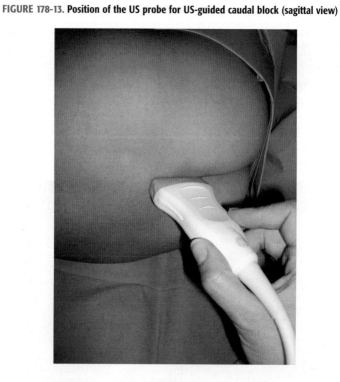

FIGURE 178-14. Longitudinal view of the sacral hiatus

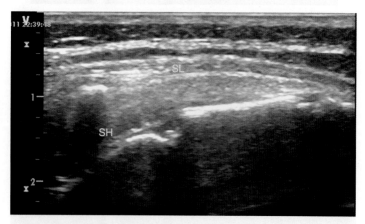

SL, sacrococcygeal ligament; SH, sacral hiatus.

Epidural Block	
Indications	Major thoracic, abdominal, or lower extremity surgical procedures associated with GA
Contraindications	Relative: VP shunts (consider prophylactic antibiotics and special attention to asepsis) and risk of compartment syndrome in lower extremities
Landmarks	Spinous processes; Tuffier's line for L4–L5/L5–S1 level; inferior angle of scapula for T6–T7 level
Patient position	Lateral decubitus with hips and knees flexed 90°
Blind technique	The same as adults, except: children are anesthetized and ES more shallow with a variable depth Depth guidelines: children >1 year = 1 mm/kg or depth (cm) = $1 + 0.15 \times$ age (years) or $0.8 + 0.05 \times$ weight (kg); mean depth in neonates = 1 cm Prefer LOR technique with saline (avoid using air b/o increased risk of venous embolism) Prefer L4–L5 or L5–S1 interspace for lumbar approach. Best angle for needle insertion is 74° pointing cephalad In younger patients, thoracic epidurals do not need as steep angles as for adults
Tests for correct needle placement	See caudal block table
UG	Ultrasound imaging can be used preprocedurally (to define angle/depth from the skin to the ES) and during block performance (spread of LA) at sacral, lumbar, and thoracic levels Use a dynamic approach changing transducer planes from axial to median longitudinal to paramedian longitudinal to guide needle and catheter placement. Does not preclude LOR technique Best "acoustic window" to the ES: infants <3 months of age; paramedian longitudinal plane and lumbar >thoracic level. *Dura mater* is better identified than *ligamentum flavum* Insert the needle midline at the chosen interspace. LOR can be seen as widening of the ES followed by ventral displacement of the *dura mater* Main limitation: difficult needle shaft and tip visualization with the tangential relationship of the needle (midline) and the transducer (paramedian longitudinal) and real-time catheter placement usually requires an assistant
Complications	See chapter 124 Hypotension and bradycardia are rare in children <8 years
LA solution	Ropivacaine 0.2% (single dose) to 0.1% (continuous infusion) or levobupivacaine 0.125–0.25%
LA dose	Single dose: 0.7–1 mL/kg (maximum of 30 mL) Continuous infusion–0.2 mg/kg/h (neonates) to 0.4 mg/kg/h (older children) PCEA–0.15 mL/kg/h infusion, bolus–0.07 mL/kg, lockout 20 min
Comments	Postoperative continuous SpO_2 monitoring is advised Average duration of infusion is 72 h

Regional anesthesia complications in addition to those mentioned above for specific techniques:

Complications Associated with RA		
Overall incidence 0.12% (6 × higher for CNB) 0.14% overall incidence with catheters versus 0.13% with single-dose techniques		
Awake versus asleep		RA performed under GA or deep sedation is considered standard of care in pediatrics
Injuries related to sensitive/motor block		Risk of masking compartment syndrome (controversial) Maintain close limb monitoring and vigilance for breakthrough pain on a previous functioning block, paresthesia, pallor, pulselessness, and paralysis (5 P's)
Systemic toxicity Seizures Cardiac toxicity Respiratory arrest	IV injection	5.6% in caudal block Epidurography can detect IV epidural catheter
	Systemic absorption	Greater risk in infants <6 months Do not exceed recommended doses of LA 0.01% with epidural continuous infusion of bupivacaine
Nerve injury Transient paresthesia with no permanent neurological injury		6/10,000 epidurals 2/1,000 PNB
Infection Greater risk with indwelling catheters Most common agent staphylococcus	CNB	Most are superficial (managed with catheter withdrawn, local skin care, and a course of antibiotics) Deep infections (epidural abscess, meningismus) are extremely rare and usually detected days after catheter withdrawal
	PNB	Cellulitis (extremely rare) Catheter colonization is common with no clinical consequence

REFERENCES

For references, please visit **www.TheAnesthesiaGuide.com**.

CHAPTER 179
Basics of Pediatric Cardiac Anesthesia

Eric P. Wilkens, MD, MPH

BASICS

- Patients with repaired cardiac congenital disease are being seen more and more often for noncardiac surgery: important to understand lesions and repairs
- Congenital heart defects have an incidence of between 4 and 50 per 1,000 live births
- Most common: ventricular septal defect (VSD):
  - Most resolve spontaneously in the first few years of life
  - Larger ventricular defects (>5 mm) have a higher rate of spontaneous closure than smaller VSDs
- Four most important physiologic pearls for congenital heart disease:
  - Know primary lesion shunt direction and lesion
    - Left-to-right shunt (noncyanotic):
      - Atrial septal defect (ASD)
      - VSD
      - Patent ductus arteriosus (PDA)
    - Right-to-left shunt (cyanotic): examples include tetralogy of Fallot, pulmonary atresia, tricuspid atresia, Ebstein anomaly
    - Complex shunt: truncus arteriosus, transposition of the great vessels, total anomalous pulmonary venous return, hypoplastic left heart syndrome
    - Obstructive lesions:
      - Aortic stenosis (AS)
      - Mitral stenosis (MS)
      - Pulmonic stenosis (PS)
      - Coarctation of the aorta
  - Know initial arterial oxygen saturation
  - Know pulmonary to systemic blood flow ratio (Qp/Qs)
  - Know the primary cardiac valve lesions (restrictive or regurgitant)
- Knowing where the blood flows and in what proportion allows the provider to try to maintain a Qp/Qs ratio appropriate for the patient
- Influencing pulmonary vascular resistance (PVR) is the most important way we have to optimize circulation in these patients
  - Carbon dioxide: hyperventilation and the resulting respiratory alkalosis decrease pulmonary resistance; hypoventilation and respiratory acidosis raise it
  - Nitrates: medications such as inhaled nitric oxide (5–40 ppm) or medications that affect the intracellular nitric oxide pathway (e.g., sildenafil) decrease PVR
  - Milrinone (an inotrope with vasodilatory effects) can decrease PVR and increase the ability of the right heart to contract
  - Inhaled or infused prostaglandins (inhaled: 5–50 µg/h; infused: start at 2 µg/h) selectively decrease PVR

- A simplified template of normal blood flow is available below (Fig. 179-3)
- Simpler procedures, such as ASD and some VSDs, are amenable to extubation in the OR. Other procedures, such as repair of PDA or repair of other lesions such as hypoplastic left heart syndrome or arterial switch procedures, involve complicated vessel and cardiac repair and are likely to require sedation and mechanical ventilation postoperatively

Different Types of Cardiac Shunts Seen in Pediatric Patients
Left-to-right shunts
These shunts result from oxygenated blood being directed from the arterial circulation into the venous circulation without crossing a capillary bed resulting in a normal SpO_2 reading, a higher than normal venous blood saturation, and a pulmonary blood flow (Qp) that is higher than the systemic blood flow (Qs). These shunts can occur anywhere from the atria to the precapillary blood vessels in end organs
Faster inhalation induction
Right-to-left shunts
These shunts result from deoxygenated blood being directed from the venous circulation into the arterial circulation without crossing a capillary bed resulting in a low, abnormal SpO_2 reading, a lower than normal venous blood saturation, and a pulmonary blood flow (Qp) that is lower than the systemic blood flow (Qs). These shunts can occur anywhere from the atria to the precapillary blood vessels in end organs
Slower inhalation induction
Mixed shunts
These shunts are associated with primarily intracardiac lesions and are the result of mixing of oxygenated and deoxygenated (arterial and venous) blood. The measured SpO_2 will vary depending on the size of the shunt, and the pulmonary and systemic blood flows. Usually the SpO_2 is lower than normal because of the mixing

Basics of cardiac development (see Figure 179-1):
- A heart in its normal arrangement and position is referred to as situs solitus
- The looping of the primitive heart tube is followed by septation and development of the heart valves
- The aorta and pulmonary artery differentiate from the truncus arteriosus when a septum develops, spiraling up the truncus to isolate these two large vessels from each other

FIGURE 179-1. Mammalian heart development

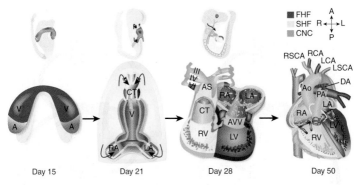

Day 15   Day 21   Day 28   Day 50

Oblique views of whole embryos and frontal views of cardiac precursors during human cardiac development are shown. (First panel) First heart field (FHF) cells form a crescent shape in the anterior embryo with second heart field (SHF) cells medial and anterior to the FHF. (Second panel) SHF cells lie dorsal to the straight heart tube and begin to migrate (arrows) into the anterior and posterior ends of the tube to form the right ventricle (RV), conotruncus (CT), and part of the atria (A). (Third panel) Following rightward looping of the heart tube, cardiac neural crest (CNC) cells also migrate (arrow) into the outflow tract from the neural folds to septate the outflow tract and pattern the bilaterally symmetric aortic arch artery arteries (III, IV, and VI). (Fourth panel) Septation of the ventricles, atria, and atrioventricular valves (AVVs) results in the four-chambered heart. V, ventricle; LV, left ventricle; LA, left atrium; RA, right atrium; AS, aortic sac; Ao, aorta; PA, pulmonary artery; RSCA, right subclavian artery; LSCA, left subclavian artery; RCA, right carotid artery; LCA, left carotid artery; DA, ductus arteriosus. Reproduced with permission from Srivastava D. Making or breaking the heart: from lineage determination to morphogenesis. *Cell.* 2006;126:1037. © Elsevier.

Fetal circulation basics (see Figures 179-2 to 179-4):
- In utero, fetal circulation relies on two major shunts to direct the majority of blood flow around the pulmonary vasculature:
  ‣ Foramen ovale in the atrial septum
  ‣ Ductus arteriosus, connecting the aorta to the pulmonary artery
- In utero, the pulmonary circulation receives approximately 10% of the right ventricular output
- Within the first breaths of ex utero, right atrial and IVC pressures decrease. PVR drops precipitously due to aeration of the lungs secondary to pulmonary arterial oxygenation responses:
  ‣ The increase in pulmonary blood flow increases left atrial pressure relative to the right, helping close the foramen ovale
  ‣ The increase in oxygen pressure in neonatal blood is the primary stimulus for the contraction (and hence closure) of the ductus arteriosus
  ‣ A third shunt, the extracardiac ductus venosus, contracts and restricts flow over the first few days of neonatal life

FIGURE 179-2. Differences in fetal and adult circulation

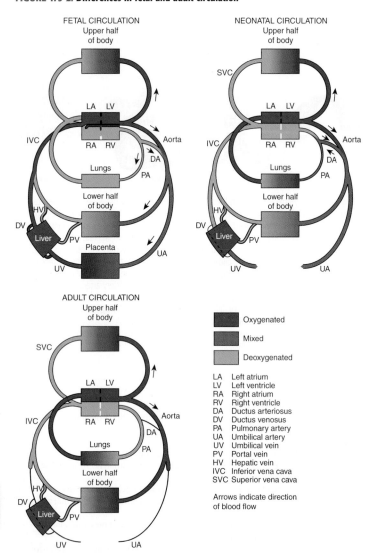

Reproduced with permission from Scott JR et al, eds. *Danforth's Obstetrics and Gynecology*. 7th ed. Philadelphia: Lippincott-Raven; 1997:149.

FIGURE 179-3. Simplified normal heart blood flow template

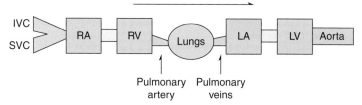

FIGURE 179-4. Shunts caused by the foramen ovale and the ductus arteriosus

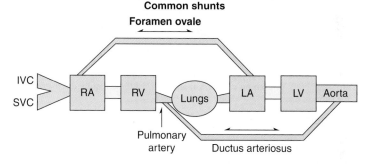

PREOPERATIVE

Preoperative concerns for a patient include the standard concerns for a pediatric patient as well as those of a patient undergoing cardiac surgery.

- *NPO status*: Possible hypovolemia and hypoglycemia, particularly in neonates, after appropriate NPO times. Consider placement of intravenous catheter and replacement with appropriate dextrose-containing crystalloid solution in the immediate preoperative period
- *Mask versus IV induction*: While mask induction is common in the pediatric congenital cardiac surgical population, the patient's acuity may necessitate an IV induction—anesthetic creams at the IV catheter site may help, as well as IM, PO, or intranasal sedatives
- *Reflux*: Neonatal and childhood reflux is common, particularly in populations that have multiple midline defects. Confirm that the patient's antacid or metoclopramide doses have been given appropriately. Reflux may be bad enough that the patient has a gastrostomy tube—if present, ensure that it is appropriately vented
- *Parent/guardian reassurance*: Appropriate counseling and assurance are an absolute necessity, especially in the neonatal population. Some patients are not diagnosed with cardiac congenital disease until birth, adding the further stress of "surprise" to the parents
- *Surgical plan*: Consult with surgeon before the procedure, if only briefly, to discuss the initial surgical repair plan, expectations for inotropic support, and plans for postoperative ventilation
- Meticulously remove any air bubbles from IV tubing, especially if any shunt is present

MONITORING

Monitoring the pediatric patient with congenital heart disease does not vary much from monitoring for other pediatric surgical procedures. Standard, accepted monitors include:

- Continuous pulse oximetry (SpO_2): two for most procedures—one above the diaphragm and one below
- Noninvasive blood pressure (NIBP) (not on the same limb as invasive blood pressure monitor)
- ECG (three-lead on very small neonates and infants, otherwise five-lead)
- End-tidal carbon dioxide monitoring ($EtCO_2$)
- Invasive blood pressure monitor: usually placed after induction. Neonatal patients may have umbilical artery catheters that surgeons may prefer be replaced with peripheral monitors. In some instances, a cutdown may have to be performed to locate the radial or femoral artery
- TEE: TEE monitors, usually with assistance of a pediatric cardiologist, can be placed in children as small as 2 kg. Other options include a small "surface" probe in a sterile sheath placed directly and intermittently on the heart by the surgeon under the direction of the cardiologist

Optional monitors:

- Central venous access: use of these monitors varies widely by institution, surgeon/ICU preference, and case type. Ranging from standard central venous access catheters in the internal jugular, subclavian, or femoral veins to umbilical vein, atrial catheters, or even no catheters at all; plans for these require discussion with the surgical team

INDUCTION

- Most patients for pediatric congenital heart surgery can safely be induced via mask induction with volatile agent
- In general, induction with 100% oxygen is acceptable, but decreasing the FiO_2 to 0.21 or as low as possible is preferred so that a patient's hypoxic pulmonary vasoconstriction reflexes are maintained
- Avoid N_2O:
  - Myocardial depressant
  - Decreases FiO_2
- Right-to-left shunt (cyanotic heart disease) will slow mask induction
- Left-to-right shunt (patients with noncyanotic heart disease) may shorten induction
- Mixed shunts will result in unpredictable induction times
- Some facilities have a policy that all pediatric congenital cardiac patients have an IV access present prior to induction
- IV induction is safe:
  - Benzodiazepine and opioid
  - With or without small doses of etomidate (0.1–0.2 mg/kg) or propofol (1–2 mg/kg)
- Administer a small dose of atropine (10–30 µg/kg) to neonates prior to induction
- Antibiotics for endocarditis prophylaxis

MAINTENANCE

- Balance of volatile agent with opioids and nondepolarizing muscle relaxant
- Plan for extubation after relatively simple repairs such as ASDs
- Expect continued intubation for the majority of cardiac surgical patients, even if positive pressure ventilation is not the best physiologic option for the patient
- Patients who rely on passive pulmonary blood flow after repair (classically patients with Glenn or Fontan shunts) may benefit from the absence of PEEP

- Discuss with the surgeon and perfusionist the use of antifibrinolytics and the optimum time to begin inotropic agents
- Patients may arrive in the operating room with collateral blood vessels that develop over time in response to chronic cyanotic disease. Collaterals present surgical problems because they increase bleeding intraoperatively and postoperatively
- Hemodynamic stability during induction, maintenance, and emergence primarily involves:
  ‣ Ratio of pulmonary to systemic blood flow (Qp/Qs)
  ‣ Kinking of shunts and coronary arteries

POSTOPERATIVE

- Postoperative concerns of these patients involve mainly the monitoring of adequate hemodynamic and ventilator issues
- Deep hypothermia and occasionally periods of circulatory arrest → diagnose and correct bleeding disorders
- Maintain appropriate intravascular fluid volume in the patient
- Patients may be extubated while on vasoactive support (milrinone, dopamine, etc.), but must be normothermic
- Patients who have their great veins (SVC and IVC) anastomosed directly to their pulmonary arterial tree rely on *passive flow* and a decreasing pressure gradient from the venous system, through the pulmonary tree, into the cardiac atrium for proper maintenance of cardiac output and oxygenation
  ‣ They are acutely sensitive to increases in PVR:
    ▪ Avoid hypercarbia (beware of sedation)
    ▪ Maintain oxygenation but avoid high FiO_2 (disturb pulmonary vasculature responsiveness)
    ▪ Avoid intravascular volume depletion
- Collaterals are another reason that patient SaO_2 may not be normal, even after a "complete" repair. The main reason for an abnormal oxygen saturation postoperatively is because of the patient's anatomy, usually with the presence of a shunt and blood mixing

PEARLS AND TIPS

- Three helpful hints when looking at congenital cardiac disease:
  ‣ Structures that do not get blood flow do not grow to normal size and function
  ‣ Structures that get too much blood flow dilate
  ‣ Ventricles that push against too much pressure or resistance thicken
- Review case goals with surgeon
- Draw a simplified diagram of patient's anatomy—both a preoperative diagram and an expected postoperative result to attach to the anesthesia machine for immediate reference intraoperatively
- Remember PVR. A normal saturation may be very bad (severe left-to-right shunt)
- Remember that low oxygen saturation in this population is normal and expected, and supplemental oxygen may result in too much pulmonary blood flow compared with systemic blood flow. Consider the result of having low systemic cardiac output with 100% saturation and sufficient or high cardiac output at a lower than normal (e.g., 86%) oxygen saturation because the cardiac output is more easily maintained in this situation; the patient is accustomed physiologically to chronic hypoxic conditions
- Remember the target saturation when weaning from cardiopulmonary bypass

Most Common Congenital Heart Lesions

Lesion	Description	Shunt type
Atrial septal defect	Naturally occurring as part of septal formation, persistent foramen ovale, or iatrogenic from surgery or catheterization procedure. In some cases an ASD may be necessary for patient survival	Predominantly left-to-right, but right-to-left and mixed can occur. Some argue there are no "true" L-to-R shunts in ASDs because the right atrium depolarizes before the left atrium in a normal sinus rhythm
Ventricular septal defect	Most common defect (17% of diagnosed congenital defects). VSDs may be single large or multiple small lesions and can occur anywhere in the ventricular septum	Predominantly left-to-right, except when the right heart is thickened and enlarged from responding to high pulmonary vascular pressures
Patent ductus arteriosus	A normal fetal structure connecting the aorta and pulmonary artery that occasionally fails to occlude physiologically shortly after birth	Usually left-to-right resulting in too much pulmonary blood flow and pulmonary hypertension
Aortic stenosis	Anomaly of aortic valve resulting in a smaller than normal orifice for blood exiting heart. Results in thickened LV and diastolic dysfunction	Not associated with any shunts
Aortic regurgitation	Anomaly of aortic valve such that there is lack of coaptation or holes in leaflets causing blood to fill heart retrograde from aorta during diastole. Results in dilated LV	Not associated with any shunts
Atrioventricular canal	Anomaly of endocardial cushion development resulting in abnormal tricuspid and mitral valves and usually a VSD	Mixed shunt, depends on pulmonary vascular resistance and systemic vascular resistance
Coarctation	A stricture of the aorta, usually distal to the ductus arteriosus. Results in diminished blood flow to body distal to stricture, often diagnosed after child becomes active (running, etc.)	Not associated with any shunts
Ebstein anomaly	A displacement of the tricuspid leaflets into the right ventricle. Almost always associated with an ASD	Mixed shunt
Hypoplastic left heart	The incomplete development of the left heart and usually aortic valve. The right heart thickens and dilates to compensate for the work of circulating to the systemic blood flow as well as the pulmonary circulation	Predominantly right-to-left
Tetralogy of Fallot	Second most common defect (12%). A constellation of anomalies including pulmonary stenosis, overriding aorta, VSD, and RV hypoplasia	Right-to-left shunt

(*continued*)

Most Common Congenital Heart Lesions (*continued*)

Transposition of great arteries	Development of aorta from the right heart and the pulmonary artery from the left heart. Not a problem in utero; the newborn quickly becomes hypoxic when the foramen ovale and ductus occlude	Mixed shunt. This diagnosis requires shunting and methods to maintain the ductus arteriosus open until definitive surgical repair can be performed. Without a shunt, there is no communication between the right and left heart circulation
Anomalous pulmonary venous return	Anomaly where some or all pulmonary veins flow into the right atrium instead of the left. Similar to transposition	Left-to-right primarily, but neonates are hypoxic because of increased oxygen extraction from the blood in the systemic circulation
Blalock–Taussig shunt	The classic repair developed on tetralogy patients. A subclavian artery (or, in modern times, an artificial graft) is placed from the aorta to the pulmonary artery to improve pulmonary blood flow	Left-to-right and a mixed shunt. Increases pulmonary blood flow over systemic blood flow and increases pulmonary vascular pressures. Patients still hypoxic from mixing of blood through VSD
Tricuspid atresia	Incomplete development of tricuspid valve, usually resulting in a persistent ASD and low pulmonary blood flow	Right-to-left predominantly
Truncus arteriosus	A rare (less than 1% of congenital cardiac lesions) anomaly where there is a single common arterial outlet for both ventricles	Predominantly left-to-right because the lesion is usually accompanied by a VSD
Mitral regurgitation	Blood flow retrograde across the mitral valve resulting in dilated left atrium and potentially increased pulmonary pressures	Not associated with any shunts
Mitral stenosis	Restriction of blood flow antegrade across the mitral valve results in increased filling pressures in left atrium	Not associated with any shunts

REFERENCES

For references, please visit **www.TheAnesthesiaGuide.com**.

PART XI

OBSTETRICS

CHAPTER 180
Physiology of Pregnancy

Imre Rédai, MD, FRCA

OVERVIEW

Overview of Physiological Changes During Pregnancy		
Mean body weight	Increases by 17% on average	Parenchymal organ hypertrophy
Oxygen demand and CO_2 production	Increased by 30–40% at term	Increase in muscle mass Fetoplacental unit
Total body fluids and electrolytes	7 L water and 900 mEq sodium is gained by term	

Cardiovascular System			
Cardiac output	By 5th week	Increase noticeable	Due to increase in heart rate
	By 12th week	35–40% over nonpregnant value	Stroke volume also increases
	End of second trimester	50% over nonpregnant value	At term both heart rate and stroke volume increased by 25% compared with nonpregnant values
Ventricular volumes	LVED increases LVES unchanged		
Contractility	Unchanged throughout pregnancy		
Filling pressures	CVP, PADP, PCWP	All unchanged compared with nonpregnant values	
Systemic vascular resistance	Reduced by 20% at term compared with nonpregnant values		
Systolic blood pressure	Minimally affected	Declines by 8% at midgestation Returns to baseline at term	

(continued)

Cardiovascular System (*continued*)		
Diastolic blood pressure	Reduced by 20% at midgestation	
	Returns close to baseline at term	Due to aortocaval compression
EKG changes	Sinus tachycardia Shortened PR QRS axis shifts initially to the right, and then to the left	
	ST depression, T-wave changes in lead III New Q wave in leads III, aVF	Do not confuse with myocardial ischemia, pulmonary embolism
Echocardiography	By 12th week	Noticeable LVH
	By term	50% increase in LV mass
	Valve annular diameters increase (except aortic valve)	94% patients have tricuspid regurgitation 27% have mitral regurgitation Aortic insufficiency is *never* normal

PHYSIOLOGY OF AORTOCAVAL COMPRESSION

The degree of compression of the aorta and inferior vena cava by the gravid uterus depends on:
- The gestational age
- The position of the pregnant woman

Effect of Gestational Age and Position on Aortocaval Compression			
13–16 weeks	First sign of IVC compression detectable		
At term	Lateral decubitus	Partial obstruction of IVC	
		No significant obstruction of aorta	
	Supine	Full or close to full obstruction of IVC	RV filling pressure drops Cardiac output reduced by 20% or more
		Noticeable compression of the abdominal aorta	20% decrease in uterine blood flow 50% decrease in lower extremity blood flow Increase in SVR
	15° left lateral tilt	Reduces but does not eliminate compression of IVC and aorta	
Supine hypotensive syndrome	Bradycardia Severe hypotension	Occurs in about 8% women at term in supine position	Combination of reduced venous return and inadequate response of the autonomic nervous system

Respiratory System			
Nasopharynx and oropharynx	Vascular engorgement	Starts as early as 7th week	
Bony thorax	AP and transverse diameters increase		Due to emergence of uterus from pelvis
Diaphragm	At rest 4 cm higher at term compared with nonpregnant state		
Tidal volume	Increased by 20% in first trimester	Due to decrease of inspiratory reserve volume	Progesterone sensitizes the respiratory center to CO_2
	Increased by 45% by term	Due to decrease in expiratory reserve volume	
Functional reserve capacity	Begins to decrease by 5th month		
	80% of nonpregnant value at term	Supine FRC is 70% of upright FRC at term	
Minute ventilation	Increased by 45% at term	Due to increase in tidal volume	RR unchanged or slightly elevated
V_D/V_T	Unchanged or slightly decreased $P_{A\text{-}a}CO_2$ gradient is minimal	Airway conductance increased by progesterone	Cardiac output increase reduces dead space ventilation
Arterial blood gases	$Paco_2$	Declines to 30–32 mm Hg by 12 weeks There is compensatory reduction in serum bicarbonate (to 20 mEq/L)	$P\bar{v}co_2$ is 34–38 mm Hg
	pH	Increases by about 0.02–0.06	
	Pao_2	Pao_2 increases to 107 mm Hg by the end of the first trimester in the upright position Drops by 2 mm Hg each following trimester	In the supine position, the Pao_2 may be considerably less

Blood, Plasma, and Red Blood Cells		
Blood volume	10% increase in the first trimester	Larger increases with multiple gestation
	30% increase in the second trimester	
	45% increase by term	
Plasma volume	15% increase in the first trimester	
	50–55% increase in the second trimester	No further increase
Red blood cell volume	Initial fall, and then returns to baseline by 16 weeks	RBC mass increase depends on iron stores and erythropoietin activity
	30% increase at term	
At term	Blood volume is 94 mL/kg	
	Plasma volume is 69 mL/kg	
	Red blood cell volume is 27 mL/kg	
Hemoglobin and hematocrit	Falls parallel with changes above At term hemoglobin is 11–12 g/dL At term hematocrit is 33–36%	
Leukocytes	Rise to 9,000–11,000/mm³	PMN rise; lymphocytes and eosinophils drop

Coagulation and Fibrinolysis

Pregnancy is a state of accelerated, compensated intravascular coagulation		Increased platelet turnover Enhanced clotting and fibrinolysis	
Platelet count	In 8% of patients is less than 150,000/mm^3	Increased production compensates for increased activation and consumption	
	In 0.9% of patients, less than 100,000/mm^3		
Coagulation factors	Factors I, VI, VIII, IX, X, XII, vWF increase	PT, aPTT shortened	
	Factors II, V remain unchanged		
	Factor XI, XIII decrease		
Fibrinolytic system	Plasmin levels rise	Increased FDP reflect enhanced fibrinolysis	

Gastrointestinal System

Esophagus	Decreased lower esophageal sphincter tone	Progesterone effect
	Intra-abdominal portion of the esophagus is displaced to the thorax	Prevents the rise in the sphincter tone which normally accompanies the increase in intragastric pressure
Stomach	Displaced upwards and to the left Rotated 45° from its normal vertical position	
	The intragastric pressure is elevated in the third trimester	
	Gastric emptying not altered at any time during pregnancy (except labor)	
The incidence of heartburn is 22%, 39%, and 72% in the consecutive trimesters		
Gastric acid	80% of women have a gastric pH <2.5	These numbers are representative throughout the whole of pregnancy
	50% of women have gastric volumes over 25 mL	
	40–50% of women have both a pH <2.5 and a residual gastric volume of >25 mL	
Small bowel	Intestinal transit time is slowed	Progesterone effect

Urinary Tract

Kidney	Enlarged in size	Return to normal by 6 months postpartum
	Glomerular filtration rate increases by 50%	
	Renal plasma flow increases by 75–85%	
	Creatinine clearance increases	
	BUN falls to 8–9 mg/dL by the end of the first trimester	
	Serum creatinine falls progressively to 0.5–0.6 mg/dL at term	
	Proximal tubular resorption of glucose is impaired leading to increased urinary glucose excretion	

GLUCOSE HOMEOSTASIS

Glucose intolerance is common (reduced tissue sensitivity to insulin):
- The main contributor is placental lactogen
- Fasting blood glucose levels are significantly lower at term
- Starvation ketosis is also exaggerated

MUSCULOSKELETAL SYSTEM

The lumbar lordosis increases with the growth of the pregnant uterus:
- Stretching of the lateral femoral cutaneous nerve may result in meralgia paresthetica
- Anterior flexion of the neck may result in brachial plexus neuropathy
- The incidence of low back pain or pelvic discomfort during pregnancy is about 50%

The incidence of carpal tunnel syndrome is increased during pregnancy.

Further Physiological Changes Relevant to Anesthetic Management			
MAC is reduced in pregnancy	The pain threshold increases near the end of pregnancy and during labor due to increased production of endogenous analgesic neuropeptides	Some studies attribute this effect to spinal cord rather than cortical action of volatile anesthetics	
Lower extremity venous capacitance	Reduced by increased sympathetic outflow	Pharmacological sympathectomy leads to more pronounced reduction in BP than in nonpregnant women	
Epidural space	IVC compression diverts blood toward the epidural venous plexus	Reducing the volume of the spinal CSF	This (and endogenous opioids) explains the increased sensitivity to neuraxial local anesthetics and opioids
	Absorption of fluids injected in the epidural space is delayed		
Plasma cholinesterase	Activity decreases by 25%	Not sufficient to affect succinylcholine	

CHAPTER 181
Physiology of Labor and the Postpartum Period

Imre Rédai, MD, FRCA

Respiratory System			
Minute ventilation during labor	75–150% increase in the first stage	Oxygen consumption may increase by 45%	Epidural anesthesia prevents changes in the first stage
	150–300% increase in the second stage	Oxygen consumption may increase by 75% Pa_{CO_2} may fall to 10–15 mm Hg Serum lactate rises	Epidural anesthesia does not prevent changes in minute ventilation, oxygen consumption and serum lactate in the second stage
Postpartum	FRC increases after birth but remains below normal for 1–2 weeks	O_2 consumption, minute ventilation, and tidal volume remain elevated till at least 6–8 weeks postpartum	

Cardiovascular System

Cardiac output in labor (between uterine contractions)	10% increase in early first stage	Increase in SV (HR unchanged)	Epidural analgesia reduces but does not fully eliminate the increases in cardiac output
	25% increase in late first stage		
	40% increase in second stage		
Systolic and diastolic blood pressures	Elevated from the late first stage	Progressive activation of the sympathetic nervous system during labor	Labor epidural analgesia attenuates these changes
Aortocaval compression (in the supine position)	20% reduction in uterine blood flow	About 8% of women may develop bradycardia and significant hypotension when lying supine (supine hypotensive syndrome)	
	50% decrease in lower extremity blood flow		
Uterine blood flow and uterine contractions during labor	Increases to 600–900 mL/min on average (50–190 mL/min preconception)	Uterine contractions augment CO and SV by an additional 15–25% (300–500 mL of blood displaced with each contraction)	
	Compression of the aorta by the uterus increases with contractions	Reduces uterine filling and increases afterload	
Immediate postpartum hemodynamics	CVP rises and cardiac output increases up to 75% of predelivery values	Relative hypervolemia and increased venous return in this period is a result of relief of caval compression and reduction of vascular capacitance, which exceeds the blood loss of labor (autotransfusion)	
Further postpartum hemodynamics	During the first hour postpartum term, CO decreases to 30% above the prelabor value; it reaches the prelabor value about 48 h postpartum CO 10% above prepregnant value at 2 weeks, returns to baseline at 12–24 weeks postpartum HR normalizes in 2 weeks Stroke volume takes much longer and is still 10% above baseline at 24 weeks LV hypertrophy regresses gradually and is still appreciable at 24 weeks		

Blood Volume

Blood volume	94 mL/kg (prepregnant value is 76 mL/kg)	Average blood loss during vaginal delivery is about 600 mL Average blood loss during Cesarean section is 1,000 mL	General anesthesia using volatile anesthetics results in a somewhat larger blood loss than regional anesthesia
Plasma volume	69 mL/kg (prepregnant value is 49 mL/kg)		
Postpartum changes	Blood volume falls to 125% of prepregnant value by the end of the first postpartum week and declines to 110% at 6–9 weeks Hb and hematocrit fall in the first 3 days, and then rise rapidly (plasma volume contraction) and reach prepregnant values at 6 weeks postpartum		

Coagulation System

At delivery	Platelet count, fibrinogen, factor VIII, and plasminogen levels fall Antifibrinolytic activity increases Clotting tests remain shortened during the first postpartum day	
Days 3–5 postpartum	Fibrinogen concentration and platelet count rises	Increased incidence of thrombotic complications
The coagulation profile returns to normal prepregnant values at 2 weeks postpartum		
During labor and the first postpartum day	Leukocyte count increases to 13,000 and 15,000/mm³	
Leukocyte count gradually decreases, but remains above prepregnant values when measured at 6 weeks postpartum		

Gastrointestinal Tract

During labor	Gastric function is slowed and gastric volume increases	Opiates administered during labor impair gastric emptying and reduce the tone of the LES Spinal or epidural fentanyl can inhibit gastric emptying	Epidural anesthesia using local anesthetics only does not delay gastric emptying during labor Low-dose epidural fentanyl infusion (≤2.5 mg/mL) has no adverse effect unless it is preceded by an epidural or intrathecal bolus
Postpartum period	Gastric emptying rate returns to normal by 18 h postpartum		Fasting gastric volumes and pH 18 h postpartum are similar to those in nonpregnant women

CHAPTER 182
Medications and Pregnancy

Imre Rédai, MD, FRCA

FDA Classification of Medications During Pregnancy	
Category A	Adequate and well-controlled human studies have failed to demonstrate a risk to the fetus in the first trimester of pregnancy (and there is no evidence of risk in later trimesters)
Category B	Animal reproduction studies have failed to demonstrate a risk to the fetus and there are no adequate and well-controlled studies in pregnant women Or Animal studies have shown an adverse effect, but adequate and well-controlled studies in pregnant women have failed to demonstrate a risk to the fetus in any trimester
Category C	Animal reproduction studies have shown an adverse effect on the fetus and there are no adequate and well-controlled studies in humans, but potential benefits may warrant use of the drug in pregnant women despite potential risks
Category D	There is positive evidence of human fetal risk based on adverse reaction data from investigational or marketing experience or studies in humans, but potential benefits may warrant use of the drug in pregnant women despite potential risks
Category X	Studies in animals or humans have demonstrated fetal abnormalities and/or there is positive evidence of human fetal risk based on adverse reaction data from investigational or marketing experience, and the risks involved in use of the drug in pregnant women clearly outweigh potential benefits

Anesthetic Medications		
	Dosing	Fetal effects
Induction agents	Dosing requirements are unchanged or mildly reduced for ultrashort-acting barbiturates and propofol (10–15%) Propofol TIVA: reduce dose by <10%	Equilibration with fetal tissues is rapid Fetal elimination strongly depends on reverse diffusion to mother Intravenous induction agents reduce fetal heart rate variability
Narcotics	Endogenous endorphin production reduces exogenous opioid requirement Peripartum oxytocin release has been implicated in reduced narcotic requirements Remifentanil has the shortest half-life in the newborn and has become a popular agent for labor analgesia when a neuraxial technique is contraindicated (usual starting dose is 0.03 µg/kg/min increased as needed to 0.1 µg/kg/min)	Narcotics reduce fetal heart rate variability Short-acting rapid-onset opioids have been reported to cause fetal bradycardia Intrathecal narcotic requirements are reduced by 30–50% when compared with nonpregnant patients There are no clear data for IV narcotic dose reduction

(continued)

Anesthetic Medications (*continued*)		
	Dosing	Fetal effects
Sedatives	Benzodiazepines are traditionally avoided in pregnant patients Dexmedetomidine has been reported for labor analgesia (insufficient data for assessment of safety of drug)	
Muscle relaxants	Sensitivity to muscle relaxants is unchanged Pseudocholinesterase activity is reduced by 30% in the pregnant patient; this has no effect on the onset and duration of succinylcholine	NMBs do not cross the placenta in significant amounts Magnesium sulfate therapy may increase sensitivity to nondepolarizing NMB (no effect on succinylcholine)
Neuromuscular reversal agents	Dosing requirements are unchanged	Neostigmine and glycopyrrolate do not cross the placenta Atropine crosses the placenta
Volatile anesthetics	MAC reduced by 30%	Volatile anesthetics reduce fetal heart rate variability
Local anesthetics	Nerves are more sensitive to local anesthetic effect (faster block onset)	Possible progesterone effect

Relevant doses of anesthetic agents are discussed in the individual chapters on anesthetic procedures for the pregnant patient:
- Uterotonics: see chapter 194
- Antihypertensive agents: see chapter 185
- Use of antibiotics: see chapter on 183
- Use of anticoagulants: see chapters 184 and 193
- Use of tocolytic agents: see chapter 192

ANESTHETIC DRUGS AND THE LACTATING MOTHER

- Relatively small amounts of anesthetic agents cross into the breast milk
- The safest advice is "pump and dump"; discard the first pumping of breast milk after a general anesthetic
- Ketorolac is safe for postpartum analgesia
- Meperidine and codeine are *not* recommended in breast-feeding mothers as they or their metabolites may accumulate in breast milk and cause neonatal respiratory depression

CHAPTER 183
Antibiotic Prophylaxis and Therapy in Obstetrics

Imre Rédai, MD, FRCA

Antibiotic therapy is guided by local pathogens. Consult your infectious diseases specialist for information and advice for best prophylactic and empirical therapy. Infected patients should get appropriate cultures sent and pathogen sensitivities determined to guide therapy.

General Guidelines		
Procedure	Prophylaxis	Comments
Uncomplicated vaginal delivery	No antibiotic	
Cesarean section	Cefazolin 2 g before incision • Delaying prophylactic antibiotics until after delivery is *no longer recommended* In patients with ruptured amniotic membranes, cefoxitin 2 g may be considered	If penicillin allergy • Clindamycin 600 mg
Antibiotic prophylaxis for patients at risk for bacterial endocarditis	Not indicated for routine vaginal deliveries and routine Cesarean sections	Select patients where antibiotic prophylaxis should be considered • Chorioamnionitis • Concomitant urinary tract infection • High-risk patients (prosthetic heart valves or conduits, unrepaired cyanotic lesions)
Group B streptococcus carriers (GBS + patients)	Penicillin 5 million U loading dose followed by 2.5 million U q4 h until delivery	If penicillin allergy, depending on culture and sensitivity • Erythromycin 500 mg q8 h • Clindamycin 600 mg q6 h
Chorioamnionitis	Empirical therapy options • Ampicillin 2 g q6 h + gentamicin 1.5 mg/kg q8 h • Cefoxitin 2 g q6 h • Ampicillin/sulbactam 3 g q6 h Continue antibiotics for at least 24 h postpartum	±Anaerobic coverage as well • Metronidazole 500 mg q8 h, or • Clindamycin 600 mg q8 h If penicillin allergy • Vancomycin 1 g q12 h + gentamicin 1.5 mg/kg q8 h ± anaerobic coverage
Acute pyelonephritis	Ampicillin 2 g q6 h and gentamicin 1.5 mg/kg q8 h Ceftriaxone 1 g q24 h	Avoid fluoroquinolones in pregnancy

REFERENCES

For references, please visit **www.TheAnesthesiaGuide.com**.

CHAPTER 184
Anticoagulation During Pregnancy

Imre Rédai, MD, FRCA

Long-term *therapeutic* anticoagulation during pregnancy is necessary for:
- History of venous thromboembolism in prior pregnancy
- History of recurrent thromboembolism
- Thrombophilias
- Mechanical heart valve prosthesis
- Certain medical conditions (Eisenmenger, severe heart failure, chronic atrial fibrillation)

Antithrombotic Agents in Pregnancy		
Medication	Characteristics	Comments
Unfractionated heparin (UFH)	Does not cross placenta Bone demineralization with long-term use Risk of HIT Does not cross into breast milk in significant amounts (safe with breast-feeding)	Reversal of anticoagulation for delivery seldom necessary If reversal is needed (usually for Cesarean delivery), titrate protamine
Low-molecular-weight heparin (LMWH)	Does not cross placenta Bone demineralization may occur with long-term use Does not cross into breast milk in significant amounts (safe with breast-feeding)	Should be converted to UFH at 36 weeks gestation In an emergency situation reversal is not complete (discuss with hematologist dose of protamine) Substitution of LMWH for warfarin in patients with mechanical heart valves remains controversial
Warfarin	Freely crosses placental barrier Fetal effects appear to be dose related rather than INR related Fetal hemorrhage may occur Neonatal hemorrhage may occur (if patient has not been converted to UFH, delivery should be via Cesarean section) Does not cross into breast milk in significant amounts (safe with breast-feeding)	Use is limited to patients with mechanical heart valves Should not be used between 6 and 13 weeks of gestation to minimize teratogenic effects Dose should be kept under 5 mg daily Switch to UFH at 36 weeks If emergency delivery is necessary, both mother and newborn should receive FFP to reverse drug effects (vitamin K onset is too slow in this clinical setting)

Anticoagulation should be restarted 6 hours following vaginal delivery and 12 hours following Cesarean delivery if there are no clinical signs of ongoing hemorrhage.

Anesthesia Considerations in the Anticoagulated Parturient

Labor analgesia	Neuraxial analgesia should not be attempted in an actively anticoagulated patient Follow neurological status throughout labor and postpartum for spinal hematoma	Neuraxial analgesia in patients on prophylactic UFH is safe UFH in intermediate and therapeutic dose should be stopped for 6 h and a normal aPTT documented before neuraxial analgesia is attempted Check platelet count if patient has received UFH for at least 4 days Prophylactic LMWH should be stopped for at least 12 h Intermediate and therapeutic LMWH should be stopped for at least 24 h Warfarin should be stopped for at least 5 days and a normal PT/INR should be documented; furthermore, time should be allowed for substitute antithrombotic agents to wear off (bleeding risk increases in patients recently converted from warfarin to UFH or LMWH)
Vaginal delivery	Risk of bleeding in mother may be increased	Evaluate patient thoroughly for potential intrapartum and postpartum hemorrhage Establish adequate venous access Consider reversing heparin effects with protamine Have 4 U PRBC cross-matched Evaluate and review airway throughout labor
Cesarean section	Neuraxial anesthesia should not be attempted in an actively anticoagulated patient Risk of bleeding in mother is increased Follow neurological status postpartum for spinal hematoma	Neuraxial anesthesia recommendations are the same as above for labor analgesia Establish adequate venous access Consider arterial line for monitoring hemoglobin and coagulation Consider reversing heparin effects with protamine Have 4 U PRBC cross-matched

REFERENCES

For references, please visit **www.TheAnesthesiaGuide.com**.

CHAPTER 185

Pregnancy-Induced Hypertension, Chronic Hypertension in Pregnancy, Preeclampsia, Eclampsia

Imre Rédai, MD, FRCA

DEFINITIONS

- Chronic hypertension:
  - ‣ Systolic blood pressure >140 mm Hg or diastolic blood pressure >90 mm Hg prior to pregnancy of before 20 weeks of gestation
  - ‣ Hypertension that persists beyond the 12th postpartum week
- Gestational hypertension:
  - ‣ New-onset hypertension after midpregnancy without proteinuria that resolves within 12 weeks postpartum
- Preeclampsia:
  - ‣ New-onset hypertension after 20 weeks gestation associated with >300 mg per day proteinuria
  - ‣ New-onset seizures in the setting of preeclampsia are defined as eclampsia
- Preeclampsia superimposed on chronic hypertension

Hemodynamic Characteristics of Hypertensive Disorders During Pregnancy[1]				
	Healthy	Early preeclampsia	Late preeclampsia	Gestational or chronic hypertension
Cardiac output	6.2	8.9	5.0	9.0
Systemic vascular resistance	1,210	1,082	1,687	922
Wedge pressure	7.5	9	13	7
Stroke volume	80	104	58	110
LVSWI	48	61	33	64
Colloid oncotic pressure	18	17	14	18

[1]No ranges are given; numbers are presented for comparison as representative values.

Chronic Hypertension		

Affects 3% of pregnant population More common in
• African Americans (up to 44%)
• Older gravidas (>12% after the age of 35)
Frequently associated with obesity, diabetes mellitus
	Maternal complications
	• Superimposed preeclampsia
	  ‣ 10–25% incidence of progression to preeclampsia
	  ‣ 2.7-fold increase in risk for severe preeclampsia
	• Placental abruption
		Commonly used oral medications[1]
		• α-Methyldopa
		• Labetalol
		  ‣ Metoprolol SR is an alternative
		• Nifedipine SR

		Less commonly used oral medications[1] • Hydrochlorothiazide • Hydralazine (oral)
	Fetal complications • IUGR/low birth rate • Fetal demise	Contraindicated in pregnancy[1] • ACEIs, ARBs, direct renin inhibitors • Propranolol (atenolol)

[1]Pharmacological options for the treatment of gestational hypertension are the same as those for chronic hypertension.

Preeclampsia

Estimated frequency in healthy nulliparous women is 2–7% Majority of cases (75%): mild, near term or intrapartum onset, negligible increase in risk for adverse outcome Frequency and severity is higher with history of • Multiple gestation • Chronic hypertension • Prior pregnancy with preeclampsia • Pregestational diabetes mellitus • Thrombophilia	Maternal complications • Placental abruption (1–4%) • Disseminated coagulopathy/HELLP syndrome (10–20%) • Pulmonary edema/aspiration (2–5%) • Acute renal failure (1–5%) • Eclampsia (1%) • Liver failure or hemorrhage (1%) • Stroke (rare) • Death (rare) • Long-term cardiovascular morbidity	Diagnosis and management is supported by adequate prenatal care Main objective remains the safety of the mother Expectant management for pre-34 weeks remains controversial
Multisystem disorder with poorly understood pathomechanism • Abnormal vascular response to placentation • Placental humoral factors (sFlt-1, sEng) cause endothelial dysfunction in mother Unique to human pregnancy Characterized by • Microvascular dysfunction • Increased SVR • Activation of inflammatory pathways • Enhanced coagulation • Increased platelet activation and aggregation • Endothelial barrier dysfunction Preeclampsia is most likely the common manifestation of a number of diseases affecting pregnant women	Fetal effects • IUGR/low birth weight • Reduced amniotic fluid • Restricted placental oxygen exchange, fetal hypoxia and neurological injury Preterm delivery	Antihypertensives • Little evidence for benefit in mild/moderate cases • Severe hypertension (>160 mm Hg systolic, >100 mm Hg diastolic) should be treated to prevent maternal end-organ damage • Hydralazine was associated with more maternal side effects and worse perinatal outcome than labetalol or nifedipine
	Maternal and perinatal outcomes in preeclampsia depend on • Gestational age at time of disease onset • Onset after 36 weeks has better outcome than onset before 33 weeks • Severity of disease • Quality of management • Presence or absence of preexisting medical disorders	Anticonvulsants • Magnesium sulfate is associated with significantly fewer seizures and better maternal outcome than diazepam, phenytoin, or a lytic cocktail Steroids • Beneficial effects of betamethasone prior to 34 weeks on fetal lung maturity and neonatal outcome • Ongoing studies on effect of steroids on HELLP syndrome Plasma volume expansion • Hypovolemia and organ underperfusion from intravascular volume depletion versus volume overload from overzealous administration of crystalloids or colloids • BNP values are markedly elevated in severe preeclampsia highly suggestive of LV dysfunction

Anesthetic Considerations in Hypertensive Disorders of Pregnancy

	Chronic hypertension or gestational hypertension	Mild or moderate preeclampsia	Severe preeclampsia
Hemodynamics	Increased cardiac output secondary to increased sympathetic tone and sodium and fluid overload	Maintained cardiac output with mildly increased systemic vascular resistance due to reduced endothelial production of NO	Reduced cardiac output and severely increased systemic vascular resistance due to a combination of endothelial dysfunction and increased sympathetic activation secondary to end-organ hypoperfusion
Circulating blood volume	Normal or slightly decreased to pregnancy	Decreased	Severely decreased
Renal function	Depends on duration and severity of disease	Mildly decreased	Severely decreased
Liver function	Normal	Usually normal	Often affected: HELLP syndrome
Coagulation system	Unaffected	Platelet count may drop due to endothelial dysfunction: checking platelet count within 6 h of neuraxial anesthesia/analgesia is recommended	Platelet count may drop due to endothelial dysfunction: checking platelet count within 6 h of neuraxial anesthesia/analgesia is recommended
CNS	Severe hypertension may cause hypertensive encephalopathy or intracerebral hemorrhage	Headaches in mild preeclampsia may herald eclamptic seizures The mechanism is likely inadequate vasoconstriction and endothelial capillary leakage in the setting of increased intracranial perfusion and pressure	Both of the two mechanisms on the left may contribute to CNS morbidity
Effects of neuraxial anesthesia[1]	Sympathectomy reduces blood pressure significantly Rate of onset determines response (spinal > epidural)	Reduction in blood pressure is often mild, even minimal, even with spinal anesthesia	Blood pressure drop can be significant due to intravascular volume depletion and underlying increased sympathetic tone

(continued)

Anesthetic Considerations in Hypertensive Disorders of Pregnancy (*continued*)

	Chronic hypertension or gestational hypertension	Mild or moderate preeclampsia	Severe preeclampsia
General anesthesia[1]	Induction of anesthesia may produce significant drop in blood pressure and uterine hypoperfusion Laryngoscopy may result in exaggerated hypertensive response	Induction of anesthesia is usually well tolerated Laryngoscopy may result in exaggerated hypertensive response Magnesium therapy may interfere with neuromuscular monitoring	Induction of anesthesia may produce significant drop in blood pressure and uterine hypoperfusion Laryngoscopy may result in exaggerated hypertensive response Magnesium therapy may interfere with neuromuscular monitoring

[1]Preeclampsia superimposed on hypertension may present with any combination of the two conditions depending on the individual contribution of the two entities to the overall clinical case.

Intravenous Treatment Options for Severe Hypertension in the Pregnant Patient

Labetalol	10–20 mg bolus repeated as needed every 10 min until desired blood pressure is reached (repeat doses may be increased by 20 mg/dose up to 80 mg) Start infusion at 2 mg/min and titrate to response Doses over 300 mg/day should be used with caution	Fetal bradycardia and hypoglycemia may occur
Nicardipine	125 μg bolus repeated every 5 min until desired blood pressure is reached Start infusion at 5 mg/h and increase by 2.5 mg/h as needed Infusion rates over 15 mg/h are not recommended	Tocolysis may happen Pulmonary edema has been associated with calcium channel antagonist use in pregnancy
Hydralazine	5 mg every 20 min up to 20 mg; dose may need to increase due to tachyphylaxis with repeat administration Start infusion at 0.5 mg/h and increase as needed every 20 min Infusion rates over 10 mg/h are not recommended	Maternal tachycardia is common
Sodium nitroprusside	0.3 μg/kg/min infusion increased by 0.5 μg/kg/min every 10 min until desired effect Doses in excess of 10 μg/kg/min are not recommended and should be used with extreme caution	Cyanide toxicity risk in mother and fetus is increased with doses over 2 μg/kg/min and infusion durations beyond 4 h Do not use without invasive BP monitoring Use of sodium nitroprusside in the pregnant patient is a *last resort*

Management of Severe Preeclampsia and Preeclampsia-Related Complications		
Eclamptic seizures	Call for help Turn patient to side to reduce risk of aspiration Protect patient from injury Protect IV access Break seizures with IV benzodiazepine or propofol • Diazepam 5–10 mg • Midazolam 2–5 mg • Propofol 50–100 mg Once seizures cease • Administer supplemental oxygen • Check fetal heart rate • Check vital signs Allow spontaneous return of consciousness Transfer to high dependency unit Load magnesium sulfate if patient is not on magnesium therapy	Tonic–clonic eclamptic seizures result in hypoxemia and combined metabolic and respiratory acidosis Fetal effects depend on duration of seizure and underlying uteroplacental insufficiency associated with preeclampsia Fetal bradycardia after an eclamptic seizure is very common; recovery should be brisk once maternal oxygenation is restored • If fetal depression remains, sustained operative delivery is indicated

HELLP syndrome	Patients presenting with epigastric or right upper quadrant pain should be screened for HELLP syndrome
	• Nausea, malaise are often associated
	Laboratory tests: thrombocytopenia with elevated AST, LDH. Prolongation of PT follows thrombocytopenia in HELLP
	Follow laboratory tests every 8 h
	Blood and platelet transfusion may be necessary
	Use of dexamethasone for treatment when platelet count is below 100,000 remains controversial
	Vaginal delivery is preferred
	If there is progressive worsening of symptoms or laboratory findings, operative delivery should be performed
	Labor analgesia options are determined by platelet count and PT/INR
	• If the platelet count is >100,000 within 8 h and the PT/INR is normal, neuraxial analgesia may be considered
	• Removal of epidural catheter should be delayed until both platelet count and PT/INR normalized after delivery
	• Cesarean section should be performed under general endotracheal anesthesia in patients with HELLP syndrome
		Hypertension, proteinuria, or both may be absent in some patients (atypical HELLP syndrome)
		Prolonged PT with hypoglycemia and hypocholesterolemia suggests acute fatty liver of pregnancy rather than HELLP; platelet count is often normal in early stages of acute fatty liver of pregnancy when PT is already markedly prolonged
		Thrombotic thrombocytopenic purpura (TTP) presents with thrombocytopenia and elevated LDH but normal liver enzymes
		Possible complications
		• Common
		  ▸ DIC
		  ▸ Placental abruption
		• Rare
		  ▸ Hepatic capsular hematoma
		  ▸ Rupture of liver
		  ▸ Renal failure
		  ▸ Pulmonary edema

(*continued*)

Management of Severe Preeclampsia and Preeclampsia-Related Complications (*continued*)

Renal failure	Low urine output in preeclampsia is common Changes in serum creatinine is a poor indicator of renal function Use of FeNa in preeclamptic oliguria is seldom useful due to the complex nature of the problem • If FeNa is suggestive of prerenal causes, fluid challenge should be performed	Combination of intravascular fluid depletion and glomerulopathy associated with preeclampsia Response to fluid boluses may not reflect on intravascular fluid status Fluid management may necessitate placement of • Central venous line if there is no evidence of heart failure • Pulmonary artery catheter if there is evidence of heart failure Indiscriminate fluid loading of preeclamptic patients may lead to pulmonary edema and hypoxemia Prolonged hypovolemia may lead to uterine hypoperfusion and fetal distress
Pulmonary edema	Relatively rare • More common in patient receiving magnesium sulfate therapy Restrict IV fluids Supplemental oxygen If necessary, positive pressure ventilation with PEEP Use of noninvasive positive pressure (CPAP, BiPAP) has been clinically successful	Combination of fluid load, poor urine output, increased capillary leakage (hypoalbuminemia), and magnesium sulfate Diuretics are seldom useful Check BNP levels or perform TTE exam of left ventricle to exclude cardiac causes

REFERENCES

For references, please visit **www.TheAnesthesiaGuide.com**.

CHAPTER 186
Nonobstetrical Surgery in the Pregnant Patient

Elena Reitman Ivashkov, MD and Imre Rédai, MD, FRCA

PREOPERATIVE CONSIDERATIONS IN THE PREGNANT PATIENT

See also chapter 180.
- Airway and airway equipment:
  - ‣ Mallampati classification may underestimate difficulty of intubation
  - ‣ Evaluate carefully neck mobility (presence of "buffalo hump" posteriorly)
  - ‣ Look at the patient supine as well as sitting (enlarged breasts, position of neck)
  - ‣ Have *extra equipment (airway cart)* immediately available when planning general anesthesia for a pregnant patient
  - ‣ *Difficult intubation* is more likely (risk increased about *4-fold*)
  - ‣ *Enlargement of lingual tonsils* (protrusion of tongue) is an important reason for Mallampati 3–4 scores: this results in reduced orohypopharyngeal junction diameter
  - ‣ Increased risk of injury resulting in *swelling and bleeding* during laryngoscopy
  - ‣ When difficulty in intubation is anticipated, the route of choice for *fiber-optic intubation is "oral"* rather than nasal
- NPO guidelines:
  - ‣ Fasting time for pregnant patients before elective cases is the same as that for the nonpregnant population
- When is a pregnant patient considered to have a full stomach?
  - ‣ Presence of *heartburn* is suggested to be indicative of reduced lower esophageal sphincter (LES) tone (<20 cm H_2O) and *potential regurgitation* during induction and mask ventilation
  - ‣ Early onset heartburn is hormonally driven
  - ‣ From about 20 weeks the enlarging uterus mechanically distorts the position of the stomach and the LES and increases intra-abdominal pressure
  - ‣ *Gastric emptying is "not" reduced* in pregnancy until advanced stages of labor
- Looking after the fetus (see detailed discussion about fetal well-being and anesthesia below):
  - ‣ Every pregnant patient should have an identified designated obstetrician with hospital privileges available before any elective surgery; in an emergency, attempts should be made to contact the on-call obstetrician
- Laboratory tests:
  - ‣ Routine laboratory tests are similar to those for the nonpregnant female: CBC to evaluate for presence of anemia. All other tests should be performed as clinically indicated
  - ‣ Ketosis and hypoglycemia are common in pregnant patients when NPO for a prolonged period of time. This is well tolerated and routine testing is *not* recommended
  - ‣ Type and screen should be done for all cases in case labor ensues; extent of maternal hemorrhage is unpredictable
- Postoperative planning:
  - ‣ Patients who are <24 weeks pregnant are recovered in the general PACU and are discharged to the general floor (fetus is not considered viable)
  - ‣ Patients who are >24 weeks pregnant are recovered and are transported to labor and delivery once stable postoperatively (monitoring, staff, and neonatology is immediately available should labor ensue)
  - ‣ ICU admission criteria are similar to those for nonpregnant patients; obstetrical input into ICU care should be arranged

CONCERNS RELATED TO PERIOPERATIVE AND LONG-TERM FETAL WELL-BEING, FETAL MONITORING DURING SURGERY

- Effect of maternal surgery on the offspring with emphasis on teratogenicity of anesthetic agents:
  - No anesthetic drug has been shown to be clearly dangerous to the human fetus
  - Incidence of stillbirth and birth defects is unchanged
  - Incidence of low birth weight is increased
  - Incidence of neural tube defects increased if surgery is in the first trimester
  - Although some agents (N_2O, benzodiazepines) have been implicated in adverse neonatal outcome, these studies have been either refuted or associated with exposure in excess of an average anesthetic
  - There is *no optimal anesthetic technique*
  - *Avoid elective surgery in the first trimester*
  - Enhanced risk of preterm labor after abdominal and pelvic surgeries, especially in cases of acute appendicitis and presence of peritonitis
  - Risk factors for preterm labor:
    - Mechanical perturbation
    - Local inflammation
- Maintaining fetal homeostasis during nonobstetrical surgery:
  - Brief periods of maternal hypoxemia and uterine hypoperfusion are well tolerated
  - Prolonged or serious maternal hypoxemia and/or hypoperfusion causes uteroplacental vasoconstriction and decreased uteroplacental perfusion
  - Fetal hypoxemia leads to acidosis and ultimately fetal death
  - Maternal hypercarbia directly results in fetal respiratory acidosis
  - Severe fetal respiratory acidosis causes fetal myocardial depression and metabolic acidosis
  - Hypercarbia causes uterine artery vasoconstriction and reduced uterine blood flow
  - Hypocarbia results in reduced uterine blood flow and can ultimately cause fetal acidosis
  - *Maintenance of normal maternal blood pressure* is of great importance:
    - Passive dependence of the uteroplacental circulation on maternal blood pressure (spiral arteries are maximally vasodilated at baseline)
    - Reduction in maternal blood pressure causes reduced uteroplacental blood flow and fetal asphyxia
  - Except under special circumstances (severe maternal renal or cardiac disease) intravenous fluid administration should be generous and appropriate to the surgical blood loss
  - *Both ephedrine and phenylephrine* are considered safe and effective vasopressors for control of maternal blood pressure during surgery
  - Maintenance of adequate maternal gas exchange under anesthesia is important:
    - Use *supplemental oxygen* with regional anesthesia even without sedation
    - Use *controlled rather than spontaneous ventilation* for cases under general anesthesia
    - When using PEEP, make sure preload and afterload changes have been corrected for with adequate fluid loading
- Perioperative fetal monitoring:
  - Fetal heart rate monitoring is practical from 18 to 22 weeks
  - Heart rate variability can be readily observed from 25 weeks
  - Outcome data supporting continuous monitoring in normal delivery are not yet available
  - The decision to use fetal monitoring should be individualized and each case warrants a team approach for optimal safety of the woman and her baby
  - Gestational age and fetal maturity guides perioperative monitoring:
    - *Nonviable fetus (<24 weeks) is usually monitored preoperatively and postoperatively*
    - *Viable fetus (>24 weeks) is commonly monitored intraoperatively as well*

- Availability of the obstetrical team before surgery should be ascertained
- All general anesthetic drugs cross the placenta to some extent
- Loss of fetal heart rate variability in the setting of general anesthesia is not always an indicator of fetal distress, but may simply be an indication of expected anesthetic effects on the fetal autonomic nervous system
- Slowing of the fetal heart rate in the operative setting is most concerning for fetal hypoxemia and acidosis, but could be also related to:
  - Fall in temperature
  - Maternal respiratory acidosis
  - Drugs that tend to slow the heart rate (opioids, beta-blockers)

REGIONAL ANESTHESIA FOR THE PREGNANT PATIENT

- Neuraxial anesthesia:
  - Lower extremity surgery
  - Pelvic and lower abdominal operations (open appendectomy, ovarian torsion)
  - Consider long-acting opioids (intrathecal preservative-free morphine) for postoperative analgesia
  - Spinal anesthesia or combined spinal epidural anesthesia is preferred to reduce total dose of the drug
  - Downward adjustment is not necessary until the third trimester (reduce dose by 30%)
  - Fluid preload may not prevent maternal hypotension
  - Maintain left lateral tilt after the second trimester
  - Treat hypotension aggressively:
    - Both phenylephrine and ephedrine are acceptable
    - Phenylephrine infusion (30–60 µg/min) started after administration of spinal anesthetic and adjusted according to response appears to get best clinical results
  - Administer supplemental oxygen
  - Fetal monitoring
  - Avoid sedation to minimize fetal exposure to drugs
  - Postoperative analgesia with epidural catheter
- Peripheral nerve blocks:
  - Good option when appropriate block is available
  - Local anesthetic maximum doses are the same as in the nonpregnant patient
  - Use US guidance to minimize drug amount and optimize block
  - Use supplemental oxygen
  - Fetal monitoring
- IVRA:
  - Not recommended
  - Large doses of local anesthetics used
  - Rapid absorption into circulation once tourniquet is released
  - Fetal drug concentrations may reach sustained high levels

GENERAL ANESTHESIA FOR THE PREGNANT PATIENT

- Induction and airway management:
  - Maintain *left lateral tilt* after the second trimester throughout
  - *Rapid sequence induction with cricoid pressure* is recommended unless hemodynamic considerations due to underlying disease process necessitate otherwise (aortic stenosis, intracranial aneurysm, etc.)
  - *Endotracheal intubation is recommended after 13 weeks* to prevent aspiration
  - However, several small clinical series suggest that routine elective cases using LMA in pregnant patients may not increase aspiration risk
  - Avoid unnecessary nasogastric tubes
  - Consider preinduction intrathecal preservative-free morphine
  - Dose requirements for induction agents are the same as in the nonpregnant population
  - Most commonly used induction agent in the United States is propofol
  - If an unexpected difficult airway is encountered, use the ASA airway algorithm

- Consider the increased vascularity of airway mucosa when manipulating the airway: when difficulty with intubation is encountered, check for ability to mask ventilate before causing excessive pharyngeal swelling with airway instrumentation
- Maintenance:
  - Both volatile anesthetics and TIVA have been successfully used to maintain anesthesia
  - FiO_2 should be adjusted to maintain maternal oxygenation
  - *$ETCO_2$ should be 31–35 mm Hg*
  - *Avoid N_2O*
  - Maternal awareness has been associated with "light" anesthesia. Use awareness monitoring (BIS, entropy, SEDLine)
  - For intraoperative fluid management see above ("maintaining fetal homeostasis during nonobstetrical surgery")
  - Volatile anesthetics suppress uterine activity if used >1 MAC, but high concentrations of volatile anesthetics may reduce mean arterial pressure and uteroplacental flow
  - All anesthetic agents reduce fetal heart rate variability
  - Fast-acting opioids may produce rapid-onset fetal bradycardia (remifentanil)
  - Muscle relaxants do not cross the placenta in clinically significant amounts
- Intraoperative monitoring:
  - ASA standard monitors, with additional monitoring as required
  - Arterial line and blood gas monitoring is not recommended for routine cases
- Emergence:
  - Always reverse neuromuscular blockade:
    - Neostigmine and glycopyrrolate do not cross the placenta
    - Atropine does cross the placenta
  - Reinflate lungs (gentle recruitment maneuver)
  - Gently suction pharynx
  - Switch to $FiO_2 = 100\%$
  - Remove endotracheal tube when the patient is awake to maximize airway protection:
    - "Deep extubation" is not recommended
  - Supplemental O_2 in recovery
- Postoperative analgesia:
  - Regional analgesia is an excellent choice
  - PCA use may reduce total narcotic drug requirements
  - Acetaminophen is safe
  - Avoid NSAIDs (concerns about premature closure of ductus arteriosus)
  - Avoid meperidine
  - Dexmedetomidine has not been tested adequately (only few case reports available)

ANESTHESIA FOR CARDIAC SURGERY IN THE PREGNANT PATIENT

- Indications:
  - Severe aortic or mitral valvular disease:
    - Valvular restriction in the setting of increased maternal blood flow demands and hypervolemia may result in clinical decompensation not responsive to medical therapy
    - Transcatheter vascular surgery offers novel therapy to avoid open heart surgery
  - Pregnancy-associated cardiomyopathy:
    - Mechanical assist devices (LVAD) have been used successfully to bridge to recovery or to heart transplantation
- Cardiopulmonary bypass:
  - Related factors that may adversely affect fetal oxygenation:
    - Nonpulsatile flow
    - Inadequate perfusion pressure
    - Inadequate pump flow

- Embolic phenomena to the uteroplacental bed
- Release of renin and catecholamines in response to cardiopulmonary bypass
▸ Use of continuous intraoperative fetal monitoring decreases fetal mortality rate
▸ *High pump flow rate (>2.5 L/min/m²) and perfusion pressure (>70 mm Hg)* are recommended to maintain uteroplacental blood flow
▸ Maintain maternal hematocrit greater than 28% to optimize oxygen-carrying capacity
▸ *Normothermic bypass* may be beneficial to the fetus
▸ Pulsatile flow may better preserve uteroplacental blood flow
▸ Changes in CO_2 tension can affect uteroplacental blood flow:
  - Alpha-stat management may be advantageous for maintenance of CO_2 homeostasis and uteroplacental blood flow

ANESTHESIA FOR NEUROSURGERY IN THE PREGNANT PATIENT

- Indications
- Bleeding saccular aneurysm or AV malformation:
  ▸ Pregnancy may increase risk of vascular rupture:
    - Stress induced by the increased cardiac output and blood volume
    - Softening of vascular connective tissue by the hormonal changes of pregnancy
  ▸ The risk of intracranial hemorrhage is increased by hypertensive conditions of pregnancy and their associated risk factors
- Brain tumor:
  ▸ Newly diagnosed brain tumor during pregnancy is rare
  ▸ Patients with undiagnosed lesions may present with increased intracranial pressure; lumbar puncture in these patients has been associated with cerebral herniation
- Head trauma:
  ▸ Traumatic head injury may result in significant catecholamine release and compromise to uterine flow
  ▸ Associated injuries may result in hypovolemia and compromised uterine flow
- Controlled hypotension:
  ▸ Controlled hypotension (high-dose volatile anesthetic, sodium nitroprusside, nitroglycerin, labetalol):
    - Reduction in uteroplacental blood flow
    - All of the above drugs cross the placenta and can induce hypotension in the fetus
  ▸ Reduction in systolic blood pressure of 25–30% or a mean blood pressure of less than 70 mm Hg will lead to reductions in uteroplacental blood flow
  ▸ *Fetal heart rate monitoring should be used under these conditions and hypotension limited to the least period of time possible*
  ▸ Nitroprusside is converted to cyanide; cyanide accumulation in the fetus has been observed with significant toxicity and fetal death:
    - If nitroprusside is used, it should be for only a short time and should be discontinued:
      ◆ If the infusion rate exceeds 0.5 mg/kg/h
      ◆ If maternal metabolic acidosis ensues
      ◆ If resistance to the agent is apparent
  ▸ Nitroglycerin has yet to be associated with adverse fetal effects:
    - Metabolized to nitrites, which can produce methemoglobinemia
- Controlled hypothermia:
  ▸ Hypothermia is used in neurosurgical anesthesia to decrease metabolic requirements in the brain and to reduce cerebral blood flow
  ▸ The usual goal is a temperature of 30°C, which will induce fetal bradycardia
  ▸ The heart rate will increase again with rewarming of the mother
- Controlled hyperventilation:
  ▸ Hyperventilation is used because decreasing carbon dioxide reduces cerebral blood flow
  ▸ During pregnancy, the normal $Paco_2$ at steady state is 30–32 mm Hg

- Vigorous hyperventilation ($Paco_2$ <25 mm Hg) may cause uterine artery vaso-constriction and leftward shift of the maternal oxyhemoglobin dissociation curve
- Potential adverse effects on the fetus:
  - Decreased placental oxygen transfer
  - Umbilical vessel vasoconstriction
- In the available clinical experience, *a healthy fetus tolerates well maternal moderate intraoperative hyperventilation ($Paco_2$ of 25–30 mm Hg)*
- Continuous intraoperative fetal heart rate monitoring should alert to compromises in fetal condition and adjustments to maternal ventilation should be made accordingly
- Diuretic therapy:
  - Diuresis is often accomplished with osmotic agents or loop diuretics to decrease brain volume both intraoperatively and postoperatively
  - These can cause significant negative fluid shifts for the fetus. Mannitol given to the mother slowly accumulates in the fetus causing fetal hyperosmolality:
    - Reduced fetal lung fluid production
    - Reduced urinary blood flow
    - Hypernatremia
  - However, in individual case reports, *mannitol in small doses of 0.25–0.5 mg/kg* has been used without ill effect to the fetus and appears safe if required
  - Furosemide is an alternative but should also be used cautiously with fetal monitoring and only if necessary

ANESTHESIA FOR LAPAROSCOPIC SURGERY IN THE PREGNANT PATIENT

- Common indications:
  - Acute appendicitis
  - Ovarian torsion
  - Cholelithiasis
  - *Whenever possible, surgery should be performed in the second trimester*
- Concerns during laparoscopic surgery for fetal well-being:
  - Direct fetal and uterine trauma
  - Fetal acidosis from absorption of insufflated carbon dioxide
  - Clinical experience using a careful surgical and anesthetic technique has been favorable: no difference in maternal and fetal outcome when compared with open surgery in >2 million cases
  - End-tidal CO_2 monitoring is sufficient and *routine ABG monitoring is "not" recommended*
  - Aortocaval compression should be avoided
  - Continuous *transabdominal intraoperative fetal monitoring may not be possible due to pneumoperitoneum*:
    - Continuous intraoperative fetal monitoring is seldom performed in patients in the second trimester
- Concerns regarding pneumoperitoneum:
  - With increased intra-abdominal pressure maternal cardiac output and thus uteroplacental perfusion may decrease
  - *Low pneumoperitoneal pressure (<12 mm Hg) should be used*

REFERENCE

For references, please visit **www.TheAnesthesiaGuide.com**.

CHAPTER 187
Labor Analgesia

Anjali Fedson Hack, MD, PhD

Stages of Labor		
Stages	Dermatomes	Definition
First	T10–L1	Uterine contractions with dilation of cervix until fully dilated
Second	S2–S4	Full dilation of cervix until delivery of infant
Third	S2–S4	Expulsion of placenta

Nonpharmacologic Methods of Pain Relief	
Method	Technique
Hypnosis	Modify perception of pain through self-hypnosis and posthypnotic suggestion
Psychoanalgesia	Reduction in maternal anxiety through controlled breathing and relaxation techniques (Dick-Read method)
Psychoprophylaxis	Reduction in pain perceptions through controlled relaxation and breathing (Lamaze)
Leboyer technique	"Birth without violence" or avoidance of birth trauma for neonate through decreasing environmental stimuli
Acupuncture	Insertion of fine needles at meridians to correct energy paths disrupted by labor
TENS	Transcutaneous electrical nerve stimulation at T10–L1 bilaterally
Water birthing	Maternal stress relief through immersion in warm bath
Aromatherapy	Stress relief in labor through inhalation of aerosolized essential oils
Touch and massage	Emotional and pain relief through therapeutic touch

SYSTEMIC MEDICATIONS AND INHALATIONAL AGENTS FOR LABOR PAIN RELIEF

See table on following page.

Systemic Medications and Inhalational Agents for Labor Pain Relief

Medication	Use and/or dosage	Comments
Opioids	Popular in first stage of labor	Maternal and fetal respiratory depression possible Decrease fetal heart rate variability
Morphine	5–10 mg IM (peak effect 1–2 h) 2–3 mg IV (peak effect 20 min)	Often used as PCA or continuous infusion
Meperidine	50–100 mg IM (peak effect 40–50 min) 25–50 mg IV (peak effect 5–10 min)	
Fentanyl	50–100 μg IM (peak effect 7–8 min) 25–50 μg IV (peak effect 3–5 min)	Short duration Use for PCA in labor analgesia has decreased since the introduction of remifentanil
Remifentanil	PCA: initial infusion 0.03 μg/kg/min; titrate to 0.1 μg/kg/min	Short half-life in plasma Use supplemental oxygen Minimizes neonatal respiratory depression
Agonist–antagonists		Limited potential for respiratory depression
Butorphanol (Stadol)	1–2 mg IM	Transient sinusoidal fetal heart rate pattern
Nalbuphine (Nubain)	5–10 mg IV	Neonatal respiratory depression
Sedatives/tranquilizers		
Phenothiazines		Anxiolytic and antiemetic
Hydroxizine (Vistaril)	25–50 mg IM	Decreases fetal heart rate variability
Promethazine (Phenergan)	25–50 mg IM	
Inhalational analgesia		
Entonox: 50% N_2O/50% O_2 (mixture not available in the United States)	Patient controlled	May be difficult to obtain precise concentration Availability of proper scavenging is often lacking

REGIONAL ANALGESIA/ANESTHESIA

Epidural analgesia:
- Analgesia provided by analgesics delivered via epidural catheter
- Most effective form of intrapartum analgesia
- Requires preanesthetic evaluation, presence of anesthesiologist, resuscitation equipment

Indications:
- Maternal request for pain relief represents sufficient condition for epidural administration (ACOG/ASA joint guidelines)

Contraindications:
- Patient refusal/inability to cooperate
- Elevated intracranial pressure/mass effect
- Soft tissue infection at epidural site

- Sepsis
- Coagulopathy
- Hypovolemia

Technique:
- Patient positioned, monitors in place
- Epidural space accessed using epidural needle
- Catheter passed through the needle, aspirated, and secured as usual
- Epidural catheter tested:
  ‣ Every dose is a test dose and should be given in a divided fashion
  ‣ Each subsequent dose of local anesthetic not to exceed 5 mL
  ‣ Intrathecal test:
    ▪ Three milliliters 1.5% lidocaine + 1:200,000 epinephrine
    ▪ Three milliliters 0.25% bupivacaine
  ‣ Intravascular test:
    ▪ Fifteen micrograms epinephrine (in 3 cm^3 1.5% lidocaine + 1:200,000) is unreliable in OB practice (variable HR, no EKG monitoring)
    ▪ One hundred micrograms fentanyl is safe and effective
    ▪ One milliliter air is effective with uniport catheters but may be unreliable with multiport catheters
- Loading the catheter:
  ‣ Ten milliliters 0.125% bupivacaine in divided doses
  ‣ Fifteen to 20 mL 0.0625% bupivacaine with 20–30 μg fentanyl

Maintenance of analgesia:
- Intermittent technique:
  ‣ Reinforcement with bolus injection every 1.5–2 hours
- Infusion technique:
  ‣ Decreased demand on physician
  ‣ Increased maternal satisfaction
  ‣ Bupivacaine (0.0625–0.125%) + 2 μg/mL fentanyl or 0.5 μg/mL sufentanil at 6–15 mL/h
  ‣ Ropivacaine (0.125–0.25%) + 2 μg/mL fentanyl or 0.5 μg/mL sufentanil at 6–12 mL/h
- Patient-controlled epidural analgesia (PCEA):
  ‣ Maternal control and satisfaction increased
  ‣ Lower concentrations of local anesthetics and opioids offer superior analgesia to local anesthetics alone
  ‣ Decreased anesthesiologist-administered boluses
  ‣ Lower average hourly dose of bupivacaine than continuous infusions

Typical PCEA Settings				
Anesthetic solution	Rate (mL)	Bolus (mL)	Lockout (min)	Hourly maximum
Bupivacaine 0.125 % + 2 μg/mL fentanyl	6	3	10	24
Bupivacaine 0.0625% + 2 μg/mL fentanyl	12	6	15	30
Ropivacaine 0.125%	6	4	19	30

Side effects:
- Hypotension:
  ‣ Volume expansion, avoidance of aortocaval compression, 5–10 mg ephedrine
- Inadequate analgesia:
  ‣ Assess catheter: is it in the space? If in doubt, replace
  ‣ Check pump and reservoir bag

- ‣ Asymmetric block: consider withdrawing catheter 0.5–1 cm, aspirate, give bolus 4–6 mL 0.125% bupivacaine with patient lying on side with poor block, and reassess
- ‣ Do not give epidural opioids to "cover up" a misplaced catheter

Monitoring following epidural:
- Record blood pressure, pulse rate, and pulse oximetry every 5 minutes for 30 minutes
- Resume routine monitoring in labor after this initial period
- Following every top-up dose check vitals every 5 minutes for 30 minutes

Complications of Regional Anesthesia		
Paresthesias	If a paresthesia persists, the catheter should be removed and inserted in another space	
	Incidence has been reported as 5–42 in 10,000 patients	
Accidental dural puncture	Rate depends on institution, practitioner experience, and characteristics of the patient population (obesity) Postdural puncture headache (PDPH) is the most common complication of accidental dural puncture (likelihood of headache with 17–18G Tuohy is 76–88%) Following accidental dural puncture, place epidural in another space. Alternatively, thread intrathecal catheter for spinal anesthetic (danger *if given epidural dose by error*) Liberal hydration, analgesics (Fioricet: acetaminophen, caffeine, butalbital), oral or IV caffeine Other measures include epidural saline, prophylactic blood patch, therapeutic blood patch (see chapter 125)	
Subdural injection	Injection of local anesthetic between dura mater and arachnoid Rare (0.1–0.82%) Increased with rotation of needle or history of prior back surgery Widespread sensory block with small amount of local anesthetic Delayed onset of weak patchy block, little motor effect, cephalad spread Hypotension common Faster resolution than epidural or subarachnoid block Self-limiting Treatment is replacement of the catheter to epidural space	
High epidural block	Excessive segmental spread from relative overdose of local anesthetic Treatment is supportive	
Accidental intravascular injection	Can lead to systemic neurotoxicity with seizures or possible cardiovascular collapse	
	Treat seizures	Assure left uterine displacement Control the airway Benzodiazepines (midazolam 1–2 mg, diazepam 5–10 mg, or propofol 10–30 mg)
	Treat cardiovascular collapse with LipidRescue	Intralipid 20% 1.5 mL/kg over 1 min Follow with infusion 0.25 mL/kg/min Continue chest compressions to circulate Intralipid Repeat bolus every 3–5 min up to 3 mL/kg until circulation restored Continue infusion until hemodynamic stability restored and increase to 0.5 mL/kg/min if BP declines Maximum dose of 8 mL/kg recommended

Labor outcome after neuraxial labor analgesia:
- No difference in duration of labor or progress of labor, incidence of forceps deliveries, cesarean sections, or NICU admissions

OTHER COMPLICATIONS OF LABOR AND DELIVERY

Backache:
- Occurs in 40% of postpartum women (regardless of whether they received an epidural)
- Increased rate of localized pain with multiple epidural attempts
- Epidural analgesia does not increase risk of ongoing back pain

Major neurologic injury during childbirth:
- Obstetric causes (1:2,000 to 1:6,400)
- Anesthesia-related causes (1:10,000)
- Bladder dysfunction
- Direct trauma to nerve roots

Neurologic Injury after Childbirth	
Cauda equina syndrome	Characterized by lower extremity and perineal numbness, sphincter dysfunction, and varying degrees of lower extremity paralysis
Transient neurologic symptoms	Aching pain in buttocks, associated with subarachnoid lidocaine, short duration of symptoms, and lithotomy position
Epidural hematoma	Following trauma to epidural vessels Requires immediate surgical decompression (within 6 h of onset of symptoms)
Epidural abscess and meningitis	Severe back pain with local tenderness, fever, leukocytosis
Adhesive arachnoiditis	Clinical irritation of structures in subarachnoid space due to contamination of spinal needles or solution
Anterior spinal artery syndrome	Anterior spinal cord ischemia Presents as motor deficit Hypotension and unfavorable anatomy are risk factors

CHAPTER 188
Combined Spinal Epidural in Obstetrical Anesthesia

Imre Rédai, MD, FRCA

BASIC IDEA

- Initial analgesia provided by intrathecal administration of an analgesic (or mixture)
- Labor analgesia is maintained using analgesic(s) delivered via an epidural catheter

TECHNIQUE (SEE CHAPTERS 121–124 FOR FIGURES)

- Epidural space accessed using an epidural needle
- A long spinal needle is passed through the epidural needle into the intrathecal compartment
- The spinal analgesic is administered and the spinal needle is withdrawn:
  ▸ Most common intrathecal doses are: 2–2.5 mg isobaric 0.25% bupivacaine or 0.2% ropivacaine with 10–20 µg fentanyl or 2–2.5 mg sufentanil
- An epidural catheter is passed via the epidural needle, aspirated, and secured as usual
- An epidural infusion is started as usual:
  ▸ Testing of the epidural catheter is not common:
    ▪ Careful aspiration for blood and CSF usually reveals intravascular or intrathecal catheter placement in multiorifice catheters
    ▪ Spinal effects are hard to differentiate from the original spinal dose
    ▪ Intravascular catheter placement testing with diluted epinephrine is notoriously poor in obstetrical patients:
      ◆ Heart rate variability at baseline is considerable due to periods of pain
      ◆ There is no EKG monitoring to assess T-wave amplitude
    ▪ Response to epidural infusion often reveals concealed intrathecal or inadvertent intravascular catheter position:
      ◆ Currently used dilute concentrations of epidural infusions are unlikely to produce rapid, dangerous cephalad spread of neuraxial blockade
      ◆ Do not bolus an "untested" catheter with a full bolus dose immediately after a CSE dose (i.e., without an infusion running for 15–20 minutes) without testing for intrathecal and intravascular placement first as it may produce inadvertent high blocks or local anesthetic toxicity
  ▸ Starting an epidural infusion straightaway allows onset of epidural analgesia by the time the spinal dose wears off
  ▸ Adjust inadequate level of initial analgesia by bolusing the epidural catheter:
    ▪ Initial doses may need to be reduced by about half
    ▪ After about 30–45 minutes, usual "top-up" boluses should have the same effect as with a routine labor epidural

Comparison with Epidural Analgesia for Labor Pain	
Combined spinal epidural	Epidural
Rapid onset	Slower onset
Good or excellent initial analgesia in most cases	Initial analgesia good or satisfactory in most cases
Overall satisfaction with labor analgesia is the same	
Good option in late first stage of labor	Sacral spread is poor; may not provide analgesia in patients presenting in advanced labor
Clear end point on insertion (CSF)	Placement is determined on subjective "feel"
Fewer failed epidural catheters in less experienced hands	
Postdural puncture headache incidence is ~0.5–1%	Postdural puncture headache incidence is ~1%
There have been recent reports of meningitis cases in healthy pregnant women	Meningitis in healthy pregnant women is exceedingly rare (no large-volume study has included cases of healthy pregnant women until now)
Maintenance of a sterile technique with cap/mask on everyone present in the room is important	
Fetal bradycardia incidence increases with dose of intrathecal narcotic (use ≤20 µg fentanyl or ≤2.5 µg sufentanil)	Fetal bradycardia with epidural narcotics has been observed
Rapid onset of sympathectomy; increased use of vasopressor agents	Slow onset of sympathectomy
Increased incidence of pruritus, nausea/vomiting with intrathecal opioids	
No difference in duration or progress of labor, incidence of forceps deliveries, Cesarean sections, or NICU admissions	

REFERENCE

For references, please visit **www.TheAnesthesiaGuide.com**.

CHAPTER 189
Anesthesia for Cesarean Section, Postoperative Analgesia Options

Imre Rédai, MD, FRCA

Cesarean section is one of the most common surgical procedures worldwide. The vast majority of these are performed under neuraxial anesthesia.

Neuraxial Anesthesia for Cesarean Section

Technique	Basics	Comments	Dose
Spinal (single shot)	Most commonly used in cases without a preexisting labor epidural in the United States Rapid onset Single shot limits duration of surgery (when combined with intrathecal fentanyl 25 μg): • 90 min with hyperbaric bupivacaine • 120 min with isobaric bupivacaine • 45 min with hyperbaric lidocaine Reliable distribution of spread	Risk of PDPH with thin blunt tip spinal needles is <1% Rapid-onset sympathectomy results in rapid drop in preload and afterload (hypotension) • Avoid in patients dependent on adequate preload and/or afterload • Have vasoactive drugs ready (phenylephrine infusion 30–60 μg/min recommended) Cephalad spread is unpredictable	Usual doses for Cesarean section: • 10.5–12 mg (1.4–1.6 mL of 0.75%) hyperbaric bupivacaine • 8–10 mg (1.6–2 mL of 0.5%) isobaric bupivacaine • 75 mg (1.5 mL of 5%) hyperbaric lidocaine • All combined with 15–25 μg fentanyl and 200–300 μg preservative-free morphine
Spinal (continuous)	Has all the advantages of the single-shot spinal Dosing can be titrated gradually Duration of block can be extended	Current lack of availability of microcatheters in the United States limits usefulness of technique (large-bore needles result in PDPH incidence of >50%) Repeat dosing of hyperbaric solutions is *not* recommended (risk of cauda equina syndrome)	Usual starting dose is 2.5 mg isobaric bupivacaine with 10 μg fentanyl Repeat every 5–10 min until adequate level is achieved

Epidural	Most commonly used when labor epidural is present Presence of adequate labor analgesia (T10 block) does not guarantee successful extension of block to surgical levels (>T5) • Once the full epidural loading dose is given and the block remains inadequate, conversion to spinal anesthesia may result in high cephalad spread (total spinal) even when the spinal dose is significantly reduced	Slower cephalad spread and limited sympathectomy produces better control of preload and afterload • Recommended technique as primary anesthetic if neuraxial block is considered in preload- or afterload-dependent patients "Patchiness" of block remains most common cause of failure	Usual doses and onset times for Cesarean section Lidocaine in newly inserted epidural catheter: 400–500 mg (20–25 mL) 2% lidocaine with 1:200,000 epinephrine in three to four divided doses–20–30 min Lidocaine in well-established labor epidural: 350–400 mg (17.5–20 mL) 2% lidocaine in three to four divided doses–10–15 min Use of adjuvant opioids is recommended • 100 µg fentanyl • 2–3 mg preservative-free morphine In an emergency situation, when rapid onset is desired, load labor epidural catheter with 540–600 mg (18–20 mL) 3% chloroprocaine in two divided doses; onset time is about 5 min Adjuvant neuraxial opioids do not have full effect when chloroprocaine is used • Reason remains unclear • Consider alternative modalities of postoperative pain control (PCA)
Combined spinal epidural	Combines advantages of the two techniques while eliminating some of the undesirable effects Consider if • Longer than usual surgery is expected (history of intra-abdominal adhesions) • Morbid obesity • Very short stature	Cephalad spread of spinal may still be rapid and extensive (have phenylephrine infusion ready)	Use of isobaric solution is recommended (difficulty in placing epidural catheter after the spinal dose may result in a saddle block) 7.5 mg (1.5 mL) isobaric bupivacaine with 15–25 µg fentanyl and 200–300 µg preservative-free morphine

• Neuraxial block above the T5 dermatome is considered to be adequate for Cesarean section.
• This is below the cardioaccelerating fibers (T1–3).
• For detailed description of individual techniques and common contraindications see chapters 121–124.

General Anesthesia for Cesarean Section

Step	Management	Comments
Induction of anesthesia	Use aspiration prophylaxis • 30 mL Bicitra or similar nonparticulate antacid • If time permits, give metoclopramide (10 mg IV) and a H_2 blocker IV Adequate preoxygenation is a *must* because of increased oxygen demand and supply and reduced FRC Rapid sequence induction with cricoid pressure is recommended unless hemodynamic considerations are a priority	Usual dose of induction agent is well tolerated and produces reliable loss of consciousness Use succinylcholine rather than a rapid-onset nondepolarizing muscle relaxant unless it is clinically indicated (MH, risk of hyperkalemia)
Airway management	Endotracheal intubation is recommended • LMA was successfully used in several small elective series and reported as rescue device when endotracheal intubation has failed Increased vascularity of airway mucosa, enlarged lingual tonsils, change of body habitus, airway edema due to prolonged pushing in labor all contribute to worse than usual intubating conditions	Evaluate airway before induction even in the most dire emergency Have backup plan and equipment available (LMA, fiber-optic scope, airway cart) Call for help if in doubt before induction!
Maintenance of general anesthesia	Volatile anesthetics relax the uterus if used >1 MAC N_2O has traditionally been used in Cesarean sections as it has no effect on uterine tone $N_2O:O_2$: • 50:50 before delivery • 60:40 after delivery TIVA (propofol) has been successfully used for anesthesia for Cesarean section; minimal reduction of dosing (8–10%), if any, is recommended Narcotics are usually withheld until after the delivery of the baby unless clinically indicated (suppression of autonomic response to airway manipulation) Use controlled ventilation to reduce airway collapse Additional muscle relaxation is seldom needed • If a nondepolarizing muscle relaxant is used, the dosing and monitoring is the same as with a nonpregnant patient	Use of inhaled anesthetics with a combined MAC of <1 may result in awareness even in pregnant patients (while pregnant patients have an increased sensitivity to inhaled anesthetics, individual variability should be considered and planned for) Ketamine (30–100 µg) is often used in place of narcotics during induction • Contrary to common belief, ketamine does have neurobehavioral effects on the newborn
Intraoperative monitoring under general anesthesia	ASA standard monitors are sufficient for healthy patients If clinically indicated, use additional monitors Keep $ETCO_2$ in the 32–36 mm Hg range	

(continued)

General Anesthesia for Cesarean Section (*continued*)		
Step	Management	Comments
Emergence	Extubate the patient awake to minimize risk of aspiration on emergence Apply supplemental oxygen	Make sure that patient maintains adequate airway and oxygenation in the recovery room Loss of airway after Cesarean section has emerged as leading cause of airway catastrophes in pregnancy in recent years
Neonatal outcome	Neonatal outcome depends on dose and duration of the anesthetic	Delivery of the newborn often coincides with the redistribution of the induction agent while the inhalational maintenance agent still has not equilibrated with the fetus • This leads to a vigorous, responsive baby A prolonged period of general anesthesia before delivery will allow for equilibration of the maintenance anesthetic in the fetus and will result in a baby born with a full general anesthetic • A period of positive pressure ventilation may be necessary to allow for elimination of the anesthetic agent • Presence of a competent neonatologist is important in these cases as the anesthesiologist's primary responsibility is the mother

- While general anesthesia is considered safe for mother and fetus (recent review of anesthesia mishaps has shown that relative risk of maternal death is no longer higher from general anesthesia than from regional anesthesia), the excellent safety record of neuraxial techniques in mothers with a variety of underlying medical conditions (including preeclampsia) and compromised uteroplacental circulation has significantly decreased the use of general anesthesia for Cesarean section in the United States
- Common indications for the use of general anesthesia for Cesarean section:
  ‣ Refusal of regional anesthesia
  ‣ Failed block (preincision or intraoperative)
  ‣ Emergency scenarios when rapid establishment of surgical anesthesia is a priority
  ‣ Coagulopathy
  ‣ Sepsis
  ‣ Hemodynamic compromise (at presentation or anticipated severe maternal hemorrhage)

▸ Coagulopathy
▸ Infection at insertion site
▸ Elevated intracranial pressure

Common Considerations for the Anesthesiologist Before and During a Cesarean Section		
Topic	Management	Comments
Blood replacement therapy	Expected blood loss during a Cesarean section is about 1,000 mL • This is well tolerated in healthy women Type and screen should be performed before all but the most urgent Cesarean sections • The obstetrician *must* document the urgency of the case if the type and screen is omitted	Blood crossmatching is recommended in patients with • Prior history of peripartum hemorrhage • Anticipated increased blood loss (multiple gestation, polyhydramnios, placenta previa, abruption, abnormal placentation) • Baseline anemia
Antibiotic prophylaxis	Cefazolin 2 g IV is most commonly used Clindamycin 600 mg ± gentamicin 1.5 mg/kg is an alternative in patients with penicillin allergy Administer antibiotics *prior to skin incision*	For detailed discussion, see chapter 183
Intraoperative positioning	Maintain 15° left uterine tilt until delivery	Reduces effects of aortocaval compression
IV access and fluid replacement therapy	At least one 18G IV is recommended Establish second IV if higher than usual blood loss is anticipated Balanced salt solutions are the most common choice Avoid rapid infusions of dextrose-containing solution as it may result in neonatal hyperglycemia	In cases with very high blood loss (placenta percreta) large-bore central venous access is mandatory
Uterotonics	Routine use of oxytocin after delivery of baby is recommended Infuse at a rate of 5–10 U in 10–15 min initially, and then adjust depending on uterine tone	Oxytocin may cause hypotension (oxytocin receptors are present on the vascular endothelium and are linked to eNOS and NO-dependent vasodilation) Hold oxytocin if cord blood is collected until collection is finished
Thromboprophylaxis	See chapter 193	
Temperature control	Labor room operating rooms are often kept at suboptimal temperatures	Use appropriate devices (forced-air warming, blankets)

Postoperative Analgesia		
Modality	Management	Comments
Oral analgesics	Acetaminophen 500–1,000 mg q6 h; maximum daily dose 4 g Ibuprofen 400 mg q8 h Percocet (acetaminophen and oxycodone) one or two q6 h; maximum eight pills a day	Avoid codeine (metabolites may accumulate in breast milk and cause neonatal depression)
Parenteral analgesics	Ketorolac 30 mg q6 h for a maximum of 2 days Morphine IV PCA	Ketorolac is safe in breast-feeding mothers Avoid meperidine
Neuraxial analgesia	Preservative-free morphine • 200–300 μg intrathecal • 2–3 mg epidural	Doses above those recommended on left increase side effects without improving postoperative analgesia Common side effects are pruritus and nausea and vomiting Urinary retention is *not* a problem as patients have urinary catheters for 24 h Respiratory depression is extremely rare with these doses
	PCEA	Keep epidural catheter postoperatively in patients where tight pain control is indicated (limited physiological cardiovascular or pulmonary reserve) and wean analgesia gradually

REFERENCE

For references, please visit **www.TheAnesthesiaGuide.com**.

CHAPTER 190
Anesthesia for Episiotomy, Perineal Laceration, and Forceps Delivery

Imre Rédai, MD, FRCA

Anesthesia for all these procedures can be successfully performed by extension of a working labor epidural. The following summary advises for cases where there is *no* labor epidural in place (or when it is failing to provide analgesia). The use of a labor epidural is briefly summarized at the end of the chapter.

Anesthesia for Episiotomy and Perineal Laceration	
Procedure/comments	Technique

Local infiltration	• 1% lidocaine or 2% chloroprocaine
	  ‣ Prior to episiotomy
	  ‣ For repair of
	    ▪ Episiotomy
	    ▪ Small lacerations

Pudendal block
• Complications and caveats:
  ‣ Failure of block
  ‣ Systemic absorption of local anesthetic can be fast
  ‣ Deep hematoma (rare but serious)
  ‣ Deep pelvic abscess, subgluteal abscess
  ‣ Operator injury. Needle is close to palpating finger in vagina
	• Use any of
	  ‣ 1% lidocaine or mepivacaine or
	  ‣ 0.5% bupivacaine or ropivacaine or 2% chloroprocaine
	  ‣ With or without epinephrine 1:200,00
	• Transvaginal approach (see Figure 190-1):
	  ‣ Insert finger in vagina and identify the ischial spine and the sacrospinous ligament. Advance needle through vaginal mucosa toward the sacrospinous ligament. Once the needle passes through the ligament (loss of resistance), administer 3–10 mL local anesthetic after careful aspiration. Use a needle guard set at 1–1.5 cm
	• Transperineal approach:
	  ‣ Insert finger in vagina and identify the ischial spine and the sacrospinous ligament. Insert needle through the skin between anus and ischial tuberosity and direct slightly inferior and lateral to the ischial spine and the ligament. Administer 3–10 mL local anesthetic after careful aspiration

Spinal anesthesia	• Saddle block
	  ‣ 50–70 mg hyperbaric lidocaine or
	  ‣ 7.5–9 mg hyperbaric bupivacaine
	  ‣ With 15–15 μg fentanyl in the sitting position
	  ‣ Keep patient sitting for 5 min
	  ‣ Pros
	    ▪ Limited spread of block (minimal lower extremity block) enhances recovery
	    ▪ Minimizes sympathectomy
	    ▪ Profound, rapid-onset block
	  ‣ Cons
	    ▪ Concerns about transient radiculopathy with hyperbaric solutions and lithotomy position
	    ▪ Uncomfortable to sit on injured part
	• Isobaric spinal anesthetic
	  ‣ 7.5–10 mg isobaric bupivacaine or
	  ‣ 30–45 mg chloroprocaine
	  ‣ Pros
	    ▪ Can be done in the lateral decubitus position
	    ▪ Lesser incidence of transient radiculopathy
	  ‣ Cons
	  ‣ Slower onset
	    ▪ More pronounced sympathectomy
	    ▪ Slower recovery of lower extremity strength

GA If regional anesthesia failed or is contraindicated	

Anatomy: pudendal nerve, S2–4 distribution.

FIGURE 190-1. Pudendal block, transvaginal approach

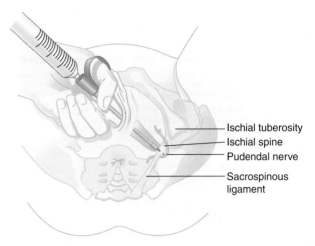

Ischial tuberosity
Ischial spine
Pudendal nerve

Sacrospinous
ligament

Anesthesia for Forceps Delivery		
Method	Management	Comments
Local infiltration	Episiotomy often performed with forceps delivery	Insufficient analgesia
Supplemental agents	N₂O, intravenous remifentanil, alfentanil, fentanyl	Moderately effective Easy to use *Avoid general anesthesia without airway protection*
Spinal anesthesia	Usually performed in the lateral decubitus position Relatively small amount of local anesthetic is sufficient (5–7.5 mg isobaric bupivacaine with 15 μg fentanyl)	Monitor patient carefully for development of hypotension, fetal bradycardia Treat hypotension aggressively
Caudal epidural	Almost never used in current practice	Injury to presenting fetal part is major concern
Perineal block	See description above	Limited to pudendal nerve Injury to presenting part is major concern
General endotracheal anesthesia	If regional anesthesia failed or is contraindicated and patient cannot tolerate procedure without intervention	

Anatomy:
• T10–L1 (uterus)
• L1–2 (vulva)
• L4–S3 (pelvic structures)
• S2–4 (perineum)
NB: Forceps is applied to the fetal head while it is still in the birth canal; vacuum extractor is applied to the visible part of the head.

USE OF LABOR EPIDURAL CATHETER FOR LACERATION REPAIR OF FORCEPS DELIVERY

- Use 3% chloroprocaine:
  - ‣ Need rapid onset
  - ‣ Duration of procedure is usually short
  - ‣ 10 to 12 mL in two divided doses 2–3 minutes apart results in adequate analgesia in 5–7 minutes
- Monitor hemodynamic changes (maternal heart rate, blood pressure)
- Make sure IV is functional before dosing the epidural
- Supplement with short-acting IV narcotics if necessary
- *Avoid general anesthesia without endotracheal intubation*
- *Encourage complex repairs in the operating room*:
  - ‣ Better access to anesthesia equipment
  - ‣ Better lighting
  - ‣ More room, more help

CHAPTER 191
Anesthesia for Cerclage

Imre Rédai, MD, FRCA

Cervical incompetence is a common cause of miscarriage. Placing a suture around the cervical os of the uterus mechanically prevents premature opening of the cervix and subsequent premature delivery of the baby.

TRANSVAGINAL CERCLAGE

- Pudendal (S2–4) and genitofemoral (L1–2) nerves supply the surgical area
- Surgical approach is transvaginal
- Lithotomy position
- Duration variable but usually less than an hour in experienced hands
- Intraoperative fetal monitoring not routinely used

Management:
- "High saddle block" is the most commonly used approach (the block has to reach T12):
  - ‣ One to 1.2 mL hyperbaric 0.75% bupivacaine
  - ‣ One to 1.2 mL hyperbaric 5% lidocaine (rarely used because of risk of TNS)
  - ‣ Patient should remain sitting for 3–5 minutes to establish saddle block
- General anesthesia is an option
- Epidural anesthesia is a poor choice as sacral sparing is common
- Adequate perioperative hydration is important to prevent increase in uterine activity
- Treat hypotension associated with spinal anesthesia aggressively:
  - ‣ Retching may result in bearing down and rupture of the amniotic membrane; this is hypotension-induced, no indication for PONV prophylaxis
- Use of intrathecal short-acting neuraxial opioids (e.g., fentanyl 25 μg) is controversial:
  - ‣ Improves intraoperative analgesia
  - ‣ Extends duration of block
  - ‣ May contribute to postoperative urinary retention
- Use of long-acting neuraxial opioids is not recommended

Comments:
- Postoperative pain is variable:
  - ‣ If the pain does not respond to common analgesics, admission may be necessary
- Urinary retention is a significant complication (patients need to void before discharge)
- Uterine contractions may follow and may require admission for hydration and bed rest

ELECTIVE REMOVAL OF CERCLAGE BEFORE ONSET OF LABOR

Management:
- The patient presents at term and the cerclage is removed
- Patient presents/returns to the labor and delivery unit when in active labor

Comments:
- This is often done without anesthesia in the office setting
- If anesthesia is indicated, a low saddle block (0.8–1 mL hyperbaric 0.75% bupivacaine or 0.8–1 mL hyperbaric 5% lidocaine) is adequate

REMOVAL OF CERCLAGE IN A PATIENT PRESENTING IN ACTIVE LABOR

- The patient presents with contractions or with ruptured membranes and is allowed to labor
- The cerclage is often removed without an anesthetic
- In this setting, if the patient is a candidate for labor analgesia, a modified combined spinal epidural is the recommended approach:
  - ‣ A low saddle dose (see above) is administered as the spinal component
  - ‣ An epidural catheter is threaded and is used to provide analgesia for labor

ABDOMINAL CERCLAGE

- Selected patients may undergo an abdominal approach for closing the cervix
- The surgical approach is usually a Pfannenstiel incision
- Duration is dependent on level of experience of surgeon (about 60–90 minutes)
- Abdominal cerclage is permanent. Delivery is by Cesarean section
- Spinal, epidural, combined spinal epidural, and GA have all been used successfully
- Usual precautions for anesthesia during second trimester (see chapter 186)
- Dosing is similar to anesthesia for Cesarean section (see chapter 189)
- May need hospital admission postoperatively for pain management, hydration, and observation for uterine contractions

CHAPTER 192
Tocolysis

M. Lee Haselkorn, MD and Imre Rédai, MD, FRCA

PRETERM LABOR

- Defined as delivery before completion of 37 weeks
- Increasing in frequency in the United States: 9.4% (1981), 10.7% (1992), 12.3% (2003), 12.8% (2006)
- Pathophysiology:
  - ‣ Excessive myometrial and fetal membrane overdistention:
    - ▪ Multiple gestation
    - ▪ Polyhydramnios
  - ‣ Decidual hemorrhage
  - ‣ Precocious fetal endocrine activity
  - ‣ Intrauterine infection or inflammation
- Clinical diagnosis: regular, painful uterine contractions + cervical dilatation or effacement
- Outcome:
  - ‣ Thirty percent diagnosed as "preterm labor" will deliver full term
  - ‣ Fifty percent hospitalized for "preterm labor" will deliver full term
  - ‣ Therapeutic interventions seldom effective in prolonging pregnancy

GOALS OF TOCOLYTIC THERAPY

- Most tocolytic drugs are only effective to prolong pregnancy for 24–48 hours
- Delay delivery to allow corticosteroid (betamethasone) delivery and effect to mature pulmonary surfactant:
  - ‣ Typical dose 12 mg IM once daily (two doses total)
  - ‣ Initial benefit at 18 hours after first dose
  - ‣ Maximum benefit at 48 hours of therapy
  - ‣ Decrease risk of neonatal respiratory distress, intraventricular hemorrhage, necrotizing enterocolitis, and perinatal death
- Permit transport of mother to regional facility

TOCOLYTIC AGENTS

See table on following page.

Tocolytic Agents

Medication	Mechanism	Efficacy	Side effects
Beta-2 agonists (terbutaline, ritodrine)	Beta-2 stimulation inhibits myosin light chain kinase via a G-protein-coupled increase in intracellular cAMP Bolus dose of terbutaline is 250 μg IV push; this achieves uterine relaxation for a few minutes duration For suppression of preterm labor an infusion is started at 2.5 μg/min and increased by 2.5 μg/min every 20 min until the contractions stopped; maximum rate is 25 μg/min Ritodrine is no longer available in the United States	Decrease immediate (within 48 h) birth rate No decrease in delivery rates at 7 days No change in perinatal or neonatal mortality	Hypotension due to beta-2-mediated vasodilation Tachycardia, atrial fibrillation/flutter Myocardial ischemia Pulmonary edema Hyperglycemia secondary to glucagon-mediated glycogenolysis and gluconeogenesis Hypokalemia/rebound hyperkalemia (intracellular transfer) Increased fetal heart rate Fetal hypoglycemia
Calcium channel blockers (nifedipine)	L-type calcium channel inhibition reduces intracellular calcium levels in uterine smooth muscle Nifedipine is the most commonly used agent Usual starting oral dose is 10–20 mg Repeat dosing and frequency is less clear • High doses have been associated with pulmonary edema	Reduce delivery rates within 7 days of treatment Reduce frequency of neonatal respiratory distress, intraventricular hemorrhage, necrotizing enterocolitis, and neonatal jaundice	Pulmonary edema (possible high-output heart failure?) Hypotension Fetal death Heart block Neuromuscular block in combination with magnesium sulfate therapy
Magnesium sulfate	Mechanism of action is poorly understood Decreases the frequency of depolarization of muscle by modulating calcium uptake, binding, and distribution High concentrations needed for effect Loading dose is 6 g (as opposed to 4 g in preeclampsia) and infusion of 2 g/h for maintenance	No difference in the risk of birth within 48 h No difference in perinatal mortality compared with placebo May have neuroprotective effects in newborn if administered to mother prior to preterm birth	Nausea, vomiting, and lethargy Volume overload Shortness of breath Pulmonary edema Chest pain Respiratory arrest Cardiac arrest Neonatal paralytic ileus Interference with neuromuscular monitoring Enhances effects of nondepolarizing NM blocking drugs

(continued)

Tocolytic Agents (*continued*)

Medication	Mechanism	Efficacy	Side effects
Prostaglandin synthesis inhibitors (indomethacin)	Inhibition of prostaglandin synthesis (PGE1, PGE2, PGF2alpha) from arachidonic acid: COX-1: constitutively present in human decidua, myometrium, and fetal membranes COX-2: inducible; increases in decidua and myometrium in term and preterm labor Indomethacin is the most commonly used drug The dose is 50 mg rectally followed by 25 mg q6 h	Reduction in birth before 37 weeks gestation Increased gestational age and birth weight	Premature closure of ductus arteriosus
Oxytocin receptor antagonists (atosiban)	Inhibition of oxytocin-mediated PIP → DAG + IP3 pathway of myosin light chain kinase activation	Do not reduce the incidence of preterm birth Do not improve neonatal outcome	Minimal maternal side effects Association with lower birth weight and increased death in first year of life has been suggested
Nitroglycerine	Relaxes uterine smooth muscle via NO-mediated mechanism Bolus dose is 125–250 µg IV push; this achieves uterine relaxation for a few minutes	Not used for therapeutic tocolysis; however, often used to induce uterine relaxation during childbirth (fetal extraction), external cephalic version, or postpartum (uterine eversion)	Hypotension Dizziness Headache Facial flushing
Volatile anesthetics	Dose-dependent relaxation of uterus Usual dose for complete uterine relaxation is about 2 MAC	Seldom used in current practice Fetal surgery under GA is most common indication Desflurane is the preferred agent for rapid onset and offset	High dose (2 MAC) results in significant cardiovascular side effects (hypotension) and may need BP support (phenylephrine, norepinephrine)

CHAPTER 193
Anticoagulation after Cesarean Section

Imre Rédai, MD, FRCA

Pregnancy increases incidence of deep vein thrombosis and venous thromboembolic disease (0.5–2/1,000 pregnancies).
- Incidence highest postpartum:
  - Increased 2- to 5-fold for deep vein thrombosis
  - Increased 15-fold for pulmonary embolism
- Cesarean section increases risk even further:
  - Two-fold increase compared with vaginal delivery

Risk Factors	
Endothelial injury	Delivery of placenta results in large surge of procoagulants Surgical intervention increases endothelial injury Smoking (>1/2 ppd) may increase risk for endothelial injury
Changes in coagulation	Coagulation factors increase, protein S and C activity decreases, antifibrinolytics increase Patients with inherited thrombophilias are at increased risk (factor V Leiden, protein S or C deficiency, AT-III deficiency, antiphospholipid antibody) Chorioamnionitis may increase risk
Venous stasis	Compression by enlarged uterus (L > R) Proximal and pelvic vein thrombosis more common Obesity, bed rest, multiple gestation are additional risk factors

Diagnostic Approach			
History	Prior history of thromboembolic disease Preexisting thrombophilias		
Physical exam	Swelling of lower extremity is common in pregnancy Left-sided thrombosis in >80% of cases		
	Dyspnea Common during pregnancy and after Cesarean section		
Radiographic evaluation	Venous thrombosis in lower extremities and pelvis	Venous compression Doppler US	Highly sensitive and specific for proximal vein thrombosis
		MRI	May help when Doppler US is equivocal Suspected pelvic vein thrombus
		Contrast venography	"Gold standard," seldom done
	Pulmonary vasculature	V/Q scan	Superior test if CXR Normal
		CT angiography	Test of choice with abnormal chest x-ray If V/Q scan is equivocal Inadequate sensitivity for subsegmental emboli

Prophylaxis	
Indicated in all patients with	One or more episode of venous thromboembolism in the past Antiphospholipid syndrome Homozygous prothrombin mutation Homozygous factor V Leiden mutation Coexisting heterozygosity for prothrombin and factor V Leiden mutations Hyperhomocysteinemia Protein S deficiency Protein C deficiency
Cesarean section in patients with *no* additional risk factors is *not* an indication for thromboprophylaxis	
One risk factor	Graduated compression stockings or pneumatic compression device *or* pharmacologic thromboprophylaxis
Multiple risk factors	Graduated compression stockings or pneumatic compression device *and* pharmacologic thromboprophylaxis

Pharmacologic Thromboprophylaxis		
SQ LMWH	Enoxaparin 40 mg q day or BID Dalteparin 5,000 U Q day or BID Tinzaparin 4,500 U Q day	Some recommend therapeutic doses in patients with past history of multiple DVT
Heparin (unfractionated; SQ)	5,000 U BID Adjusted dose: start with 5,000 U BID and titrate to anti-Xa activity (therapeutic if anti-Xa is 0.1–0.3 U/mL); usual range is 5,000–10,000 U twice daily. Measure anti-Xa 6 h after every other dose	Some recommend therapeutic doses in patients with past history of multiple venous thromboembolism
Warfarin	Start after heparin; overlap for at least 5 days Therapeutic range: INR 2–3	Warfarin does not get excreted in breast milk in significant amounts

- Usually started 6 hours after Cesarean delivery unless there is concern for ongoing postpartum hemorrhage
- Graduated compression stockings or pneumatic compression device should be used in the meantime, starting in the preoperative period
- Should continue for 4–6 weeks postpartum

Therapeutic Anticoagulation after Cesarean Section		
IV heparin Most common initial therapy Once established, transition to SQ heparin, LMWH, or warfarin for ease of administration	Staring dose 80 U/kg Maintenance 18 U/kg/h	Titrate to aPTT (this is laboratory specific: check institutional range) Check aPTT every 6 h until in range, and then every 12 h
SQ heparin	Divide total daily IV dose by two and administer that amount every 12 h	Check aPTT every 6 h after dose until in range
LMWH (SQ)	Enoxaparin 1 mg/kg BID Dalteparin 200 U/kg q day or 100 U/kg BID Tinzaparin 175 U/kg q day	Titrate to anti-Xa levels: 0.6–1 IU/mL for twice a day dosing 1–2 IU/mL for once-daily dosing Draw samples following the third consecutive dose, 6 h after the drug is given Adjust up or down by 20%

- Usually started 12 hours after Cesarean delivery unless there is concern for ongoing postpartum hemorrhage (some institutions wait 24 hours in patients with mechanical heart valves)
- Graduated compression stockings or pneumatic compression device should be used in the meantime, starting in the preoperative period

REFERENCE

For references, please visit **www.TheAnesthesiaGuide.com**.

CHAPTER 194
Peripartum Hemorrhage

Imre Rédai, MD, FRCA

- Severe hemorrhage happens in about 6.7/1,000 deliveries:
  - ‣ Seventeen percent of maternal deaths are due to hemorrhage in the United States
  - ‣ Maternal hemorrhage is the leading cause for maternal death in developing countries

CHANGES IN VITAL SIGNS ASSOCIATED WITH MATERNAL HEMORRHAGE

See table on following page.

Changes in Vital Signs Associated with Maternal Hemorrhage	
Changes in vital signs	Estimated blood loss (% of total blood volume)
None	Up to 15–20%
Tachycardia (<100 bpm) Mild hypotension Peripheral vasoconstriction	20–25%
Tachycardia (100–120 bpm) Hypotension (SBP 80–100 mm Hg) Restlessness Oliguria	25–35%
Tachycardia (>120 bpm) Hypotension (SBP <60 mm Hg) Altered consciousness Anuria	>35%

ANTEPARTUM HEMORRHAGE

- *Trivial bleeding*:
  - Occurs in about 6% of pregnancies
  - Usually secondary to cervicitis. Important to exclude more serious scenarios
  - No bleeding is trivial in the pregnant patient until serious causes have been excluded
- *Placental abruption*:
  - Occurs in 10% of pregnancies
  - May occur at any gestational age
  - Known risk factors:
    - Hypertension
    - Smoking
    - Advanced maternal age
    - Cocaine
    - Trauma
    - PROM
    - History of previous abruption
  - May be complicated by:
    - Amniotic fluid embolism
    - Uterine rupture
    - Coagulopathy
  - IUGR, fetal malformations are common
  - Presents with:
    - Vaginal bleeding (often concealed)
    - Uterine tenderness
    - Increased uterine activity
  - Ultrasound exam often diagnostic but may miss small abruptions
  - Tocolytic therapy in preterm patients is controversial
  - FHR monitoring is essential
  - Mode of delivery is determined by:
    - Condition of mother
    - Condition of fetus
  - Labor and vaginal delivery:
    - If coagulation studies normal, epidural analgesia is *not* contraindicated
    - Place two large IVs
    - Monitor hemodynamic status closely
  - Cesarean section:
    - Often emergent
    - General anesthesia in most cases

- Aggressive volume resuscitation is a must; large-bore venous access may necessitate central venous cannulation
  - If necessary, place an arterial line to guide therapy
  - Uterine atony, rapidly developing coagulopathy may worsen hemorrhage
  - Consider postdelivery ICU admission of unstable patients
- *Placenta previa*:
  - Prior uterine trauma is often associated
  - Painless vaginal bleed is often first sign
  - Up to 10% may have associated abruption
  - Diagnosed by ultrasonography
  - MRI may be helpful if uterine wall invasion is suspected
  - Avoid vaginal examination
  - Expectant management with admission to hospital
  - Optimal tocolytic is still debated:
    - $MgSO_4$ worsens maternal hypotension
  - IUGR is common
  - Always abdominal delivery
  - All patients should be evaluated on arrival
  - Place at least one large-bore IV
  - Send labs, type, and crossmatch (2 U PRBC)
  - Start volume resuscitation if indicated
  - Double setup if vaginal examination is necessary
  - Cesarean section:
    - Increased risk of bleeding even during elective case
    - Place second IV before start
    - Order a minimum of 4 U PRBC in actively bleeding patients
    - Consider general anesthesia for patients presenting with significant hypovolemia

THE "DOUBLE SETUP"

- In case of uncertainty as the source of hemorrhage in a patient with known placenta previa it may become necessary to perform a vaginal examination
- The patient is prepped and draped as for a Cesarean section with a team ready to perform an emergency abdominal delivery should the hemorrhage become threatening
- An obstetrician then performs the vaginal examination
- An anesthesiologist is always present, ready to induce GA in case of an emergency:
  - Full history, physical exam, labs should be available at the time of the double setup
  - Two large-bore IVs in situ
  - A total of 4 U PRBC should be immediately available
  - All equipment checked, all monitoring applied on the patient
  - Preoxygenation
  - Induction medications in-line on the IV
  - Help available to apply cricoid pressure and manage potentially life-threatening hemorrhage

INTRAPARTUM HEMORRHAGE

- *Retained placenta*:
  - Placental expulsion incomplete beyond 30 minutes after birth of baby
  - Cause often remains unknown:
    - Prior history of retained placenta
  - Increased risk of hemorrhage and infection
  - Cord traction with oxytocin stimulation is first step
  - Manual exploration and evacuation in the labor room follows
  - If necessary, completed in the OR
  - Residual placental fragments may need D&C
  - Thin-walled postpartum uterus may get perforated
  - Assess hemodynamic status

- ‣ Neuraxial anesthesia is preferred if hemodynamic status is adequate
- ‣ IV sedation is *not* recommended: protective airway reflexes may be lost
- ‣ Uterine relaxation can be provided with IV nitroglycerine (50–500 μg bolus)
- ‣ Have uterotonic agents ready after completion of evacuation of the retained placenta
- ‣ Historically, potent inhalational agents were used for uterine relaxation
- *Abnormal placental adherence (accreta, increta, percreta)*:
  - ‣ Strong association with placenta previa and prior C/S:
    - ▪ No prior C/S: 5%
    - ▪ One prior C/S: 10%
    - ▪ More than one prior C/S: up to 40% risk of abnormal placental adherence
  - ‣ Prior history of retained placenta or abnormal adherence
  - ‣ High degree of suspicion in patients with placenta previa
  - ‣ US and MRI have about 30–35% predictive capability for accreta, much better for percreta
  - ‣ Small areas can be oversewn or excised during surgery (uterine conservation)
  - ‣ High probability of Cesarean hysterectomy
  - ‣ Operative blood losses can be very high:
    - ▪ Forty percent of cases require >10 U PRBC
  - ‣ Mortality remains significant
  - ‣ Use of interventional radiology techniques is advocated but remains controversial
  - ‣ Consider general anesthesia for elective cases
  - ‣ Cases diagnosed intraoperatively:
    - ▪ Consider converting to GA
    - ▪ Appropriate means of volume resuscitation *must* be established before surgery proceeds if bleeding is still under control
  - ‣ Arterial line, large-bore central IV access mandatory
  - ‣ Blood and coagulation factor supply must be adequate (20 U PRBC, 20 U FFP, 12 U platelets initial order; maintain stock throughout case and postoperatively)
  - ‣ Appropriate infusions of vasopressor agents should be available
  - ‣ Have calcium replacement therapy available in view of potential massive transfusion
  - ‣ Have laboratory support available (point-of-care lab equipment)
  - ‣ Admit to ICU postoperatively if bleeding has not been controlled adequately
- *Uterine rupture*:
  - ‣ Previous uterine surgery
  - ‣ Direct trauma to the uterus
  - ‣ Incidence is about 1% when labor attempted after prior Cesarean section (TOLAC)
  - ‣ Fetal mortality is up to 35%
  - ‣ Diagnosis is based on:
    - ▪ Sudden abdominal pain
    - ▪ Fetal distress
    - ▪ Hypotension, tachycardia
    - ▪ Cessation of labor
    - ▪ Change in shape of abdomen
  - ‣ Emergent abdominal delivery:
    - ▪ Cesarean hysterectomy is common
  - ‣ General anesthesia with rapid sequence induction
  - ‣ Aggressive volume resuscitation
  - ‣ Sometimes desperate cases may result in favorable outcome!
- *Uterine inversion*:
  - ‣ Rare (1:5,000–10,000)
  - ‣ "Shock is out of proportion with hemorrhage":
    - ▪ Hemorrhage is usually severely underestimated
  - ‣ Treatment is early replacement (i.e., repositioning) of uterus followed by uterotonic drugs to firm up uterus

- ‣ Uterine relaxation may be necessary for successful replacement:
  - ▪ A total of 125–250 μg nitroglycerine IV push
  - ▪ This may result in further significant drop in blood pressure
- ‣ Aggressive volume resuscitation
- ‣ Vasopressor agents
- ‣ General anesthesia may be necessary if the patient does not have working neuraxial labor analgesia

POSTPARTUM HEMORRHAGE

- Significant postpartum hemorrhage (defined as a 10% decrease in the hemoglobin) occurs in about 10% of patients
- Severe postpartum hemorrhage (hemoglobin: 5.8–7.7 g/dL; tachycardia: HR >115 and hypotension SBP >85 mm Hg, DBP >55 mm Hg) has been associated with myocardial injury
- *Uterine atony*:
  - ‣ Factors associated with uterine atony:
    - ▪ Macrosomia
    - ▪ Twin pregnancy
    - ▪ Multiparity
    - ▪ Uterine leiomyomata
    - ▪ History of postpartum hemorrhage
    - ▪ Fetal demise
    - ▪ Chorioamnionitis
    - ▪ Precipitous labor
    - ▪ Prolonged labor
    - ▪ Uterine overstimulation
    - ▪ Tocolytic therapy
    - ▪ General anesthesia
    - ▪ Amniotic fluid embolism
    - ▪ Placental abruption
  - ‣ Medical management: uterotonics:
    - ▪ Oxytocin:
      - ♦ Do not bolus undiluted oxytocin IV while there is ongoing hemorrhage
      - ♦ Typical starting dose is 5–10 U infused over 10 minutes
    - ▪ Prostaglandins
    - ▪ PGE1 analog (misoprostol, Cytotec); dose: 1 mg rectally
    - ▪ PGE2 (dinoprostone, Cervidil, Prostin E2)
    - ▪ 15-Methyl PGF2-α (carboprost, Hemabate®); dose 250 μg IM q30 minutes:
      - ♦ Contraindicated in patients with reactive airway disease
      - ♦ Causes significant nausea and vomiting
    - ▪ Ergot alkaloids
    - ▪ Methylergonovine (Methergine®); dose 200 μg IM q15–20 minutes or 10–20 μg IV repeated q2–3 minutes:
      - ♦ Use with caution in hypertensive patients
      - ♦ Avoid in patients with reactive vasculopathies (Prinzmetal angina, Raynaud's, Buerger's) and with vulnerable vascular structures (unclipped cerebral aneurysm, diabetic retinopathy, Marfan's)
  - ‣ Surgical management:
    - ▪ Packing the uterine cavity
    - ▪ Bakri balloon (an occlusive balloon shaped to resemble the uterine cavity
    - ▪ B-Lynch suture (compressive suture shaped around the body of the uterus)
    - ▪ Embolization
    - ▪ Uterine artery ligation
    - ▪ Hysterectomy
  - ‣ Assess hemodynamics promptly:
    - ▪ Maternal blood loss is severely underestimated (see table above)

- ‣ Establish adequate vascular access:
  - ▪ At least two large-bore peripheral lines
  - ▪ If peripheral access is difficult, consider using US
  - ▪ Consider central line
- ‣ Consider arterial line for hemodynamic monitoring and repeat blood draws
- ‣ Order blood products:
  - ▪ Order FFP early; coagulopathy is very common
- ‣ Provide adequate analgesia and anesthesia for obstetrical interventions
- • *Genital trauma*:
  - ‣ Vaginal hematoma:
    - ▪ Associated with instrumental delivery
    - ▪ Often insidious
    - ▪ Rectal pressure may direct attention
    - ▪ Anesthesia for a perineal procedure is recommended (most commonly a saddle block or extension of a labor epidural)
  - ‣ *Vulvar hematoma*:
    - ▪ Eighty percent appears soon after delivery
    - ▪ Vulvar pain
    - ▪ Most commonly the labor epidural is used for exploration and repair
  - ‣ *Retroperitoneal hematoma*:
    - ▪ Least common, most dangerous
    - ▪ Few clinical signs except for blood loss
    - ▪ Often discovered late postpartum
    - ▪ If exploration is necessary, commonly performed under general anesthesia

TRANSFUSION THERAPY IN THE PREGNANT PATIENT

- • Overall incidence:
  - ‣ Transfusion for NSVD is about 1.1%
  - ‣ C/S is about 3.5%
  - ‣ Urgent (no crossmatch, O Rh negative blood) 0.8/1,000
- • Oxygen delivery in most patients remains adequate if Hb is >7 g/L
- • In patients with negative antibody screen, further crossmatch is rarely contributory
- • Extent of maternal hemorrhage is almost always underestimated
- • Two hemorrhagic disorders often coexist in the same patient
- • Awareness of possibility of hemorrhage, planning, and coordinated action is key
- • Call for help early:
  - ‣ Early involvement of the anesthesia team in maternal hemorrhage significantly improves outcome
- • Coagulopathy may develop early in the course of hemorrhage in pregnant women

REFERENCE

For references, please visit **www.TheAnesthesiaGuide.com**.

CHAPTER 195
Fetal HR Monitoring

Ruchir Gupta, MD

FETAL HR DECELERATION TYPES

See table on following page.

Deceleration	Etiology	Clinical situation	Appearance
Early	Fetal head compression	During sterile vaginal examinations In second stage of labor when pushing During application of internal FHR electrode CPD After rupture of amniotic sac Vertex presentations	
Variable	Cord compression		
Late	Uteroplacental insufficiency	Excessive uterine contractions Maternal hypotension Maternal hypoxemia (asthma, pneumonia) Reduced placental exchange as in: Hypertensive disorders, diabetes, IUGR abruption	

Reproduced from Hon EH. *An Atlas of Fetal Heart Rate Patterns.* New Haven: Harty Press; 1968.

Significance of the Various Patterns	
Reassuring patterns (positive outcomes, fetal well-being)	Mild variable decelerations (<30 s with rapid return to baseline) Early decelerations Accelerations without any other significant changes
Nonreassuring, or "warning," patterns suggest decreasing fetal capacity to cope with the stress of labor	Decrease in baseline variability Progressively worsening tachycardia (>160 bpm) Decrease baseline FHR Intermittent late decelerations with good variability
Patterns suggesting fetal compromise	Persistent late decelerations, with decreasing variability Variable decelerations with loss of variability, tachycardia, or late return to baseline Absence of variability Profound bradycardia

CHAPTER 196

Twin Pregnancy, Breech Presentation, Trial of Labor after Cesarean Birth: Anesthetic Considerations for Patients Attempting Vaginal Birth

Imre Rédai, MD, FRCA

- Maternal and neonatal morbidity is increased in these scenarios when compared with singleton vertex vaginal delivery
- Vaginal delivery is preferred in appropriate patients when obstetrical expertise is available, backed up by adequate hospital facilities including presence and expertise of an anesthesiologist

TWIN PREGNANCY

- Favorable presentations:
  - ‣ First twin has to be vertex
  - ‣ Version or breech extraction may be necessary if presentation is not vertex–vertex
- Preterm delivery common:
  - ‣ Sixty percent of twin pregnancies are delivered by Cesarean section in the United States
- Intrapartum fetal heart rate monitoring may be difficult
- Intrapartum complications may necessitate conversion to Cesarean section:
  - ‣ Nonreassuring fetal heart rate
  - ‣ Failed delivery of second twin
  - ‣ Cord prolapse
  - ‣ Abruption of placenta
- Delivery is often in the OR or in designated labor room with easy access to the OR

- Epidural analgesia is strongly recommended:
  ‣ Good labor analgesia
  ‣ Augmentation of analgesia for version or breech extraction (8–10 mL 3% chloroprocaine or 2% lidocaine with 1:200,000 epinephrine)
  ‣ Conversion to surgical anesthesia if urgent Cesarean delivery is indicated (15–20 mL 3% chloroprocaine)
  ‣ Administer supplemental oxygen during second stage of labor
- Presence of an anesthesiologist for delivery is recommended:
  ‣ Provide continued analgesia
  ‣ Intervene with IV medications if necessary
  ‣ Uterine relaxation
  ‣ Uterotonics
  ‣ Induce general anesthesia if fetal emergency

BREECH PRESENTATION

- The deciding factor in the choice of vaginal or Cesarean delivery is most commonly the experience and skill of the obstetrician
- Facilities for emergent Cesarean delivery must be immediately available
- Urgent conversion to Cesarean delivery:
  ‣ Nonreassuring fetal heart rate
  ‣ Cord prolapse
  ‣ Failed second stage (pushing past 30 minutes)
  ‣ Fetal head entrapment
- Epidural analgesia is strongly recommended
- Anesthesiologist should be immediately available in case of emergency obstetrical intervention

TRIAL OF LABOR AFTER CESAREAN BIRTH (TOLAC)

- The risk of uterine rupture during TOLAC is estimated at about 1%
- ACOG guidelines recommend TOLAC in facilities with staff present or immediately available to perform emergency care
- Most women with low transverse incision are candidates for TOLAC:
  ‣ Induction of labor and oxytocin augmentation are allowed; prostaglandins are not recommended
- Uterine rupture should be suspected if:
  ‣ Acute onset, severe abdominal pain
  ‣ Sudden fetal bradycardia
  ‣ Sudden change in shape of abdomen
  ‣ Maternal circulatory shock
  ‣ Vaginal bleeding
- Epidural analgesia is strongly recommended:
  ‣ Epidural analgesia may ameliorate pain of uterine rupture
  ‣ Premature urge to push is diminished by good labor analgesia; this reduces pressure on uterine scar
  ‣ Conversion to surgical anesthesia is possible
- General anesthesia is often necessary in frank rupture of the uterus and delivery of fetus in abdominal cavity
- Associated maternal hemorrhage is often significant

PART XII

CRITICAL CARE

CHAPTER 197
Central Venous Access

Manuel Corripio, MD

INDICATIONS

- Hemodynamic monitoring (CVP, PAC insertion)
- Administration of fluids that cannot be administered peripherally:
  ‣ Hypertonic fluids
  ‣ Vasoactive drugs (vasopressors)
  ‣ Total parenteral nutrition (TPN)
- Aspiration of air emboli
- Insertion of transcutaneous pacing leads
- Continuous renal replacement therapy in ICU
- Impossible peripheral IV access

CONTRAINDICATIONS

- Renal cell tumor extending into right atrium
- Fungating tricuspid valve endocarditis
- Anticoagulation (relative contraindication), platelets <50,000
- Ipsilateral carotid endartectomy (internal jugular [IJ] cannulation if not US-guided)

PREPARATION

- Hygiene:
  ‣ Proper hand hygiene and use *maximal barrier precautions* including gown, mask, and gloves and a large sterile drape or multiple drapes covering a large area
- Skin:
  ‣ Chlorhexidine (alcohol solutions rather than aqueous) associated with lower bloodstream infection rates than povidone–iodine or alcohol-based preparations
  ‣ Adequate local anesthetic infiltration (unless under GA)
- Adequate sedation as appropriate
- Protect bed in ICU ("chucks" to avoid soiling sheets with skin prep or blood)
- Trendelenburg position (as tolerated) for IJ/subclavian lines to:
  ‣ Increase venous pressure and reduce risk of air embolism
  ‣ Increase size of veins
- Know anatomy:
  ‣ Relative position of IJ vein to carotid artery (Figure 197-1)

FIGURE 197-1. Position of IJ vein relative to the carotid artery (at the center of the circle) with the patient's head rotated 30° toward the opposite side

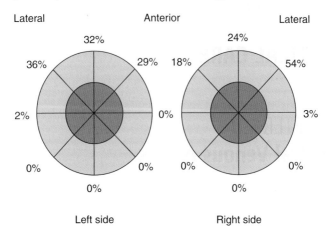

Adapted from Maecken T, Marcon C, Bomas S, Zenz M, Grau T. Relationship of the internal jugular vein to the common carotid artery: implications for ultrasound-guided vascular access. *Eur J Anaesthesiol.* 2011;28(5):351–355.

PROCEDURE

- Typical procedure using landmarks:
  - Patient supine, arms alongside body
  - Ascertain landmarks
  - Use finder needle (20G) to obtain venous blood (not used for subclavian access)
  - Leave finder needle (and syringe) in place, and use its direction as a guide to insert the introducer needle (16G)
  - When venous blood is aspirated in the syringe, remove finder needle
  - Ensure free blood flow, and then transduce pressure to ascertain venous placement:
    - Some syringes (Raulerson) allow direct transduction (and guidewire insertion) through the plunger, without having to disconnect the syringe
    - Otherwise, disconnect needle from syringe. Occlude needle to avoid air embolism
    - Insert guidewire and exchange needle for angiocath
    - Connect sterile IV tubing and hold tubing down to have blood flow 5-10 cm into the tubing. Then hold tubing up. The blood should oscillate a few centimeters above the skin puncture (venous pressure in cm H_2O) but not fill the tubing (arterial puncture). Alternatively, measure pressure using a piezoelectric transducer
  - Insert wire to about 20 cm. Avoid inserting too far as this may trigger ventricular arrhythmias
  - *Never let go of wire end* to avoid losing it into the vein
  - Insert dilator over guidewire; nick skin with blade and push dilator into the vein. *Do not insert dilator more than half its length* (risk of vein injury)

- Remove dilator while maintaining wire in place
- Insert catheter over wire. *Ensure to have wire exit at the proximal end of the catheter before inserting tip of catheter into skin*
- Push catheter over guidewire
- Flush lines by aspirating with a saline-filled syringe to fill line with blood, and then injecting saline and clamping *while injecting* to avoid blood getting into the line and clotting
- Secure at typically 15 cm at skin for right-sided IJ and subclavian lines, and 17 cm for left-sided lines
- Obtain CXR as soon as convenient; the tip should be at the junction between SVC and RA; if tip in RA, pull catheter back, as this may lead to RA perforation

FIGURE 197-2. Seldinger technique for central venous line insertion

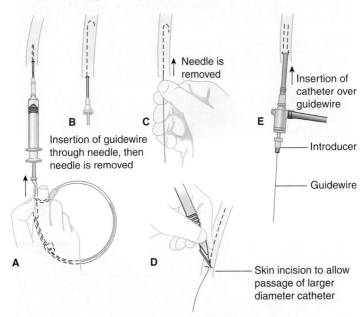

US guidance is becoming standard of care. Decreases complications (even though RCTs conflicted)
- Vein seen as compressible hypoechoic structure (Figures 197-3 and 197-4)
- If available, at least scan intended site prior to prepping to locate vein (ascertain patency as proximal as possible), artery, and any other structure that might be injured

FIGURE 197-3. Landmarks for ultrasound-guided central line placement in the internal jugular vein

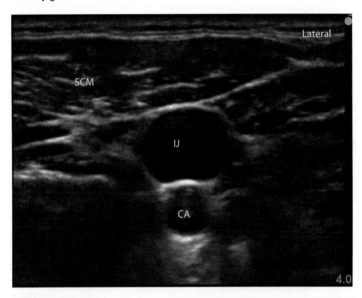

Internal jugular vein visible, deep to the sternocleidomastoid muscle, and superficial to the carotid artery. IJ, internal jugular vein; CA, carotid artery; SCM, sternocleidomastoid muscle.

FIGURE 197-4. Same view as Figure 197-3 with compression of the internal jugular vein by the ultrasound probe

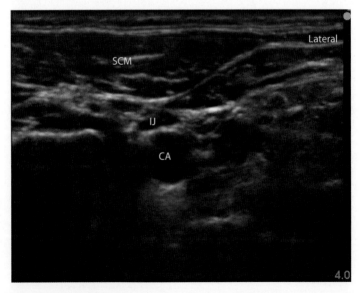

IJ, internal jugular vein; CA, carotid artery; SCM, sternocleidomastoid muscle.

- If using US guidance for procedure:
  - Use long sterile sheath for probe
  - Position IJ in center of field
  - Insert needle out-of-plane slowly, using "hen-pecking" motion to ascertain the position of its tip, while maintaining negative pressure in the syringe
  - When venous blood is aspirated, insert guidewire
  - Slide US probe proximally. The guidewire can usually be seen in the vein, especially if the probe is rotated 90° to have a long-axis view of the vein (Figure 197-5). Shaking the wire can help to locate it
  - Then proceed as above

FIGURE 197-5. Internal jugular vein seen in long axis with an intraluminal guidewire

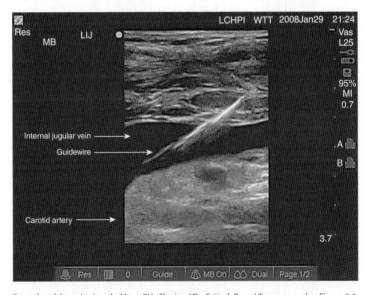

Approaches to Central Venous Line Insertion			
Approach	Landmarks	Advantages	Risks/Issues
IJ central approach	Puncture at the apex of the triangle between two heads of SCM Aim: lateral to CA if palpated; otherwise, nipple in men, sagittal or slightly lateral in women Angle 20–30° toward floor	Easy landmarks in most people	Pneumothorax Carotid artery puncture
IJ anterior approach	• Puncture at the anterior border of the SCM, 6–8 cm above clavicle • Separate carotid from SCM with free hand • Introduce needle between carotid and SCM • Aim: sagittal toward feet or slightly lateral, angle 45° toward floor	Easy landmarks = carotid pulse and anterior SCM High in the neck → lower risk of pneumothorax	Higher risk of carotid puncture Catheter/dressing site in facial hair in men Uncomfortable for awake patient as catheter high in the neck
IJ posterior approach	Puncture site is posterolateral to the SCM and immediately cephalad to where the sternocleidomastoid is crossed by the external jugular vein, or 4–6 cm from clavicle The needle should be directed beneath the muscle (deep to the muscle's deep surface) and advanced in an anterior and caudad direction toward the sternal notch Aim: posterior aspect of ipsilateral sternoclavicular joint Angle 20–30° **toward ceiling** (anterior)	Lower risk of pneumothorax and of carotid puncture	Posterior border of SCM less obvious, especially in obese patients Risk of thoracic duct damage on the left Risk of brachial plexus injury if poor landmarks (too posterior)

Subclavian	Puncture 1 cm below the clavicle, at either • Junction medial 1/3–central 1/3 (medial puncture increases risk of pneumothorax, especially on R) • Midpoint between sternoclavicular and acromioclavicular joints (lateral puncture increases risk of arterial or brachial plexus injury) Aim: toward contralateral shoulder, or toward operator's finger in suprasternal notch Angle 20–30° toward floor (45° leads straight into lung) Forcibly depress the soft tissues in order to insert the needle at a 20° angle **under** the clavicle	• Bony landmarks • Patent even if hypovolemic • Clean site (no drooling, away from tracheostomy) • Comfortable for awake patient	• Higher risk of pneumothorax (?) • Steep learning curve • Difficult to compress if bleed (can catheterize axillary vein [slightly more distal] under US guidance) • Kinking possible during cardiac surgery (sternal retraction), or with Vascath for CRRT (poor flow) • Malposition possible with wire and line going up ipsilateral IJ, or across into innominate vein and contralateral SC
Femoral	• Puncture 1 cm medial to the femoral pulse • 2–3 cm below the inguinal ligament ▸ Aim: sagittal toward head, slightly medial ▸ Angle 30–40° toward floor	Easy landmark = femoral pulse Low rate of complications, no CXR needed	"Dirty" area, higher risk of line sepsis (controversial) Risk of retroperitoneal bleed Guidewire difficult to pass if major ascites
Peripheral upper extremity vein	Cannulate basilic or cephalic vein and thread line into central position	Easy vein cannulation but occasional difficult central access More comfortable for patient Low rate of complications	Malposition common Long line, slow flow (infusion and aspiration, e.g. if air embolism)

SCM, sternocleidomastoid muscle; IJ, internal jugular vein; CA, carotid artery. Directions are given referring to the patient in standard anatomical position.

FIGURE 197-6. Landmarks for IJ cannulation

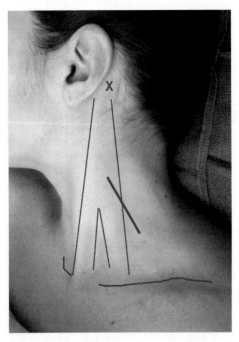

X marks the mastoid; the two heads of the SCM muscle are highlighted, as is the clavicle and the sternal notch. In blue, the typical position of the external jugular vein (EJ).

FIGURE 197-7. Needle insertion site and direction for central approach to IJ

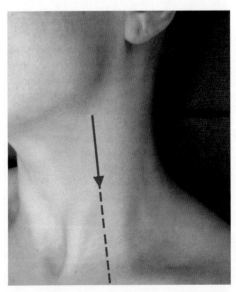

FIGURE 197-8. Needle insertion site and direction for anterior approach to IJ

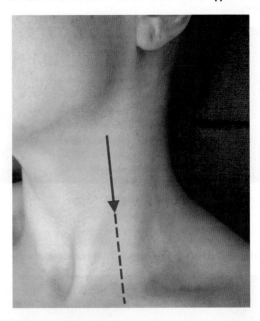

FIGURE 197-9. Needle insertion site and direction for posterior approach to IJ

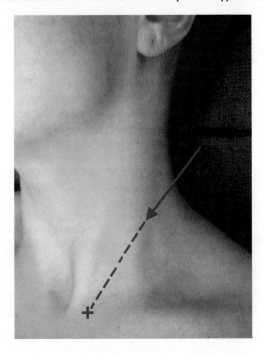

FIGURE 197-10. Needle insertion site and direction for posterior approach to IJ (lateral view)

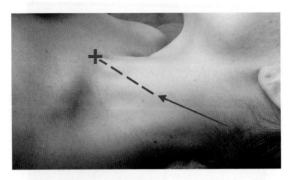

Note that the needle is aimed slightly anterior (toward the ceiling).

FIGURE 197-11. Needle insertion sites for subclavian vein cannulation

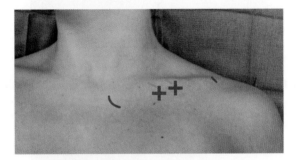

Points shown correspond to 1 cm below the midpoint of the clavicle and the junction between medial one third and lateral two thirds.

FIGURE 197-12. Needle aim for subclavian vein cannulation

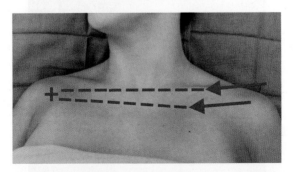

The needle inserted at any of the two possible sites is directed toward the contralateral shoulder.

FIGURE 197-13. Schematic illustration of the need to forcibly depress the soft tissues caudad to the clavicle in order to insert the needle (dashed arrow) at a "flat" angle, about 20°, between clavicle and first rib. Inserting the needle at a 45° angle (solid arrow) leads into the pleura.

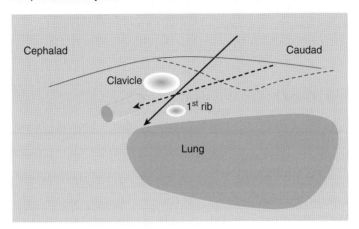

PEARLS AND TIPS FOR CVC ACCESS

- Maintain aseptic conditions at all times
- Trendelenburg position for IJ/subclavian lines
- Insert the needle at a flat angle under the clavicle for subclavian cannulation
- Continuously occlude needle and catheter hub to decrease the risk of air embolism
- Line to stay in place more than 5–7 days: consider antibiotic-impregnated catheter:
  ‣ Patient with no major risk of severe mechanical complications:
    ▪ Subclavian access
  ‣ Major risk, failure of the first attempt:
    ▪ Consider US guidance
    ▪ IJ or femoral access; tunneling?
- Less than 5–7 days, PAC, hemodialysis:
  ‣ Mechanical >infectious complications:
    ▪ IJ or femoral access
- Care:
  ‣ Meticulous site care
  ‣ Change infusion system every 48–72 hours
  ‣ Low-dose anticoagulants (heparin, LMWH): controversial
  ‣ Remove CVC as soon as no longer needed
  ‣ No routine catheter change

COMPLICATIONS

- Immediate:
  ‣ Bleeding
  ‣ Arrhythmias
  ‣ Air embolism
  ‣ Nerve injury (brachial plexus)
  ‣ Pneumothorax, hemothorax
  ‣ Thoracic duct injury (left side of neck)
- Delayed:
  ‣ Infection
  ‣ Venous thrombosis
  ‣ Catheter migrations
  ‣ Myocardial perforation

Complications of Central Venous Access	
Complication	Preferred access to avoid complication
Infection (2–10%)	Subclavian (SC) > IJ ≥ femoral (F)
Thrombosis (2–40%)	SC > IJ > F
Mechanical complications (2–4%)	F > IJ ≥ SC
Failures and malposition (0–3%)	F > IJ ≥ SC

Relative Rating of Approaches to Central Venous Access					
	Basilic/ cephalic	External jugular	Internal jugular	Subclavian	Femoral
Ease of vein cannulation	1	3	2	5	3
Success rate (e.g., pulmonary artery catheter placement)	4	5	1	2	3
Long-term use	4	3	2	1	5
Immediate complications	1	2	4	5	3
Delayed complications	1	3	4	2	5

1, best or easiest; 5, worst or most difficult.

REFERENCES

For references, please visit **www.TheAnesthesiaGuide.com**.

CHAPTER 198
Shock

Nirav Mistry, MD and Adel Bassily-Marcus, MD, FCCP, FCCM

TABLE 198-1 Differentiating Different Types of Shock							
Type of shock	MAP	PAWP	CO	SVR	SvO$_2$	Lactic acid	Contractility on echo
Hypovolemic	↓	↓	↓	↑	↓	↑	Small hyperkinetic LV
Distributive	↓	↔↓	↔↑	↓	↔↑	↑	↑ or ↓
Cardiogenic	↓	↑	↓	↑	↓	↑	↓
Obstructive	↓	↔↑	↓	↑	↓	↑	PE: large hypokinetic RV Tamponade: RV diastolic collapse

MAP, mean arterial pressure; PAWP, pulmonary artery wedge pressure; CO, cardiac output; SVR, systemic vascular resistance; SvO$_2$, mixed venous oxygen saturation; LV, left ventricle; RV, right ventricle; PE, pulmonary embolism.

FIGURE 198-1. Stepwise approach to the patient in shock

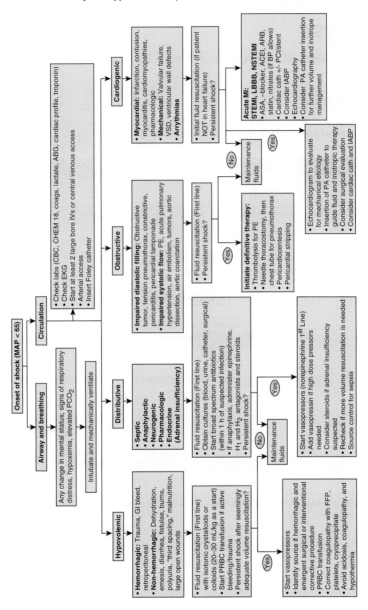

CHAPTER 199
Sepsis

Nirav Mistry, MD and Adel Bassily-Marcus, MD, FCCP, FCCM

DEFINITIONS

- Systemic inflammatory response syndrome (SIRS): systemic response to any inflammatory/infectious etiology (see Table 199-1)

TABLE 199-1　SIRS Criteria (Need 2 Out of 4)
• WBC >12,000/mL, <4,000/mL, or >10% immature bands
• HR >90/min
• Temperature >38.5°C or <35°C
• RR >20 breaths/min, or $Paco_2$ <32 mm Hg

FIGURE 199-1. Diagnostic workup of sepsis

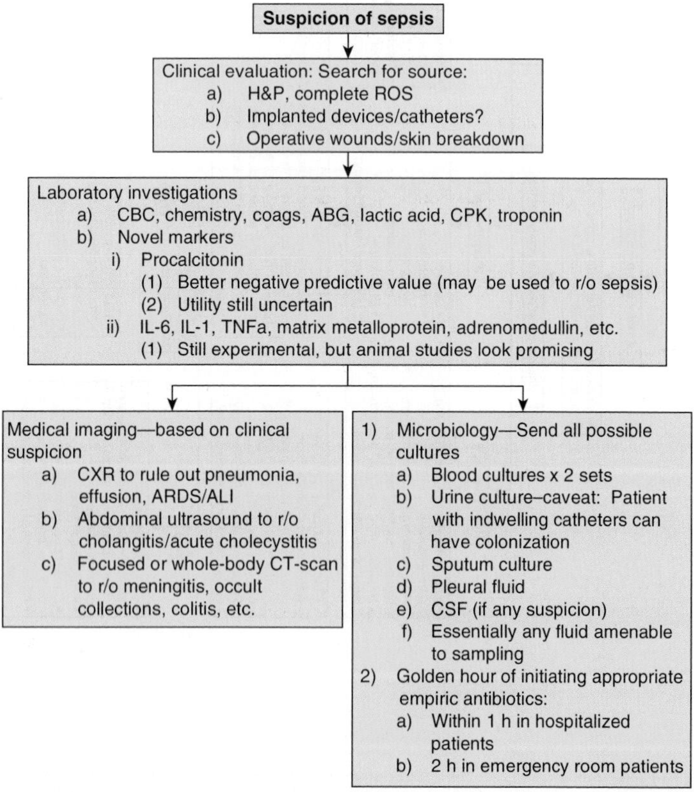

- Sepsis: definite infectious etiology with a resultant systemic response (at least two or more SIRS criteria)
- Severe sepsis → sepsis with acute organ dysfunction
- Septic shock → sepsis-induced hypotension refractory to fluid resuscitation and evidence of end-organ damage including lactic acidosis, oliguria, or altered mental status
- *Mortality ranges from 28% to 50%*

Management of Severe Sepsis or Septic Shock	
Initial resuscitation (first 6 h)	
Patients with hypotension, lactic acid >4 mmol/L require immediate resuscitation	
Goals	• Mean arterial pressure ≥65 mm Hg • Urine output ≥0.5 mL/kg/h • Central venous pressure (CVP) 8–12 mm Hg (controversial benefit) • Central venous oxygen saturation ≥70% or mixed venous ≥65% (controversial benefit)
Crystalloids and colloids equally effective	• Challenges of 1,000 mL of crystalloid or 300–500 mL of colloid over 30 min • May require larger volumes in patients with persistent hypotension with vasopressors • Bicarbonate therapy contraindicated in patients with hypoperfusion-induced lactic acidosis and pH ≥7.15
Blood product transfusion	• Transfuse packed red blood cells to target Hb ≥7 (may require higher targets in patients with special circumstances [myocardial ischemia, etc.]) • Avoid plasma or platelet administration unless active bleeding or planned procedure
Vasopressors	• Start if shock persists despite fluid resuscitation (20–30 mL/kg) to keep MAP ≥60–65 mm Hg • Vasopressors, including norepinephrine and dopamine, should be administered via central venous catheter • Vasopressin (0.03 U/min), phenylephrine, or epinephrine may be added if shock unresponsive to initial vasoactive medications • Arterial catheter use recommended for hemodynamic monitoring • Dobutamine recommended in patients with myocardial dysfunction
Source control and antibiotics	• Identify infectious etiology within 6 h of presentation • Evaluate and implement measures of source control (abscess drainage, tissue debridement, etc.) • Remove infected intravascular devices • Culture all available specimens • Start broad-spectrum antibiotics within the first hour as sepsis and septic shock recognized ▸ Combination therapy should be used in patients with suspected *Pseudomonas* infection or who are otherwise immunocompromised
Mechanical ventilation in patients with ALI/ARDS	• Tidal volume of 6 mL/kg (ideal body weight) • Maintain plateau pressures ≤30 cm H_2O • Increase PEEP as needed to avoid lung collapse at end-expiration and to avoid oxygen toxicity with high FiO_2 levels • Allow $Paco_2$ to rise to minimize plateau pressures and tidal volumes • Keep head of bed elevated to at least 30° (30–45°), unless contraindicated • Institute weaning protocols and daily assessment for SBT to liberate patients from mechanical ventilation • Use conservative fluid strategy • Some advocate against PAC in patients with ALI/ARDS: no survival benefit, increased risk of infection, health care costs, and risk of nonfatal cardiac arrhythmias

(continued)

Management of Severe Sepsis or Septic Shock (*continued*)	
Recombinant human activated protein C (drotrecogin alfa [activated]) withdrawn from the market in 10/2011 due to lack of efficacy in the PROWESS-SHOCK trial	
Steroids	• May consider starting in patients with shock refractory to fluid resuscitation and vasopressor therapy (refractory shock: increasing doses of vasopressors, add vasopressors to maintain MAP >65 mm Hg) • Start with hydrocortisone (preferred steroid) dose of 200–300 mg/day • ACTH stimulation test is not recommended prior to starting steroids • Do not treat sepsis with steroids unless hypotension present or patient's medical status necessitates the use of steroids (prior steroid use, endocrine disorder, etc.)
Glycemic control	• Intravenous insulin should be used for correcting severe hyperglycemia in critically ill patients • Most recent evidence suggests intensive insulin therapy may lead to worse outcomes • Monitor glucose closely and aim to maintain plasma glucose levels ≤180 mg/dL
Sedation/ analgesia	• For critically ill mechanically ventilated patients, use sedation protocols • Sedation may be intermittent or as a continuous infusion • Allow for daily sedation interruption to awaken patients • Neuromuscular blockers should be avoided unless refractory hypoxemia in ARDS. Monitor response using train-of-fours
Stress ulcer prophylaxis	Use H_2 blockers or PPI
VTE prophylaxis	• No difference between low-dose unfractionated heparin or low-molecular-weight heparin • If heparin is contraindicated, mechanical compression devices can be used

REFERENCES

For references, please visit **www.TheAnesthesiaGuide.com**.

CHAPTER 200
Acute Myocardial Infarction, Complications and Treatment

Awais Sheikh, MD and Roopa Kohli-Seth, MD

DIAGNOSIS OF ACUTE MI

- *Clinical*: new angina, increasing angina, or angina at rest. Diaphoresis, hypotension, new MR murmur, pulmonary edema or rales, JVD
- *EKG (Figures 200-1 and 200-2)*: ST segment elevation (≥0.2 mV in men or ≥0.15 mV in women in leads V2–V3 and/or ≥0.1 mV in other leads) or depression (>0.05 mV in two contiguous leads), T-wave inversion, new blocks especially LBBB
- *Echo*: wall motion abnormality, new MR (papillary muscle dysfunction)
- *Lab*: cardiac enzymes (troponin) serially STAT (for baseline) and q6 hours × 3
- *DDx*:
  ‣ Elicit cocaine use
  ‣ PE, aortic dissection: CT angiography to rule out

NB: See chapter 5 for more details on EKG changes.

FIGURE 200-1. Electrocardiographic signs of ischemia

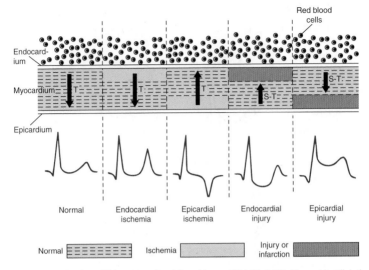

Patterns of ischemia and injury. Reproduced from Morgan GE, Mikhail MS, Murray MJ. *Clinical Anesthesiology*. 4th ed. Figure 20-3. Available at: http://www.accessmedicine.com. Copyright © The McGraw-Hill Companies, Inc. All rights reserved.

INITIAL MANAGEMENT

- Oxygen 2–4 L/min by NC; attach monitors and get IV access
- NTG 0.4 mg sublingual × 3; if no relief, then morphine 2–4 mg IV; repeat q5–15 minutes
- Beta-blockers such as metoprolol 25 mg PO if no CHF, hypotension, or bradycardia. If hypertensive, give IV metoprolol 5 mg q5 minutes up to three times
- Aspirin 160–325 mg non-enteric coated, ideally chewable
- Atorvastatin 80 mg PO stat if not on statin

ST ELEVATION MI (STEMI)

- **PCI within 90 minutes of presentation.** Call cardiology stat
- Fibrinolysis within 30 minutes of presentation if known PCI not possible within 90 minutes, symptoms <12 hours, and no contraindications (ICH, ischemic stroke <3 months, cerebral AVMs or malignancy, aortic dissection, bleeding diathesis or active bleeding, except menses; head trauma <3 months)
- Antiplatelet therapy (in addition to aspirin):
  ‣ Prasugrel 60 mg: with PCI and no risk of bleeding
  ‣ Or clopidogrel 600 mg. Discuss with cardiologist
- Glycoprotein IIb/IIIa inhibitor in consultation with cardiologist
- Give anticoagulant therapy to all patients:
  ‣ *Unfractionated heparin (UFH)*:
    ▪ PCI with GP IIb/IIIa inhibitor: 50–60 U/kg IV bolus then infusion for aPTT 50–75 s
    ▪ Without GP IIb/IIIa inhibitor: 60–100 U/kg IV bolus (maximum 4,000 U)
- *Enoxaparin*: for non-PCI patients with normal kidney function load with 30 mg IV bolus and 1 mg/kg SC q12 hours. UFH preferred in ESRD patients

FIGURE 200-2. Location of MI (coronary supply, myocardium) and corresponding EKG leads

A
Normal blood supply

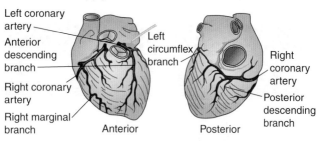

Typical EKG leads

B
Relative frequency, 50%

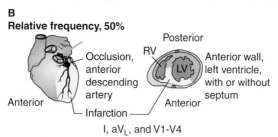

I, aV$_L$, and V1-V4

C
Relative frequency, 30%

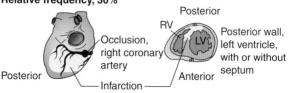

(RV: V3R, V4R, V5R, III and aV$_F$)
Inferior: II, III, aV$_F$

D
Relative frequency, 20%

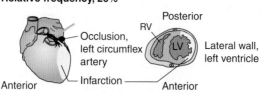

V$_5$ or V$_6$ V7-V9, with reciprocal ST
depression in leads V$_2$ or V$_3$

UNSTABLE ANGINA (UA) OR NON-STEMI

- Give antiplatelet therapy (in addition to aspirin): prasugrel 60 mg—with PCI and no risk of bleeding or clopidogrel 600 mg. Discuss with cardiologist
- Glycoprotein IIb/IIIa inhibitor in consultation with cardiologist
- Give anticoagulant therapy in all patients:
  ‣ *UFH* is preferred: PCI—give 50–60 U/kg IV bolus followed by 12 U/kg/h IV (goal aPTT 50–75 seconds)
  ‣ Or *enoxaparin*: for non-PCI patients with normal kidney function load with 30 mg IV bolus and 1 mg/kg SC q12 hours. UFH preferred in ESRD patients
  ‣ Or *fondaparinux* 2.5 mg SC daily

COCAINE-RELATED ACS

- Alleviate anxiety with lorazepam 2–4 mg IV every 15 minutes
- Beta-blockers contraindicated

COMPLICATIONS OF ACUTE MYOCARDIAL INFARCTION

- *Acute congestive heart failure:*
  ‣ Primary cause of in-hospital mortality after MI
  ‣ S3, S4 gallop, rales, hepatojugular reflux, extremity perfusion, and edema
  ‣ Obtain TTE to assess LV function, chest x-ray
  ‣ *Treatment:*
    ▪ Decrease preload: IV furosemide or IV nitroglycerin
    ▪ Decrease afterload: IV nitroglycerin or IV ACE inhibitor
    ▪ Avoid nitroprusside due to coronary steal
    ▪ If still symptomatic, use inotropes
- *Cardiogenic shock:*
  ‣ Due to acute HF, VSD, MR, free wall rupture, tamponade, cardiotomy
  ‣ Also due to excessive negative inotrope and vasodilator use
  ‣ Continuous chest pain, SOB, diaphoresis, confusion, pallor, cyanosis
  ‣ S3 gallop, MAP <60 mm Hg, oliguria <0.5 mL/kg/h, CI <2.2 L/min/m^2, PAWP >18 mm Hg
  ‣ Chemistry, cardiac enzymes, ECG, chest x-ray, ECHO with color Doppler
  ‣ *Treatment:*
    ▪ Keep MAP >65 mm Hg: IV fluids and vasopressors
    ▪ Correct O$_2$ and pH with ETT ventilation
    ▪ Intra-aortic balloon counterpulsation (IABP): increases aortic diastolic pressure, coronary flow, CO and decreases O$_2$ consumption and ischemia. *Contraindication:* AI/aortic dissection
    ▪ Ventricular assist device
    ▪ Definitive treatment: revascularize coronaries, valve repair
- *Pulmonary edema:*
  ‣ Usually associated with LV failure
  ‣ SOB, tachypnea, tachycardia, hypoxia, crackles, HTN
  ‣ Chest x-ray, echocardiogram. Cardiac PAWP >18 mm Hg versus noncardiac PAWP <18 mm Hg
  ‣ *Treatment:*
    ▪ Decrease preload: IV furosemide or IV nitroglycerin, morphine, nesiritide
    ▪ O$_2$, ETT ventilation
    ▪ Increase MAP and SVR by vasopressors
    ▪ Increase CO by inotropes or IABP
- *Cardiogenic shock due to right-sided MI:*
  ‣ Not uncommon with inferior MI. Usually responsive to treatment
  ‣ JVD, hepatojugular reflex, lower extremity edema. No pulmonary congestion
  ‣ Chest x-ray, ECHO, ECG, PA catheter: increased RAP, RA/PAOP ≥0.8 (Nl 0.5)

- ▸ *Treatment*:
  - IV fluid resuscitation to RAP 10–15
  - Increase CO by inotropes, IABP; last resort = RV assist device (poor prognosis)
  - Increase MAP, SVR by vasopressors
  - Maintain AV synchrony by AV pacer if rhythm other than sinus
  - Decrease PVR by inhaled nitric oxide (20–40 ppm) and epoprostenol (IV 1–2 ng/kg/min; increase q15 minutes by 2 ng/kg/min until side effects or response plateaus; usual dose: 25–40 ng/kg/min)
  - Definitive treatment is early revascularization
- • *Mechanical complications of acute myocardial infarction*:
  - ▸ *Acute MR*:
    - Papillary muscle dysfunction, rupture, chordal rupture, LV dilatation, or aneurysm
    - Hypotension, pulmonary edema, hyperactive precordium, systolic murmur
    - Echocardiogram with color Doppler. PAOP: giant V waves
    - *Treatment*:
      - ◆ Avoid bradycardia as it increases the duration of diastole and hence regurgitation
      - ◆ Decrease preload: IV furosemide or IV nitroglycerin
      - ◆ Avoid increasing afterload (ETT, surgical stimulation): deep sedation, vasodilators
      - ◆ Excessive volume expansion worsens MR
      - ◆ Increase CO by inotropes and IABP
      - ◆ Definitive treatment is surgical repair
  - ▸ *Acute VSD*:
    - Not common, usually within first 14 days
    - Hypotension, predominant RV failure, harsh holosystolic murmur
    - Echocardiogram with color Doppler
    - PA catheter: all pressures increased, increased pulmonary flow, and decreased systemic flow
    - *Treatment*:
      - ◆ Similar to acute MR (see above)
  - ▸ *Free wall rupture*:
    - Often within 7 days. Major cause of sudden cardiac death, PEA, tamponade. Often fatal
    - Acute pulmonary edema, cardiogenic shock
    - Echocardiogram with color Doppler
    - *Treatment*:
      - ◆ Closed-chest CPR useless as no forward flow
      - ◆ Volume resuscitation
      - ◆ Inotropes
      - ◆ Pericardiocentesis, emergent sternotomy
      - ◆ Often fatal
- • *Arrhythmias*: due to ANS hyperstimulation, electrolyte imbalance, and ischemia:
  - ▸ *Treat as appropriate (see chapters 5, 15, 16, and 222)*
  - ▸ *Accelerated idioventricular rhythm* ("slow VT"): rarely seen outside of MI:
    - Wide complex, rate 60–100
    - Usually benign with reperfusion
    - If treatment required: atropine to increase sinus rate
- • *Other complications of MI*:
  - ▸ *Hypovolemia*:
    - Often also due to prior diuretic use, decreased PO intake, vomiting
    - Hypotension, vascular collapse, dry mucous membranes
    - Monitor O_2, PAWP, and CO
    - IVF cautiously up to PAWP 20 mm Hg
    - Eventually CO plateaus and congestion appears with decreasing oxygenation
  - ▸ *Recurrent chest pain*:
    - Often due to recurrent ischemia and needs revascularization

- ‣ *Pericarditis*:
  - ▪ Cautious anticoagulation due to hemopericardial tamponade risk
- ‣ *Thromboembolism*:
  - ▪ LV thrombus needs anticoagulation for 3–6 months to prevent embolization
- ‣ *LV aneurysm*:
  - ▪ Noncontractile outpouching leads to CHF, embolism, and arrhythmias
  - ▪ Surgery
- ‣ *Pseudoaneurysm*:
  - ▪ Free wall rupture contained by pericardium and organized thrombus
  - ▪ Surgery to prevent extension and tamponade

REFERENCES

For references, please visit **www.TheAnesthesiaGuide.com**.

CHAPTER 201
Anaphylaxis

Alexandra P. Leader, MD, Ryan Dunst, MD, and Michael H. Andreae, MD

BASICS

- Potentially lethal allergic reaction
- Rapid onset, from minutes to hours after exposure
- Generally requires a prior sensitization to antigen; can occur on first exposure due to cross-reactivity among drugs/products
- Pathophysiology: type I hypersensitivity reaction involving multiple organ systems
  - ‣ IgE-mediated mast cell degranulation with release of stored histamine, proteases, proteoglycans, and platelet-activating factor (PAF); followed by production of proinflammatory prostaglandins and leukotrienes
  - ‣ Histamine, prostaglandin, and leukotriene receptors elicit changes in vascular permeability and tone, bronchial smooth muscle contraction, and coagulability, and may produce angioedema, urticaria, bronchoconstriction, and DIC; PAF can further contribute to anticoagulation and constriction of bronchial smooth muscle
- Clinically indistinguishable from anaphylactoid reactions, that is, "pseudoanaphylaxis" (non-IgE-mediated, no prior sensitization, nonspecific histamine release)
- Incidence 1/3,500–20,000 anesthetic procedures; higher mortality rate in perioperative anaphylaxis than anaphylaxis in other settings
- Early signs often unrecognized and undertreated in anesthetized patients; cutaneous signs masked by surgical draping
- May be biphasic with recurrence of symptoms 8–10 and up to 72 hours after initial occurrence
- Requires immediate treatment and resuscitation
- Death from upper airway edema, bronchial obstruction, circulatory collapse
- Comorbidities with high risk of poor outcomes: asthma/COPD and CV disease
- Four grades:
  1. Cutaneomucosal generalized signs: rash, urticaria
  2. Moderate multivisceral involvement: hypotension, tachycardia, bronchial hyperreactivity
  3. Severe, life-threatening multivisceral involvement: MI, severe bronchospasm
  4. Cardiorespiratory arrest

NB: Cutaneous signs can be delayed or absent.

Clinical Features of Anaphylaxis/Anaphylactoid Reactions and Differential Diagnosis		
System	Clinical features	Differential
Mucocutaneous	Pruritus, flushing, erythema, acute urticaria, angioedema	Carcinoid syndrome, contact or cholinergic urticaria, medication-induced vasodilation
Respiratory	Laryngeal edema, hoarseness, bronchospasm, hypersecretion, increased peak airway pressure, decreased O_2 saturation	Malignant hyperthermia, asthma, aspiration, mucous plug, mainstem intubation, recurrent laryngeal nerve injury, post-extubation stridor
Cardiovascular	(Pre)syncope, tachycardia/bradycardia, hypotension, dysrhythmia, cardiovascular collapse, cardiac arrest	Vasovagal reaction, arrhythmia, MI, PE, tension pneumothorax, tamponade, shock
Hematologic	Disseminated intravascular coagulation (DIC)	Transfusion reaction, hemorrhage

Causative Agents	
NMBAs	50–70% of perioperative anaphylaxis; 60–70% cross-reactivity (no absolute contraindication to all NMBAs, if allergy testing available); more common in females (75% of NMBA-related reactions)
Latex	Higher risk of sensitivity in health care workers and with multiple past surgeries (prior exposures to antigen), history of spina bifida, allergy to tropical fruits (bananas, kiwi, avocado, papaya, mango, passion fruit), chestnut allergy
Antibiotics	Penicillins, cephalosporins, carbapenems, monobactams, vancomycin, sulfonamides
Local anesthetics	Rare and occurring mostly with amino ester local anesthetics (reaction to amino ester local anesthetic metabolite *para*-aminobenzoic acid [PABA])
Others	Colloids, protamine (diabetics receiving NPH insulin), radiology contrast dye (not an iodine allergy, no correlation to seafood allergy), hypnotics (primarily barbiturates), opioids

PREOPERATIVE: PREVENTION

- Elicit risk factors for allergy to medications, latex, foods
- If patient had an anaphylactic reaction during a prior anesthetic:
  ‣ Prefer regional if possible
  ‣ If GA, avoid NMBAs and histamine-releasing medications (e.g., morphine); use propofol, inhalation agents; prefer non-histamine-releasing opioids (fentanyl, hydromorphone)
  ‣ No preoperative tests have been shown to reliably identify medications to avoid
  ‣ No benefit in premedicating allergic patients with H_1 or H_2 blockers
  ‣ If possible, administer antibiotics in the OR, with full monitoring, prior to anesthetic induction

INTRAOPERATIVE: TREATMENT

- Immediate discontinuation of suspected drug or antigen; discontinuation of anesthetic drugs if anaphylaxis occurs on induction or if circulatory collapse present
- Prompt administration of *epinephrine* to correct hypotension and enable bronchial smooth muscle relaxation; also stop mast cell degranulation and factor release:
  - ‣ Initial epinephrine bolus 5–10 µg IV if patient hypotensive; 0.1–0.5 mg IV epinephrine bolus if cardiorespiratory arrest; subsequent 1–20 µg/min IV epinephrine infusion, as needed
  - ‣ For cardiovascular collapse or arrest, give epinephrine 1–3 mg IV over 3 minutes; initiate ACLS protocol
  - ‣ *No contraindications to epinephrine* in setting of anaphylaxis
  - ‣ Delay in treatment with epinephrine may predispose to biphasic, protracted, and fatal anaphylaxis
  - ‣ **Avoid high-dose epinephrine in patient with mild symptoms due to risk of causing MI and/or CVA**
  - ‣ If beta-blocker therapy, higher doses of epinephrine may be needed; glucagon 1–2 mg IV q 5 minutes followed by infusion 0.3–1 mg/h has been anecdotally reported to bypass blockade of beta-adrenergic receptors
- Maintain airway; administer 100% oxygen; immediate tracheal intubation if any evidence of laryngeal edema or airway compromise
- Inform surgical team; cancel, accelerate, or terminate surgical procedure
- 2 to 4 L of IV crystalloid for intravascular volume replacement/expansion
- Add norepinephrine (start at 0.1 µg/kg/min) if epinephrine continuous IV infusion requirements >8–10 µg/min
- Raise lower extremities to improve venous return; use military antishock trousers (MAST) if available; limited efficacy due to increased vascular permeability
- Adjunctive pharmacologic therapy:
  - ‣ Bronchodilator: albuterol ± ipratropium bromide nebulizer (7.5 mg albuterol ± 0.5 mg ipratropium bromide)
  - ‣ Glucocorticoids to prevent late phase reactions: hydrocortisone 200 mg IV q6 hours
  - ‣ Antihistamines: diphenhydramine 25–50 mg IV and ranitidine 150 mg IV. (There is no evidence to support antihistamines in anaphylaxis; they are still part of many treatment algorithms, however.)
- Consider blood draw to measure tryptase in serum/plasma/clotted blood, ideally within 30 minutes of reaction; if decision made to stop resuscitation, draw blood prior to interruption of CPR

POSTOPERATIVE: OBSERVATION, DIAGNOSIS, AND SECONDARY PREVENTION

- Monitor in ICU or PACU for further hemodynamic instability; consider delayed extubation as persistence of airway edema possible
- Consider extending antihistamine and steroid treatment for 3 days to minimize likelihood of further reaction
- Refer patient to allergy specialist for further testing and management
- Diagnostic testing:
  - ‣ Serum tryptase level; elevated in anaphylaxis, obtain within 3 hours of onset, does not differentiate anaphylactic from anaphylactoid reaction
  - ‣ Serum histamine level; transiently elevated in anaphylaxis, metabolized in blood within 60 minutes of reaction
  - ‣ In vitro serum test (e.g., RAST) to detect IgE antibodies to specific antigen; high specificity, low sensitivity for most drugs
  - ‣ In vivo skin test (prick or intradermal technique) ± patch testing; high predictive value in setting of previous anaphylaxis, done in a monitored setting 4–6 weeks after anaphylactic reaction
  - ‣ It is possible to desensitize patients to achieve temporary tolerance of antigen via incremental increases in antigen exposure

REFERENCES

For references, please visit **www.TheAnesthesiaGuide.com**.

CHAPTER 202
Lung Anatomy for Fiber-Optic Bronchoscopy

Constantin Parizianu, MD and Roopa Kohli-Seth, MD

Approach: nasal/oral (if not intubated) or via ETT/LMA/tracheostomy tube.

Indications: therapeutic/diagnostic/intubation aid.

The airways follow a branching tree pattern of approximately 23 generations from the trachea to the alveolar sacs. Only four to five can be visualized via bronchoscopy.

Segmentation of the Lungs			
Right lung		Left lung	
Lobes (3)	Segments (10)	Lobes (2)	Segments (8)
Upper lobe	Apical	Upper lobe	Apicoposterior
	Posterior		
	Anterior		Anterior
Middle lobe	Medial		Superior lingula
	Lateral		Inferior lingula
Lower lobe	Superior	Lower lobe	Superior
	Medial basal		Anteromedial basal
	Anterior basal		
	Lateral basal		Lateral basal
	Posterior basal		Posterior basal

The lingula on the left corresponds to the right middle lobe. There are multiple variations, especially within the basal segments.

FIGURE 202-1. Upside-down schematic of the tracheobronchial tree

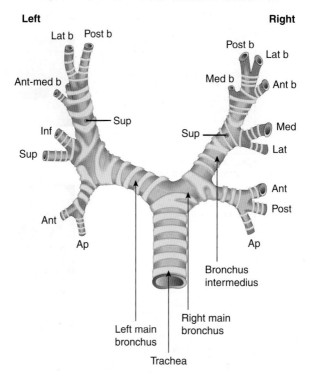

Bronchoscopic View of the Tracheobronchial Tree

Trachea	From the inferior margin of the cricoid cartilage to the main carina Dimensions: length–newborns ~5.7 cm; adults ~11 cm for males and 10 cm for females Diameter–newborns ~4–5 mm; adults ~2.5 cm Anterior wall (cartilaginous)–18–24 incomplete cartilaginous rings, open posteriorly Posterior wall (membranous)–trachealis muscle	Figure 202-2 Anterior rings Posterior wall
Main carina	Sharp anteroposterior cartilaginous ridge at the bifurcation of the trachea	Figure 202-3 Carina Left main bronchus Right main bronchus
Right mainstem bronchus	Short, approximately 2 cm, runs more vertically than the left mainstem bronchus, it diverges at a 25–30° angle from midline A foreign body will most likely enter here	
Right upper lobe	The first branch off the lateral side of the right mainstem bronchus It quickly trifurcates into three segments: apical, anterior, and posterior	Figure 202-4 Apical segment Anterior segment Posterior segment
Bronchus intermedius	The distal continuation of the right mainstem bronchus past the origin of the RUL It runs for 2 cm and it bifurcates into the RML and RLL	Figure 202-5 Right middle lobe Right lower lobe basilar segments Right lower lobe superior segment

(continued)

Bronchoscopic View of the Tracheobronchial Tree (*continued*)

Right middle lobe	It originates from the anterior and medial wall of the distal bronchus intermedius It further bifurcates into the middle and lateral segments	Figure 202-6 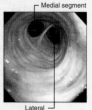
Right lower lobe	Its superior segment takes off from the distal bronchus intermedius, on the posterior aspect, opposite from the origin of the RML Descending past the superior segment, you will encounter the four basilar segments. First the medial basal segment (medial origin), and the other three segments on the lateral side in the A–L–P order: anterior, lateral, and posterior basal	Figure 202-7 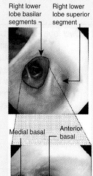
Left mainstem bronchus	Diverges at a 45° angle from the midline It is longer (4–5 cm) and narrower than the right mainstem bronchus Distally, there is the left mainstem carina, which marks the bifurcation into the LUL and LLL	Figure 202-8 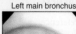 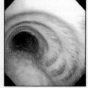 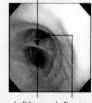

Bronchoscopic View of the Tracheobronchial Tree *(continued)*		
Left upper lobe	Appears superior to the left mainstem carina It further subdivides into the lingular division and superior division The lingular division (medial takeoff) further divides into the superior and inferior lingular segments The superior division divides into the apicoposterior and anterior segment	Figure 202-9
Left lower lobe	It starts inferior and posterior to the left mainstem carina The superior segment takes off first from the posterior wall Below this point, the LLL divides into the three basal segments: anteromedial, lateral, and posterior basal	Figure 202-10

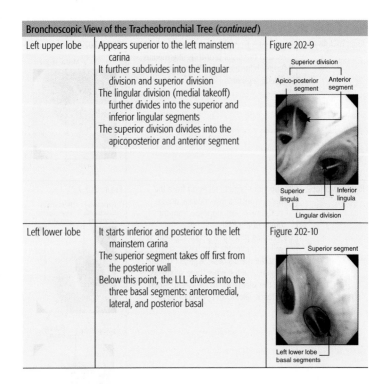

Pointers: the easiest navigation is with the operator standing at the head of the patient, and the patient supine. Use the tracheal rings to orient yourself; keep the rings at 12 o'clock, anteriorly. Keep the bronchoscope in the middle of the airway. Every time you are not sure of your location, return to the carina.

REFERENCES

For references, please visit **www.TheAnesthesiaGuide.com**.

CHAPTER 203
ICU Ventilator Modes

Constantin Parizianu, MD and Roopa Kohli-Seth, MD

BASIC SETTINGS

Tidal volume (V_T)	Initially choose 8–10 mL/kg IBW Avoid high volumes to prevent barotrauma $\uparrow V_T = \uparrow$ MV and $\downarrow$ Paco$_2$ and $\uparrow$ pH If ARDS/ALI is present, use 6 mL/kg IBW
Respiratory rate (RR)	12–14 breaths/min usually adequate $\uparrow$ RR = $\uparrow$ MV and $\downarrow$ Paco$_2$ and $\uparrow$ pH, but beyond a certain point, dead space ventilation and risk of breath stacking
Fraction of inspired oxygen (FiO$_2$)	Start at 1.0 and taper down quickly to achieve a goal Pao$_2$ of >60 mm Hg and O$_2$ saturation of >90%
Inspiratory flow	Usually 40–60 L/min $\uparrow$ Flow = $\downarrow$ inspiratory time and $\uparrow$ expiratory time, thus $\downarrow$ I:E ratio Useful in obstructive airways disease to decrease auto-PEEP, be careful though about the increase in peak airway pressure
Positive end-expiratory pressure (PEEP)	Typically set at 5 cm H$_2$O $\uparrow$ PEEP (up to 20–24 cm H$_2$O) = $\uparrow$ oxygenation in ALI/ARDS May lead to decreased venous return/hypotension, increased plateau pressure/barotrauma, may increase ICP (in theory)

IBW, ideal body weight; ARDS, acute respiratory distress syndrome; ALI, acute lung injury; I:E ratio, inspiratory to expiratory ratio; ICP, intracranial pressure.

INSPIRATORY PHASE VARIABLES

- Trigger: What signals the ventilator to initiate the inspiration?
  - Time or patient effort (pressure or flow)
- Target (limit): What limits/governs the airflow during inspiration?
  - Pressure or flow or volume (not time)
- Termination (cycle): What signals the ventilator to stop the inspiration?
  - Time or pressure or flow or volume

TYPES OF BREATHS

- Mandatory—The machine triggers and/or cycles the breath
- Spontaneous—Patient triggered and cycled (the patient determines the V_T); may be assisted or unassisted
- Assisted—The patient triggers the spontaneous breath and the machine does at least some of the work. The airway pressure rises above the baseline pressure (e.g., pressure support ventilation)

Types of Breaths					
	Volume control	Volume assist	Pressure control	Pressure assist	Pressure support
Trigger	Time	Patient	Time	Patient	Patient
Target (limit)	Flow	Flow	Pressure	Pressure	Pressure
Termination (cycle)	Volume	Volume	Time	Time	Flow

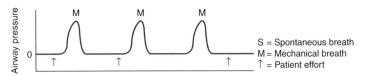

Modes: CMV   AC/VC   SIMV   APRV   CA/PC   PSV

- Volume-cycled ventilation:
  ‣ *Controlled mechanical ventilation (CMV)*—rarely used nowadays in the ICU
    Time triggered, preset RR and V_T, the patient cannot trigger any extra breaths
    The patient should be heavily sedated/paralyzed
  ‣ *Assist control/volume control (AC/VC)*—most common mode

FIGURE 203-1. Controlled mechanical ventilation

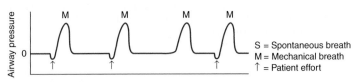

Reproduced from Morgan GE, Mikhail MS, Murray MJ. *Clinical Anesthesiology*. 4th ed. Figure 49-1.
Available at www.accessmedicine.com.

Time and patient triggered, preset RR and V_T. Patients can trigger additional set tidal volumes; they do not necessarily need to be sedated or paralyzed. Beware of hyperventilation and respiratory alkalosis.

FIGURE 203-2. Assist control/volume control

Reproduced from Morgan GE, Mikhail MS, Murray MJ. *Clinical Anesthesiology*. 4th ed. Figure 49-1.
Available at www.accessmedicine.com.

▸ *Intermittent mandatory ventilation (IMV)/synchronized intermittent mandatory ventilation (SIMV)*—may also be used as a weaning mode (not routinely used today, may actually prolong the weaning process)

IMV: time-triggered mandatory breaths, preset RR and V_T. In between breaths, the patient can take additional spontaneous assisted breaths with a chosen pressure support (the V_T varies with the effort).

May lead to breath stacking (mandatory breath on top of a spontaneous breath).

SIMV: similar to IMV, but the mandatory breaths are machine (time) or patient triggered, providing synchrony with the patient's effort and eliminating breath stacking.

FIGURE 203-3. Intermittent mandatory ventilation (IMV) and synchronized intermittent mandatory ventilation (SIMV)

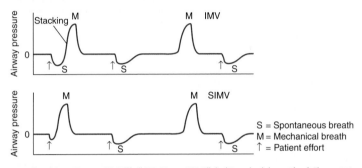

- Flow-cycled ventilation:
  ▸ *Pressure support ventilation (PSV)*—can be used as a weaning mode. The patient should not be too sedated: if the patient is not initiating breaths, the machine would not provide any breaths (actually, all modern machines have apnea alarms that will trigger mandatory machine breaths). Assisted spontaneous breaths are patient triggered, pressure limited, flow cycled
  ▸ No RR or V_T to be set. The pressure support (above PEEP) is set and should overcome the resistance of the ventilator tubing. The higher the pressure support, the lower the work of breathing
  ▸ If the pressure support is set to zero, then this mode becomes continuous positive airway pressure (CPAP), which is a spontaneous unassisted breathing mode with no ventilator cycling

FIGURE 203-4. Pressure support

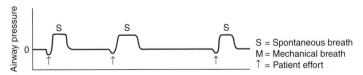

- Time-cycled ventilation:
  - *Assist control/pressure control ventilation (AC/PC)*—aimed at reducing the peak airway pressures. Time/patient triggered, pressure limited, time cycled. Set the inspiratory pressure, RR, inspiratory time, and PEEP. The V_T varies depending on the airway resistance and patient effort. May lead to hypercapnia, which could be "permissive."
  - *Pressure-regulated volume control (PRVC)*—aimed at minimizing the airway/plateau pressure. Somewhat similar to AC/VC; set RR and V_T, but the flow rate is constantly adjusted by the ventilator to deliver the V_T at the lowest possible peak pressure
  - *Airway pressure release ventilation (APRV)*—may be useful in ALI/ARDS

    Alternates a high CPAP for a set longer duration and a low CPAP for a shorter duration (release). Results in an inverse I:E ratio. The pressure gradient and the lung stiffness determine the V_T.

    It is time triggered, pressure limited, time cycled. Spontaneous unassisted breathing is possible at any point, but more often during the high airway pressure interval (because it is longer). Avoid in severe obstructive airways disease. May cause barotraumas.

FIGURE 203-5. Airway pressure release ventilation

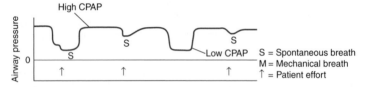

  - *Bilevel* (different from the noninvasive bilevel positive airway pressure [BiPAP])

    Similar to APRV; set RR, high and low airway pressure, but more conventional I:E ratio. Spontaneous breathing may occur at any point, but more often during the lower airway pressure interval.

    Other modes: high-frequency oscillatory ventilation, adaptative support ventilation, mandatory minute ventilation, noninvasive ventilation (CPAP, bilevel positive airway pressure).

REFERENCES

For references, please visit **www.TheAnesthesiaGuide.com**.

CHAPTER 204
ARDS

Yan Lai, MD, MPH and Michael H. Andreae, MD

DEFINITION AND DIAGNOSIS

- Acute onset and progression within *hours*
- *Respiratory*: *N*ot cardiogenic clinically or by echo. PA occlusion pressure (wedge) <18 cm H_2O
- *Distress*: *Decreased oxygenation*:
  - ‣ Pao_2/FiO_2 <200 mm Hg
  - ‣ <300 for ALI regardless of PEEP
- *Syndrome*:
  - ‣ Mortality with current management still 25–50%
  - ‣ Survivors suffer from significant morbidity and reduced quality of life because of respiratory sequelae such as chronic infections and tracheostomy
  - ‣ Pulmonary HTN and RV failure may be present:
    - ▪ Acute RV failure on echo: RV dilation and paradoxical septum motion

COMMON ETIOLOGIES (MORTALITY RATES)

- *Sepsis* (30%)
- Aspiration (36%)
- Trauma (11%)
- TRALI and others (burns and toxic fumes, drug overdose, drowning, acute pancreatitis)

MANAGEMENT

- Treat underlying cause if possible (especially sepsis)
- Sedate as little as possible
- Respiratory management:
  - ‣ *First goal*: Avoid secondary lung injury with hyperinflation:
    - ▪ Low tidal volume ventilation (6 mL/kg IBW):
      - ◆ VC and PCV same efficacy. Watch TV and maintain plateau pressure (Ppl) <30 cm H_2O (add 0.2 second inspiratory pause to measure Ppl)
      - ◆ *Absolute mortality risk reduction from 40% to 31% with NNT = 11*
  - ‣ *Second goal*: Optimize oxygenation and V/Q matching:
    - ▪ Place arterial line and titrate to Pao_2 >60 with incremental PEEP up to 12 first and then increasing FiO_2
  - ‣ *Third goal*: Permissive hypercapnia (accept $Paco_2$ up to 60 mm Hg):
    - ▪ RR up to 30 if needed, but watch auto-PEEP with risk of breath stacking
    - ▪ No indication to $NaHCO_3$ with respiratory acidosis
- Troubleshooting: when the goals are difficult to achieve:
  - ‣ *Recruitment maneuver* to reopen atelectatic areas of lungs:
    - ▪ Set APL valve to 40, squeeze bag to achieve peak airway pressures of 40 cm H_2O, hold for 30 seconds (8–12 seconds probably sufficient), and repeat a few times
    - ▪ May transiently improve oxygenation by opening collapsed alveoli (but also by reducing pulmonary shunt by decreasing cardiac output)
    - ▪ Watch for hypotension (usually brief, due to decrease in venous return) and pneumothorax
    - ▪ Contraindicated if elevated ICP

- *Conservative fluid* strategy (ARDSNet trial in ICU setting):
  - Guided strictly by CVP, PAOP, urine output, MAP, cardiac output, and capillary refill
  - Elaborate treatment algorithm using fluid boluses, KVO fluid, dopamine, or furosemide
  - Conservative strategy improved lung function and shortened mechanical ventilation without increasing nonpulmonary organ failures
- *No proven* mortality benefit but can be considered:
  - *Prone position*: Improves oxygenation, but does not reduce mortality
  - *Steroids*: May shorten course and decrease fibrosis if given <7 days (methylprednisolone 2 mg/kg per day), but may worsen mortality if given >2 weeks into ARDS. Avoid combining with NMB (risk of critical illness myo/neuropathy)
  - *Inhaled nitric oxide*: Improves oxygenation but not survival. May be useful with refractory hypoxemia, severe pulmonary hypertension, or RV failure
  - *Inhaled surfactant/prostaglandins, ECMO* for intractable hypoxemia
  - *Nutritional support*: Avoid hypophosphatemia; reduce CO_2 with increased lipid proportion in diet
  - *PA catheter* not useful

ANESTHETIC MANAGEMENT

- Use pressure-controlled-volume-guaranteed (PCVG) mode if available to optimize V_t to 6–8 mL/kg IBW while limiting P_{aw} to 40 cm Hg and $P_{plateau}$ to 30 cm Hg with paralysis. Otherwise, use PCV mode. Consider using ICU ventilator + TIVA
- Start with PEEP of 10 cm H_2O, but watch for hypotension from reduced venous return secondary to increased intrathoracic pressure
- Start with FIO_2 100% and titrate down to maintain Pao_2 >60
- Frequent recruitment maneuvers if Pao_2 <60
- Permissive hypercapnia to $Paco_2$ <60. Increase RR if $Paco_2$ >60
- Restrict fluids (<10 mL/kg/h) and transfusion (<5 U PRBC or FFP) as clinically tolerated
- Maintain minimal anesthetic depth as tolerated
- Watch PAP and CVP; consider TEE to evaluate for pulmonary hypertension and RV failure. Treat with vasopressors, diuresis, inhaled NO
- Watch for signs of pneumothorax

REFERENCES

For references, please visit **www.TheAnesthesiaGuide.com**.

CHAPTER 205
Status Asthmaticus

Awais Sheikh, MD and Roopa Kohli-Seth, MD

Medical emergency when bronchospasm is refractory to bronchodilator and steroids in the ED.

HISTORY

High-risk predictors:
- Previous severe exacerbation (e.g., intubation or ICU admission for asthma)
- Two or more hospitalizations for asthma in the past year
- Three or more ED visits for asthma in the past year

TABLE 205-1	Special Considerations for Anesthesia
Emergent surgery	Aggressive O_2, beta-2-agonist, IV steroid therapy
Preoperative	Sedate with benzodiazepines Anticholinergic only if profuse secretions or using ketamine Avoid H_2 antagonist due to unopposed H_1-triggered bronchospasm
Induction	Propofol and ketamine are bronchodilators Sevoflurane is the most potent bronchodilator among volatile agents (but clinical significance unclear) Avoid atracurium, mivacurium, morphine, meperidine (histamine release)
Intraoperative	Bronchospasm due to intubation, high spinal, pain, surgical stimulus Assess: wheezes, high peak pressure, low exhaled V_T, rising E_TCO_2 Treatment: • Deepen anesthesia: IV propofol, increase volatile agent concentration • Rule out other causes: tube kinking, secretions, bronchial intubation, pulmonary edema, embolism, or pneumothorax • Beta-2-agonist MDI in the inspiratory limb of the breathing circuit • IV steroids
Postoperative	Anticholinergic agent prevents bronchospasm before anticholinesterase Deep extubation (consider Bailey maneuver [replacement of ETT by LMA in patient under GA breathing spontaneously] if no risk of regurgitation) and lidocaine IV 1–2 mg/kg to prevent bronchospasm on emergence

- Hospitalization or ED visit for asthma in the past month
- Using >2 canisters of short-acting beta-2-agonist per month
- Attack while under systemic steroids, or recent discontinuation of steroids
- Difficulty perceiving asthma symptoms or severity of exacerbations, noncompliance

PHYSICAL

Signs of severity:
- Cyanosis, profuse sweating, mental status changes
- Bradycardia, hypotension, pulsus paradoxus >15 mm Hg
- Accessory muscle use, silent chest, difficulty speaking, inability to lie down
- Peak expiratory flow rate (PEFR) <200 L/min and/or <40% predicted/usual value
- FEV1 <40% of predicted is an ominous sign in an adult
- Room air SpO_2 <92%, PaO_2 <60 mm Hg, $Paco_2$ >45 mm Hg

TREATMENT

See Table 205-2 for drug dosages.
- Oxygen: keep SaO_2 ≥92% (>95% in pregnancy)
- Inhaled nebulized beta-2-agonist: albuterol
- Inhaled nebulized anticholinergic agent: ipratropium bromide, along with albuterol
- Steroids: methylprednisolone, dexamethasone, or hydrocortisone, IV, IM, or even PO:
  ‣ Give steroids early as peak action delayed by 3–4 hours
- Monitor K; replete as needed: both beta-agonists and steroids cause hypokalemia
- If high-risk predictors, signs of severity, no improvement after first treatment, transfer to ICU
- Magnesium sulfate IV if no resolution after 1 hour of continuous nebulization and steroids, or as first line if signs of severity
- Terbutaline or epinephrine (never both) after 1 hour of nebulization and steroids
- Heliox-driven albuterol nebulization after 1 hour of continuous nebulization and steroids. It decreases work of breathing and improve ventilation (but may lower O_2)
- Ketamine is sometimes helpful when everything else fails before intubation

TABLE 205-2 Drugs Used in Status Asthmaticus

Class	Drug	Dose
Inhaled beta-2-agonist	Albuterol	Intermittent nebulization: 2.5–5 mg q20 min × 3, and then 2.5–10 mg q1–4 h prn 4–8 puffs q20 min up to 4 h, and then q1–4 h prn Continuous nebulization: for persistent symptoms, 10–15 mg/h
Anticholinergic agent	Ipratropium bromide	500 µg q20 min × 3, and then prn or 4 MDI puffs q20 min up to 3 h
Corticosteroid	Methylprednisolone	IV 40–80 mg q6–24 h
	Dexamethasone	IV 6–10 mg q6–24 h
	Hydrocortisone	IV 150–200 mg q6–24 h
Calcium influx inhibitor	Magnesium sulfate	IV 2 g × 1 over 10 min
Systemic beta-2-agonists	Epinephrine 1:1,000 (1 mg/mL)	0.3–0.5 mg sq q20 min × 3 100 µg IV if hemodynamic collapse
	Terbutaline (1 mg/mL)	0.25 mg sq q20 min × 3
General anesthetic	Ketamine	IV bolus 0.5–1 mg/kg over 2 min, followed by infusion of 0.5–2 mg/kg/h

- Intubate with rapid sequence if:
  - Lethargic
  - Unable to maintain airway
  - Slow respiratory rate
  - Pco_2 normal or high
- If intubated:
  - V_t 5–7 mL/kg, RR 6–8/min, I:E 1:3 or 1:4 (avoid breath stacking)
  - Maintain PAP <40 cm H_2O and Ppl<20 cm H_2O
  - Permissive hypercapnia
  - FiO_2 for SpO_2 ≥94%
  - Deep sedation; avoid NMB, especially if steroids administered (risk of myoneuropathy)
  - In extreme cases, administer volatile agent (sevoflurane) in ICU

NO ROLE FOR THE FOLLOWING AGENTS

Intravenous beta 2-agonists, methylxanthines, antibiotics (unless documented infection), aggressive hydration, chest physical therapy, mucolytics, sedation (unless intubated).

REFERENCES

For references, please visit **www.TheAnesthesiaGuide.com**.

CHAPTER 206
Pulmonary Embolism

Arif M. Shaik, MD and Adel Bassily-Marcus, MD, FCCP, FCCM

INTRODUCTION

- *Lower extremities DVT found in 70% of patients with PE*
- *PE is life-threatening in critically ill patients with a 30% mortality rate*

DIAGNOSIS

A. Clinical assessment

Modified Geneva Score	
Factor	Points
Age ≥65	1
Surgery/fracture within 1 month	2
Active malignancy	2
Hemoptysis	2
Previous DVT or PE	3
Unilateral lower limb pain	3
HR 75–94	3
HR ≥95	5
Pain on deep palpation of lower limb, unilateral edema	4

Probability of PE:
- 0–3 points: low probability (8%)
- 4–10 points: intermediate probability (28%)
- ≥11 points: high probability (74%)

- *High index of suspicion*: Any patient with immobilization with above symptoms should be evaluated
- Intraoperative or postoperative: long bone fracture repair with unexplained symptoms should be evaluated for fat emboli
- Complicated vaginal or Cesarean delivery patients evaluated for amniotic fluid embolization

B. Diagnostic tests

- EKG: classic signs of *right heart strain* demonstrated by an *S1–Q3–T3* pattern (Figure 206-1) are observed in *only 20% of patients* with proven PE
- Arterial blood gas shows slight alkalosis and *raised alveolar–arterial oxygen gradient*
- Increased cardiac markers (BNP, troponin T and I): suggest RV strain; perform echo; discuss thrombolysis

FIGURE 206-1. Classic EKG pattern in PE

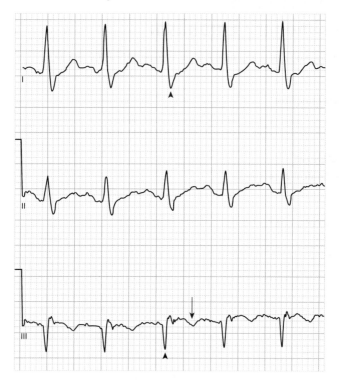

S wave is apparent in lead I (blue arrowhead), Q wave in lead III (black arrowhead), and inverted T wave in lead III (blue arrow). Reproduced from Knoop KJ, Stack LB, Storrow AB, Thurman RJ. *The Atlas of Emergency Medicine*. 3rd ed. Figure 23-47B. Available at: http://www.accessmedicine.com. Copyright © The McGraw-Hill Companies, Inc. All rights reserved.

C. Imaging

- *Chest x-ray*: usually *normal* in PE, occasional atelectasis, consolidation, and elevated hemidiaphragm with lung infarcts seen
- *CT angiography* (CTA) is the initial imaging modality of choice for stable patients, *sensitivity 96–100%, specificity 89–98%*
- *Ventilation–perfusion (V/Q) scans* should be used only when CT is not available or if the patient has a contraindication to intravenous contrast; only useful if normal chest x-ray. Preferable if pregnancy (controversial)
- *Lower extremities Doppler ultrasound* to rule out DVT
- *Echocardiography*: may demonstrate right ventricular dysfunction in acute PE, predicting a higher mortality and possible benefit from thrombolytic therapy. TEE can visualize large thrombus in pulmonary artery

FIGURE 206-2. Algorithm if clinical suspicion of PE

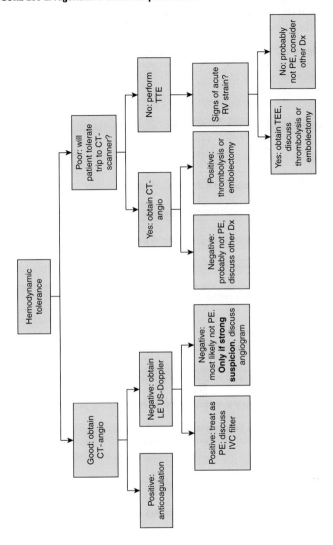

TREATMENT

A. Initial (O$_2$, vasopressors if needed)

- Anticoagulation (AC) reduces mortality and is considered a primary therapy for PE:
  - *Empiric AC is considered if index of suspicion is high and no contraindication, IV heparin, SC LMWH, or SC fondaparinux can be started before diagnosis is confirmed*

"Standard" Dosing of Anticoagulants for PE		
IV heparin	80 U/kg bolus, and then 18 U/kg infusion Titrate for PTT between 60 and 80 s	Prefer in unstable patients as short duration of action
Enoxaparin (Lovenox®)	1.5 mg/kg SC daily	
Tinzaparin (Innohep®)	175 IU/kg SC daily	
Fondaparinux (Arixtra®)	5/7.5/10 mg SC daily	
Rivaroxaban (Xarelto®)	15 mg PO BID or TID × 3 weeks, followed by 20 mg PO q day	Not FDA approved

- AC reduces the mortality rate of PE because it *slows or prevents clot progression* and *reduces the risk of further embolism*
  - Prompt effective AC has been shown to *reduce the overall mortality rate from 30% to less than 10%*
  - *Absolute contraindications to AC*:
    - *Recent intracerebral bleed (<3 weeks)*
    - *Recent GI bleed (<2 weeks)*
    - *HIT* (treat with direct thrombin inhibitors)
- The decision to use *fibrinolytic therapy* depends on severity of the PE, prognosis, and risk of bleeding:
  - Thrombolytic therapy is recommended for two groups of patients:
    - *Hemodynamic instability*
    - *Right heart strain/failure on echo*
  - Typically tPA 100 mg infusion over 2 hours, or 0.6 mg/kg (maximum 50 mg) over 15 minutes
  - Contraindications to tPA:
    - Absolute:
      - History of hemorrhagic stroke
      - Active intracranial neoplasm
      - Recent (<2 months) intracranial surgery or trauma
      - Active internal bleeding
    - Relative:
      - Bleeding diathesis
      - Recent serious gastrointestinal bleeding
      - Uncontrolled severe HTN (SBP >200 mm Hg or DBP >110 mm Hg)
      - Nonhemorrhagic stroke within prior 2 months
      - Surgery within the previous 10 days
      - Thrombocytopenia (<100,000 platelets/mm^3)
- Catheter clot fragmentation and aspiration:
  - Specialized center, same indications as thrombolysis
- Surgical embolectomy: last resort, high mortality
- IVC filter is an option if AC is contraindicated, for example, fall risk or active bleeding

B. Long term

- *Warfarin* can be started after 1 day on IV or SC therapeutic AC:
  - ▸ Continue heparin for the first 5–7 days of warfarin therapy, regardless of INR, to allow time for depletion of procoagulant vitamin K–dependent proteins
  - ▸ Six months of AC reduces rate of recurrence by 50% compared with 6 weeks
  - ▸ Long-term AC indicated for patients with a permanent underlying risk factor and recurrent DVT or recurrent PE
  - ▸ Duration of treatment differs with different situations:
    - ▪ Upper extremity DVT: AC for ≥3 months
    - ▪ *Lower extremity DVT and PE*

Long-Term Anticoagulation Following DVT and PE		
Cause	Duration of treatment	Further considerations
Reversible cause for DVT	3 months	
First isolated distal DVT–no triggering factor	3 months	
First DVT and/or PE–no triggering factor	3 months	Evaluate at the end of treatment risk–benefit ratio for long-term therapy
First DVT–proximal or PE–no triggering factor	Long term	Long term recommended if no bleeding risk and good anticoagulation monitoring is achievable
Second DVT and/or PE–no triggering factors	Long term	
DVT and/or PE with cancer	LMWH for first 3–6 months of long term	Continue until cancer in remission

- In *pregnant patients*, once diagnosis is confirmed, start SC LMWH or IV heparin:
  - ▸ SC LMWH should be stopped 24–36 hours prior to delivery and restarted 12 hours after C-section and 6 hours after vaginal delivery if no bleeding concern
- In geriatric patients, exercise caution using SC LMWH as it is renally cleared; adjust dosing according to creatinine clearance

REFERENCES

For references, please visit **www.TheAnesthesiaGuide.com**.

CHAPTER 207
Acid–Base Abnormalities

Aditya Uppalapati, MD, Sumit Kapoor, MD, and Roopa Kohli-Seth, MD

Three essential questions to answer in a critically ill patient with acid–base disorder:
• What disorder does the patient have?
• How severe is the disorder?
• What is the underlying etiology?

Basic Terminology and Normal Values	
Alkalemia	Arterial pH >7.45
Acidemia	Arterial pH <7.35
Alkalosis	Abnormal process or condition that lowers arterial pH
Acidosis	Abnormal process or condition that raises arterial pH
pH	7.35–7.45
$Paco_2$	40 mm Hg (35–45)
Pao_2	100 mm Hg
HCO_3	24 mEq/L (22–26)
Anion gap $(Na - [Cl + HCO_3])$	8–12
Albumin	4 mg/dL

Major Consequences		
Organ system	Acidemia	Alkalemia
Cardiovascular	Impairment of cardiac contractility Arteriolar dilatation Hypotension Attenuation of cardiovascular responsiveness to catecholamines Increased sensitivity and decreased threshold for arrhythmias Increased pulmonary vascular resistance	Arteriolar constriction Reduction in coronary blood flow Decreased threshold for arrhythmias
Respiratory	Hyperventilation Decreased strength of respiratory muscles and promotion of muscle fatigue Respiratory failure	Hypoventilation Hypercapnia and hypoxemia
Metabolic	Inhibition of anaerobic glycolysis Hyperkalemia Insulin resistance Reduction in ATP synthesis	Stimulation of anaerobic glycolysis Hypokalemia Decreased ionized calcium Hypomagnesemia Hypophosphatemia
Cerebral	Inhibition of metabolism and cell volume Regulation, altered mental status	Reduction in cerebral blood flow Seizures Altered mental status Tetany

EVALUATING ACID–BASE ABNORMALITIES

Knowing the clinical scenario is important for a correct interpretation of acid–base abnormalities.

There are two main approaches.
- *Henderson–Hasselbalch approach (traditional approach)*—relates pH to P_{CO_2} and HCO_3:

$$pH = 6.1 + \log \left[\frac{HCO_3}{0.03} \times P_{CO_2} \right]$$

Does not take into account changes in non-bicarbonate buffers such as phosphate, albumin, etc.
- *Stewart approach (physicochemical or quantitative approach)*—the Stewart approach takes into account the other components of the extracellular fluid. It is mostly useful in critically ill patients:
  - Strong ions are completely dissociated at physiologic pH:
    - The strong ion difference (SID) = (Na + K + Ca + Mg) − (Cl − other strong anions) = 40–44 mEq/L
  - SID is balanced by an equivalent amount of "buffer base," mostly HCO_3, albumin, and phosphate:
    - Albumin and phosphate are weak acids and are measured as A_{TOT}
    - While usually not significant, they can affect the acid–base balance in critically ill patients:
      - Hypoalbuminemia results from malnutrition, hepatic failure, and/or hemodilution
      - Hypophosphatemia can result from malnutrition, refeeding, and hemodilution
        - *Hypoalbuminemia and hypophosphatemia will result in metabolic alkalosis*
      - *Hyperphosphatemia* occurs from renal failure and *will worsen metabolic acidosis*
  - The major source of acid in the body is CO_2. Most of the H+ produced by the dissociation of H_2CO_3 (CO_2 binding to water) is buffered by hemoglobin
  - Two principles apply:
    - Electrical neutrality: all positively charges = all negatively charges
    - Mass conservation, taking into account strong ions, buffer bases, and P_{CO_2}

GENERAL APPROACH TO ACID–BASE DISORDERS EVALUATION (HENDERSON–HASSELBALCH)

Five steps (see Figure 207-1):
1. Determine arterial pH (acidemia or alkalemia)
2. Identify the primary acid–base abnormality (metabolic/respiratory)

FIGURE 207-1. Algorithm for evaluating acid–base disorders (steps 1 and 2)

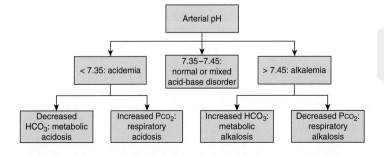

3. If respiratory disturbance, is it acute or chronic?
4. Ensure that actual compensation matches calculated compensation, and that measured base excess (BE) matches calculated BE
5. Determine etiology:
   - If metabolic acidosis present, calculate anion gap (AG)
   - If AG metabolic acidosis, calculate corrected bicarbonate to determine if there is a triple disorder
   - If metabolic alkalosis, measure urine chloride

Step 3: clinical context determines whether respiratory disturbance is acute or chronic.

Step 4: compensation for acid–base abnormalities.

Acid-Base Disorders		
Disorder	Primary abnormality	Compensation (usually incomplete)
Metabolic acidosis	Increased H^+	Expected $Pco_2 = 1.5 \times HCO_3 + (8 \pm 2)$ (Winters formula)
Metabolic alkalosis	Increased HCO_3	Expected $Pco_2 = 0.7 \times HCO_3 + (20 \pm 5)$
Respiratory acidosis (acute)	Increased CO_2	For every 10 increase in Pco_2 above 40, HCO_3 increases by 1 mEq/L pH change by $0.008 \times (Pco_2 - 40)$
Respiratory acidosis (chronic)	Increased CO_2	For every 10 increase in Pco_2 above 40, HCO_3 increases by 3.5 mEq/L pH change by $0.003 \times (Pco_2 - 40)$
Respiratory alkalosis (acute)	Decreased CO_2	For every 10 decrease in Pco_2 below 40, HCO_3 decreases by 2 mEq/L pH change by $0.008 \times (40 - Pco_2)$
Respiratory alkalosis (chronic)	Decreased CO_2	For every 10 decrease in Pco_2 below 40, HCO_3 decreases by 5 mEq/L pH change by $0.003 \times (40 - Pco_2)$

Compare measured and predicted values to evaluate for mixed disorders. If, for example, a patient with metabolic acidosis has a measured pH that is higher than calculated, there is a superimposed respiratory alkalosis.

Base excess (BE) is defined as the number of milliequivalents of acid or base that would be needed to titrate 1 L of blood to pH 7.40 at 38°C while the Pco_2 is held constant at 40 mm Hg. Standardized base excess (SBE) uses serum instead of whole blood to eliminate hemoglobin as a buffer.

Base Excess for Various Acid–Base Disorders	
Disorder	Standard base excess (SBE)
Metabolic acidosis	≤−5 (change in P_{CO_2} = change in SBE)
Metabolic alkalosis	≥+5 (change in P_{CO_2} = 0.6 × change in SBE)
Respiratory acidosis (acute)	0
Respiratory acidosis (chronic)	0.4 × (P_{CO_2} − 40)
Respiratory alkalosis (acute)	0
Respiratory alkalosis (chronic)	0.4 × (P_{CO_2} − 40)

Step 5: etiologies of acid–base abnormalities.

Etiologies of Acid-Base Abnormalities	
Metabolic acidosis	Anion gap: MUDPILES—*m*ethanol, *u*remia (renal failure), *d*iabetic ketoacidosis, *p*araldehyde, *i*sopropyl alcohol, *l*actic acidosis (sepsis, ischemia, hypoperfusion, shock, drugs [propofol, linezolid, metformin]), *e*thanol, *s*alicylates, starvation ketoacidosis Non-anion gap: excessive normal saline resuscitation, gastrointestinal (diarrhea or other intestinal losses [ileostomy]), renal (renal tubular acidosis, carbonic anhydrase inhibitors)
Metabolic alkalosis	GI: gastric suction, vomiting Renal: contraction alkalosis, loop and thiazide diuretics, primary mineralocorticoid excess, alkali administration
Respiratory acidosis	Alveolar hypoventilation: obesity, COPD, severe asthma, pneumothorax, laryngospasm, flail chest, CNS lesions, drugs (sedatives, analgesics), malignant hyperthermia, thyroid storm, burns, excessive caloric intake
Respiratory alkalosis	Pain, anxiety, ischemia, stroke, sepsis, fever, CHF, pulmonary edema, drugs (progesterone, salicylates)

FIGURE 207-2. Evaluation of metabolic acidosis (steps 5a and b)

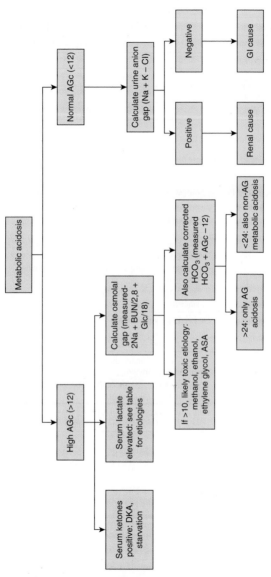

AG, anion gap; $AG = Na - [Cl + HCO_3]$. AGc, corrected anion gap; $AGc = AG + 2.5 \times (4.4 - [albumin\ in\ g/dL])$. Also look at phosphate levels. If the corrected HCO_3 is less than normal (<22 mEq/L), then there is an additional metabolic acidosis present. Corrected HCO_3 values over 26 mEq/L reflect a coexisting metabolic alkalosis (i.e., "triple disorder" with metabolic acidosis, compensatory respiratory alkalosis, and coexisting metabolic alkalosis or non-AG metabolic acidosis).

Step 5c: evaluation of metabolic alkalosis.

Evaluation of Metabolic Alkalosis	
Chloride sensitive (urine Cl <20 mEq/L)	Chloride resistant (urine Cl >40 mEq/L)
GI acid loss: NG suction, vomiting, rectal adenoma, congenital Cl losses in stool	Hypertensive: renovascular hypertension, hyperaldosteronism, Liddle syndrome, licorice ingestion
Renal acid loss: postdiuretic, posthypercapnic, citrate, penicillins	Normotensive: diuretics, Bartter and Gitelman syndromes, administration of alkali

TREATMENT

Metabolic acidosis:
- Treatment focused on reversing the pathogenesis of endogenous acid production and eliminating the excess acid
- Identify the source of the acidosis
- Diabetic ketoacidosis: IV regular insulin and IV fluids (see chapter 210)
- Lactic acidosis due to shock—treat shock state (septic, circulatory)
- Metformin-related lactic acidosis: associated with renal failure; initiate early renal replacement therapy (eliminate metformin and replace renal function)
- Alkalinization using bicarbonate:
  ‣ Almost *no indication* except:
    ▪ Associated life-threatening disorder (e.g., hyperkalemia)
    ▪ To facilitate toxic removal (e.g., alkaline diuresis in salicylate intoxication)
    ▪ In cases of renal or GI bicarbonate loss (non-AG metabolic acidosis, oral citrate solutions also used for chronic therapy of non-AG acidosis)
  ‣ Especially NOT indicated if lactic acidosis secondary to shock: no benefit

Metabolic alkalosis:
- If possible, stop alkali administration, d/c diuretics; stop NGT suction
- Correct hypokalemia, hypercalcemia, hypovolemia
- Chloride-sensitive metabolic alkalosis responds to replacement of chloride deficit with normal saline. Potassium chloride can be used when hypokalemia also present
- In severe, symptomatic metabolic alkalosis, pH >7.6, hemodialysis may be indicated
- *No indication for acid administration* (ammonium chloride, chlorhydric acid); acetazolamide occasionally to reduce bicarbonate in chronic respiratory insufficiency

Respiratory acidosis:
- Treat underlying disorder
- Supplemental O_2 if hypoxemia also present
- Increase effective alveolar ventilation through either reversal of the underlying cause or, if required, mechanical ventilation
- Decrease Pco_2 gradually in chronic respiratory acidosis as rapid correction of Pco_2 may cause severe alkalemia

Respiratory alkalosis:
- Treat underlying disorder
- In psychogenic hyperventilation, rebreathing air into a bag increases the Pco_2

REFERENCES

For references, please visit **www.TheAnesthesiaGuide.com**.

CHAPTER 208
Continuous Renal Replacement Therapy

Krunal Patel, MD and Roopa Kohli-Seth, MD

BASICS

- Continuous renal replacement therapy (CRRT) permits fluid and solute removal with greater hemodynamic stability than intermittent hemodialysis
- Two principles underlie CRRT:
  - ▸ Diffusion: net movement of solute across semipermeable membrane from high concentrated compartment to low concentrated compartment. Dialysis is a diffusive process
  - ▸ Convection: movement of solute across semipermeable membrane due to transmembrane pressure gradient (also known as solvent drag). Hemofiltration is a convective process

INDICATIONS

- Fluid overload
- Refractory hyperkalemia
- Severe acidosis
- Uremic symptoms
- Heart failure

ADVANTAGES OF CRRT OVER REGULAR HEMODIALYSIS

- More effective for fluid removal in hemodynamically unstable patient
- Corrects abnormalities as they evolve, so better control of uremia, electrolyte, and acid–base balance
- Facilitates administration of parental nutrition and obligatory intravenous medication as well as allowing continuous ultrafiltration
- Less effect on intracranial pressure

Four Main Types of CRRT (See Figure 208-1)		
1	Slow continuous ultrafiltration (SCUF)	• No dialysate and replacement fluid required • Large fluid removal via ultrafiltration
2	Continuous venovenous hemofiltration (CVVH)	• Solute removed by convection • Dialysis solution is not used; instead a large volume of replacement fluid is infused either inflow or outflow of bloodline
3	Continuous venovenous hemodialysis (CVVHD)	• Solute removed by diffusion • Dialysis solution is passed through the dialysate compartment of filter in opposite direction of blood flow
4	Continuous venovenous hemodiafiltration (CVVHDF)	• Solute removed by diffusion and convection • Uses dialysate and replacement solution

NB: Arterial access is no longer used because of high complication rate.

FIGURE 208-1. Diagrams of the four main types of renal replacement therapy

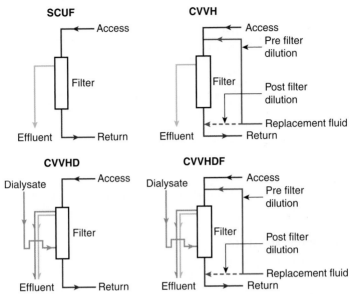

Technical Considerations	
Access	• Right internal jugular vein is preferred over any other central venous access as it is straight to superior vena cava • Femoral and subclavian accesses tend to kink and decrease flow
Replacement fluid	• It is added either prefilter or postfilter of CVVH or CVVHDF circuit • Predilution (adding replacement fluid before filter) is better as it minimizes filter clotting and reduces downtime for CVVH machine • Either lactate- or bicarbonate-buffered CVVH or CVVHDF found equivalent degrees of correction of acidosis at 24 h, but lactate buffer cannot be used in lactic acidosis, hepatic failure, or liver transplant patient • Most commonly used fluids are Plasma-Lyte and 0.45% normal saline with 100 mEq/L of bicarbonate
Anticoagulation	• Filter clotting is most frequent cause of therapy interruption in CRRT • There is no universally accepted anticoagulation • Unfractionated heparin is the most common agent for anticoagulation as it is easy to manage, easy to reverse, and inexpensive. Avoid if HIT • LMWH; not superior to unfractionated heparin • Citrate; avoid in hepatic failure, can cause hypocalcemia and, metabolic alkalosis • Prostacyclin; can cause systemic hypotension • No anticoagulation, for example, in liver transplant patient with high INR

Complications of CRRT	
Access	• Thrombosis • Infection • Bleeding
Circuit-related complication	• Air embolism • Disconnection/hemorrhage • Clotting • Kinking • Membrane hypersensitivity reaction
Therapy-related complication	• Decreased level of calcium, magnesium, and phosphorus • Hypothermia • Overanticoagulation/citrate intoxication.

There is no difference regarding either technical aspects or complications for performing CVVH in the OR. Major indications for CRRT are also the same: refractory electrolyte disturbance, acidosis, and volume overload. A dedicated CRRT nurse must be in the OR for continuous monitoring.

DRUG DOSING ADJUSTMENT

• Drug clearance is highly dependent on the method of renal replacement, filter type, and flow rate. Monitor pharmacologic response, signs of adverse reactions due to drug accumulation, as well as drug levels in relation to target trough (if appropriate)
• Propofol and midazolam do not require adjustment
• Little data exist on opioids and NMB. They are most likely not significantly affected by CRRT. However, effects should be monitored and dosing adjusted as needed
• Adjustment tables for antibiotics are available

REFERENCES

For references, please visit **www.TheAnesthesiaGuide.com**.

CHAPTER 209
Transurethral Resection of the Prostate (TURP) Syndrome

Sonali Mantoo, MD and Roopa Kohli-Seth, MD

BASICS

Transurethral resection of the prostate (TURP) syndrome is the result of complex changes in intravascular volume, solute, and neurophysiologic function.

TURP syndrome has been reported after endoscopic procedures performed under irrigation:
- Transurethral resection of the prostrate and bladder tumors
- Diagnostic cystoscopy
- Percutaneous nephrolithotomy
- Other ureteroscopic procedures
- Endometrial ablation
- Arthroscopy

PATHOPHYSIOLOGY

The acute changes in intravascular volume and plasma solute concentrations occur as a result of irrigation fluid entering the intravascular space through the prostate venous plexus or more slowly absorbed from the retroperitoneal and perivesical spaces.

Risk Factors for TURP and Prevention Measures	
Factors associated with irrigating fluid absorption	**Prevention measures**
• Length of procedure	• Limit duration of surgery to <60 min
• Hypotonic irrigating fluid • Absorption >1 L of glycine solution is associated with an increased risk of symptoms (5–20% of the TURP)	• Use isoosmotic fluids for irrigation • Bipolar TURP is performed using NS as irrigant
• Intravesical pressure >30 mm Hg resulting from high irrigating pressure (governed by the height of the irrigation bag above the prostatic sinuses)	• Limit the position of the irrigation bag to maximum 60 cm above the surgical field to minimize hydrostatic pressure of the fluid (controversial) • Perform TURP under low pressure irrigation (<2 kPa)
• Number of persistently open venous prostate sinuses increases the surface area from where absorption can take place	• Minimize exposure to open venous sinuses by careful surgical resection • Limit extent of bladder distension by frequent drainage of the bladder (to avoid increased absorption through open venous sinuses) • Maintain adequate blood pressure and therefore normal periprostatic venous pressure • Preferably operate on glands <45 g

INCIDENCE

Older studies report incidence between 0.5% and 8% with a mortality of 0.2–0.8%. Newer studies have shown lower incidence rates of 0.78–1.4% with much lower mortality rates

SIGNS AND SYMPTOMS

Syndrome can start from 15 minutes to 24 hours after procedure starts. Indicators of volume gain are:
- Serum sodium dilution
- CVP trending up
- Plasma electrolyte concentrations (lower magnesium and calcium)
- Transthoracic impedance change
- Weight gain

Clinical Manifestations of TURP Syndrome		
Central nervous system	Cardiovascular and respiratory systems	Metabolic and renal systems
• Restlessness	• Hypertension	• Hyponatremia
• Headache	• Tachycardia	• Hyperglycinemia
• Confusion	• Tachypnea	• Intravascular hemolysis
• Convulsions	• Hypoxia	• Acute renal failure
• Coma	• Frank pulmonary edema	
• Visual disturbances	• Hypotension	
• Nausea, vomiting	• Bradycardia	

If 1% ethanol marker is added to irrigation fluids, fluid absorption during TURP can be diagnosed by measuring the ethanol concentration in the patient's breath. This technique is not used routinely.

ANESTHESIA AND TURP

GA and regional anesthesia result in comparable outcomes.

However, spinal anesthesia is the technique of choice:
- May reduce the risk of pulmonary edema
- Decreases blood loss
- Permits early detection of mental status changes
- Reduces CVP, potentially resulting in greater absorption of irrigating fluid

Once TURP syndrome has been detected, the following steps should be undertaken:
- Terminate the procedure
- Insert CVL and A-line
- Assess volume status
- Assess neurological status
- Check electrolyte and pertinent laboratory markers
- Prepare for intubation if necessary
- Start treatment of hyponatremia and related symptoms (see below)

Treatment of TURP Syndrome		
Symptoms	Cause	Treatment
Hyponatremia Hypervolemia Hypertension	• Excess absorption of irrigating fluids during TURP • These are usually the earliest manifestations	• Furosemide • Replete calcium and magnesium • Treat severe hyponatremia (serum sodium <120 mmol/L) with hypertonic 3% saline • Rate of correction of sodium = 0.5 mEq/h • Place patient in reverse Trendelenburg position to limit risk of cerebral edema
Hyperammonemia Encephalopathy	• These occur as a result of glycine administration	• Supportive care • Administer arginine, which acts in the liver, prevents hepatic release of ammonia, accelerating its conversion to urea
Hyperglycinemia Temporary blindness Nausea, vomiting, headache, malaise	• Harmless in plasma, can be fatal in the brain • Glycine inhibits neurotransmitters in the retina, spinal cord, and midbrain	• Consider magnesium for seizures when glycine used during TURP • Vision returns to normal within 24 h (half-life of glycine is 85 min)
Seizures	• Hyponatremia • Hyperglycinemia • Hyperammonemia	• Treat underlying cause, supportive care as needed • Consider magnesium • Correction of electrolytes • Benzodiazepines to abate the acute episode

PEARLS AND TIPS

• Incidence and mortality of TURP syndrome has been decreasing over the last 40 years
• Monitor serum sodium, serum osmolality, and volume status during procedures
• Use isoosmotic fluids for irrigation
• Supportive care is the mainstay of treatment

REFERENCES

For references, please visit **www.TheAnesthesiaGuide.com**.

CHAPTER 210
Diabetic Ketoacidosis

Krunal Patel, MD and Roopa Kohli-Seth, MD

INTRODUCTION

• DKA is defined by a lack of insulin or an excess of hyperglycemic hormones leading to an inability by the tissues to use glucose. This leads to lipolysis and the synthesis of ketoacids that will be used as fuel. Ketoacids will trigger metabolic acidosis and polyuria leading to severe dehydration

- Triggering factors:
  - ▸ Inaugural in DM1 (common, revealing about 10% of DM1) or DM2 (rare)
  - ▸ Noncompliance or iatrogenic (inadequate insulin coverage, steroids, beta-agonists)
  - ▸ Infection or inflammation (e.g., pneumonia, UTI, foot ulcer, abdominal [appendicitis, cholecystitis, pancreatitis, etc.])
  - ▸ MI
  - ▸ Pregnancy
  - ▸ Trauma
- Mortality in DKA is primarily due to the underlying precipitating illness and only rarely due to the metabolic complications of hyperglycemia or ketoacidosis. The prognosis of DKA is substantially worse at the extremes of age and in the presence of coma and hypotension
- DKA can present as severe, pseudosurgical abdominal pain. Accurate diagnosis will prevent unnecessary surgery

PATHOPHYSIOLOGY AND CLINICAL FEATURES (SEE FIGURE 210-1)

FIGURE 210-1. Pathophysiology and clinical features of DKA

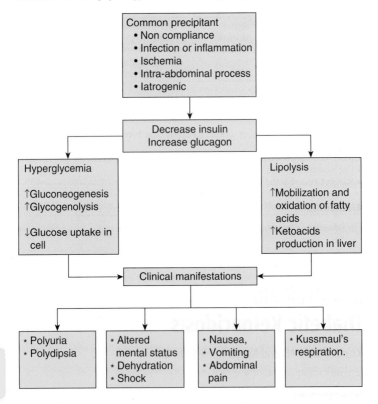

Management of DKA:

Management of Diabetic Keto-Acidosis
Fluids
• Average fluid deficit in DKA is 6 L
• If clinically hypovolemic (hypotension, tachycardia), start with 500–1,500 mL of colloid bolus
• Initial fluid should be NS bolus 10–15 mL/kg
• After that, change to 1/2 NS with 20 mEq/L potassium
• Ongoing intraoperative blood and fluid losses should be replaced as usually
• Once blood sugar dropped to 250 mg/dL and anion gap is still present, fluid can be changed to D5W with 1/2 NS. This will allow insulin administration to reduce ketone without causing hypoglycemia
Insulin
• Regular insulin 10 U IV bolus followed with an infusion at (blood glucose/150) U/h
• If glucose <90, do not stop insulin but rather increase IV glucose administration
• When patient resumes PO alimentation, consider changing to SQ insulin
Electrolytes
• Follow electrolytes closely every 4–6 h (every 2 h at very beginning) until anion gap closed
• Potassium; need usually 10–15 mEq/h for at least first 4 h, irrespective of initial potassium level, for a goal 4–5 mEq/L, as potassium will shift back to intracellular compartment because of insulin, and lead to hypokalemia if uncorrected
• Phosphate goal should be 1–2 mg/dL
• Magnesium goal should be 2 mEq/L
Acidosis
• Typically will correct itself with insulin treatment
• Administer bicarbonate only if pH <7.0 or hemodynamic instability (rare)
Triggering factor
• Diagnose and treat
Other
• Consider thromboprophylaxis depending on risk
• Education to prevent recurrence

REFERENCES

For references, please visit **www.TheAnesthesiaGuide.com**.

CHAPTER 211
Hyperosmolar Hyperglycemic State (HHS)

Zafar A. Jamkhana, MD, MPH and Roopa Kohli-Seth, MD

DEFINITION

Acute medical emergency seen in type 2 DM characterized by:
- Impaired mental status
- Hyperglycemia (plasma glucose >600 mg/dL)
- Hyperosmolality (serum osmolality >320 mOsm/kg)
- Dehydration
- pH >7.30
- HCO_3^- >15 mEq/L
- No ketoacidosis or severe ketosis

Initial presentation of DM in 20% of patients.

Mortality 30–50%.

ETIOLOGY

Precipitating factors are:
- Acute infection 30–40% (pneumonia, UTI, sepsis)
- CVA
- MI
- Acute pancreatitis
- Renal failure
- Thrombosis
- Severe burns
- Hypothermia
- Trauma
- Subdural hematoma
- Endocrine (acromegaly, thyrotoxicosis, Cushing syndrome)
- Drugs (β-blockers, calcium channel blockers, diuretics, steroids, and TPN)

PATHOPHYSIOLOGY (FIGURE 211-1)

Ketone production is minimal as pancreas still retains ability to secrete insulin to prevent fatty acid lipolysis.

CLINICAL FEATURES

- Elderly individual with type 2 DM
- Nausea/vomiting
- Muscle weakness and cramps
- Polyuria, and then oliguria
- Slight hyperthermia common; if >38°C, suspect infection
- Confusion, lethargy, seizures, hemiparesis, and coma

LABORATORY FINDINGS

- Extreme hyperglycemia (>1,000 mg/dL) is sufficient for diagnosis
- Serum osmolality >320 mOsm/kg with higher osmolality leading to worse impairment of mental status. (Osmotic concentration is referred to as *osmolality when expressed in milliosmoles/kilogram of solvent* and as *osmolarity when expressed in milliosmoles/liter of solvent.*)

FIGURE 211-1. Pathophysiology of HHS

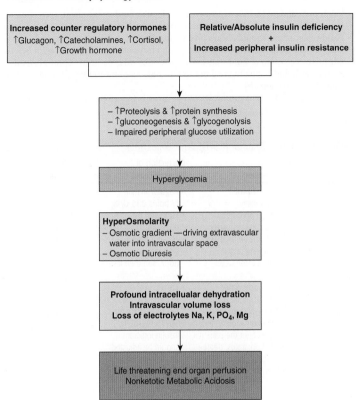

- Effective serum osmolality calculated as:
  - $2(Na^+ + K^+) + (mg/dL\ of\ glucose/18) + (BUN/2.8)$ can give a quick assessment
- Urine ketones are absent, which distinguishes from DKA
- Serum Na^+ concentration is usually normal or elevated because of severe dehydration
- Serum K^+ concentration is initially frequently high and goes down with treatment
- Wide anion gap due to mild metabolic acidosis (multifactorial but HCO_3^- >15 mEq/L)
- Prerenal renal insufficiency

SEVERITY ASSESSMENT

- Overall mortality ranges from 10% to 20%
- Mortality rate increases with age and higher levels of osmolality
- Mortality directly associated with age: 10% in patients <75 years and 35% in patients >75 years
- Degree of dehydration should be assessed with decrease in body weight, tachycardia, oliguria, and hypotension
- A complete neurological assessment with subsequent frequent assessments should be done

MANAGEMENT

- Goals of treatment include aggressive intravascular fluid replacement, correction of hyperglycemia, electrolyte replacement, and supportive care
- Fluid replacement should always precede insulin replacement
- Care should be taken to avoid pitfalls. Insulin infusion should not be begun before adequate correction of fluid status or with K$^+$ <3.5 mEq/dL or hypophosphatemia
- Also care should be maintained not to lower glucose by >100 mg/dL/h for risk of osmotic encephalopathy
- Adequate subcutaneous insulin should be given before stopping insulin infusion

Management of hyperosmolar hyperglycemic state (HHS):

Management of Hyperosmolar Hyperglycemic State (HHS)			
	Fluid replacement	Correction of hyperglycemia	Electrolyte management
Initial management	• NS 15–20 mL/kg/h initially, until BP and organ perfusion normalize • Then, subsequent fluid management should focus on free water replacement • **Total body water deficit may be as high as 100–200 mL/kg**; estimation should take into account the patient's hydration status, degree of hyperglycemia, level of renal function	• **Regular insulin IV bolus 0.15 U/kg** • **Followed by 0.1 U/kg/h** • Monitor **blood glucose every hour**, and then less often once stable • Ideally, goal is to **decrease the blood glucose by 50–75 mg/dL/h**; insulin infusion should be adjusted accordingly with doubling of insulin dose if blood sugar does not fall by 50 mg/dL in first hour	• If serum K$^+$ <3.3 mEq/L, hold insulin and give **40 mEq of K$^+$ (two thirds as KCl and one third as KPO$_4$)**; repeat if needed until K$^+$ is >3.3 mEq/L • If serum K$^+$ is between 3.3 and 5 mEq/L, K can be added as **20–30 mEq in each liter of IV fluid** with a goal to keep serum K$^+$ at 4–5 mEq/L • If serum K$^+$ is ≥5 mEq/L, do not administer K$^+$ and check potassium level every 2–4 h
Transitional management	• Change to **0.45% saline at reduced rate** • Once serum glucose is between 250 and 300 mg/dL, change IV fluid to **5% dextrose with 0.45% saline** • Goal of fluid replacement: **half of the estimated deficit given over 8 h, followed by the other half replaced over 16 h** • **Serum osmolality should not decrease by more than 3 mOsm/kg/h** to minimize the risk of cerebral edema	• Once blood glucose concentration reaches target of <250 mg/dL, decrease insulin infusion rate to **0.05 U/kg/h** and add dextrose to fluid infusion • Follow blood glucose every 4 h and give SC sliding scale insulin accordingly • Once stable, start PO diet; administer long-acting insulin at 0.2–0.3 U/kg or patient's home dose either NPH or glargine insulin	• Check electrolytes frequently (insulin infusion shift K intracellularly, loss through diuresis): possible severe deficit in K, Mg, and PO$_4$ • Phosphate should be adequately replaced if levels are low, before symptoms of cardiac/respiratory dysfunction are seen • Magnesium should be replaced if levels are low

SUPPORTIVE CARE

- High risk of thromboembolism: subcutaneous heparin 5,000 U q8 hours or LMWH
- Treat underlying precipitating cause
- No benefit to prophylactic antibiotic coverage
- Frequent neurological exams should be done in patients who present with neurological symptoms. If seizures are seen at presentation, avoid phenytoin as it inhibits endogenous insulin secretion and is ineffective in HHS

COMPLICATIONS

- Pancreatitis
- Rhabdomyolysis
- Thromboembolism
- Acute gastric dilatation
- Cerebral edema:
  - ▸ Headache, lethargy, and depressed mental status. Very low risk in adults
  - ▸ No single factor identified as predictor of cerebral edema
  - ▸ Currently recommended to lower blood glucose at a rate of 50–75 mg/dL/h and limit fluid replacement to <50 mL/kg in the first 4 hours
  - ▸ Typically treated with hyperventilation, hypertonic saline, mannitol, and ICP monitoring
- Pulmonary edema, ARDS, and hyperchloremic metabolic acidosis can result from overaggressive hydration

REFERENCES

For references, please visit **www.TheAnesthesiaGuide.com**.

CHAPTER 212
Critical Illness–Related Corticosteroid Insufficiency (CIRCI)

Nirav Mistry, MD and Adel Bassily-Marcus, MD, FCCP, FCCM

INTRODUCTION

- Critical illness–related corticosteroid insufficiency (CIRCI) is defined as inadequate corticosteroid activity for the severity of the patient's illness

TABLE 212-1	Etiology, Symptoms, and Diagnosis of Adrenal Insufficiency in Critically Ill Patients

- Etiology
  - Structural damage to adrenals
  - Drugs
  - Primary and secondary etiologies
  - Reversible hypothalamic–pituitary–adrenal dysfunction
- Clinical manifestations
  - Primarily results in shock refractory to fluids and vasopressors
  - Consider in patients with progressive ALI/ARDS
  - Possible eosinophilia and hypoglycemia
  - Uncommonly–hyponatremia and hyperkalemia
- Diagnosis
  - ACTH stimulation test no longer recommended
  - Random cortisol level <10 µg/dL
  - Alternative: cosyntropin stimulation test
    - Check cortisol level before 250 µg cosyntropin administration and then 30 and 60 min after
    - Diagnostic if change in cortisol is <9 µg/dL (difference between pre- and post-cosyntropin administration)

- Possible complications from corticosteroid therapy:
  - Immune suppression
  - Increased risk of infections (wound, nosocomial)
  - Impaired wound healing
  - Hyperglycemia
  - Myopathy
  - Psychosis
  - Hypokalemic metabolic acidosis
  - Further HPA and glucocorticoid receptor suppression

FIGURE 212-1. Algorithm for the management of patient with suspected critical illness–related corticosteroid insufficiency (CIRCI)

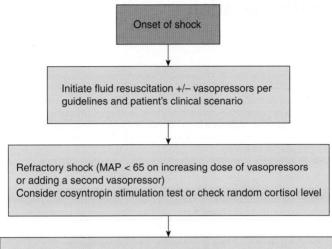

Onset of shock

Initiate fluid resuscitation +/− vasopressors per guidelines and patient's clinical scenario

Refractory shock (MAP < 65 on increasing dose of vasopressors or adding a second vasopressor)
Consider cosyntropin stimulation test or check random cortisol level

Start empiric therapy while awaiting test results
1. Hydrocortisone IV 50 mg every 6 h or 100 mg every 8 h or bolus of 100 mg followed by continuous infusion at 10 mg/h
2. Severe ARDS: methylprednisolone 1 mg/kg/d can be used
3. Continue for ≥ 7 days before tapering every 2–3 days in small steps (≥14 days in ARDS) (controversial)
4. Fludrocortisone (oral) is optional
5. Dexamethasone should not be used — lacks mineralocorticoid effect

REFERENCES

For references, please visit **www.TheAnesthesiaGuide.com**.

CHAPTER 213
Caustic Ingestion

Jennifer Alt, MD

TYPES

- Acids—cause immediate coagulative necrosis. Usually self-limiting injury
- Alkalis—cause liquefactive necrosis resulting in deeper penetration and more extensive injury. Neutralization by the tissues themselves will terminate reaction
  - *NB*: Alkalis are typically odorless and tasteless, which can lead to consumption of larger volumes than acids
  - Alkalis also cause blood vessel thrombosis, which can worsen necrosis

Common Caustic Substances Ingested	
	Found in
Alkali	
Sodium hydroxide	Industrial chemicals, drain openers, oven cleaners
Potassium hydroxide	Drain openers, batteries
Calcium hydroxide	Cement, hair relaxers, and perm products
Ammonium hydroxide	Hair relaxers and perm products, dermal peeling/exfoliation, toilet bowl cleaners, glass cleaners, fertilizers
Lithium hydroxide	Photographic developer, batteries
Sodium tripolyphosphate	Detergents
Sodium hypochlorite	Bleach
Acid	
Sulfuric acid	Car batteries, drain openers, explosives, fertilizer
Acetic acid	Printing and photography, disinfectants, hair perm neutralizer
Hydrochloric acid	Cleaning agents, metal cleaning, chemical production, swimming pool products
Hydrofluoric acid	Rust remover, glass and microchip etching, jewelry cleaners
Formic acid	Model glue, leather and textile manufacturing, tissue preservation
Chromic acid	Metal plating, photography
Nitric acid	Fertilizer, engraving, electroplating
Phosphoric acid	Rustproofing, metal cleaners, disinfectants

USUAL AREAS OF INJURY

- Oropharynx/nasopharynx
- Esophagus
- Larynx
- Trachea

FACTORS AFFECTING SEVERITY OF INJURY

- Amount of caustic fluid ingested
- Type of caustic (pH)

- Concentration
- Duration of contact with mucosa—if vomiting, duration of contact will be lengthened

INITIAL ASSESSMENT

- *The main issues to decide are:*
  - ‣ *Should the patient be intubated?*
  - ‣ *Is there an indication for immediate surgical intervention?*
  - ‣ *Is there an indication for early (before 6 hours) esophagoscopy?*
- History—type and amount of caustic ingested. ±Vomiting? If pediatric ingestion, parents should bring container of caustic ingested for correct identification
- Symptoms:
  - ‣ Hoarseness, stridor, dyspnea → indicate airway injury
  - ‣ Odynophagia, drooling, refusal of food → indicate orophayngeal/nasophayngeal and esophageal injury
  - ‣ Abdominal pain and peritoneal signs: immediate CXR and abdominal x-ray to r/o intraperitoneal or mediastinal air
  - ‣ Substernal chest pain, abdominal pain, rigidity → indicate profound injury or perforation of esophagus/stomach
  - ‣ Signs of perforated viscus, peritonitis, mediastinitis, or hemodynamic instability: immediate surgical evaluation
  - ‣ Criteria for emergent surgery:
    - ▪ Presence of shock
    - ▪ Disseminated intravascular coagulation
    - ▪ Need for hemodialysis
    - ▪ Acidosis (arterial pH <7.22 or base excess <−12)
    - ▪ Grade 3 esophageal injury (see below) seen on endoscopy (controversial)
- Physical exam—injury to lips, chin, hand, clothing, mouth, and pharynx
  - ‣ *Note*: Absence of injury to mouth/pharynx is *not* predictive of esophageal or laryngeal injury
  - ‣ If airway stable—examine pharynx and hypopharynx with flexible fiber-optic scope

AIRWAY MANAGEMENT

Patients with caustic ingestions should always be considered "difficult airways".
- Respiratory distress and stridor indicate pharyngeal or laryngotracheal injuries
- Place oral/nasal airway early in management prior to rapid worsening of airway edema
- Consider administration of dexamethasone (10 mg IV) to counteract upper airway edema
- *Intubate if symptomatic, or if massive ingestion, even without symptoms*
- Awake oral intubation using flexible fiber-optic scope is preferred
  - ‣ *Surgical backup should always be available* for emergent cricothyroidotomy/ tracheotomy as tissue friability, bleeding, and edema may make intubation impossible
  - ‣ Avoid long-acting paralytics as airway edema and muscle relaxation may make mask ventilation impossible
  - ‣ Contraindicated: blind nasotracheal intubation—can exacerbate airway injury
  - ‣ Last resort only: LMA, Combitube, retrograde intubation, bougies—can worsen oropharyngeal injury

GI MANAGEMENT

- Drink water/milk—if done immediately, may lead to dilution of chemical. Not to exceed 15 mL/kg so as not to increase risk of emesis. Controversial, numerous authors strongly recommend *against* it. No evidence of effectiveness in humans
- *No* induced emesis (ipecac), charcoal, or gastric lavage—will expose esophagus to further injury
- *No* neutralizing agents—may cause exothermic reaction leading to thermal injury

- *No* blind nasogastric/orogastric tube insertion—may worsen injuries or perforate tissue. Tubes are sometimes placed at the end of endoscopy in patients with severe circumferential burns as a stent to keep the esophagus open
- Esophagoscopy—should be done in first 48 hours, but no earlier than 6 hours, except if a complication supervenes. After 48 hours, structural weakness of tissue may have developed and lead to iatrogenic perforation:
  ‣ Degree of injury—by esophagoscopy:
    ▪ Grade 1—superficial
    ▪ Grade 2—transmucosal. Use of steroids indicated to prevent stricture formation
    ▪ Grade 3—transmural. Immediate surgical evaluation

SYSTEMIC TOXICITY

- All caustics cause tissue injury/shock leading to lactate production and anion gap acidosis
- Acids cause gap and non-gap acidosis, hemolysis, coagulopathy, renal failure:
  ‣ Hydrofluoric acid: free fluoride ion complexes with body calcium and magnesium $\rightarrow$ calcium chelation and cell death $\rightarrow$ severe hypocalcemia, hypomagnesemia, hyperkalemia, acidosis, and ventricular dysrhythmias
  ‣ Sulfuric acid: anion gap metabolic acidosis
  ‣ Hydrochloric acid: non-anion gap acidosis

EVOLUTION OF INJURY

- Acute phase—immediate damage to mucosa, typically occurs within the first 24 hours
- Latent phase—over the next several weeks. Late complications:
  ‣ Stenosis, strictures (especially Grade 2/3 following alkali ingestion)
  ‣ Delayed perforation
  ‣ Esophageal carcinoma (risk increased 100-fold)
  ‣ Dysphagia
  ‣ Esophageal motility abnormalities
  ‣ Gastric outlet obstruction (primarily associated with acid ingestion)
  ‣ Pancreatic or intestinal injury

REFERENCES

For references, please visit **www.TheAnesthesiaGuide.com**.

CHAPTER 214
Upper Gastrointestinal Bleeding

Oriane Gardy, MD, Eric Cesareo, MD, David Sapir, MD,
and Karim Tazarourte, MD

EPIDEMIOLOGY

80% ulcer, gastric >duodenal.

15% esophageal varices.

5% Mallory–Weiss or angiodysplasia.

DIAGNOSIS

Presentation:
- Hematemesis 75%
- Melena in 20%
- Hematochezia (red blood per rectum) 5%

Differential diagnosis: hemoptysis, bleeding from mouth.

In case of hypovolemic shock without exteriorized bleeding, remember to insert a nasogastric tube.

Assessment of Blood Loss Severity			
Blood loss (mL)	<750	750–1,500	1,500–2,000
SBP	Normal	Normal	≤90 mm Hg
MAP	Normal	Normal	<60 mm Hg
HR (min⁻¹)	<100	≥100	>120
RR (min⁻¹)	14–20	20–30	30–40
Neurologic status	Normal	Anxious	Confused

Markers of severity—*BLEED*:
- Ongoing *bleeding*
- *Low* SBP
- *Elevated* PT
- *Erratic* mental status
- Comorbid *disease*

MANAGEMENT (FIGURE 214-1)

- *Resuscitation goals*:
  - MAP 60 mm Hg and SpO_2 ≥95%:
    - Administer crystalloids (LR)
    - Start norepinephrine (2–5 μg/min infusion) if BP goal not reached after 1,000 mL LR
  - Transfuse RBC if Hct <24% (or 30 if h/o CAD [or high likelihood: elderly, long-standing DM, etc.]):
    - Use clinical judgment to transfuse RBC without waiting for labs if obviously massive bleed or poorly tolerated
  - Transfuse FFP if RBC given. Start with 1 U FFP/3 U RBC, but if >10 U RBC, give 1 U FFP/1 U RBC

FIGURE 214-1. Algorithm for the management of upper GI bleed

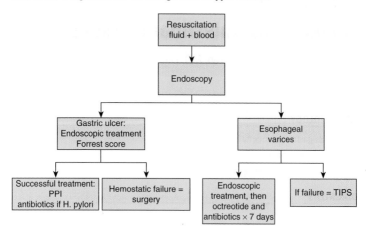

- *EGD:*
  - ‣ Insert NGT/OGT; perform irrigation with saline, GT to gravity
  - ‣ EGD performed when the patient is stabilized:
    - ▪ In the first 6 hours if active bleeding
    - ▪ Otherwise in the first 12 hours
  - ‣ Erythromycin 250 mg IV in 20 minutes, 30 minutes before EGD, to promote gastric emptying (controversial)
  - ‣ Intubate if refractory shock or altered consciousness
- *Ulcer/gastritis:*
  - ‣ During EGD: ulcer *sclerosis*, *epinephrine* injection, *clips* if needed
  - ‣ The *Forrest score assesses* the prognosis and the recurrence risk of bleeding in gastric ulcer case

Forrest Score for Gastric Ulcers				
Forrest	Endoscopic view	Frequency (%)	Risk of recurrence (%)	Mortality (%)
III	Clean ulcer	40	<5	<5
IIc	Hemorrhagic spot	20	10	0–10
IIb	Adherent clot	15	20	5–10
IIa	Visible vessel	15	45	10
Ib	Diffuse bleeding	14	10	10
Ia	Pulsatile bleeding	12	90	10

- ‣ If Forrest IIa or Ia, start *PPI infusion*: for example, omeprazole 80 mg IV bolus, and then 8 mg/h infusion × 48 hours
- ‣ Consider *surgery* if:
  - ▪ Unable to stop bleeding on EGD
  - ▪ Diameter >2 cm
  - ▪ Posterior bulb location
- ‣ Consider *embolization* if unable to stop bleeding on EGD *and* focal (not diffuse) bleeding
- ‣ If *H. pylori* on biopsies, treat with *two antibiotics + PPI* (consult GI)

- *Esophageal varices rupture*:
  - ‣ *Treat bleeding*:
    - *Banding* or *sclerotherapy* during EGD (give cefazolin 1–2 g IV)
    - *Octreotide* 25 μg/h (no bolus) to be continued for 2–5 days
    - *Antibiotics*: norfloxacine 400 mg PO BID × 7 days
    - If unsuccessful, consider *repeat EGD*
    - If bleeding still persists: *TIPS*
    - Blakemore/Linton balloon: rarely used nowadays
  - ‣ *Once bleeding stopped*:
    - Prevent *hepatic encephalopathy* (lactulose, neomycin, or rifamixin)
    - Consider evacuating *ascites*
    - Prevent rebleeding: *propranolol* 80–160 mg per day (goal: limit HR increase to 25%)

REFERENCES

For references, please visit **www.TheAnesthesiaGuide.com**.

CHAPTER 215
Acute Pancreatitis

Zafar A. Jamkhana, MD, MPH and Roopa Kohli-Seth, MD

INCIDENCE

5 to 40 per 100,000 with overall mortality of 1.5 per 100,000; severe forms, however, can have a mortality >30%.

ETIOLOGIES

- Alcohol (men)
- Biliary (women): ultrasound, endoscopic ultrasound (before ERCP)
- Trauma (abdominal, surgical, post-ERCP)
- Metabolic (hypertriglyceridemia, uremia, hypothermia, hypercalcemia)
- Infections (EBV, mumps, HIV, HBV, mycoplasma, *Campylobacter*, *Legionella*)
- Drugs (steroids, sulfonamides, azathioprine, NSAIDs, diuretics, didanosine, etc.)
- Autoimmune (PAN, SLE, TTP)
- Toxins (methanol, organophosphates, scorpion venom)
- Pancreatic tumors
- Idiopathic

PATHOPHYSIOLOGY

Inappropriate activation of trypsin leads to activation of protease activated receptor-2 (PAR2) and activation of other pancreatic enzymes. It results in out of proportion inflammation of pancreas leading to a SIRS-like response.

DIAGNOSIS

Abdominal pain + lipase >3 times normal is sufficient for diagnosis.

Negative type-2 trypsinogen in urine (stick) virtually eliminates Dx of pancreatitis.
- *Clinical features*:
  - ‣ Abdominal pain typically radiating to the back
  - ‣ Nausea, vomiting
  - ‣ Abdominal distension

- ‣ Jaundice
- ‣ Fever
- ‣ Tachycardia
- ‣ Hypotension
- ‣ Cullen's sign (hemorrhagic discoloration of the umbilicus)
- ‣ Grey-Turner's sign (hemorrhagic discoloration of the flanks)
- *Laboratory findings*:
  - ‣ Increased serum amylase >3 times upper limit of normal (returns to normal in 2–4 days)
  - ‣ Increased serum lipase (more sensitive and specific, remains elevated 10–14 days)
  - ‣ Increased CRP (more frequent association with pancreatic necrosis, 24- to 48-hour latency period)
  - ‣ IL-6, procalcitonin, and polymorphonuclear elastase could be used
- *Radiologic findings*:
  - ‣ *X-ray*: duodenal ileus, sentinel loop sign, colon cutoff sign, pleural effusion (especially left side)
  - ‣ *Ultrasonography*: more sensitive to identify gallstones, biliary ducts. Difficult to assess pancreas. Endoscopic ultrasound of use when other modalities fail or cannot be used to assess biliary disease and guide therapy
  - ‣ *CT scan*: contrast-enhanced CT gold standard to diagnose pancreatitis. Useful to assess necrosis, abscess, fluid collections, hemorrhage. Indicated if dilemma in diagnosis/complications. Recommended to delay until 48–72 hours or repeat at this time if initial obtained on presentation. Not of much use if disease mild. Carries risk of contrast nephropathy
  - ‣ *MRI*: useful when CT contraindicated

SEVERITY ASSESSMENT

- Pancreatitis deemed severe if local complications (necrosis, abscess, pseudocyst) or organ failure
- Multiple classifications and criteria are available to assess severity
- Ranson's criteria (Table 215-1) have the disadvantage of requiring 48 hours to assess and cannot help at-risk patients in initial assessment
- The 2004 International Consensus Guidelines to assess severe acute pancreatitis on presentation (Table 215-2) are also helpful
- Balthazar's classification (Table 215-3) assesses pancreatic necrosis based on CT criteria

TABLE 215-1 Ranson's Criteria
On admission
• Age >55 years
• Blood glucose >200 mg/dL
• WBC >16,000/mm³
• LDH >350 IU/L
• AST >250U/L
At 48 h
• Serum Ca <8 mg/dL
• Pao$_2$ <60 mm Hg
• Base deficit >4 mEq/L
• ↑ BUN ≥5 mg/dL
• ↓ Hct ≥10%
• Fluid sequestration >6 L
Mortality
• 0–2 → 5%
• 3–4 → 20%
• 5–6 → 40%
• 7–8 → 100%

TABLE 215-2 Risk Factors for Severe Acute Pancreatitis
• Presence of organ failure and/or local complications (such as necrosis)
• Clinical manifestations
‣ Obesity (BMI >30)
‣ Hemoconcentration (Hct >44%)
‣ Age >70 years
• Organ failure
‣ Shock
‣ Pao$_2$ <60
‣ Renal failure (Cr >2 mg%)
‣ GI bleeding
• ≥3 Ranson's criteria
• APACHE II score >8

TABLE 215-3	Severity Grading Based on CT Scan (Balthazar Score)		
Grade	CT findings	Points	Pancreatitis necrosis
A	Normal pancreas	0	No necrosis (0 patient)
B	Enlargement of pancreas focal or diffuse (contour irregularities, enhancement)	1	<30% (2 patients)
C	Findings in B with peripancreatic inflammation	2	30–50% (4 patients)
D	Findings in B or C with fluid collection in a single location with/without localized gas bubbles	3	>50% (6 patients)
E	Findings in B or C with ≥2 fluid collections and/or gas bubbles in or adjacent to pancreas	4	

Severity index (total points)	Complications (%)	Mortality (%)
<3	8	3
4–6	35	6
7–10	92	17

MANAGEMENT

- Supportive care is the main goal of treatment, along with early identification of patients with/or at risk for severe acute pancreatitis to be monitored in ICU
- Main treatable etiology is biliary. Urgent ERCP (within 24 hours of admission/72 hours of onset of symptoms) with sphincterotomy is recommended in patients with obstructive jaundice, confirmed gallstone pancreatitis. Also useful to prevent recurrence from remaining gallstones. Consider cholecystectomy once resolved
- Mild pancreatitis:
  ‣ Admit to regular floor
  ‣ Oral alimentation as tolerated
  ‣ Analgesia (APAP, IV PCA, no NSAIDs)
- Severe pancreatitis: admit to ICU, treat complications:
  ‣ Adequate fluid resuscitation up to 10 L of crystalloid with frequent assessment of intravascular volume status. Hypotension frequently due to vasodilation, with norepinephrine drug of choice
  ‣ ARDS at admission or delayed: mechanical ventilation support with low tidal volume strategy
  ‣ Assess intra-abdominal hypertension with close monitoring of urine output and airway pressures, treated with gastric decompression, sedation, neuromuscular relaxation, and if needed surgical intervention
  ‣ Enteral nutrition is recommended with jejunal route of feeding preferred. Parenteral feeding to be used when enteral feeds not tolerated. Adequate glycemic control is of utmost importance. Lipids are not contraindicated unless hypertriglyceridemia present
  ‣ Renal failure often prerenal. Need for RRT of poor prognosis
  ‣ Routine use of *prophylactic antibiotics* or selective decontamination of gut in pancreatic necrosis is *not recommended*. In case of infected pancreatic necrosis, imipenem (±aminoglycoside) is the drug of choice. CT-guided FNAB with staining and culture to diagnose sterile versus infected necrosis
  ‣ Open surgical debridement/necrosectomy recommended in presence of infected necrosis/abscess, with timing of it primarily dependent on the clinical picture with recommendation to delay it 2–3 weeks if possible to allow demarcation of necrosis. Debridement of sterile necrosis is not recommended
  ‣ Monitor for vascular complications such as bleeding from splanchnic pseudoaneurysms, portal vein thrombosis, hemorrhage, and hematomas. Treatment of bleeding involves X-ray-guided catheter-directed balloon tamponade/coil embolization as needed

REFERENCES

For references, please visit **www.TheAnesthesiaGuide.com**.

CHAPTER 216
Agitation, Delirium, Delirium Tremens

Ronaldo Collo Go, MD and Roopa Kohli-Seth, MD

DEFINITION

Delirium—acute fluctuating disturbance of consciousness accompanied by alteration of cognition.

EPIDEMIOLOGY

Postoperative delirium in elderly undergoing elective surgery: 11%.

Postoperative delirium more common in vascular surgery and long-lasting oral surgery.

One in 10 Americans consumes excess alcohol and is at risk for withdrawal. The risk for delirium is doubled in this population.

RISK FACTORS

Preoperative: age >70, preexisting cognitive impairment, alcohol abuse, narcotics and drug use, previous history of delirium.

Peroperative: significant blood loss, pain, hypoxia; anesthetic agents—ketamine, opioids, benzodiazepines, metoclopramide, anticholinergics, droperidol; possible influence of intraoperative embolization (e.g., joint replacement).

Postoperative: major surgery, perioperative hypoxia.

PATHOGENESIS

Acute cerebral dysfunction in relation to neurotransmitter disturbance, particularly anticholinergic, melatonin, norepinephrine, and lymphokines.

DIAGNOSIS

Confusion Assessment Method (CAM) in ICU and Intensive Care Delirium Screening Checklist (ICDSC) can be used to detect delirium in patients. However, mechanical ventilation and/or sedation make utilization of these screening tools challenging. In addition, medications for sedation might induce or treat symptoms of delirium.

Confusion Assessment Method	
Feature 1: acute onset or fluctuating change in baseline mental status in the past 24 h as evidenced by sedation scale, Glasgow coma scale, or other delirium assessment?	Yes or no
Feature 2: inattention test	Yes or no
Feature 3: altered level of consciousness—if RASS is other than alert and calm	Yes or no
Feature 4: disorganized thinking	Yes or no
Feature 1 plus 2 and either 3 or 4 = CAM–ICU positive	

The Intensive Care Delirium Screening Checklist	
1 point for each positive finding; score ≥4 indicates delirium	
• Altered level of consciousness • Inattention • Disorientation • Hallucination, delusion, or psychosis	• Psychomotor agitation or retardation • Inappropriate speech or mood • Sleep/wake cycle disturbance • Symptom fluctuation

TREATMENT

Nonpharmacologic treatment might benefit patients preoperatively and postoperatively.
- Daily orientation—increase exposure to daylight, clocks in rooms
- Reduce sleep deprivation
- Decrease unnecessary sedatives or antipsychotics
- Avoid use of restraints
- Encourage early mobilization; physical therapy and occupational therapy
- Early family contact

PHARMACOLOGIC TREATMENT

- After ensuring adequate ventilation and perfusion, treat any underlying acid base disturbances or electrolyte abnormalities. Physostigmine (0.5–2 mg IV) may reverse postoperative delirium due to anticholinergics
- For patients with history of substance abuse, detoxification is beneficial prior to surgery
- For prevention of the effects of stress on the hypothalamic–pituitary–adrenal axis (HPA axis), morphine 15 µg/kg/h is initiated prior to induction of anesthesia
- For patients with known alcohol use disorder, treatment is symptom-based during perioperative state:
  ‣ Benzodiazepines for agitation and seizures
  ‣ Clonidine or dexmedetomidine for autonomic symptoms
  ‣ Neuroleptics (haloperidol or risperidone) for hallucinations
  ‣ Premedication:
    ▪ Long-acting benzodiazepine before the surgery or short-acting benzodiazepine on the morning of surgery
    ▪ After induction of anesthesia, clonidine 0.5 µg/kg/h, haloperidol up to 3.5 mg per day, ketamine 0.5 mg/kg
  ‣ Prevention of Wernicke encephalopathy:
    ▪ Thiamine 200 mg per day × 3–5 days

- Nicotine use disorder (NUD):
  - Detoxification 4–6 weeks before or after surgery
  - Nicotine replacement therapy (patch)
  - Postoperative—physostigmine as cholinergic agent (1.5 mg IV, and then 1 mg/h for 24 hours)
  - Beware of postoperative nausea and vomiting, particularly if no perioperative nicotine replacement therapy
- Drug use disorder:
  - Lofexidine (titrate before surgery, 0.4–0.8 mg per day)
  - Clonidine 0.075 mg per day; increase up to 0.3 mg per day in two to four doses or start with patches from 0.1 to 0.3 per day
  - Methadone 30 mg per day (in two oral doses, increased by 10 mg per day; IV dose is half of PO)
  - Alpha-2 agonist titration following induction of anesthesia
- Geriatric population:
  - Ketamine 0.5 mg/kg on induction associated with lower incidence of postoperative delirium

REFERENCES

For references, please visit **www.TheAnesthesiaGuide.com**.

CHAPTER 217
Trauma Anesthesia

Satyanarayana Reddy Mukkera, MD, MPH and Roopa Kohli-Seth, MD

Polytrauma: several lesions, of which at least one is a vital risk.

Principles of Trauma Patient Management

Perform immediate triage: assess severity of trauma
Ensure availability of needed teams/imaging for adequate management (neurosurgery, CT surgery, vascular surgery, orthopedics, CT, MRI, etc.)
Multidisciplinary approach, importance of having a team leader
Concurrent therapy (ABC) and diagnosis (H&P, imaging studies)
Time is of the essence (first hour = golden hour)

Management Steps for Polytrauma Patient

Triage
Stabilization/workup on arrival
Airway, breathing
Circulation/heme
Neurological
After initial workup/stabilization
Secondary treatment round, depending on lesions identified

TRIAGE

Severity criteria (Vittel, 2002): any of these require transfer to trauma center (except patient factors, which are evaluated on a case-by-case fashion):

- Vital signs:
  ‣ GCS <13
  ‣ SBP <90 mm Hg
  ‣ SpO_2 <90%
- High-energy trauma:
  ‣ Ejection from vehicle
  ‣ Another person died in the same vehicle
  ‣ Fall >6 m (about 20 ft)
  ‣ Patient thrown or crushed
  ‣ No helmet/seatbelt
  ‣ Blast
- Lesion itself:
  ‣ Penetrating trauma of head, neck, thorax, etc
  ‣ Limb amputation or ischemia
  ‣ Pelvis fracture
  ‣ Severe burn and/or smoke inhalation
- Management:
  ‣ Need for mechanical ventilation
  ‣ Fluid resuscitation >1,000 mL and/or pressors and/or military antishock trousers (MAST)
- Patient:
  ‣ Age >65
  ‣ CHF, CAD, respiratory insufficiency
  ‣ Pregnancy (especially second and third trimesters)
  ‣ Bleeding diathesis or anticoagulants

Major mortality criteria:
- SpO_2 <80% or unobtainable (76% mortality)
- SBP <65 mm Hg (65% mortality)
- GCS = 3 (62% mortality)

STABILIZATION/WORKUP ON ARRIVAL

- Document basic information:
  ‣ NIBP, HR, SpO_2, $EtCO_2$ if intubated, temperature
  ‣ GCS, pupil size and reactivity, moving lower extremities; full neuro exam before any sedative given
  ‣ Finger stick for blood glucose, point-of-care Hct
- *At least two large-bore IVs*
- Consider *CVL and/or A-line*; prefer femoral access unless abdominal trauma or B/L LE trauma; insert both lines side-by-side; use 5 Fr arterial catheter (can be used for arteriogram); draw labs when inserting lines:
  ‣ Chem 7, CBC, coags, LFTs, troponin, alcohol/drugs, β-HCG (if female), ABO-Rh for blood bank
- Give *tetanus booster shot*
- If open fracture, start Abx, for example, cefazolin 2 g IV, and then 1 g q8 hours (if allergy, clindamycin 600 mg IV, and then 600 mg q6–8 hours); add 5 mg/kg per day of gentamycin if Gustilo grade III open fracture (crushed tissue and contamination, with or without vascular compromise)
- Consider *analgesia*; however, no sedation without intubation
- *Portable CXR and pelvic AP film* (if pelvic Fx, *do not insert Foley*)
- Focused Assessment with Sonography in Trauma (*FAST*: rule out intraperitoneal fluid) and *thoracic U/S* to r/o hemothorax and/or pneumothorax
- B/L *transcranial Doppler* if available: Vd on MCA <20 cm/s, pulsatility index >1.2 suggest increased ICP
- Consider *OGT* to avoid further aspiration of gastric contents/blood (no NGT until skull base fracture ruled out)

AIRWAY, BREATHING

- *Do not blindly trust ETT in situ*; check position and B/L breath sounds, CXR
- Assess airway for difficult intubation: LEMON:
  - *Look*: obesity, micrognathia, evidence of previous head and neck surgery or irradiation, dental abnormalities (poor dentition, dentures, large teeth), a narrow face, a high and arched palate, a short or thick neck, and facial or neck trauma
  - *Evaluate*: 3–3–2 rule:
    - Mouth opening at least three (of the patient's) fingerbreadths
    - Mentum to hyoid bone at least three fingerbreadths
    - Hyoid to thyroid cartilage at least two fingerbreadths
  - *Mallampati*
  - *Obstruction*: stridor, foreign bodies, etc
  - *Neck* mobility
- Intubate if:
  - GCS <8
  - Facial trauma
  - Respiratory distress
  - Shock
  - Need for emergent surgery or significant analgesia
- Rapid sequence intubation with etomidate + succinylcholine or rocuronium preferred. Avoid propofol or benzodiazepines due to risk of profound hypotension especially in underresuscitated patient
- Full stomach, use cricoid pressure (despite controversial efficacy)
- Assume cervical instability if:
  - Unconsciousness/intoxicated
  - Blunt head injury
  - Complaint of neck or back pain
  - Weakness of any extremity
- In these patients, only use jaw thrust maneuver if needed. Do not extend or rotate neck. Fiber-optic bronchoscopic intubation should be considered. Manual in-line stabilization by another person is necessary while intubating. Intubation in awake patients with head trauma can increase ICP: consider risk/benefit ratio
- In order to remove a cervical collar:
  - *Clinically cleared* if awake, alert, not intoxicated, follow commands, and:
    - No complaint of neck pain at rest
    - No tenderness to palpation over the cervical vertebrae
    - Painless, active range of motion of the C-spine to 45° to each side
  - *Radiographically cleared*:
    - If altered mental status; obtain 3 C-spine x-rays:
      - Lateral view showing C7–T1
      - A–P view
      - Open-mouth odontoid
    - Even if no fracture or dislocation on good quality films, *keep collar* until clinically cleared
  - If protracted alteration of mental status—obtain CT scan. Ligamentous injuries can be missed on CT scan. In these cases MRI is needed to safely clear cervical spine
  - *Radiographically suspicious*: if a fracture is seen, obtain CT scan. If not possible, maintain cervical immobilization
  - *Flexion and extension views* are useful for excluding ligamentous injury in patients who have neck pain and no evidence of unstable injury on the screening films
- Be ready for surgical airway: cricothyroidotomy faster than tracheostomy
- Inspection, palpation, and auscultation for breath sounds bilaterally are important to exclude pneumothorax, flail chest, cardiac tamponade. Percutaneous needle decompression may be needed initially, followed by chest tube placement
- Ventilation: maintain SpO_2 >95% and $EtCO_2$ around 30–35 mm Hg

CIRCULATION/HEME

- Staple scalp bleeder, tamponade epistaxis
- Consider MAST if patient hypotensive, intubated, without intrathoracic bleeding
- Best resuscitation fluid in trauma is blood. Use crystalloids along with blood as it becomes available. Intraoperative blood savage is an option if no contamination of blood noted. Crossmatched blood is ideal but uncrossmatched O negative blood should be available for life-threatening hemorrhage
- Avoid dextrose-containing solutions as they can worsen neurologic outcome
- Prevent hypothermia (fluid warmer, increased room temperature, forced-air warmer)
- Maintain MAP 60–65 until bleeding controlled, using fluids, and then if needed after 1,500 mL, norepinephrine (start at 1 μg/min)
- Aim to maintain Hgb >7 (10 if active angina or acute myocardial ischemia/infarction)
- Hemorrhagic shock is the most common cause of hypotension, but not the only one
- Refractory shock should evoke tamponade (distended neck veins, narrow pulse pressure, muffled heart sounds, worsening hypotension, and equalization of pressures on PA catheter). Emergent pericardiocentesis is needed
- Consumptive coagulopathy from large bleed and/or DIC from massive tissue injury. Give 1 U FFP for each 3 U RBC. A 1:1:1 ratio of RBC:FFP:platelets should be considered in massive transfusions (>12 U RBC); correct ionized calcium
- If uncontrollable hemorrhage, consider activated FVII (200 μg/kg, possibly administer 100 μg/kg after 1 hour)

NEUROLOGICAL (IF HEAD TRAUMA)

- Unilateral or bilateral *mydriasis* is the first sign of brain herniation. Treat with hyperventilation (EtCO$_2$ to 20 mm Hg), hypertonic saline (30 mL of 23% saline over 10 minutes via central line), or mannitol (20% solution: 1.3 g/kg IV bolus)
- When available, 23% hypertonic saline is preferred over mannitol. Elevate HOB to 30° and keep in midline to promote CSF drainage. Intracranial pressure monitoring, if available, can be helpful. Control agitation, pain, and shivering as they can increase ICP
- *Maintain MAP 90–100*, unless concurrent bleeding (then MAP 60 until emergent surgical hemostasis)
- Maintain PT >60%, platelets >100 × 10^9/L
- *Avoid hyperthermia, hypoxemia, and hypotension*
- *Perform rectal exam* to assess sphincter tone if patient unconscious to r/o spinal cord lesion

AFTER INITIAL WORKUP/STABILIZATION

- If stable or stabilized, send patient to radiology:
  - *Head CT* without contrast
  - *Whole-body CT with contrast* (mastoid to ischium)
  - Spine reconstruction from CT, any other bone x-ray needed
  - If pelvic fracture, perform retrograde urethrogram; if urethral rupture, insert suprapubic catheter
- If unstable, move patient to OR for hemostasis

SECONDARY TREATMENT ROUND, DEPENDING ON LESIONS IDENTIFIED

Damage control if patient unstable:
- Pack bleeders
- External-fixator on fractures
- Thoracotomy if hemothorax >1 L and/or output >150 mL/h
- Exploratory-lap if intraperitoneal fluid with hemodynamic instability
- Surgical limb hemostasis/amputation and/or embolization
- Craniotomy if impending herniation

OTHER LESIONS

- High spinal cord injury causes spinal shock, manifested as hypotension, bradycardia, and areflexia. High-dose steroids to reduce cord edema, and dopamine for spinal shock are preferred treatment
- Hypoxia can be due to pulmonary contusion/pneumothorax/hemothorax. Severe hemoptysis from lung contusion may require DLETT to isolate contused lung. Major bronchial ruptures also require one-lung ventilation to avoid air leaks into pulmonary circulation
- Hypoxia could also be due to TRALI from blood products. Treatment is supportive with high FiO_2
- Follow urine output, lactate, and potassium. K can severely be elevated due to acidosis and after major crush injuries. Rhabdomyolysis from severe crush injuries can lead to renal failure. Treat with aggressive hydration
- Fat embolism is associated with long bone fractures, recognized by sudden hypoxia, tachycardia, and hypotension. Diagnosed by fat in urine and elevation of serum lipase
- Severed limbs or digits can be reattached until up to 20 hours if kept cooled. Nerve/plexus block (continuous if possible) recommended for reimplantation
- Do not focus on the obvious; always look for other injuries as well. Blunt trauma patients have multiple injuries in head, thorax, abdomen, pelvis, and extremities
- At the end, do tertiary survey looking at skin and all other areas for unnoticed injuries

REFERENCES

For references, please visit **www.TheAnesthesiaGuide.com**.

CHAPTER 218
Burn Injury

Jean Charchaflieh, MD, DrPH, FCCM, FCCP

PREOPERATIVE CARE

Immediate resuscitation: follow the primary and secondary surveys of Advanced Trauma Life Support (ATLS).

PRIMARY SURVEY: A, B, C, D, E (AIRWAY, BREATHING, CIRCULATION, DISABILITY, EXPOSURE)

- Airway:
  - ‣ Intubate early: airway edema can progress rapidly
  - ‣ Use ETT with ID ≥8 mm to allow subsequent bronchoscopy
  - ‣ Unconscious patient ⇒ full stomach and unstable neck
  - ‣ Succinylcholine safe during the first 24–48 hours, and then contraindicated up to 18 months after major burn
- Breathing:
  - ‣ Inhalation injury is the leading cause of death during the acute phase
  - ‣ Three components:
    - Thermal: hot smoke burns mucous membranes ⇒ edema ⇒ obstruction (more in upper airway since smoke cools as it moves distally)
    - Chemical: smoke components toxic by themselves ⇒ alveolar damage
    - Systemic: carbon monoxide (CO) and cyanide (CN) can displace oxygen (O_2) from hemoglobin (Hb), leading to tissue hypoxia

‣ Face mask 100% O_2; consider hyperbaric O_2 for patients with neurologic symptoms and carboxyhemoglobin (HbCO) levels >25%
‣ Suspect CN poisoning in comatose patients with HbCO <30%, particularly if high (>80%) $S\overline{v}O_2$ and metabolic acidosis:
  ▪ 100% O_2
  ▪ Full and prolonged CPR as needed
  ▪ Sodium thiosulfate (150 mg/kg over 15 minutes IV infusion)
‣ Circumferential chest wall injury: consider escharotomy
• Circulation:
  ‣ During the first 24 hours, use one of the common formulas for fluid resuscitation

| Fluid Resuscitation for the First 24 Hours | |
Adults (Parkland formula)	Children (Evans formula)
LR at 4 mL × %TBSA × kg over 24 h Give first half of total fluids in first 8 h and second half in next 16 h	LR at 1 mL/kg/TBSA% burn + colloid at 1 mL/kg/TBSA% burn + D5W at 2 L/m²/24 h Treat burns that are on second day as 50% TBSA as 50% TBSA burns On second day, give 50% of first day

‣ Estimate adequacy of resuscitation by U/O:
  ▪ Adults: ≥0.5 mL/kg/h
  ▪ Children: ≥1 mL/kg/h
  ▪ Myoglobinuria: ≥2 mL/kg/h (consider adding $NaHCO_3$ to IV fluids)
‣ Also Hct ≤50%, serum Na ≤150 mEq/L, serum albumin ≥2 g/dL, urine Na ≥40 mEq/L, SBP ≥100 mm Hg, HR ≥120
‣ After 24 hours, use 5% or 25% albumin to keep albumin ≥2 g/dL
‣ Monitor for abdominal compartment syndrome (IAP ≥25 mm Hg) whenever IV fluid volumes ≥20 L
• Disability:
  ‣ GCS score in all trauma patients
  ‣ Assess for spinal cord injury (SCI)
  ‣ Consider CO and CN poisoning as causes of coma
• Exposure:
  ‣ Perform head-to-toe examination on a fully exposed patient while protecting from hypothermia
  ‣ Assess for any associated injury
  ‣ Assess burn injury taking into consideration burn size and depth as well as patient age (see Figure 218-1)
  ‣ For thermal injury, follow the 6 C's approach:
    ▪ Clothing: remove nonsticking clothing
    ▪ Cooling: with clean water
    ▪ Cleaning: with nonalcoholic solution such as chlorhexidine
    ▪ Chemoprophylaxis: with topical antibiotic cream
    ▪ Covering: with gauze impregnated with petroleum jelly and wrapped with absorbent gauze
    ▪ Comforting (pain relief): with analgesics
  ‣ For chemical burns, brush off dry chemical powder, rinse with water for 30 minutes (irrigate eye for 8 hours), and then treat according to causative agent
  ‣ For electrical burns:
    ▪ Internal injury (eye, heart, nerve, muscle) can far exceed external skin injury
    ▪ CPK and K^+ levels
    ▪ Monitor EKG for arrhythmias
    ▪ Myoglobinuria: maintain UO ≥2 mL/kg/h and add 50 mEq $NaHCO_3$ plus 12.5 g mannitol to each 1 L IV fluids
    ▪ High-voltage injury, measure compartmental intramuscular pressure (IMP) and perform fasciotomy if >30 mm Hg or neurovascular compromise

FIGURE 218-1. Lund and Browder method of calculating the percentage of burned body surface area

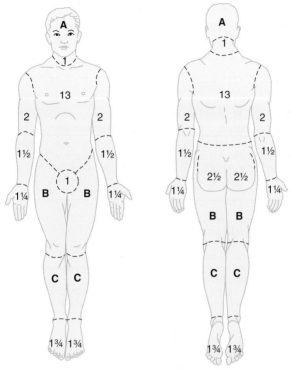

Relative percentages of areas affected by growth

	Age		
Area	10	15	Adult
A = half of head	5½	4½	3½
B = half of one thigh	4¼	4½	4¾
C = half of one leg	3	3¼	3½

SECONDARY SURVEY

- Quick medical history using the **AMPLE** mnemonic (*a*llergies, *m*edications, *p*ast illness/pregnancy, *l*ast meal, *e*vents/environment related to injury)
- Detailed head-to-toe physical examination
- Laboratory and imaging studies as appropriate based on clinical picture
- Treat any detected injuries
- Refer patient with major burn injury to a burn center

INTRAOPERATIVE CARE

Monitoring:
- Consider needle electrodes for EKG monitoring
- Consider reflectance pulse oximetry if no site is available for absorbance oximetry
- Use $EtCO_2$ monitoring to adjusting minute ventilation to match the hypermetabolic state
- Temperature monitoring is necessary to prevent and treat hypothermia
- Invasive monitoring of BP + CVL/PAC is required for most cases

Induction:
- Inhalation induction is possible if no preoperative IV access
- Avoid succinylcholine after 1–2 days: risk of hyperkalemic cardiac arrest

Maintenance:
- Anesthetic and analgesic requirements are increased by two to three times:
  ‣ Hypermetabolism
  ‣ Intense pain
  ‣ Increased volume of distribution
  ‣ Muscle relaxants: proliferation of extrajunctional NM receptors
- Limitations on regional anesthesia:
  ‣ Platelet dysfunction
  ‣ Extensive wound area
  ‣ Need for harvest areas
- Prevent heat loss:
  ‣ Increase room temperature to ≥28°C (83°F)
  ‣ Warm IV fluids and inhaled gases
  ‣ Use forced air blankets
- Basal body temperature (BBT) increases by 0.03°C per 1% TBSA burned (normal BBT of 50% TBSA burn patient is 38.5°C)
- Minimize blood loss:
  ‣ Early excision and grafting
  ‣ Prevent hypothermia and hypertension
  ‣ Topical thrombin, topical fibrin glue, topical epinephrine, subcutaneous epinephrine, and IV triglycyl-lysine-vasopressin (TGLVP)
- Tangential excision (best aesthetic results) $\Rightarrow$ enormous blood loss (0.2 mL/cm^2 or 20 mL/1% TBSA burn) versus fascial excision (less bleeding)
- Minimize blood transfusion by preoperative EPO and acute hemodilution

Emergence:
- Keep intubated if postoperative ICU care, intraoperative fluids administration ≥10–15 L, scheduled surgery within 1 day, persistent airway edema, inhalation injury, or vasopressor/inotrope requirements
- Spraying harvest site with 2% lidocaine reduces postoperative opioid requirements

POSTOPERATIVE CARE

- Very high analgesic requirements (burn injury, high metabolic rate)
- Up to 50% of patients require psychiatric consult due to preexisting conditions (≥30% of burned children have history of abuse, psychiatric or behavioral problems) or postburn problems (up to 45% of all burn patients develop PTSD)
- Infection is leading cause of death past the acute phase of injury
- Immunosuppression
- Prophylactic systemic antibiotics perioperatively but not routinely for nonsurgical patients
- All burn patients should receive tetanus prophylaxis
- Nutrition: major burn has the highest metabolic and catabolic state of any disease state (up to 2.5 BMR):
  ‣ Enteral nutrition is the preferred route and can be started within hours of initial resuscitation
  ‣ Intolerance to enteral nutrition may be an early sign of sepsis and is associated with increased mortality

- Caloric requirements:
  - In adults: *Curreri* formula (25 kcal/kg) + (40 kcal/TBSA% burn)
  - In children: *Galveston* formula (1,800 kcal/m^2) + (1,300 kcal/m^2 burned)
- Supply proteins as 1.2–2 g/kg per day, or as a calorie/nitrogen ratio (CNR) of 150 for minor burns and 100 for major burns
- Provide protein supplementation to maintain positive nitrogen balance (NB) between 0 and 4 g per day (NB = [protein intake (g) × 16%] - [UUN + 4])
- If TPN is used, measure serum TG levels 4 hours after stopping lipid infusion, and hold for level >250 mg/dL
- Calculate H$_2$O imbalance and correct accordingly:
  - H$_2$O deficit = 0.6 × weight (kg) × ([plasma Na/140] − 1)
  - H$_2$O excess = 0.6 × weight (kg) × (1 − [plasma Na/140])
- Supply trace elements such as copper, selenium, and zinc and vitamins A, B, C, and E

PROGNOSIS OF BURN INJURY

- Improved critical care and early excision and grafting of full-thickness (deep second degree and third degree) burns has greatly improved survival and functional recovery of burn patients
- Three main factors of mortality: age, burn size, and inhalation injury

TABLE 218-1 Probability of Death	
Risk factors[1]	Probability of death (%)
0	0.3
1	3
2	33
3	90

[1]Risk factors:
- Age >60 years
- Burn >40% TBSA
- Inhalation injury present

REFERENCES

For references, please visit **www.TheAnesthesiaGuide.com**.

CHAPTER 219
Toxicology

Satyanarayana Reddy Mukkera, MD, MPH and Roopa Kohli-Seth, MD

INITIAL STEPS

- Airway with specific care on cervical spine immobilization (unless trauma has been excluded)
- Breathing, oxygenation, and need for intubation
- Circulation—fluid resuscitation and continuous cardiac monitoring
- Decontamination of GI—only if ingestion within 1 hour
- Elimination of toxin—antidotes, charcoal hemoperfusion, hemodialysis
- History—past medical and psychiatric history, prescription drugs, empty bottles found and pill count, time of ingestion
- Examination—a quick, but detailed exam focusing at identifying a toxidrome to narrow on the toxin ingested (multiple drug ingestion common)

Always check pupils, temperature, and GCS along with vitals to identify toxic syndrome.

Most Common Toxic Syndromes			
Drugs	**Syndrome**	**Symptoms**	**Treatment**
Organophosphates, nerve agents	Cholinergic	DUMBELS[1] **Constricted pupils**	Antidote: pralidoxime, atropine
Atropine, benztropine, tricyclic antidepressants, antihistamines	Anticholinergic	Flushed dry skin, fever, **dilated pupils**, psychosis, seizures, HTN, tachycardia, urinary retention, ileus	Antidote: physostigmine (do not use if EKG changes or seizures occur) Seizures: benzodiazepines
Cocaine, MDMA (Ecstasy), phencyclidine (PCP), amphetamines, caffeine, decongestants (ephedrine), theophylline	Sympathomimetic (adrenergic)	Fever, HTN, tachycardia, **dilated pupils**, seizures, diaphoresis	Sedation: benzodiazepines HTN control: labetalol (avoid beta-blockers)
Morphine, fentanyl, Percocet, heroin, methadone	Opiate	Hypothermia, **constricted pupils**, bradycardia, hypotension, respiratory and CNS depression	Antidote: naloxone
Benzodiazepines, barbiturates, Ambien, chloral hydrate, diphenhydramine, antipsychotics	Sedative–hypnotic	Slurred speech, altered mental status, respiratory and CNS depression—apnea, hypotension, hypothermia	Alkaline diuresis for barbiturates Flumazenil only for acute BZD overdose Hemodialysis

[1]DUMBELS—*d*iaphoresis/*d*iarrhea, *u*rination, *m*iosis, *b*ronchospasm/*b*ronchorrhea/*b*radycardia, *e*mesis, *l*acrimation, *s*alivation.

Hyperthermic Syndromes

Neuroleptic malignant syndrome (NMS)	T >40°C, rigidity, delirium, seizures, autonomic instability, elevated CPK	Overdose of neuroleptic drugs, metoclopramide, haloperidol	Treatment: bromocriptine
Malignant hyperthermia (MH) (see chapter 223)	Hyperthermia, rigidity	Anesthetic agents—succinylcholine, halothane	Treatment: dantrolene
Serotonin syndrome	Irritability, flushing, tremor, myoclonus, diarrhea, diaphoresis	Overdose of SSRI or SSRI with MAO inhibitor	Treatment: cyproheptadine, and benzodiazepines if seizure

- Laboratory investigations: CBC, Chem-7, blood glucose, anion gap, osmolar gap, PT/PTT/INR, LFTs, drug levels (*acetaminophen, salicylate, digoxin, phenytoin, valproate, phenobarbital, lithium, theophylline* as per history; quantitative levels useful for these drugs as they will change management), urine tox screen, alcohol level
- EKG—rate, rhythm, ORS duration, QTc interval
- CXR and abdominal x-ray to look for radio-opaque drugs (iron, heavy metals, and enteric-coated drugs) or packets of illicit drugs

Antidotes

Toxin	Antidote
Chloroquine	Sodium bicarbonate 1–2 mEq/kg for QRS >120 ms Diazepam 2 mg/kg
Cyanide (sodium nitroprusside drip)	Hydroxocobalamin (converts cyanide and forms cynocobalamin) Sodium thiosulfate (enhances conversion to sodium thiocyanite) Sodium nitrite (induces methemoglobinemia)
Oral hypoglycemic medications	Dextrose IV (D50 50 mL IV) + glucagon (1–2 mg IV/IM/SQ) Octreotide (2–10 μg/kg IV q12 h), diazoxide (oral)
Methemoglobinemia	Methylene blue (1–2 mg/kg IV over 5 min, q30 min PRN)
Acetaminophen	*N*-Acetylcysteine
Organophosphates/carbamate	Pralidoxime + atropine
Ethylene glycol/methanol	Fomepizole
Beta-blocker	Glucagon
Calcium blockers	Calcium
Benzodiazepines	Flumazenil
Opioids	Naloxone
Carbon monoxide	100% O_2, hyperbaric O_2
Iron	Deferroxamine
TCA, cocaine/salicylate	Sodium bicarbonate
Arsenic/mercury/lead	Dimercaprol (BAL)
Isoniazid	Pyridoxine
Digoxin	Digoxin immune Fab
Anticholinergic	Physostigmine

Supportive therapy is sufficient for most toxic ingestions.

Patients without pulse or with arrhythmias should be managed as per ACLS protocol.

DECONTAMINATION

- Induction of vomiting is not recommended in a hospital setting
- Activated charcoal can be used if ingestion <1 hour; contraindicated for volatile toxins and if altered consciousness (risk of aspiration). Drugs that are not absorbed by charcoal include acids/alkali, lithium, iron, pesticides, and alcohols
- Whole bowel irrigation (with polyethylene glycol)— for toxins not absorbed by charcoal or ingested packets of illicit drugs

ELIMINATION

- Hemoperfusion or hemodialysis:
  ‣ Drugs cleared by hemodialysis: *LET ME SAV* (mnemonic!)—*l*ithium, *e*thylene glycol, *t*heophylline, *m*ethanol, *s*alicylates, *a*tenolol, *v*alproic acid
- Multiple-dose activated charcoal—for removing drugs with enterohepatic circulation, for example, carbamazepine, phenobarbital, quinine, theophylline, sotalol
- Alkalinization (sodium bicarbonate): salicylates, barbiturates, myoglobin, methotrexate

IMPORTANT/COMMON POISONINGS

Acetaminophen:
- Depletes glutathione stores, active metabolite toxic to liver (Figure 219-1) and kidney
- *Treatment*:
  ‣ IV *N*-Acetylcysteine (20-hour protocol) as early as possible (within 8 hours) for maximal effect. Plot drug levels on nomogram to identify the severity
  ‣ Peak liver dysfunction occurs within 2–4 days with coagulopathy, encephalopathy, acidosis, and renal failure
  ‣ Consider liver transplant for refractory/severe cases

Acetylcysteine Administration Protocol		
Recommended sequential doses[1]	Dose according to patient's weight (g)	
	70 kg	110 kg[2]
150 mg/kg in 200 mL over first 15 min	10.5	16.5
50 mg/kg over next 4 h in 500 mL	3.5	5.5
100 mg/kg over next 16 h in 1,000 mL	7	11
Total dose (300 mg/kg in 20 h)	21	33

[1]Acetylcysteine in D5W administered IV.
[2]A ceiling weight of 110 kg is recommended when calculating the dosage for obese patients.

Aspirin/salicylates:
- Toxic dose is 200 mg/kg. Chronic toxicity has a high mortality rate of 25% versus 1% for acute toxicity
- Tinnitus, hyperventilation, hyperthermia at initial stages followed by cerebral edema and seizures; renal failure leading to death can occur at very high doses
- *Treatment*: gastric decontamination, alkalinization of urine, and hemodialysis

FIGURE 219-1. Hepatotoxicity as a function of acetaminophen level and time of ingestion

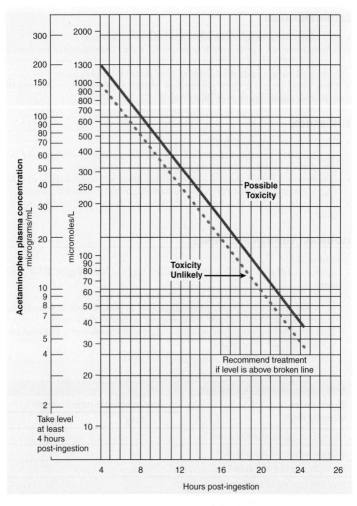

Beta-blockers:
- Bradycardia, hypotension, hypoglycemia, altered consciousness
- *Treatment*:
  ‣ Glucagon is administered as bolus of 5–10 mg IV over 1 minute followed by infusion at 1–10 mg/h if patient's HR improves after the initial bolus
  ‣ Dilute in NS (the diluent provided by the manufacturer contains phenol)
  ‣ Refractory cases are treated with vasopressors, pacer, IABP

Calcium channel blockers:
- Bradycardia, hypotension but hyperglycemia:
  ‣ Exception—dihydropyridine class drugs (e.g., amlodipine and nimodipine) cause hypotension and reflex tachycardia
- *Treatment*: IV calcium, fluids, vasopressors, insulin + glucose

Methemoglobinemia:
- Occurs when metHb >1% of Hb
- Drugs that induce metHb: dapsone, benzocaine, nitrites (e.g., nitroprusside), chloroquine, and cyclophosphamide
- Symptoms range from skin discoloration to headache, fatigue, dizziness, seizures, coma, and death as the concentration of metHb increases
- *Treatment*: IV methylene blue (1–2 mg/kg) over 3–5 minutes, repeat every 30 minutes until symptoms resolve

Digoxin:
- Early: bradycardia
- Late: complete heart block and escape rhythm; tachycardia; nausea/vomiting, vision disturbances with yellow-green haloes around lights, and hyperkalemia:
  ‣ EKG: slowed AV conduction, increased automaticity, multiple PVCs, and ventricular arrhythmias (indication for Digibind, i.e., anti-digoxin antibodies)

Tricyclic antidepressants:
- Rapidly absorbed, lipophilic drugs
- Cardiac: tachycardia, hypotension
- Neurologic: altered mental status, seizures, coma
- EKG: prolonged ORS interval and QTc interval. Right-axis deviation:
  ‣ QRS >40 milliseconds in aVR and S wave in I and aVL are early signs
- *Treatment*:
- Alkalinization of urine with sodium bicarbonate (1–2 mEq/kg IV)
- Hyperventilation
- Benzodiazepines for seizures (do not use phenytoin in TCA overdose)
- Treat hypotension with fluids and vasopressors
- Lidocaine is the drug of choice for TCA-induced ventricular arrythmias

Toxic alcohols:
- Methanol metabolized to formic acid → blindness, acidosis, seizures
- Ethylene glycol metabolized to glycolic and oxalic acid → toxic to CNS (seizures), kidney (acute renal injury by crystallization of oxalate), and heart (myocardial dysfunction due to severe acidosis) leading to pulmonary edema
- Both cause elevated anion gap and osmolar gap
- Isopropyl alcohol: no anion gap but elevated osmolar gap; causes hemorrhagic gastritis and ketonuria
- *Treatment*:
  ‣ Inhibit alcohol dehydrogenase by fomepizole: loading dose of 15 mg/kg IV followed by a 10 mg/kg IV bolus q12 hours. After 48 hours, the dose should be increased to 15 mg/kg q12 hours. For both ethylene glycol and methanol, patients are treated until serum levels fall to <20 mg/dL
  ‣ Refractory acidosis requires dialysis. Follow anion and osmolar gap
  ‣ Administer thiamine, pyridoxine, and folate to enhance metabolism of toxins

REFERENCES

For references, please visit **www.TheAnesthesiaGuide.com**.

PART XIII

RAPID REFERENCE

CHAPTER 220
Important Formulae

Ruchir Gupta, MD

FLUIDS AND ELECTROLYTES

Allowable blood loss (ABL): weight (kg) $\times$ EBV $\times$ ($H_{initial} - H_{final}$)/ H_{avg}.

Total body deficit of HCO_3: weight (kg) $\times$ (deviation from 24) $\times$ ECF.

Anion gap: Na + (Cl + HCO_3).

Normal 8–16.

$$H_2O \text{ deficit} = 0.6 \times (\text{weight in kg}) \times \left(\left[\frac{\text{plasma Na}}{140} \right] - 1 \right).$$

$$H_2O \text{ excess} = 0.6 \times (\text{weight in kg}) \times \left(1 - \left[\frac{\text{plasma Na}}{140} \right] \right).$$

Perfusion to Various Body Compartments		
Compartment	Body mass in adults (%)	Cardiac output (%)
Vessel-rich group (brain, heart, liver, kidneys)	10	75
Muscles	50	19
Fat	20	5
Vessel-poor group (bone, tendons)	20	1

RESPIRATORY

TABLE 220-1 Respiratory Formulae and Equations

Fick equation: VO_2 (O_2 consumption) (N: 250 mL/min)	$CO \times (CaO_2 - CvO_2)$	CO: cardiac output CaO_2: arterial oxygen content CvO_2: venous oxygen content
Alveolar gas equation	$PAo_2 = (PB - 47)FIO_2 - Paco_2/RQ$	PB: barometric pressure PA: alveolar pressure RQ: respiratory quotient (0.8 on a typical diet) Pa: arterial pressure FIO_2: fraction of inspired O_2
A–a gradient	$PAo_2 - Pao_2$	
O_2 content (N: 20 mL O_2/dL)	$CaO_2 = 1.39(Hb \times SaO_2) + (Pao_2 \times 0.003)$	CaO_2: arterial oxygen content Pao_2: arterial oxygen content Hb: hemoglobin
Shunt fraction (N: 5%)	$\dfrac{\dot{Q}_s}{\dot{Q}_t} = \dfrac{CcO_2 - CaO_2}{CcO_2 - CvO_2}$	CcO_2: end capillary O_2 content CaO_2: arterial oxygen content CvO_2: mixed venous oxygen content
Oxygen delivery (N: 400–660 mL/min/m²)	$DO_2 = CO \times CaO_2$	
Oxygen extraction	$(CaO_2 - CvO_2)/CaO_2$	
Bohr's equation (physiologic dead space) Normal 25–30%	$\dfrac{\dot{V}_D}{\dot{V}_T} = \dfrac{P_{aCO_2} - P_{eCO_2}}{P_{aCO_2}}$	P_{eCO_2}: mixed expired CO_2

Compliance	Dynamic compliance = $\dfrac{V_T}{PAP - PEEP}$ Static compliance = $\dfrac{V_T}{P_{plat} - PEEP}$	PAP: peak airway pressure P_{plat}: plateau pressure
Time constant definition	Total compliance × airway resistance	
Fractional SaO_2	$\dfrac{Oxyhemoglobin}{Oxyhemoglobin + reduced\ Hb + HbCO + metHb} \times 100$	SaO_2: oxygen saturation of hemoglobin in the arterial blood
Laplace's law	$T = PR/W$	T: tension W: wall thickness
Boyle's law	$P_1V_1 = P_0V_0$, i.e, the PV product is constant	T: temperature P: pressure V: volume
Ideal gas law	$PV = nRT$	P: pressure V: volume n: number of moles of gas R: universal gas constant = 8.31 J/moles/kg T: temperature

Adapted from *Schwartz's Principles of Surgery*, Table 13-3.

Cardiac Formulae		
Parameter	Formula	Normal range
Cardiac index	CO/BSA	2.2–4.2 L/min/m^2
Stroke volume index	SV/BSA	40–70 mL/beats/m^2
Left ventricular stroke work index	SI × 0.0136(MAP − PAOP)	46–60 g m/beat/m^2
Right ventricular stroke work index	SI × 0.0136(PA − CVP)	30–65 g m/beat/m^2
Stroke volume	CO × 1,000/HR	40–80 mL
Pulmonary artery systolic pressure	Measured	20–30 mm Hg
Pulmonary artery diastolic pressure	Measured	4–12 mm Hg
Central venous pressure	Measured	1–8 mm Hg
Pulmonary artery occlusion pressure ("wedge")	Measured	6–12 mm Hg
Systemic vascular resistance	(MAP − CVP)/CO × 80	800–1,400 dyne s cm^5
Pulmonary vascular resistance	(PA − PAOP)/CO × 80	100–150 dyne s cm^5

CHAPTER 221
Commonly Used Phrases in the Operating Room

Arthur Atchabahian, MD and Ruchir Gupta, MD

COMMONLY USED PHRASES IN THE OPERATING ROOM

See table on following page.

Commonly Used Phrases in the Operating Room											
English	Open your eyes	Breathe normally through your mouth and nose	Take a deep breath	This is oxygen	Squeeze my hand	Lift up your head off the bed and keep it up	Do you have any pain?	Please do not move	I am going to insert an IV	Lie down on your back	Sit down facing this direction	Bend your back like the letter C, a shrimp, or an angry cat	Relax your shoulders
Spanish	Abre los ojos AH-breh lohs OH-khohs.	Respire normalmente por la boca y la nariz. res-PEE-reh nohr-mahl-MEN-the pohr lah BOH-kah ee lah nah-REES	Respire profundo. res-PEE-reh proh-FOON-doh.	Eso es oxígeno. EH-soh ehs oh-KSEE-kheh-noh.	Apriete mi mano. ah-pree-YEH-the mee MAH-noh.	Levante la cabeza de la cama y la mantiene arriba. leh-BAHN-the lah kah-BEH-sah deh lah KAH-mah ee lah mahn-TYEH-neh ahr-REE-bah.	¿Tiene dolor? TYEH-neh doh-LOHR?	Por favor no se mueva. pohr fah-BOHR noh seh MWEH-bah.	Voy a poner un suero. BOY ah poh-NEHR oohn SWEH-roh.	Acuestase boca arriba. ah-KWESS-tah-seh BOH-kah ahr-REE-bah.	Asientase mirando en esa direccion. ah-SYEN-tah-seh mee-RAHN-doh en EH-sah dee-reh-rehk-SYOHN.	Doble la espalda como la letra C, un camaron o un gato enojado. DOH-bleh lah ess-PAHL-dah KOH-moh lah LEH-trah seh, oon kah-mah-ROHN oh oon GAH-toh eh-noh-KHAH-doh.	Relaje los hombros. reh-LAH-kheh los OHM-brohs.
French	Ouvrez les yeux. ooh-VREH leh ZYUH.	Respirez normalement par la bouche et le nez. rehs-pee-REH nohr-mahl-MAHN pahr-lah-boosh-eh-luh-NEH.	Respirez profondément. rehs-pee-REH proh-fohn-deh-MAHN.	C'est de l'oxygène. seh-duh-loh-ksee-ZHEHN.	Serrez ma main. seh-REH-mah-MEHN.	Levez la tête du lit et maintenez-la en l'air. luh-VEH lah teht dyoo lee eh mehn-tuh-NEH-lah ahn lehr.	Avez-vous mal? ah-VEH voo-MAHL?	Ne bougez pas, s'il vous plaît. nuh boo-ZHEH pah seel-voo-PLEH.	Je vais vous poser une voie veineuse. zhuh veh voo poh-ZEH yoon vwah-veh-NUHZ.	Couchez-vous sur le dos. koo-sheh-VOO syoor luh DOH.	Asseyez-vous en regardant dans cette direction. ah-seh-yeh-VOO ahn-ruh-gahr-DAHN dahn seht dee-rehk-SYOHN.	Courbez le dos comme la lettre C, une crevette ou un chat en colère. koor-beh-luh-DOH kom lah-lehtr-SEH, yoon-kruh-VEHT oo uhn-shah-ahn-koh-LEHR.	Détendez vos épaules. deh-tahn-DEH voh-zeh-POHL.

(continued)

Commonly Used Phrases in the Operating Room (continued)

English	Open your eyes	Breathe normally through your mouth and nose	Take a deep breath	This is oxygen	Squeeze my hand	Lift up your head off the bed and keep it up	Do you have any pain?	Please do not move	I am going to insert an IV	Lie down on your back	Sit down facing this direction	Bend your back like the letter C, a shrimp, or an angry cat	Relax your shoulders
Haitian Creole	Ouvri zye ou oo-VREE zee-YEH OOH	Respire nòmalman nan bouch ak nen ou Rehs-pee-REH nohr-mahl-MAHN nan boosh ak nen OOH	Pran yon gwo souf Prahn yohn groh SOOHF	Sa se oksijen Sa say oak-SEE-jehn	Peze men mwen peh-ZEH men MU-wen	Leve tèt ou nan kaban nan epi kembe tèt ou anlè Leh-VEH tet ooh nahn ka-BAN-N nahn eh-pee kem-beh tet ooh ahn-LEH	Èske ou santi doulè? Ess-KEH ooh san-TEE du-LEH?	Tanpri, pinga fè mouvman Tan-PREE, pin-GA feh moov-MAhN	Mwen pral mete yon seròm pou ou Mwen prahl meh-TEH yon seh-ROHM pooh ooh	Kouche sou do ou Kooh-SHEH sooh DOH ooh.	Chita epi gade bò isit Shee-TAH eh-PEE ga-DEH boh eh-SEET	Pliye dou tankou lèt C, yon kribich, ou byen yon chat ki fache Plee-YEH doh ooh tahn-KOOH leht SEH, yon kree-BEECH, ooh byen yon chat KEE fa-SHEH	Lage zepol ou yo LAH-geh zeh-POHL ooh yoh.
Italian	Apra gli occhi. AH-prah lyee OHK-kee.	Respiri normalmente con naso e bocca. rehs-PEE-ree nohr-mahl-MEN-the kohn NAH-soh eh BOHK-kah.	Faccia un respiro profondo. FAHTCH-tchah oohn res-PEE-roh proh-FOHN-doh.	Questo è ossigeno. KWESS-toh eh ohs-see-JEH-noh.	Stringa la mia mano. STREEN-gah lah myah MAH-noh.	Alzi la testa dal letto e mantengala alzata. AHL-tsee lah TES-tah dahl LEHT-toh eh mahn-TEHNG-gah-lah AHL-tsah-tah.	Sente alcun dolore? sehn-TEH ahl-KOON doh-LOH-reh?	Per favore non si muova. per-fah-VOH-reh nohn-see-MWOH-vah.	Sto per inserire un ago per una flebo. stoh-pehr-in-seh-REER-leh pehr-oo-nah-FLEH-boh.	Si stenda supino/a. STEN-dah soo-PEE-noh/soo-PEE-nah.	Si sieda verso questa direzione. see SYEH-dah VEHR-soh KWEHS-tah dee-reh-TSYOH-neh.	Pieghi la schiena a forma di C o come se fosse un gamberetto o un gatto infuriato. PYEH-ghee lah SKYEH-nah ah FOHR-mah dee-CHEE oh koh-MEH seh FOHS-she oon gahm-beh-REHT-toh oh oon GAHT-toh een-foo-RYAH-toh.	Rilassi le spalle. ree-LAHS-see leh SPAHL-leh.

German	Machen Sie die Augen auf MAH-khuhn-zee dee OW-guhn OWF.	Atmen Sie normal durch Mund und Nase AHT-muhn-zee nohr-MAHL doorsh moont oont NAH-zuh.	Tief einatmen TEEF AYN-aht-muhn	Das ist Sauerstoff dahs ist ZOWUHR-shtohf.	Drücken Sie meine Hand DRUH-kuhn-zee meye-nuh HAHNT.	Heben Sie den Kopf an und halten Sie diese Position HEH-buhn-zee den KOPF ahn oont HAHL-tuhn zee dee-zuh poh-zee-tsyohn.	Haben Sie Schmerzen? HAH-buhn-zee SHMEHRTS?	Bitte nicht bewegen BIT-tuh neesht buh-WEH-guhn.	Ich werde jetzt eine intravenöse Punktion durchführen eesh vehr-duh yetst ahy-nuh een-trah-veh-NUH-zuh poonk-TSYOHN DOORSH-fyoo-ruhn.	Legen Sie sich auf den Rücken LEH-guhn-zee-zeesh owf den RUH-kuhn.	Setzen sie sich in diese Richtung hin ZEH-tsuhn-zee-zeesh een dee-zuh REESH-toong hin.	Krümmen sie ihren Rücken wie der Buchstabe C, eine Gamele oder einen Katzenbuckel KRUH-muhn-zee ee-ruhn RUH-kuhn vee dee BOOKH-shtah-buh TSEH, ay-nuh GAHR-neh-luh oh-duhr ay-nuhn KAH-tsuhn-boo-kuhl.	Entspannen Sie ihre Schultern. ENT-shpah-nuhn-zee ee-ruh SHOOL-turn.
Mandarin	睁开你的眼睛。 Zhēng kāi nǐ de yǎnjīng.	正常呼吸 — 通过你的嘴和鼻子。 Zhèngcháng hūxī — tōngguò nǐ de zuǐ hé bízi.	深呼吸。 Shēnhūxī.	这是气氧。 Zhè shì yǎngqì.	用力握着我的手。 Yònglì wòzhe wǒ de shǒu.	抬起你的头，并保持这个姿势。 Tái qǐ nǐ de tóu, bìng bǎochí zhège zīshì.	你有任何疼痛吗？ Nǐ yǒu rènhé téngtòng ma?	请不要动。 Qǐng bùyào dòng.	我现在进行静脉注射。 Wǒ xiànzài jìnxíng jìngmài zhùshè.	请躺下。 Qǐng tǎng xià.	坐下望这边。 Zuò xià wàng zhè biān.	请将你背部弯成为字母C，一只虾，或一只好愤怒的猫儿。 Qǐng jiāng nǐ bèibù wān chéngwéi zìmǔ C, yī zhǐ xiā, huò-zhǐ hǎo fènnù de māo er.	放松你的肩膀。 Fàngsōng nǐ de jiānbǎng.

(continued)

English	Open your eyes	Breathe normally through your mouth and nose	Take a deep breath	This is oxygen	Squeeze my hand	Lift up your head off the bed and keep it up	Do you have any pain?	Please do not move	I am going to insert an IV	Lie down on your back	Sit down facing this direction	Bend your back like the letter C, a shrimp, or an angry cat	Relax your shoulders
Cantonese	打開眼睛。 Da hoi an jing.	用口同鼻正常呼吸。 Yong hau tong bei jing seng fu cup.	深呼吸。 Sum fu cup.	依d保氧氣。 Yi di hai yeung hei.	榨我隻手。 Jar or chek sau.	從床上抬起頭，並保持姿勢。 Chung chong cern toy hei tau, bing bo chee zi sai	你痛唔痛呀？ Lei tong ng tong ar?	請唔好郁。 Ching ng ho yuk.	我依家會進行靜脈注射。 Or yi ka wui jun hang jing mug chu sei.	用背脊訓低。 Yong bui jet fun dai.	坐低望依面。 Chor dai mong e min.	請將你既背脊彎成為字母C，一隻蝦，或者一隻好嬲既貓。 Ching chum lei gei bui jet wan sing wai zi mou see, wak jei yat zek ha, wak jei yat zek ho lou gei mao.	放鬆你既膊頭 Fong song lei gei bok tou.
Hindi	आप अपनी आंखें खोलो Aap apnee aakhe kholo	अपने मुंह और नाक के माध्यम से सामान्य रूप से सांस लो Apne muh or nak ke madhyam se samanya rup se saas lo	एक गहरी सांस लो Ek gehri saas lo	यह ऑक्सीजन है Yeh oxygen hai	मेरा हाथ दबाओ Mera hath dabao	अपना सिर बिस्तर से उपर करो और उपर ही रखो Apna sar bistar se upar karo aur upar hee rakho	क्या आप को दर्द हो रहा है? Kya aap ko durd ho raha hae?	कृपया हिलना मत Kripya hilna mat	मैं एक आई वी (IV) लगाने जा रहा हूँ Me ek IV lagane ja raha hu	अपनी पीठ पर लेट जाओ Apne peet par let jao	बैठिये इस तरफ देखिये Bethiye is taraf dekhiye	अपनी पीठ को झुकाये जो अक्षर (सी) की तरह या गुस्साई बिल्ली की तरह लगे Apni peet ko jhukaye jo akshar (C) ki tarah ya gusai billi ki tarah lage	अपने कंधों को आराम से नीचे करिये Apne kandho ko aaram se neeche kariye

Korean	당신의 눈을 여십시오. Nun te seo	당신의 입을 통해 해서 일반호흡을 하십시오. Sum si seyo	심호흡을 하고 가십시오. Gip he sum siseyo	이것 은산소이다. San so so ovida	나의 손을 쥐세 십시오. Son jap es eyo	당신의 머리를 침대 뒤쪽에서 위로 올려고그것을 들어올리십시오. Muri du seo	당신은 어디 통이 있는가? Apuseyo	움직이 지 말라. Um Ji Ji Ma Se Yo	나는 IV를 삽 입하기 위하여 피고하 고있다. Jusa Nop Ni Da	당신 의 뒤 에누 우십 시오. Nue Seyo	앉아서 쪽으로 를향해한 을직면한. Yu Gi Bo Go An E Seyo	평지 C, 세우 또 는 정반고양이 같이 악의 신의 뒤를 구부리십시오. Huri Gu Bu Ri Se Yo	당신의 어깨를 이완하 십시오. Aque Hina Su Ma Se Yo
Russian	Откройте глаза. aht-KROY-tyeh gluh-ZAH.	Дышите нормально через рот и нос. DEE-shee-tyeh nahr-MAHL-nuh CHE-ruhs roht ee nohs.	Глубокий вдох. gloo-BOH-kee vdohkh.	Этот кислород. EH-tuht kees-lah-ROHT.	Сожмите руку. sahzh-MEE-tyeh ROO-koo.	Приподнимите голову. pree-puhd-nee-MEE-tyeh GOH-luh-voo.	Вам что-то болит? vahm SHTOH-tuh bah-LEET?	Не двигайтесь. NYEH dvee-G-EYE-tyehs.	Поставлю вам капельницу. pahs-TAHV-lyoo vahm kah-pehl-NEE-tsoo.	Ложитесь на спину. lah-ZHEE-tyehss nuh-SPEE-noo.	Садитесь лицом в эту сторону. sah-DEE-tyess LYEE-tsuhm veh-TOO STOH-ruh-noo.	Согните спину, как злая кот. sahg-NEE-tyeh SPEE-noo kahk ZLAH-yah KOHSH-kuh.	Опустите плечи. ah-pooh-STEE-tyeh PLYEH-chee.
Arabic	افتح عينيك Eftah eineik	تنفس بشكل طبيعي عبر أنفك وفمك Tanafass bishakl tabeeeye	خذ نفساً عميق Khoz nafass ameek	هذا اوكسجين Hatha oxygeen	اضغط على يدي Edgat ala eidy	ارفع رأسك عن الوسادة واستمر في رافعها Irfae raasak an el wesada wa estamer fei rafeiha	هل تشعر بأي ألم Hal tashour be ay alam'	لا تتحرك Men fadlak la tataharrak	سأقوم بإدخال أنبوب الوريد Saakoum be edkhal onboub fe alwareed	نم على ظهرك Nam ala thahrak	اجلس ووجهك في هذا الاتجاه Igless wa wajhak fe hatha al etigah	نم على جانبك ودم روكبك ناحو صدرك Nam ala janbak wa dom rokabak naho sadrak	ارخي كتفيك Irkhy katifayk

Capitals indicate the stress. Mandarin transliteration uses pinyin. For others, an approximate (American) English pronunciation is given. Capitals mark the stress. "kh" stands for a velar fricative, like the Spanish j in José, or the Scottish ch in loch.

CHAPTER 222
BLS/ACLS/PALS

Ruchir Gupta, MD

Note: All figures have been reproduced from *Circulation*. 2010;122(18 Suppl3).

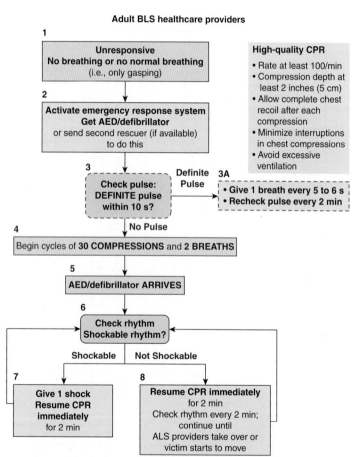

Adult BLS healthcare providers

1
> Unresponsive
> No breathing or no normal breathing
> (i.e., only gasping)

2
> Activate emergency response system
> Get AED/defibrillator
> or send second rescuer (if available)
> to do this

3
> Check pulse:
> DEFINITE pulse
> within 10 s?

Definite Pulse → **3A**
> • Give 1 breath every 5 to 6 s
> • Recheck pulse every 2 min

No Pulse

4
> Begin cycles of **30 COMPRESSIONS** and **2 BREATHS**

5
> AED/defibrillator ARRIVES

6
> Check rhythm
> Shockable rhythm?

Shockable | Not Shockable

7
> Give 1 shock
> Resume CPR
> immediately
> for 2 min

8
> Resume CPR immediately
> for 2 min
> Check rhythm every 2 min;
> continue until
> ALS providers take over or
> victim starts to move

High-quality CPR
- Rate at least 100/min
- Compression depth at least 2 inches (5 cm)
- Allow complete chest recoil after each compression
- Minimize interruptions in chest compressions
- Avoid excessive ventilation

Note: The boxes bordered with dashed lines are performed by healthcare providers and not by lay rescuers.

Reproduced with permission from American Heart Association. Guidelines for cardiopulmonary resuscitation and emergency cardiovascular care, Part 4: Adult basic life support. *Circulation.* 2005;112:IV-19. © 2005 American Heart Association, Inc.

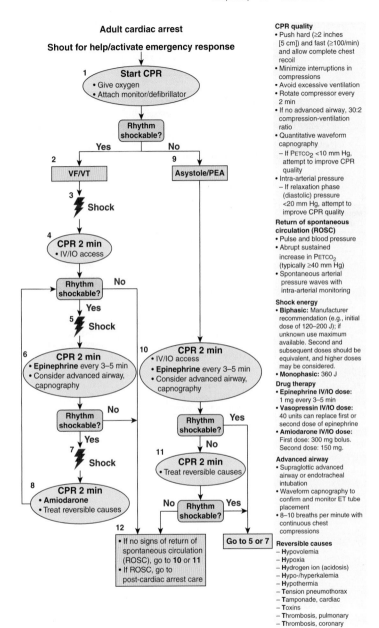

Adult cardiac arrest

Shout for help/activate emergency response

1 Start CPR
- Give oxygen
- Attach monitor/defibrillator

Rhythm shockable?

Yes → **2 VF/VT**

No → **9 Asystole/PEA**

3 Shock

4 CPR 2 min
- IV/IO access

Rhythm shockable? No

Yes

5 Shock

6 CPR 2 min
- Epinephrine every 3–5 min
- Consider advanced airway, capnography

Rhythm shockable? No

Yes

7 Shock

8 CPR 2 min
- Amiodarone
- Treat reversible causes

10 CPR 2 min
- IV/IO access
- Epinephrine every 3–5 min
- Consider advanced airway, capnography

Rhythm shockable? Yes

No

11 CPR 2 min
- Treat reversible causes

Rhythm shockable? No → / Yes → **Go to 5 or 7**

12
- If no signs of return of spontaneous circulation (ROSC), go to **10** or **11**
- If ROSC, go to post-cardiac arrest care

CPR quality
- Push hard (≥2 inches [5 cm]) and fast (≥100/min) and allow complete chest recoil
- Minimize interruptions in compressions
- Avoid excessive ventilation
- Rotate compressor every 2 min
- If no advanced airway, 30:2 compression-ventilation ratio
- Quantitative waveform capnography
  – If P_{ETCO_2} <10 mm Hg, attempt to improve CPR quality
- Intra-arterial pressure
  – If relaxation phase (diastolic) pressure <20 mm Hg, attempt to improve CPR quality

Return of spontaneous circulation (ROSC)
- Pulse and blood pressure
- Abrupt sustained increase in P_{ETCO_2} (typically ≥40 mm Hg)
- Spontaneous arterial pressure waves with intra-arterial monitoring

Shock energy
- **Biphasic:** Manufacturer recommendation (e.g., initial dose of 120–200 J); if unknown use maximum available. Second and subsequent doses should be equivalent, and higher doses may be considered.
- **Monophasic:** 360 J

Drug therapy
- **Epinephrine IV/IO dose:** 1 mg every 3–5 min
- **Vasopressin IV/IO dose:** 40 units can replace first or second dose of epinephrine
- **Amiodarone IV/IO dose:** First dose: 300 mg bolus. Second dose: 150 mg.

Advanced airway
- Supraglottic advanced airway or endotracheal intubation
- Waveform capnography to confirm and monitor ET tube placement
- 8–10 breaths per minute with continuous chest compressions

Reversible causes
– Hypovolemia
– Hypoxia
– Hydrogen ion (acidosis)
– Hypo-/hyperkalemia
– Hypothermia
– Tension pneumothorax
– Tamponade, cardiac
– Toxins
– Thrombosis, pulmonary
– Thrombosis, coronary

Adult bradycardia
(with pulse)

1

Assess appropriateness for clinical condition.
Heart rate typically <50/min if bradyarrhythmia.

2

Identify and treat underlying cause

- Maintain patent airway; assist breathing as necessary
- Oxygen (if hypoxemic)
- Cardiac monitor to identify rhythm; monitor blood pressure and oximetry
- IV access
- 12-lead ECG if available; don't delay therapy

3

**Persistent bradyarrhythmia
causing:**

- Hypotension?
- Acutely altered mental status?
- Signs of shock?
- Ischemic chest discomfort?
- Acute heart failure?

4

No → **Monitor and observe**

Yes

5

Atropine
If atropine ineffective:
- Transcutaneous pacing
   OR
- **Dopamine** infusion
   OR
- **Epinephrine** infusion

6

Consider:
- Expert consultation
- Transvenous pacing

Doses/details

Atropine IV dose:
First dose: 0.5 mg bolus
Repeat every 3–5 min
Maximum: 3 mg

Dopamine IV infusion:
2–10 mcg/kg per min

Epinephrine IV infusion:
2–10 mcg per min

Reproduced with permission from Neumar RW, et al. Part 8: Adult advanced cardiovascular life support. *Circulation*. 2010;122(18 Suppl 3):S729. © 2010 American Heart Association, Inc.

Adult tachycardia
(with pulse)

1

Assess appropriateness for clinical condition.
Heart rate typically ≥150/min if tachyarrhythmia.

2

Identify and treat underlying cause
- Maintain patent airway; assist breathing as necessary
- Oxygen (if hypoxemic)
- Cardiac monitor to identify rhythm; monitor blood pressure and oximetry

3

Persistent tachyarrhythmia causing:
- Hypotension?
- Acutely altered mental status?
- Signs of shock?
- Ischemic chest discomfort?
- Acute heart failure?

Yes →

4

Synchronized cardioversion
- Consider sedation
- If regular narrow complex, consider adenosine

No ↓

5

Wide QRS?
≥0.12 s

Yes →

6

- IV access and 12-lead ECG if available
- Consider adenosine only if regular and monomorphic
- Consider antiarrhythmic infusion
- Consider expert consultation

No ↓

7

- IV access and 12-lead ECG if available
- Vagal maneuvers
- Adenosine (if regular)
- β-blocker or calcium channel blocker
- Consider expert consultation

Doses/details

Synchronized cardioversion
Initial recommended doses:
- Narrow regular: 50–100 J
- Narrow irregular: 120–200 J biphasic or 200 J monophasic
- Wide regular: 100 J
- Wide irregular: defibrillation dose (NOT synchronized)

Adenosine IV dose:
First dose: 6 mg rapid IV push; follow with NS flush.
Second dose: 12 mg if required.

Antiarrhythmic infusions for stable wide-QRS tachycardia

Procainamide IV dose:
20–50 mg/min until arrhythmia suppressed, hypotension ensues, QRS duration increases >50%, or maximum dose 17 mg/kg given.
Maintenance infusion: 1–4 mg/min. Avoid if prolonged QT or CHF.

Amiodarone IV dose:
First dose: 150 mg over 10 min. Repeat as needed if VT recurs. Follow by maintenance infusion of 1 mg/min for first 6 h.

Sotalol IV dose:
100 mg (1.5 mg/kg) over 5 min.
Avoid if prolonged QT.

Reproduced with permission from Neumar RW, et al. Part 8: Adult advanced cardiovascular life support. *Circulation*. 2010;122(18 Suppl 3):S729. © 2010 American Heart Association, Inc.

Acute coronary syndromes

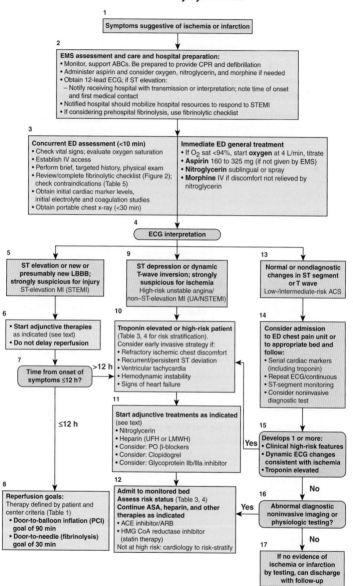

1

Symptoms suggestive of ischemia or infarction

2

EMS assessment and care and hospital preparation:
- Monitor, support ABCs. Be prepared to provide CPR and defibrillation
- Administer aspirin and consider oxygen, nitroglycerin, and morphine if needed
- Obtain 12-lead ECG; if ST elevation:
  – Notify receiving hospital with transmission or interpretation; note time of onset and first medical contact
- Notified hospital should mobilize hospital resources to respond to STEMI
- If considering prehospital fibrinolysis, use fibrinolytic checklist

3

Concurrent ED assessment (<10 min)
- Check vital signs; evaluate oxygen saturation
- Establish IV access
- Perform brief, targeted history, physical exam
- Review/complete fibrinolytic checklist (Figure 2); check contraindications (Table 5)
- Obtain initial cardiac marker levels, initial electrolyte and coagulation studies
- Obtain portable chest x-ray (<30 min)

Immediate ED general treatment
- If O₂ sat <94%, start **oxygen** at 4 L/min, titrate
- **Aspirin** 160 to 325 mg (if not given by EMS)
- **Nitroglycerin** sublingual or spray
- **Morphine** IV if discomfort not relieved by nitroglycerin

4

ECG interpretation

5

ST elevation or new or presumably new LBBB; strongly suspicious for injury
ST-elevation MI (STEMI)

9

ST depression or dynamic T-wave inversion; strongly suspicious for ischemia
High-risk unstable angina/non–ST-elevation MI (UA/NSTEMI)

13

Normal or nondiagnostic changes in ST segment or T wave
Low-/intermediate-risk ACS

6

- Start adjunctive therapies as indicated (see text)
- Do not delay reperfusion

7

Time from onset of symptoms ≤12 h?   >12 h

≤12 h

10

Troponin elevated or high-risk patient (Table 3, 4 for risk stratification). Consider early invasive strategy if:
- Refractory ischemic chest discomfort
- Recurrent/persistent ST deviation
- Ventricular tachycardia
- Hemodynamic instability
- Signs of heart failure

11

Start adjunctive treatments as indicated (see text)
- Nitroglycerin
- Heparin (UFH or LMWH)
- Consider: PO β-blockers
- Consider: Clopidogrel
- Consider: Glycoprotein IIb/IIIa inhibitor

12

Admit to monitored bed
Assess risk status (Table 3, 4)
Continue ASA, heparin, and other therapies as indicated
- ACE inhibitor/ARB
- HMG CoA reductase inhibitor (statin therapy)
Not at high risk: cardiology to risk-stratify

14

Consider admission to ED chest pain unit or to appropriate bed and follow:
- Serial cardiac markers (including troponin)
- Repeat ECG/continuous ST-segment monitoring
- Consider noninvasive diagnostic test

15

Develops 1 or more:
- Clinical high-risk features
- Dynamic ECG changes consistent with ischemia
- Troponin elevated

Yes →

No

16

Abnormal diagnostic noninvasive imaging or physiologic testing?   Yes →

No

17

If no evidence of ischemia or infarction by testing, can discharge with follow-up

8

Reperfusion goals:
Therapy defined by patient and center criteria (Table 1)
- Door-to-balloon inflation (PCI) goal of 90 min
- Door-to-needle (fibrinolysis) goal of 30 min

Reproduced with permission from American Heart Association. Guidelines for cardiopulmonary resuscitation and emergency cardiovascular care, Part 8: Stabilization of the patient with acute coronary syndromes. *Circulation*. 2005;112:IV-89. © 2005 American Heart Association, Inc.

PEDIATRIC LIFE SUPPORT

Pediatric BLS healthcare providers

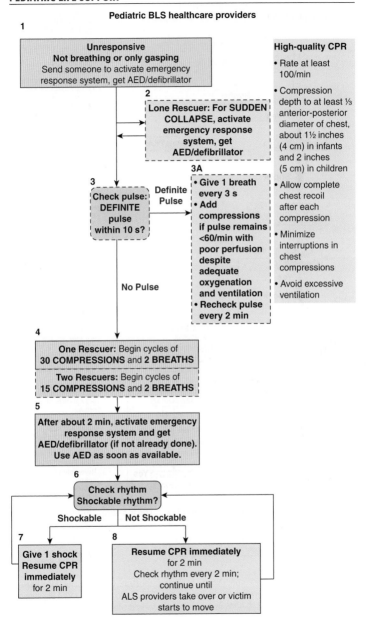

High-quality CPR

- Rate at least 100/min

- Compression depth to at least ⅓ anterior-posterior diameter of chest, about 1½ inches (4 cm) in infants and 2 inches (5 cm) in children

- Allow complete chest recoil after each compression

- Minimize interruptions in chest compressions

- Avoid excessive ventilation

1
Unresponsive
Not breathing or only gasping
Send someone to activate emergency response system, get AED/defibrillator

2
Lone Rescuer: For SUDDEN COLLAPSE, activate emergency response system, get AED/defibrillator

3
Check pulse: DEFINITE pulse within 10 s?

Definite Pulse →

3A
- **Give 1 breath every 3 s**
- **Add compressions if pulse remains <60/min with poor perfusion despite adequate oxygenation and ventilation**
- **Recheck pulse every 2 min**

No Pulse

4
One Rescuer: Begin cycles of 30 COMPRESSIONS and 2 BREATHS
Two Rescuers: Begin cycles of 15 COMPRESSIONS and 2 BREATHS

5
After about 2 min, activate emergency response system and get AED/defibrillator (if not already done). Use AED as soon as available.

6
Check rhythm Shockable rhythm?

Shockable | **Not Shockable**

7
Give 1 shock Resume CPR immediately for 2 min

8
Resume CPR immediately for 2 min
Check rhythm every 2 min; continue until ALS providers take over or victim starts to move

Note: The boxes bordered with dashed lines are performed by healthcare providers and not by lay rescuers.

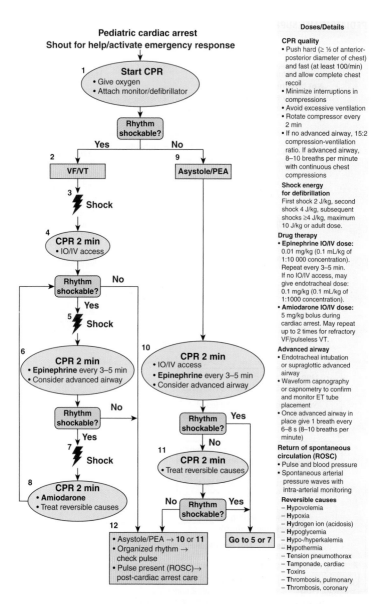

Pediatric cardiac arrest
Shout for help/activate emergency response

1 Start CPR
- Give oxygen
- Attach monitor/defibrillator

Rhythm shockable?

Yes / No

2 VF/VT

9 Asystole/PEA

3 Shock

4 CPR 2 min
- IO/IV access

Rhythm shockable?
No / Yes

5 Shock

6 CPR 2 min
- **Epinephrine** every 3–5 min
- Consider advanced airway

Rhythm shockable?
No / Yes

7 Shock

8 CPR 2 min
- **Amiodarone**
- Treat reversible causes

10 CPR 2 min
- IO/IV access
- **Epinephrine** every 3–5 min
- Consider advanced airway

Rhythm shockable?
Yes / No

11 CPR 2 min
- Treat reversible causes

Rhythm shockable?
No / Yes

12
- Asystole/PEA → **10** or **11**
- Organized rhythm → check pulse
- Pulse present (ROSC)→ post-cardiac arrest care

Go to 5 or 7

Doses/Details

CPR quality
- Push hard (≥ ⅓ of anterior-posterior diameter of chest) and fast (at least 100/min) and allow complete chest recoil
- Minimize interruptions in compressions
- Avoid excessive ventilation
- Rotate compressor every 2 min
- If no advanced airway, 15:2 compression-ventilation ratio. If advanced airway, 8–10 breaths per minute with continuous chest compressions

Shock energy for defibrillation
First shock 2 J/kg, second shock 4 J/kg, subsequent shocks ≥4 J/kg, maximum 10 J/kg or adult dose.

Drug therapy
- Epinephrine IO/IV dose: 0.01 mg/kg (0.1 mL/kg of 1:10 000 concentration). Repeat every 3–5 min. If no IO/IV access, may give endotracheal dose: 0.1 mg/kg (0.1 mL/kg of 1:1000 concentration).
- Amiodarone IO/IV dose: 5 mg/kg bolus during cardiac arrest. May repeat up to 2 times for refractory VF/pulseless VT.

Advanced airway
- Endotracheal intubation or supraglottic advanced airway
- Waveform capnography or capnometry to confirm and monitor ET tube placement
- Once advanced airway in place give 1 breath every 6–8 s (8–10 breaths per minute)

Return of spontaneous circulation (ROSC)
- Pulse and blood pressure
- Spontaneous arterial pressure waves with intra-arterial monitoring

Reversible causes
- Hypovolemia
- Hypoxia
- Hydrogen ion (acidosis)
- Hypoglycemia
- Hypo-/hyperkalemia
- Hypothermia
- Tension pneumothorax
- Tamponade, cardiac
- Toxins
- Thrombosis, pulmonary
- Thrombosis, coronary

Pediatric bradycardia
with a pulse and poor perfusion

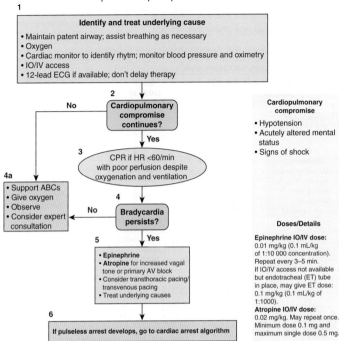

1

Identify and treat underlying cause
- Maintain patent airway; assist breathing as necessary
- Oxygen
- Cardiac monitor to identify rhytm; monitor blood pressure and oximetry
- IO/IV access
- 12-lead ECG if available; don't delay therapy

2
No → **Cardiopulmonary compromise continues?**
↓ Yes

3
CPR if HR <60/min with poor perfusion despite oxygenation and ventilation

4a
- Support ABCs
- Give oxygen
- Observe
- Consider expert consultation

No ←
4
Bradycardia persists?
↓ Yes

5
- Epinephrine
- Atropine for increased vagal tone or primary AV block
- Consider transthoracic pacing/transvenous pacing
- Treat underlying causes

6
If pulseless arrest develops, go to cardiac arrest algorithm

Cardiopulmonary compromise
- Hypotension
- Acutely altered mental status
- Signs of shock

Doses/Details

Epinephrine IO/IV dose:
0.01 mg/kg (0.1 mL/kg of 1:10 000 concentration). Repeat every 3–5 min. If IO/IV access not available but endotracheal (ET) tube in place, may give ET dose: 0.1 mg/kg (0.1 mL/kg of 1:1000).

Atropine IO/IV dose:
0.02 mg/kg. May repeat once. Minimum dose 0.1 mg and maximum single dose 0.5 mg.

Reproduced with permission from American Heart Association. Guidelines for cardiopulmonary resuscitation and emergency cardiovascular care, Part 12: Pediatric advanced life support. *Circulation*. 2005;112:IV-167. © 2005 American Heart Association, Inc.

Pediatric tachycardia
with a pulse and poor perfusion

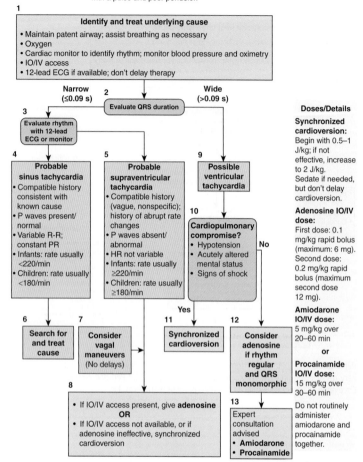

1
Identify and treat underlying cause
- Maintain patent airway; assist breathing as necessary
- Oxygen
- Cardiac monitor to identify rhythm; monitor blood pressure and oximetry
- IO/IV access
- 12-lead ECG if available; don't delay therapy

2 Evaluate QRS duration

Narrow (≤0.09 s)   Wide (>0.09 s)

3 Evaluate rhythm with 12-lead ECG or monitor

4
Probable sinus tachycardia
- Compatible history consistent with known cause
- P waves present/ normal
- Variable R-R; constant PR
- Infants: rate usually <220/min
- Children: rate usually <180/min

5
Probable supraventricular tachycardia
- Compatible history (vague, nonspecific); history of abrupt rate changes
- P waves absent/ abnormal
- HR not variable
- Infants: rate usually ≥220/min
- Children: rate usually ≥180/min

9
Possible ventricular tachycardia

10
Cardiopulmonary compromise?
- Hypotension
- Acutely altered mental status
- Signs of shock

No

Yes

6
Search for and treat cause

7
Consider vagal maneuvers
(No delays)

11
Synchronized cardioversion

12
Consider adenosine if rhythm regular and QRS monomorphic

8
- If IO/IV access present, give **adenosine** OR
- If IO/IV access not available, or if adenosine ineffective, synchronized cardioversion

13
Expert consultation advised
- **Amiodarone**
- **Procainamide**

Doses/Details

Synchronized cardioversion:
Begin with 0.5–1 J/kg; if not effective, increase to 2 J/kg. Sedate if needed, but don't delay cardioversion.

Adenosine IO/IV dose:
First dose: 0.1 mg/kg rapid bolus (maximum: 6 mg). Second dose: 0.2 mg/kg rapid bolus (maximum second dose 12 mg).

Amiodarone IO/IV dose:
5 mg/kg over 20–60 min

or

Procainamide IO/IV dose:
15 mg/kg over 30–60 min

Do not routinely administer amiodarone and procainamide together.

Reproduced with permission from Neumar RW, et al. Part 8: Adult advanced cardiovascular life support. *Circulation*. 2010;122(18 Suppl 3):S729. © 2010 American Heart Association, Inc.

CHAPTER 223
Malignant Hyperthermia

Ghislaine M. Isidore, MD

BASICS

- Inherited pharmacogenetic disorder, autosomal dominant
- Myopathy with defective Ca^{2+} release at the sarcoplasmic reticulum within the muscle fiber, setting off a cascade of events on exposure to volatile anesthetics and depolarizing muscle relaxants
- Potentially lethal, but mortality nowadays <5%

WHO IS AT RISK?

- Patients with known MH history
- Diagnosed family members
- Patients with "central core disease" and periodic hyperkalemic paralysis
- Administration of succinylcholine and volatile anesthetics to patients with muscular dystrophies can trigger rhabdomyolysis difficult to distinguish from MH. Volatile anesthetics and depolarizing muscle relaxant should be used cautiously in these patients
- Some individuals with history of clinical MH and positive in vitro contracture test (IVCT) may develop heat or exercise intolerance, but there is no evidence of the reverse, that is, no increased risk of MH in patients with a history of exertional rhabdomyolysis (ER) or exertional heat illness (EI)

TRIGGERS OF MH

- *All volatile anesthetics* and *succinylcholine* can trigger MH
- Complete information about previous anesthetics, including complications or adverse events, must be obtained
- *NB*: A patient can develop MH despite having undergone prior anesthetics with triggering agents in the past *without* having developed MH

ANESTHESIA IN MH-SUSCEPTIBLE PATIENT

- The apprehensive patient must be reassured during the perioperative evaluation
- Types of anesthesia and alternatives must be explained, including usage of safe drugs and adequate monitoring
- If any suspicion of neuromuscular disease, consultation with a geneticist, neurologist, pediatric specialist should be sought
- It is debatable whether or not further tests such as creatine kinase or blood gas analysis are required following the evaluation
- Prophylaxis with dantrolene is not required
- As per guidelines, decontaminate the anesthesia machine, that is:
  ‣ Remove vaporizers
  ‣ Change all removable parts of the machine in contact with volatile anesthetics (soda lime, fresh gas outlet hose)
  ‣ Wash circuit with 100% oxygen at a gas flow of 10 L/min for 10 minutes
- Avoid triggering agents (volatile anesthetics, succinylcholine)
- What is safe: nitrous oxide, barbiturates, propofol, etomidate, benzodiazepines, nondepolarizing muscle relaxants, and neostigmine
- Regional anesthesia is safe and is preferred as an alternative

- Standard monitors: pulse oximetry, BP, ECG, capnometry, and continuous measurement of temperature should be standard. Invasive monitoring only if otherwise clinically indicated
- With appropriate planning, MH patients can have surgery in ambulatory surgical facilities

SIGNS AND SYMPTOMS

Early signs may be acute, or subtle and slow to progress.
- Increase in expired CO_2 (most sensitive and early sign):
  ‣ Respiratory acidosis
  ‣ Then rapidly mixed acidosis with increased arterial lactate
- Muscle rigidity:
  ‣ Very specific but inconstant; can be limited to masseter spasm
- Rhabdomyolysis:
  ‣ Elevated serum K, Ca
  ‣ Increased serum and urine myoglobin
  ‣ Delayed increase in CK, peak at 24 hours
  ‣ DIC
- Hyperthermia:
  ‣ Late sign
  ‣ Can progress very quickly (1°C/5 minutes)
- Other, less specific:
  ‣ Tachycardia, dysrhythmia
  ‣ Tachypnea
  ‣ Cyanosis, skin mottling
  ‣ Dark blood in surgical field; however, typically normal SpO_2

MAIN DIFFERENTIAL DIAGNOSES

- Thyroid storm
- Pheochromocytoma

TREATMENT

- Communicate with surgical team; terminate surgery; if impossible, continue using nontriggering agents
- Discontinue triggers; remove vaporizers; not necessary to change the whole circuit, CO_2 absorber, etc
- Call for help; have MH kit brought to room
- Monitor core temperature (if not already monitoring)
- Hyperventilate (two to three times normal minute ventilation) with 100% O_2; use high flows (>10 L/min)
- Administer dantrolene 2.5 mg/kg (mix 20 mg vial [containing 3 g mannitol] in at least 60 mL sterile water); repeat until there is no sign of MH; up to 30 mg/kg might be necessary, although 95% of cases resolve with less than 5 mg/kg
- Insert CVL and arterial line
- Aggressive fluid resuscitation with NS
- Administer sodium bicarbonate based on ABG (typically 2–4 mEq/kg)
- Cool aggressively:
  ‣ Administer 15 mL/kg cold saline IV; repeat up to three times
  ‣ Cool using iced saline into stomach, bladder, rectum, surgical field (except chest)
  ‣ Use forced-air blanket without warming
  ‣ Aim for 38°C; avoid inducing hypothermia
- If arrhythmia unresponsive to correction of acidosis and hyperkalemia, use antiarrhythmic of choice but:
  ‣ Avoid calcium channel blockers (can increase hyperkalemia and cause cardiovascular collapse)
  ‣ Lidocaine or procainamide should not be given if a wide QRS complex arrhythmia is likely due to hyperkalemia; this may result in asystole

- Treat hyperkalemia:
  - Hyperventilation
  - D50 + insulin (10 U regular insulin in 50 mL D50, repeat as needed)
  - If EKG changes, give 1 g $CaCl_2$ over 10 minutes
- Monitor U/O; maintain above 2 mL/kg/h using fluid resuscitation and mannitol if needed
- Any cardiac arrest on induction (using succinylcholine) in a child is presumed due to a subclinical myopathy until proved otherwise. Treat as acute hyperkalemia ($CaCl_2$, bicarbonate, etc.)
- Blood studies: electrolytes, CK, LFTs, BUN, lactate, glucose, coagulation profiles including platelet count; serum hemoglobin and myoglobin
- Urine hemoglobin and myoglobin

POSTOPERATIVE MANAGEMENT

- Admit to ICU for at least 24 hours:
  - MH will recur in about one third of cases
  - Monitor temperature, EKG, SpO_2, $EtCO_2$ (if intubated), BP by A-line, U/O
- Continue dantrolene 1 mg/kg IV every 6 hours for at least 24 hours and up to 72 hours, and then 4 mg/kg po every 6 hours for 24 hours
- Treat myoglobinuria
- Labs: at least every 6 hours, monitor ABG, CK, K, Ca, myoglobinemia, myoglobinuria, PT/PTT
- Genetic testing, and/or muscle biopsy for IVCT using the halothane–caffeine test
- Family counseling at a certified MH center
- Fill out form for North American MH Registry (NAMHR) on www.mhreg.org

CONTENTS OF THE MH KIT

- Dantrolene—36 vials (typically 18 in OR and 18 in pharmacy)
- Sterile water for injection USP (without a bacteriostatic agent). Store as vials, not bags, to avoid accidental IV administration of this hypotonic solution
- Sodium bicarbonate (8.4%)—50 mL × 5
- Furosemide 40 mg/ampule × 4 ampules
- Dextrose 50%—50 mL vials × 2
- Calcium chloride (10%) 10 mL vial × 2
- Regular insulin 100 U/mL × 1 (*refrigerated*)
- Lidocaine for injection, 100 mg/5 mL or 100 mg/10 mL in preloaded syringes. Amiodarone (150 mg/3 mL; seven vials) is also acceptable
- NG tubes (sizes appropriate for patient population)
- Irrigation syringes (60 mL × 2) with adapter for NG irrigation
- A minimum of 3,000 mL of *refrigerated* cold saline solution for IV cooling
- Large sterile Steri-Drape (for rapid draping of wound)
- Large clear plastic bags for ice × 4
- Small plastic bags for ice × 4
- Bucket for ice
- Test strips for urine analysis
- Syringes (3 mL) for blood gas analysis or ABG kits × 6
- Urine collection container for myoglobin level
- Blood specimen tubes (each set should have two pediatric and two large tubes):
  - For CK, myoglobin, SMA 19 (LDH, electrolytes, thyroid studies)
  - For PT/PTT, fibrinogen, fibrin split products, and lactate
  - CBC, platelets
  - Blood gas syringe (lactic acid level)

REFERENCES

For references, please visit **www.TheAnesthesiaGuide.com**.

Acronyms and Abbreviations

A-Fib	Atrial fibrillation	AS	Aortic stenosis
AAA	Abdominal aortic aneurysm	ASA	American Society of Anesthesiologists/ Acetylsalicylic acid
ABG	Arterial blood gas(es)		
ACA	Anterior cerebral artery	ASAP	As soon as possible
ACE	Angiotensin converting enzyme	ASD	Atrial septal defect
		ASIS	Anterior-superior iliac spine
ACEI, ACE-I	Angiotensin converting enzyme inhibitor	ASRA	American Society of Regional Anesthesia
ACh	Acetylcholine	AST	Aspartate aminotransferase
ACLS	Advanced cardiac life support	ATLS	Advanced trauma life support
ACS	Acute coronary syndrome	ATN	Acute tubular necrosis
ACT	Activated clotting time	ATP	Adenosine triphosphate
ACTH	Adrenocorticotropic hormone	AV block	Atrio-ventricular block
ADH	Antidiuretic hormone	AV node	Atrio-ventricular node
ADP	Adenosine diphosphate	AVF	Arterio-venous fistula
AED	Automated external defibrillator	AVM	Arterio-venous malformation
AF, Afib	Atrial fibrillation	AVNRT	Atrio-ventricular nodal reentrant tachycardia
AH	Autonomic hyperactivity		
AHA/ACC	American Heart Association/ American College of Cardiologists	BBB	Bundle branch block
		BID	Twice a day
		BIPAP, BiPAP	Bilevel positive airway pressure
AI	Aortic insufficiency		
AICD	Automated implantable cardiac defibrillator	BLS	Basic life support
		BMI	Body mass index
ALI	Acute lung injury	BMR	Basal metabolic rate
ALT	Alanine aminotransferase	BMS	Bare metal stent
AMI	Acute myocardial infarction	BNE	Bilateral neck exploration
ANH	Acute normovolemic hemodilution	BNP	Brain natriuretic peptide
		BP	Blood pressure
ANS	Autonomic nervous system	BPH	Benign prostate hypertrophy
APAP	Acetaminophen	C1-INH	C1-esterase inhibitor
aPTT	Activated prothrombin time	CA	Carotid artery
AR	Aortic regurgitation	CABG	Coronary artery bypass graft
ARB	Angiotensin receptor blocker	CAD	Coronary artery disease
ARDS	Acute respiratory distress syndrome	CAR	Cerebral autoregulation
		CASP	Carotid artery stump pressure
ARF	Acute renal failure/acute respiratory failure		

CBC	Complete blood count
CBF	Cerebral blood flow
CBV	Cerebral blood volume
CEA	Carotid endarterectomy
CHD	Congenital heart disease
CHF	Congestive heart failure
CI	Cardiac index
CIRCI	Critical illness–related corticosteroid insufficiency
CK	Creatine kinase
CM	Cardiomyopathy
$CMRO_2$	Cerebral metabolic rate of oxygen consumption
CMV	Controlled mechanical ventilation/Cytomegalovirus
CN	Cranial nerve
CNB	Central neuraxial block
CNS	Central nervous system
CO	Cardiac output/carbon monoxide
COPD	Chronic obstructive pulmonary disease
COX	Cyclo-oxygenase
CPAP	Continuous positive airway pressure
CPB	Cardiopulmonary bypass
CPD	Cephalo-pelvic disproportion
CPK	Creatine phosphokinase
CPNB	Continuous peripheral nerve block(s)
CPP	Cerebral perfusion pressure
CPR	Cardio-pulmonary resuscitation
Cr	Creatinine
CRP	C-reactive protein
CRPS	Complex regional pain syndrome
CRRT	Continuous renal replacement therapy
CSE	Combined spinal-epidural
CSF	Cerebrospinal fluid
CSHT	Context-sensitive half-time
CVA	Cerebrovascular accident
CVC	Central venous catheter
CVL	Central venous line
CVP	Central venous pressure
CVVH	Continuous veno-venous hemofiltration
CVVHD	Continuous veno-venous hemodialysis

CVVHDF	Continuous veno-venous hemodiafiltration
CXR	Chest radiograph
D/C	Discontinue, discontinuation, discharge, discharged
DA	Dopamine
DBP	Diastolic blood pressure
DDAVP	Desmopressin
DES	Drug-eluting stent
DI	Diabetes insipidus
DIC	Disseminated intra-vascular coagulation
DKA	Diabetic ketoacidosis
DL	Direct laryngoscopy
DLCO	Diffusion capacity of the lung for carbon monoxide
DLETT	Double-lumen endotracheal tube
DLT	Double-lumen endotracheal tube
DM	Diabetes mellitus
DT	Delirium tremens
DTR	Deep tendon reflex
DVT	Deep vein thrombosis
EBV	Ebstein-Barr virus
ECF	Extracellular fluid
ECG	Electrocardiogram
ECMO	Extra-corporeal membrane oxygenation
ECT	Electroconvulsive therapy
EEG	Electroencephalogram
EF	Ejection fraction
EGD	Esophagogastroduodenoscopy
EJ	External jugular (vein)
EKG	Electrocardiogram
EMG	Electromyogram
EMI	Electromagnetic interference
EMLA	Eutectic mixture of local anesthetics
ENT	Ear, nose, and throat
EOM	Extra-ocular muscle(s)
EPO	Erythropoietin
ERCP	Endoscopic retrograde cholangiopancreatography
ERV	Expiratory reserve volume
ESRD	End-stage renal disease
ESU	Electrosurgical unit
ET	Endotracheal

EtOH, ETOH	Ethanol, alcohol
ETT	Endotracheal tube
FDA	Food and Drug Administration
FDP	Fibrin degradation products
FEV1/FVC	Forced expiratory volume in one second/forced vital capacity
FFP	Fresh frozen plasma
FGF	Fresh gas flow
FICB	Fascia iliaca compartment block
FOB	Fiberoptic bronchoscope
FOI	Fiberoptic intubation
FRC	Functional residual capacity
FSBG	Finger stick blood glucose
FTT	Failure to thrive
G6PD	Glucose-6-phosphate dehydrogenase
GA	General anesthesia
GABA	Gamma-aminobutyric acid
GCS	Graduated compression stockings/Glasgow coma scale
GERD	Gastro esophageal reflux disease
GETA	General endotracheal anesthesia
GFR	Glomerular filtration rate
GH	Growth hormone
GI	Gastro intestinal
GU	Genitourinary
HAE	Hereditary angioedema
Hb, Hgb	Hemoglobin
HbA1c	Glycosylated hemoglobin
HCM	Hypertrophic cardiomyopathy
Hct	Hematocrit
HD	Hemodynamic/hemodialysis
HELLP syndrome	Hemolysis, elevated liver (enzymes), low platelet syndrome
HHNK	Hyperglycemic hyperosmolar nonketotic coma
HHS	Hyperosmolar hyperglycemic state
HIT	Heparin-induced thrombocytopenia
HITTS	Heparin-induced thrombocytopenia and thrombosis syndrome
HR	Heart rate
HRT	Hormone replacement therapy
HSS	Hypertonic saline solution
HTN	Hypertension
HTx	Hemothorax
I:E	Inspiratory to expiratory (ratio)
IABP	Intra-aortic balloon pump
IBW	Ideal body weight
IC	Intracardiac
ICA	Internal carotid artery
ICD	Implantable cardioverter defibrillator
ICH	Intracranial hemorrhage
ICP	Intracranial pressure
ICU	Intensive care unit
IDDM	Insulin-dependant diabetes mellitus
IHD	Ischemic heart disease
IJ	Internal jugular
IM	Intramuscular
INR	International normalized ratio
IO	Intraosseous
IOP	Intraocular pressure
IPC	Intermittent pneumatic compression
IPF	Idiopathic pulmonary fibrosis
ITP	Idiopathic thrombocytopenic purpura
IUGR	Intra-uterine growth restriction
IV	Intravenous
IVC	Inferior vena cava
IVCT	In-vitro contracture test (for malignant hyperthermia)
IVF	Intravenous fluid(s)
IVRA	Intravenous regional anesthesia
JVD	Jugular vein distension
KIU	Kallikrein Inhibitor Unit
KVO	(To) keep vein open
LA	Local anesthetic
LBBB	Left bundle branch block
LDH	Lactate dehydrogenase
LDUH	Low-dose unfractionated heparin
LED	Light-emitting diode
LES	Lower esophageal sphincter
LFCN	Lateral femoral cutaneous nerve

LLA	Lower limit of autoregulation
LMA	Laryngeal mask airway
LMWH	Low-molecular-weight heparin
LOR	Loss of resistance
LOS	Length of stay
LP	Lumbar puncture
LR	Lactated Ringer's solution
LRD	Living related donor
LRI	Lower respiratory infection
LSC	Left subclavian
LUL	Left upper lobe
LV	Left ventricle
LVAD	Left ventricular assist device
LVEF	Left ventricular ejection fraction
LVH	Left ventricular hypertrophy
LVOT	Left ventricular outflow tract
MAC	Monitored anesthesia care/minimum alveolar concentration
MAI	*Mycobacterium avium-intracellulare*
MAO	Monoamine oxidase
MAOI	Monoamine oxidase inhibitor
MAP	Mean arterial pressure
MCA	Middle cerebral artery
MDI	Metered-dose inhaler
MEN	Multiple endocrine neoplasia
MEP	Motor evoked potential
MG	Myasthenia gravis
MH	Malignant hyperthermia
MI	Myocardial infarction
MIBG	Methyl-iodo-benzyl-guanidine
MIP	Minimally invasive parathyroidectomy
MMA	Methyl methacrylate
MR	Mitral regurgitation
MRI	Magnetic resonance imaging
MRSA	Methicillin-resistant staphylococcus aureus
MS	Mitral stenosis/multiple sclerosis
MTB	*Mycobacterium tuberculosis*
MVP	Mitral valve prolapse
N/V	Nausea/vomiting
Nd:YAG	Neodynium-doped yttrium-aluminum garnet (laser)
NDMR	Non-depolarizing muscle relaxant
NGT	Nasogastric tube
NIBP	Non-invasive blood pressure
NICU	Neonatal intensive care unit
NIDDM	Non-insulin-dependant diabetes mellitus
NIF	Negative inspiratory force
NIHSS	NIH Stroke Scale
NIPPV	Non-invasive positive pressure ventilation
NIRS	Near-infrared spectroscopy
NKHC	Non-ketotic hyperosmolar coma
NMB	Neuromuscular blocker/blockade
NMBA	Neuromuscular blocking agent
NMJ	Neuromuscular junction
NPO	Nil per os (nothing by mouth)
NRB	Non-rebreather (mask)
NS	Neurostimulation/nerve stimulation/normal saline
NSAIDs	Non-steroidal anti-inflammatory drugs
NSVD	Normal spontaneous vaginal delivery
NTG	Nitroglycerin
NTP	(Sodium) nitroprusside
NVM	Nerve to the vastus medialis (branch of the femoral nerve)
NYHA	New York Heart Association
OAA	Oral antiplatelet agent
OCP	Oral contraceptive pill
OGT	Oro-gastric tube
OLV	One-lung ventilation
OOP	Out-of-plane (ultrasound-guided needle approach)
OPCAB	Off-pump coronary artery bypass
OR	Operating room
ORIF	Open reduction and internal fixation
ORT	Orthodromic reentrant tachycardia
OSA	Obstructive sleep apnea
PAC	Pulmonary artery catheter
PACU	Post anesthesia care unit
PADP	Pulmonary artery diastolic pressure
PAN	Panarteritis nodosa

PAOP	Pulmonary artery occlusion pressure (= "wedge")		PT	Physical therapy
PAP	Pulmonary artery pressure		PTA	Percutaneous transluminal angioplasty
PAWP	Pulmonary artery wedge pressure (old term for PAOP)		PTH	Parathormone
PCA	Patient-controlled analgesia/ posterior cerebral artery		PTT	Partial thromboplastin time
			PTU	Propylthiouracil
PCEA	Patient-controlled epidural analgesia		PTx	Pneumothorax
			PVB	Paravertebral block
PCI	Percutaneous coronary intervention		PVD	Peripheral vascular disease
			PVR	Pulmonary vascular resistance
PCN	Penicillin		QD	Quaque die (every day)
PCNT	Posterior cutaneous nerve of the thigh		RA	Rheumatoid arthritis
			RAST	Radioallergosorbent test
PCP	Pneumocystis carinii pneumonia/phencyclidine		RBBB	Right bundle branch block
			RBC	Red blood cell
PCV	Pressure-controlled ventilation		RIJ	Right internal jugular (vein)
			RLN	Recurrent laryngeal nerve
PCWP	Pulmonary capillary wedge pressure (old term for PAOP)		RR	Respiratory rate
			RRT	Renal replacement therapy
PDA	Patent ductus arteriosus		RSI	Rapid sequence intubation
PDPH	Post-dural puncture headache		RUQ	Right upper quadrant
PE	Pulmonary embolism		RV	Right ventricle
PEEP	Positive end-expiratory pressure		RWMA	Regional wall motion abnormalities
PetCO$_2$	End-tidal partial pressure of carbon dioxide		SA node	Sino atrial node
			SAH	Subarachnoid hemorrhage
PFO	Patent foramen ovale		SAM	Systolic anterior motion (of the anterior leaflet of the mitral valve)
PFT	Pulmonary function test			
PICU	Pediatric intensive care unit			
PIP	Peak inspiratory pressure		SBP	Systolic blood pressure
PJRT	Paroxysmal junctional reciprocating tachycardia		SC	Subcutaneous
			SCD	Sudden cardiac death/ sequential compression device
PM	Pacemaker			
PNB	Peripheral nerve block		SCh	Succinylcholine
PNS	Peripheral nervous system/ peripheral nerve stimulation/ stimulator		SCI	Spinal cord injury
			SCM	Sternocleidomastoid (muscle)
			SCPP	Spinal cord perfusion pressure
PO	Per os (by mouth)			
PONV	Postoperative nausea and vomiting		SDU	Step-down unit
			SIADH	Syndrome of inappropriate antidiuretic hormone secretion
PPI	Proton pump inhibitor(s)			
PPN	Partial parenteral nutrition			
PPV	Positive pressure ventilation		SID	Strong ion difference
PR	Per rectum		SIMV	Synchronized intermittent mechanical ventilation
PRBC	Packed red blood cells			
PRN	Pro re nata (as needed)		SIRS	Systemic inflammatory response syndrome
psi	Pounds per square inch			
PSIS	Posterior-superior iliac spine		SLETT	Single-lumen endotracheal tube
PSV	Pressure support ventilation			
PT	Prothrombin time		SNP	Sodium nitroprusside

SNRI	Serotonin–norepinephrine reuptake inhibitor	TNT	Trinitrotoluene (an explosive)
SQ	Subcutaneous	TOF	Train of four
SSEP	Somatosensory evoked potentials	TOLAC	Trial of labor after cesarean birth
SSRI	Selective serotonin reuptake inhibitor(s)	tPA	Tissue plasminogen activator
		TPN	Total parenteral nutrition
STEMI	ST-elevation myocardial infarction	TPVS	Thoracic paravertebral space
		TRALI	Transfusion-related acute lung injury
SV	Stroke volume		
SVC	Superior vena cava	TSH	Thyroid-stimulating hormone
SVR	Systemic vascular resistance	TT	Thrombin time
SVT	Supraventricular tachycardia	TTE	Trans thoracic echocardiogram
TAA	Thoracic aortic aneurysm(s)		
TAAA	Thoraco-abdominal aortic aneurysm(s)	TTP	Thrombotic thrombocytopenic purpura
TAP	Transversus abdominis plane (block)	TURP	Transurethral resection of the prostate
TBI	Traumatic brain injury	U/O	Urine output
TBSA	Total body surface area	UFH	Unfractioned heparin
TBW	Total body weight	UG	Ultrasound guidance
TCA	Tricyclic antidepressant	ULA	Upper limit of autoregulation
TCD	Transcranial Doppler	UO, UOP	Urine output
TEE	Transesophageal echocardiogram	URI	Upper respiratory infection
		US	Ultrasound
TEF	Tracheoesophageal fistula	UTI	Urinary tract infection
TEG	Thromboelastogram/ thromboelastography	V-fib	Ventricular fibrillation
		V/Q	Ventilation/perfusion
TES	Transcutaneous electrical stimulation	VBAC	Vaginal birth after Cesarean
		VC	Vocal cord/vital capacity
TF	Tissue factor	VCV	Volume-controlled ventilation
THA/THR	Total hip arthroplasty/ replacement	Vd	Volume of distribution
		VIP	Venous infusion port
TIA	Transient ischemic attack	VMA	Vanillylmandelic acid
TID	Three times a day	VP shunt	Ventriculo-peritoneal shunt
TIPS	Transjugular intrahepatic portosystemic shunt	VS	Vital signs
		VSD	Ventricular septal defect
TKA/TKR	Total knee arthroplasty/ replacement	VT	Ventricular tachycardia
		Vt	Tidal volume
TLC	Total lung capacity	VTE	Venous thromboembolism
TLC	Triple-lumen catheter	vWF	von Willebrand's factor
TMJ	Temporomandibular joint	WFNS	World Federation of Neurological Surgeons
TNF	Tumor-necrosing factor		
TNS	Transient neurologic symptoms	WPW	Wolff-Parkinson-White

INDEX

Page references followed by *f* indicate figures and followed by *t* indicate tables.